ADVERSE DRUG REACTIONS: MECHANISMS AND MANAGEMENT

Dr. Shubham Sewariya and
Dr. Snigdha Singh

ALLIED
HEALTH
PRESS

Adverse Drug Reactions: Mechanisms and Management

Authors: **Dr. Shubham Sewariya and Dr. Snigdha Singh**

Allied Health Press
4164 Lakeshore Road
Burlington ON L7L 1A4
Canada
www.alliedhealthpress.com
Email: orders@arclereducation.com

ISBN: 978-1-77956-840-3

Allied Health Press publishes wide variety of books and eBooks. For more information about Allied Health Press and its products, visit our website at www.alliedhealthpress.com

ABOUT THE AUTHORS

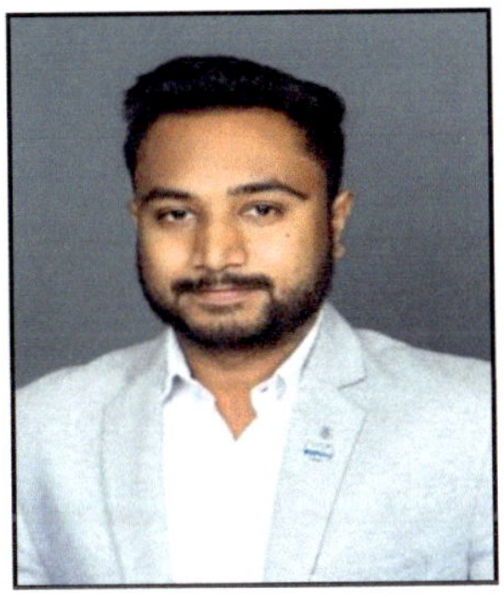

Dr. Shubham Sewariya is a Research Scientist at the University of Delhi, India, with expertise in medicinal chemistry and drug discovery. His research focuses on developing novel anticancer drug leads by combining synthetic chemistry, biological insights, and computational approaches. He holds an Integrated BS–MS degree in Chemistry from the Indian Institute of Science Education and Research (IISER), Thiruvananthapuram, and has completed his Ph.D. jointly at University of Delhi and the University of Lancashire, UK. His doctoral work centers on the discovery and development of secondary metabolites, including noscapinoids and coumarins, as potential anticancer agents. Dr. Sewariya has received several prestigious fellowships and awards, including the Commonwealth Split-site PhD Scholarship (2023–24) funded by the UK Foreign, Commonwealth & Development Office, the CSIR Senior Research Fellowship, and the INSPIRE SHE Fellowship from Department of Science and Technology, Govt of India. He has also presented his work at international platforms such as the American Chemical Society (ACS) conferences in San Francisco and Chicago. With more than a dozen peer-reviewed publications, his contributions span synthetic chemistry, nanomedicine, and biophysical studies, particularly in designing intelligent nanocarriers and molecular probes for cancer therapy. Beyond the laboratory, Dr. Sewariya is deeply committed to advancing translational research that bridges science and medicine for the betterment of human health.

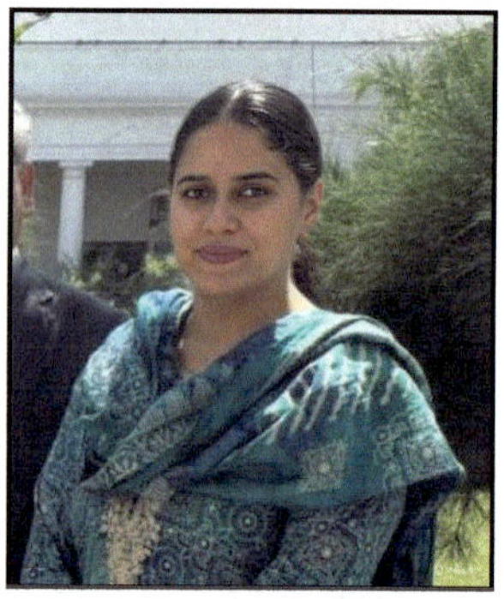

Dr. Snigdha Singh is an accomplished researcher and educator in medicinal chemistry and nanoscience, currently serving as Assistant Professor in the Department of Chemistry at the University of Delhi and Deputy Director of the Institute of Nano Medical Sciences, University of Delhi. With a distinguished academic trajectory and extensive international research exposure, she has established herself as a leading young scientist in the field of chemical and biomedical research.

She earned her Ph.D. in Medicinal Chemistry from the University of Delhi (2021), under the supervision of Prof. Ramesh Chandra, where her thesis focused on the synthesis and development of novel heterocycles and their biological evaluation. Prior to that, she completed her M.Tech. in Chemical Synthesis and Process Technologies (CSPT) at the University of Delhi with first division (2016) and her B.Sc. (Hons) in Chemistry from Hindu College, University of Delhi (2013), graduating with top merit distinctions. Her academic excellence was recognized early with a merit fellowship and multiple university-level awards.

Dr. Singh's professional journey reflects a unique blend of teaching, research, and leadership roles. Beyond her faculty appointment, she has served as Resident Tutor at Ambedkar-Ganguly Students House for Women, and has held prestigious international positions, including Postdoctoral Associate at Rensselaer Polytechnic Institute (USA), Guest Scientist at Humboldt University (Germany), and Visiting Scientist at Lobachevsky University (Russia). She was also selected as an Indo-UK Newton Bhabha Scholar at the University of Oxford and an Indo-Italy Exchange Scholar at the University of Siena, further expanding her global research collaborations.

Her research contributions span drug design, nanostructures for biomedical applications, and innovative drug delivery systems. She has published extensively in high-impact journals such as ACS Sustainable Chemistry & Engineering, RSC Advances, Bioorganic & Medicinal Chemistry, and Inorganic Chemistry Communications, alongside several book chapters and authored textbooks. She is also a co-inventor on an international patent related to hydroxyethylamine-based piperazine compounds (2022). In addition, she has mentored Ph.D. candidates and supervised more than 27 graduate and postgraduate students.

Dr. Singh's work has been recognized through numerous honors, including the Indo Asian Young Women Researcher Award (2024), Young Researcher in Medicinal Chemistry Award (2024), and the Teacher Excellence Award (2023). She has received multiple international travel fellowships and was ranked 19th All-India in the UGC-CSIR NET Examination (2017).

An active member of leading scientific societies such as the Royal Society of Chemistry, American Chemical Society, and Indian Science Congress Association, Dr. Singh also serves as a reviewer for several international journals. Her career reflects a deep commitment to advancing chemical sciences while fostering global academic exchange and mentoring the next generation of researchers.

Brief Table of Contents

Detailed Table of Contents

CHAPTER 3

CHAPTER 4

CHAPTER 5

Drug Hypersensitivity Reactions 145

CHAPTER 6

Drug-Induced Liver Injury (DILI) 183

CHAPTER 7

Drug-Induced Nephrotoxicity 219

CHAPTER 10

Dermatological Reactions to Drugs 327

CHAPTER 11

Pharmacogenomics and ADRs 363

CHAPTER 14

Prevention and Risk Minimization in Drug Use 473

CHAPTER 15

Regulatory and Ethical Aspects of Drug 509

LIST OF FIGURES

PREFACE

Adverse drug reactions (ADRs) are a significant drug development and clinical practice problem. With the increasing heterogeneity of therapeutics and increasingly heterogeneous patient populations, the risk of unwanted effects increases. They can range from trivial discomfort to life-threatening reactions, with implications that extend beyond personal harm to include public health systems and therapeutic trust. Understanding why these events occur, who is at the highest risk, and how to identify early warning signs is crucial for optimizing patient outcomes and fostering confidence in pharmacotherapy.

The evolution of pharmacology, molecular biology, and epidemiology during the past few decades has given insight into many of the mechanisms by which drugs can cause adverse reactions. Holes remain, however, in being able to anticipate idiosyncratic reactions or to have clinical protection from laboratory findings. The uniqueness of human physiology, coupled with the dynamic interaction between genetic, environmental, and comorbid factors, means that a single drug may produce varied responses in different patients. Bridging the chasm between these disparate bodies of evidence requires an integrative solution—one that combines mechanistic insight, population-level proof, and practical management solutions. This book, *Adverse Drug Reactions: Mechanisms and Management*, aims to consolidate the existing knowledge on the mechanisms of adverse reactions and their optimal prevention or minimization.

It offers a single source for clinicians, researchers, and regulatory scientists, providing both basic and current data in a format that is immediately usable. Following the chapter sequence, readers will move sequentially from the initial definition and epidemiology to molecular mechanisms, clinical syndromes, and ultimately to detection, prevention, and ethical control measures. Chapter 1 introduces the background of ADRs, defines terminology, categorizes reaction types, and describes their clinical and economic impact. It lays the groundwork by distinguishing Type A (anticipated) and Type B (unanticipated) reactions and outlining systems for causality evaluation and reporting. Chapter 2 examines the incidence and distribution of adverse drug reactions (ADRs) in various settings. Demographic, genetic, co-existent disease, and health system determinants of risk factors and influencing reaction rates are all discussed. Epidemiologic methods of surveillance and data interpretation are clarified, providing readers with the tools necessary for field analysis.

Chapter 3 describes the Type A reaction mechanism, in which pharmacologic activity at therapeutic doses results in a quantitatively predictable side effect. It covers dose-response relationships, drug accumulation, and the impact of organ impairment on drug clearance, with examples from frequently used medications.

Chapter 4 discusses the mechanisms of Type B reactions, which involve the usual doses but occur through uncommon pathways. Immune-mediated reactions, metabolic idiosyncrasies, and off-target receptor interactions are discussed, highlighting how these unanticipated events can evade standard monitoring rules.

Chapter 5 covers drug hypersensitivity reactions (DHRs), immediate (e.g., anaphylaxis) and delayed presentation (e.g., Stevens-Johnson syndrome). Immunological mechanisms are described, along with diagnostic testing (e.g., skin prick tests and patch tests) and treatment regimens, including desensitization protocols.

Chapter 6 addresses drug-induced liver injury (DILI) and covers one of the most hepatotoxic organ-specific ADRs. It covers hepatocellular, cholestatic, and mixed pattern injuries, covers biomarkers and imaging agents employed for diagnosis, and reviews existing guidelines on monitoring and rechallenge after recovery.

Chapter 7 discusses drug-induced nephrotoxicity, with both acute and chronic kidney injury syndromes being outlined. Direct tubular toxicity, glomerular injury, and immune complex deposition are the pathogenetic mechanisms. Laboratory and imaging studies, along with early detection and renal dose adjustment, are emphasized as key measures.

Chapter 8 describes cardiovascular and hematologic ADRs such as QT prolongation, arrhythmias, thromboembolism, and blood dyscrasias. This chapter discusses pathophysiologic mechanisms, including drug-receptor interactions in cardiac tissue and immune-mediated marrow suppression, as well as risk assessment and management.

Chapter 9 describes neurological and psychiatric ADRs, from extrapyramidal side effects and seizures to mood change and cognitive impairment. It addresses mechanisms such as neurotransmitter imbalance, penetration of the blood-brain barrier, and drug-drug interaction in the central nervous system (CNS).

Chapter 10 describes dermatological drug reactions, ranging from morbilliform eruptions and photosensitivity to fixed drug eruptions. The chapter discusses clinical classification systems, biopsy strategies, and pragmatic management steps, such as determining whether to use topical versus systemic therapy.

Chapter 11 discusses the future of pharmacogenomics in relation to adverse drug reactions (ADRs), explaining how genetic variations in drug-metabolizing enzymes, transporters, and receptors alter the response to drugs. Examples of cases demonstrate dosing recommendations and personalized therapy plans that utilize genomic information to inform treatment decisions.

Chapter 12 discusses polypharmacy and drug interactions, a rising issue as patients, particularly geriatric patients, are being placed on numerous medications. Pharmacokinetic and pharmacodynamic drug interactions are covered, along with recommendations for reconciling medications and addressing computer alarms.

Chapter 13 discusses the detection and monitoring of adverse drug reactions (ADRs), ranging from spontaneous reporting schemes to active surveillance programs. Signal detection algorithms, real-time monitoring tools, and the role of the electronic health record (EHR) in safety oversight are featured.

Chapter 14 discusses prevention and risk-reduction strategies, including prescriber education, patient counseling, and technological solutions such as computerized physician order entry (CPOE). It discusses whether black box warnings, risk assessment and mitigation strategies (REMS), and pharmacist reviews of medications are adequate.

Chapter 15 explores drug safety from both regulatory and ethical perspectives. It covers the activities of national and international agencies concerning licensing, labeling, and surveillance of drugs, as well as ethical issues—such as post-marketing study design, informed consent in high-risk populations, and innovation versus patient protection.

The target audience for the book is healthcare professionals (HCPs)—doctors, pharmacists, nurses, and clinical researchers seeking an academic textbook on adverse drug reaction (ADR) mechanisms and management. Regulatory officials and policymakers will also benefit from the chapters on epidemiology, prevention, and ethics. Graduate students in pharmacology, toxicology, and public health can utilize the book as both a teaching manual and a reference.

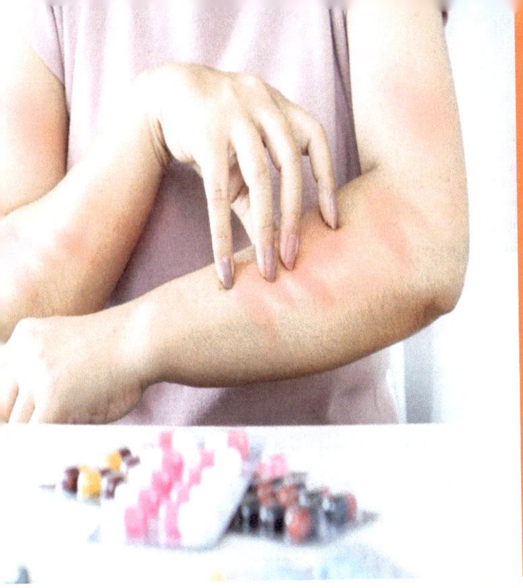

Chapter 1

INTRODUCTION TO ADVERSE DRUG REACTIONS (ADRS)

Contents

Introduction

Adverse drug reactions (ADRs) are a serious issue in pharmacology, manifesting themselves in the form of any unwanted or harmful reaction to a medication administered within regular doses. Some ADRs are just nausea and tiredness, but others can be much more serious, including anaphylaxis and organ failure. ADRs are defined by the World Health Organization (WHO) as side effects that appear in normal doses when a drug is used for the prevention, diagnosis, or treatment of a disease, and the side effects are more significant than the drug's positive effects. Healthcare providers need to know the meaning and types of ADRs to address patient safety. Most significantly, the recent augmented use of biosimilars, such as bevacizumab for treating non-small cell lung cancer, underscores the highest possible importance of monitoring ADRs from novel drugs (Zhang et al., 2024). It is essential in clinical practice to find and report ADR so that drug safety can be improved. Sometimes, the side effects are expected based on the drug's usual effects, but sometimes they happen without warning and do not always depend on the dose. The FDA and other regulatory agencies urge healthcare providers to report any adverse events to improve the safety of drugs. For example, a case of non-overt disseminated intravascular coagulation caused by obinutuzumab highlights the importance of recognizing signals in ADR management. In this case, a careful examination revealed an association between the drug and the side effect, highlighting the dynamic nature of drug safety evaluation in clinical practice (Valdiserra et al., 2023). In addition, ADRs can have an impact on both patient safety and the development of healthcare policies and practices. The cost of ADRs remains a problem, as it leads to increased hospital stays, higher healthcare costs, and reduced productivity. Dealing with this issue effectively requires cooperation among healthcare workers, scientists, and the drug regulatory bodies when developing plans for control and prevention. With the evolving landscape of pharmacotherapy, defining and identifying ADRs are imperative to ensure that the therapeutic interventions do not do more harm than good and thus safeguard patient welfare in an increasingly complex healthcare environment (Zhang et al., 2024) (Figure 1.1).

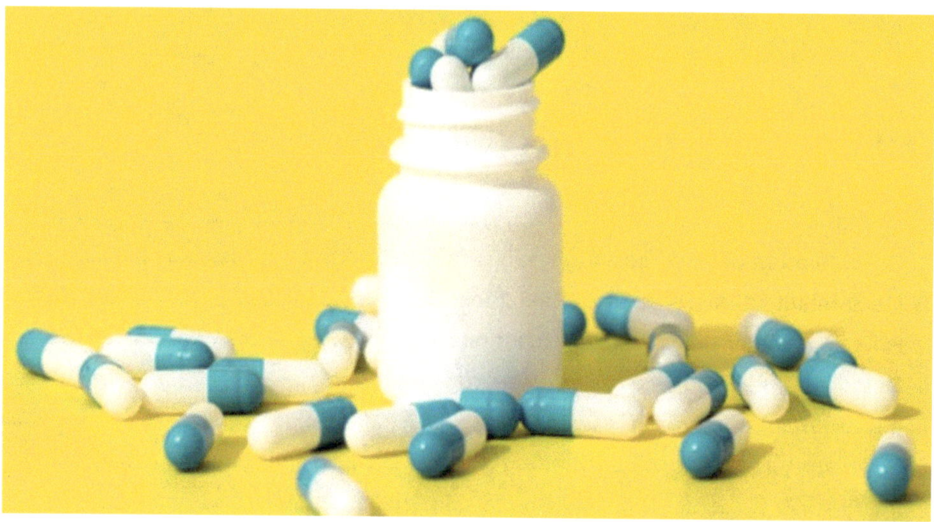

Figure 1.1. Adverse drug reactions.

Source: https://pharmainfonepal.com/wp-content/uploads/2021/04/Adverse-Drug-Reaction-ADR-1140x570.png.

Explanation of ADRs

ADRs pose a significant problem in modern medicine, as they impact not only patient safety but also treatment efficiency. ADRs are drug-induced and may destroy patients' health as well as complicate the process of therapy. A patient may experience anything from slight symptoms such as rash or nausea to lethal conditions such as anaphylaxis or organ failure. Understanding how ADRs come about is essential to doctor because it allows them to recognize at-risk patients and prevent problems. Moreover, the fact that genes affect a person's reaction to medicine confirms the importance of personalized medicine. Through this method, ADRs can be reduced, resulting in better health outcomes and more effective drugs for people. Categorization of ADRs into several categories aids in understanding their complexities. Generally, ADRs can be classified into two types: type A (augmented) and type B (idiosyncratic) reactions. Type A reactions are anticipated and dose-related, commonly arising as a consequence of the pharmacological action of the drug, e.g., sedation caused by antihistamines. In contrast to type A, type B reactions are unforeseen and not a result of the usual drug effects, thereby demonstrating the complexity of patients' responses to drugs. One such demonstration of the dual nature of drug effects is the widely used anticonvulsant valproic acid (VPA). While an extremely effective drug for epilepsy, it may produce hypersensitivity reactions (HSRs) or hepatotoxicity in vulnerable patients (Romoli et al., 2018). Understanding these categorizations enhances the prescribing of medications and ensures patient safety. Promoting rational use of medicine is vital to reduce the frequency of ADRs in medicine practice. Improper or unsystematic use of medication can exacerbate the incidence of ADRs and create excessive healthcare costs, as ineffective drugs necessitate additional interventions and prolong the length of patient stay (Ofori et al., 2016). In addition, when healthcare providers, patients, and decision makers work together, it helps in ensuring a safe environment for drug consumption. Proper education of healthcare providers and counseling training guarantees that all are informed about the possible effect of drugs and what to look out for. With these interventions applied in the practice of medicine, clinicians can choose the best treatment regimens, patients are better educated on their health, and comply with their medications, with better health and fewer ADRs.

Types of ADRs

ADRs in pharmacology can be categorized into types, wherein each refers to a distinct drug-harm relationship. Type A ADRs, or predictable or pharmacologic reactions, occur due to the known pharmacological properties of the drug. Type A reactions are usually dose-dependent and can often be avoided by adjusting the dose or by other treatments. For example, over-anticoagulation with bleeding can be designated as a Type A reaction. Healthcare providers need to be aware of these anticipated side effects because it can inform safer prescribing and enhance patient outcomes. The frequency of occurrence commonly highlights the requirement for therapeutic drug concentration monitoring, especially for drugs with narrow therapeutic indices. Conversely, Type B ADRs or idiosyncratic responses are unexpected and do not lend themselves easily to correlation with the drug's pharmacologic properties.

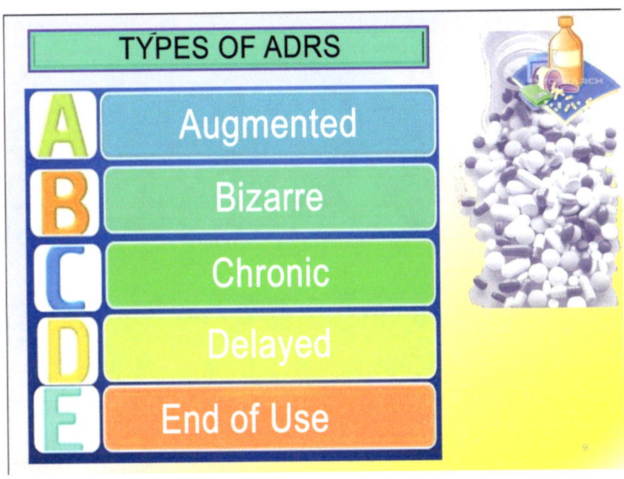

Figure 1.2. Types of adverse drug reaction.

Source: https://slideplayer.com/slide/17575169/104/images/9/Types+of+adrs+Augmented+or+exaggerated.jpg.

Such responses generally arise as a result of individual patient variables, such as genetic or environmental factors, making them particularly challenging to anticipate or prevent. For instance, the occurrence of Stevens-Johnson syndrome (SJS) as a side effect of certain antibiotics illustrates how immune-mediated responses may cause severe adverse effects. Patients younger than 50 have been shown to experience higher frequencies of these types of reactions, highlighting the complexities associated with pharmacotherapy. Understanding the basis of Type B ADRs is crucial for the safe prescribing of drugs, particularly when considering the variability of genetic factors and individual physiology in patients. Lastly, the differentiation of cutaneous and systemic ADRs further explains the variety of adverse effects to which patients may be subjected. Cutaneous ADRs such as rashes or urticaria constitute a prominent class of ADRs, as reflected by the results that highlight their frequency with antibiotic use. Of cutaneous adverse drug reactions (CADRs) in the study conducted recently, 55.5% were brought about by antibacterial drugs, and another significant percentage (14.6%) was brought about by nonsteroidal anti-inflammatory drugs (NSAIDs). Identification of CADR prevalence will enable clinicians to predict better and manage such reactions, particularly among those patients who are on long-term antibiotic therapy. Research into CADRs not only raises awareness about drug safety but also informs pharmacovigilance activities, leading to refining therapy strategies in clinical practice (Panneerselvam et al., 2019; Pandey et al., 2025) (Figure 1.2).

Importance of Understanding ADRs

The importance of being aware of ADRs cannot be overstated in the current healthcare environment, particularly with the increasing complexity of pharmacological therapies. ADRs are a big problem for both the patient and the practitioner since they can result in serious health issues or death. It is crucial for healthcare professionals to recognize the signs and symptoms of ADRs to effectively manage and minimize risks.

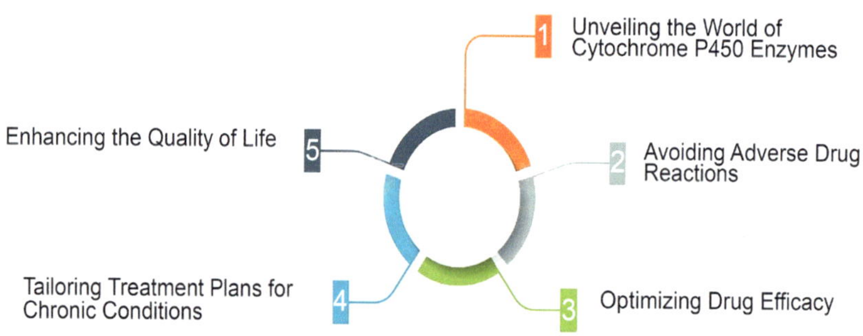

Figure 1.3. Importance of understanding adverse drug reaction.

Source: https://fastercapital.co/i/CYP-Testing--Assessing-Enzyme-Levels-for-Optimized-Drug-Therapy-update--Introduction-to-CYP-Testing-and-Its-Importance-in-Drug-Therapy.webp.

Moreover, when patients are informed, they can participate in better reporting and become aware of the possible risks associated with their treatment. Therefore, understanding ADRs improves patient safety and encourages everyone in healthcare to pay close attention, which in turn helps treatments work more effectively and holds individuals more accountable. Knowing how patient awareness affects the performance of pharmacovigilance systems is also very important in ADR. To detect patterns and create prevention plans for ADRs, it is vital to report all the data properly. In particular, patients' knowledge about the dangers of ADRs is found to be lacking in relation to the Portuguese Pharmacovigilance System. It can dissuade patients from reporting ADRs and lead to underreporting of significant drug-related events (Joaquim et al., 2023). When patients understand how to spot and report ADRs, clinicians can collect better data and make the use of drugs safer. Greater awareness helps protect each patient and also directs the development of population health programs. Also, teaching healthcare professionals (HCPs) and patients about the possible dangers of ADRs is very beneficial. For instance, medical students who indulge in self-medication would be found with poor knowledge of potential ADRs with their medication, as revealed by a study performed on third-year MBBS students where knowledge of ADRs with respect to drugs used by them was described by only 45.16% (Burute et al., 2016). It demonstrates that formal training in medicine and patient care is crucial. Filling the knowledge gap enables patients to make better decisions about their health and medicines, as well as increase the influence of pharmacovigilance in healthcare. Understanding ADRs is the first step in making healthcare safer and more knowledgeable, with the well-being of patients as its main goal (Figure 1.3).

1.1. Classification of Adverse Drug Reactions (ADRs)

The classification of ADRs is important in understanding and managing the complexity surrounding drug treatment. ADRs are classified according to several characteristics, including the manner in which they cause harm, the time at which they occur, the extent of harm they cause, and the patients on whom they act. The most common system of classification is based on the nature of the reaction, which is divided into Type A (augmented) and Type B (bizarre) reactions. The behavior of Type A reactions is dose-dependent and is usually linked with the drug's pharmacological profile. Type B reactions are different in each person and are not characterized by the quantity of drug taken or how it works within the body. This general categorization not only assists in the identification of potential drug issues by HCPs but is also a foundation for developing pharmacovigilance measures and patient safety, emphasizing ongoing observation of drug effects (Girgis et al., 2024). Moreover, more recent research highlights the severity of ADRs and their outcomes. A comparison study between reported suspected ADRs on antiseizure medication indicated that the majority of these reactions were ranked as severe and were likely to lead to critical complications such as hospitalization or death (Girgis et al., 2024). These findings underscore the need to differentiate between multiple outcomes when summing up ADRs. Severe ADRs affect the health of patients and can also change the choice and treatment of drugs. The system, therefore, needs to consider the clinical significance of such reactions, especially in individuals with a higher risk of experiencing a serious outcome. It is essential to use such classifications in clinical practice and drug monitoring to limit the risks caused by drug therapy. It is becoming increasingly the norm for medical professionals to employ reflection in the prescription of medicine, as both Type A and Type B responses are possible based on each patient's past. Early detection of adverse reactions is achievable with the help of strong monitoring systems, and better patient outcomes are feasible. Acknowledgment of the ADR classification not only facilitates better decision-making in prescribing processes but also provides regulatory agencies with a better framework upon which to enhance drug safety practice and promote successful pharmacovigilance (Suraj et al., 2023). Ultimately, better classification and management of ADRs play a key role in developing safer healthcare.

1.1.1. Type A (Augmented) Reactions

Type A (Augmented) reactions are a significant category of ADRs that occur as a predictable result of the pharmacological action of a drug. The dose of drug taken causes reactions and are generally because the drug acts on the body in an over-exuberant manner, not because of something idiosyncratic to the person. Increased doses of warfarin will cause the patient to bleed excessively, resulting in increased effects of the drug. Type A reactions should be recognized by care practitioners as this predisposes them to anticipate possible ADRs linked to the patient's personal factors and drug interactions. For this reason, close observation of patients and dosage adjustment can prevent these harmful outcomes and increase treatment efficacy.

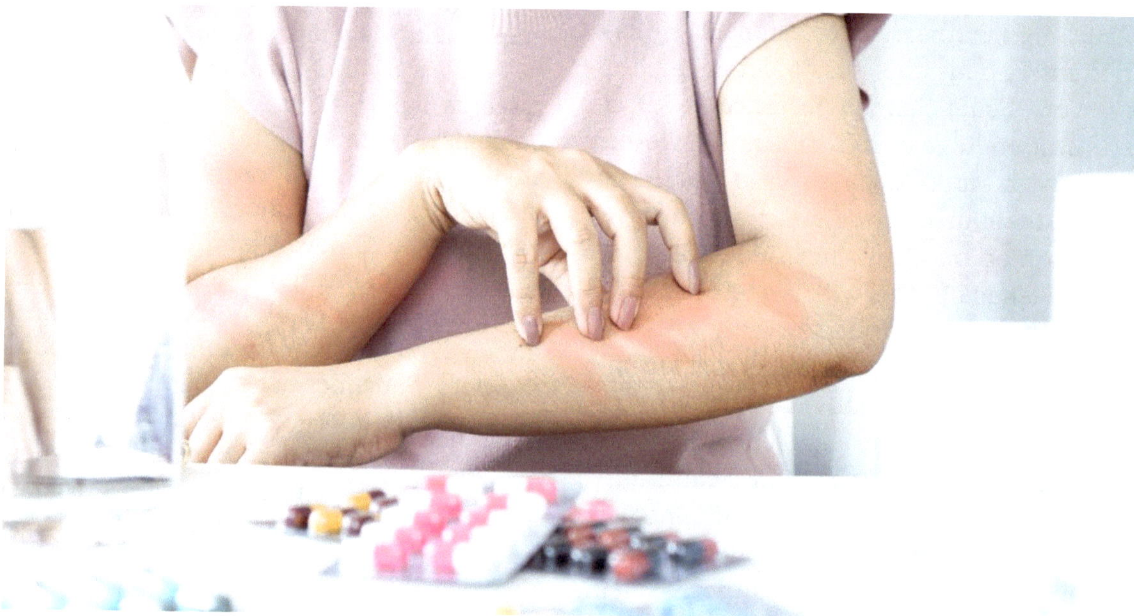

Figure 1.4. Type A (augmented) reactions.

Source: https://fastceforless.com/wp-content/uploads/2024/01/Adverse-Effects-and-Allergic-Reactions.jpg.

Second, increasing amounts of clinical data are being made more manageable. With electronic medical records (EMRs) and health sensors collecting vast amounts of data, clinicians are increasingly well-positioned to analyze patterns that lead to improved responses through advanced data analysis and machine learning (ML) algorithms. Due to this approach, patients who are at risk of developing Type A reactions can be identified early on, even before symptoms appear. Additionally, with the aid of big data, doctors can deliver medicine tailored to specific needs, reducing the likelihood of Type A Adverse reactions and increasing the success rate of therapy. As a result, utilizing data-driven methods can make drug therapy safer and more effective, benefiting patients' wellness and health. In healthcare when dealing with Type A reactions, one needs to listen to enhancing rules and educating people. The creation of drug effect tracking devices, such as continuous glucose monitoring (CGM) systems, illustrates the potential for enhanced drug response and the necessity of intervention by authorities to ensure that these devices are reliable and accurate. With the advancement of medical technology in the future, there must be regulation by authorities to ensure that these systems enable patients to take medicine in a safe manner and notify healthcare providers of important information. The intricacy of the management of type A reactions highlights the need for a collaborative effort between clinicians, pharmacists, and technology designers to enhance therapeutic interventions positively, tackling challenges related to treatment compliance as well as patient safety in innovative treatments (Bergenstal et al., 2017; Danieletto et al., 2018) (Figure 1.4).

1.1.2. Type B (Bizarre) Reactions

Type B (Bizarre) Reactions are a significant issue within ADRs, particularly because they are unpredictable and typically severe. Unlike type A reactions, which are dose-dependent and predictable, type B reactions arise from rare, idiosyncratic pharmacological reactions that vary significantly among individuals. Type B reactions could be the result of genetic idiosyncrasies or hypersensitivity and result in effects that are not only unpredictable but also potentially fatal. One of the most exemplary cases is the incidence of chloramphenicol-induced bone marrow aplasia, which is dose-related and is reported with an incidence of 1 in every 30,000 patients. The unpredictability of Type B reactions makes clinical practice more difficult since practitioners are unable to predict the side effects, suggesting the significance of increased awareness and knowledge on the part of medical personnel of such reactions (Mart et al., 2018). The clinical relevance of Type B reactions is fundamental because they most often necessitate immediate adjustments to a patient's treatment regimen. Due to their severity, the reactions can require the halt of some drugs or the application of additional therapeutic interventions to reverse their implications. For instance, with antimicrobial therapy that causes unexpected HSRs, it can require intensive care or other forms of treatment. This research has shown that these reactions are amplified at times by polypharmacy, wherein the concomitant administration of several drugs increases the likelihood of harmful interactions. Combination therapy involving antipsychotics and sedatives recently resulted in severe respiratory failure in some patients, which reflects the urgent requirement of observant monitoring of drug interactions and patient reaction, especially regarding possibly hazardous combinations (Adhikari et al., 2009). To combat the challenge emanating from Type B reactions, robust drug surveillance and reporting systems are necessary. The WHO promotes the systematic collection of ADR data to facilitate enhanced identification of such reactions. As serious as these reactions are, ADR reporting remains suboptimal in most areas, hindering efforts to understand and mitigate the risk factors for Type B reactions. Such systems, supported by programs for voluntary reporting of healthcare practitioners, can considerably increase the knowledge and control of such adverse events. Thus, continuous education and vigilant monitoring become essential components of care, yielding safer prescribing behaviors and improved patient outcomes in cases of unpredictable Type B reactions (Mart et al., 2018).

1.1.3. Other Classifications and Their Significance

ADRs can be classified in various ways to provide a clearer understanding of their function and impact on patient safety. A significant difference divides ADRs into Type A (expected) and Type B (idiosyncratic) reactions. Type A reactions are dose-dependent and classically related to the pharmacological action of a drug, representing approximately 80% of all ADRs. On the other hand, Type B reactions are more complex and often unpredictable, and could be due to genetic heterogeneity or environmental factors. Awareness of this distinction is crucial for healthcare workers, as it influences both drug selection and patient follow-up. As with the case of anti-infective agents' situations, specific demographic and clinical characteristics are to blame for the predisposing factors of severe ADRs. The classification of ADRs is particularly pertinent to successful prevention activities (Sittiphan et al., 2025). Another important classification pertains to the organ or system upon which ADRs exert their effects, i.e., gastrointestinal, dermatologic, or neurologic responses. Such a classification places the authority in the hands of medical professionals to identify patterns and relationships between some classes of drugs and the type of ADRs to which they are prone. For example, leukotriene receptor antagonists produce significant neuropsychiatric side effects; this finding calls for added vigilance for psychiatric complications among patients taking montelukast and zafirlukast compared to standard asthma medications (Khan et al., 2024). By categorizing ADRs by involved organ systems on a systematic level, clinicians can more effectively prioritize risk management interventions, optimize treatment regimens, and enhance patient education regarding possible side effects. Categorization of ADRs also enables the identification of susceptible patient populations with elevated rates of severe reactions. Data show that age, gender, ethnicity, and patient history are key drivers of both the frequency and severity of ADRs. For instance, in Thailand, data indicated that the elderly and individuals with a previous history of drug allergy had substantially higher risk of developing severe ADRs from anti-infective therapy (Sittiphan et al., 2025). This population-based approach highlights the relevance of individualized pharmacotherapy because clinicians can implement monitoring strategies for at-risk populations. The multifaceted classification of ADRs highlights not just the intricacy of drug interactions but also the need for clinicians to develop a proactive and educated approach to reducing the risks of pharmacotherapy and maximizing overall patient safety.

1.2. Mechanisms of Adverse Drug Reactions

The research on ADRs reveals different reasons for side effects in some individuals toward drugs. The central element of such mechanisms is the body's pharmacological reaction, which is often influenced by factors such as family, surroundings, and pre-existing medical conditions. Because enzymes, transporters, and receptors have polymorphisms, different individuals may react differently to a single drug. Because of this heterogeneity, some ADRs could happen in a non-predictable way, exhibiting the interrelationship of drugs and each person's body. In addition, researching adverse reactions to COVID-19 vaccines has underscored the importance of understanding these mechanisms. For example, the European Database of Suspected Adverse Drug Reaction provides evidence of heightened severity of adverse reactions following vaccination, particularly in elderly patients, thereby illustrating how patient characteristics influence drug response and safety profiles (Monta, 2022). Researchers also focus on the immune system's response to drugs. There exist immune checkpoint medications such as ipilimumab that have been linked with side effects to different parts of the body. Their ability to stimulate the immune system is possibly the reason why such drugs lead to increased risks of autoimmunity. For example, immune-related complications such as colitis, hepatitis, and dermatitis show how altering the immune system can result in serious and unexpected side effects. The additional evidence requires more sensitivity and vigilance from health practitioners to monitor for these less frequent but critical reactions (Wanchoo et al., 2017).

Determining the sources of ADRs can enable the formulation of drugs that result in high outcomes with less risk. Furthermore, the assessment of ADR mechanisms is of special interest in learning how drugs interact in the body systems. Such interactions have the potential to significantly affect drugs, making it more likely to experience damaging outcomes from consuming more drugs at once. When two drugs are taken simultaneously, their interactions can alter how they are absorbed, distributed within the body, metabolized by the liver, and excreted, potentially resulting in unexpected side effects. It is imperative to learn how these interactions occur, because elderly people often take more than one medication at the same time for their various illnesses. Examples of studies examining vaccine side effects reveal that the body's immune and systemic responses are based on the interaction between the vaccine and the body. By explaining such intricate mechanisms, researchers can devise ways to mitigate risks and enhance patient safety under pharmacotherapy, ultimately paving the way for more personalized and effective medicine (Monta, 2022) (Figure 1.5).

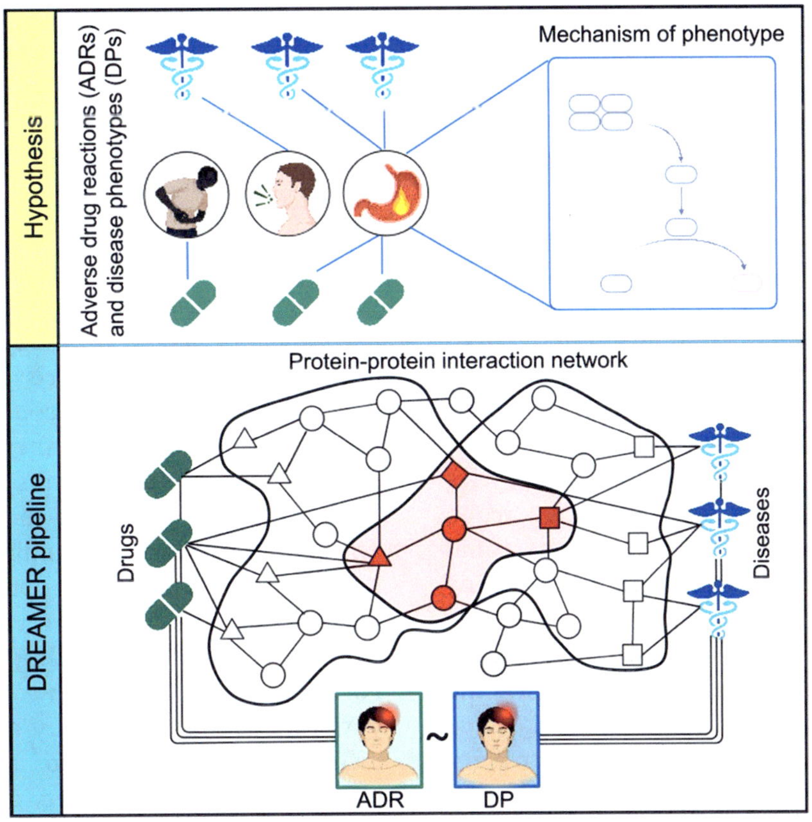

Figure 1.5. Mechanisms of adverse drug reactions.

Source: https://www.cell.com/cms/10.1016/j.crmeth.2025.100990/asset/91863168-2c33-47dc-a6ce-e383cb8d4e5d/main.assets/fx1_lrg.jpg.

1.2.1. Pharmacological Mechanisms

ADRs usually result from the pharmacological mechanisms inherent to drug interactions with biological systems. They are either predictable and dose-related (type A) or unpredictable and not related to the dose (type B). Acute tubular necrosis (ATN) is a type A reaction that usually happens when the drug's concentration exceeds what has been deemed safe. This can be seen in older patients who generally administer several medications, hence subjecting them to higher numbers of ADRs. Indeed, a significant number of reports of ADR demonstrate probable inappropriate medications (PIMs) that cause such adverse effects, highlighting the importance of correct management of pharmaceutical care systems in elderly patients (Jiang et al., 2025). Type B reactions are more complex to manage during pharmacotherapy than the usual predictable reactions. Some reactions, such as acute interstitial nephritis (AIN) or crystal-induced nephropathy, as well as others, frequently happen irrespective of the dosage of the drug. Drug-induced acute kidney injury (DI-AKI) is a good example of these unforeseen mechanisms, particularly in inpatient settings under exposure to nephrotoxic substances. Complications such as genetic issues or immune response reactions can complicate the control of ADRs. Research indicates nephrotoxic medications, such as vancomycin, are most frequently linked with DI-AKI, hence necessitating vigilance when such treatments are given concerning renal function monitoring (Garcia et al., 2024). Being cognizant of such mechanisms helps you better understand risk factors for ADRs. You must understand how drugs function to mitigate the impact of ADRs. Initiatives in pharmacovigilance are necessary since they enable the discovery and evaluation of ADRs using data collected in clinics. The surveillance allows medical professionals to observe how various drugs produce some adverse effects, enabling them to select safer medications. For instance, knowledge that certain combinations of drugs, such as aspirin and clopidogrel, enhance the risks of bleeding is central to prescribing protocols, especially for geriatric patients (Jiang et al., 2025). Secondly, the enactment of protocols to minimize PIMs and drug-drug interactions is essential to improve patient' outcomes and medication safety, as health professionals work to balance the advantages of medications against the hazards of side effects.

1.2.2. Genetic Factors Influencing ADRs

Increased recognition of genetic causes as a source of ADRs indicates the complex character of pharmacogenomics in modern practice. Genetic differences between individuals can significantly influence a patient's response to treatment, i.e., drug metabolism, effectiveness, and safety profiles. For example, polymorphisms in genes encoding drug-metabolizing enzymes, such as cytochrome P450 enzymes, can lead to variations in drug plasma levels and potentially increase ADR risks. The hidden relationship between these genetic variations and side effects justifies taking into account individual genetic factors when drugs are administered, since certain genotypes expose patients to either therapeutic failure or unacceptable side effects. As pharmacogenomic research progresses, it becomes increasingly crucial that genetic screening forms a part of clinical practice to tailor the drug therapy in line with one's genetic profile to minimize ADRs. Research has proved that specific populations are more likely to have a higher prevalence of certain genetic variants influencing drug responses. For example, studies show that populations with differentiated ancestry of origin can have differential frequencies of drug metabolism alleles such that drug safety and efficacy differ among demographic groups. Genetic factors are particularly important for drugs with narrow therapeutic indices, so that small variations in drug concentration can lead to significant adverse outcomes. Furthermore, simultaneous administration of two or more drugs, common in elderly people, can contribute to the risk of ADRs, with the impact of genetic factors. In such a multimodal context, adopting a patient-specific strategy of medication management that incorporates genetic testing, along with traditional clinical assessment, is necessary to promote patient safety and optimize therapeutic effects, particularly in vulnerable populations. Pre-emptive pharmacogenetic testing is a promising tool for limiting the incidence of ADRs and their associated healthcare costs. By identifying genetic variants that affect drug response before treatment, healthcare providers can choose specific medications or adjust dosing according to the patient's genetic makeup. Such foresight can be viewed as reducing the occurrence of major ADRs considerably, as documented by research findings that cite genetic testing as assisting in the selection of the correct therapy and enhancing patient adherence to treatment regimens.

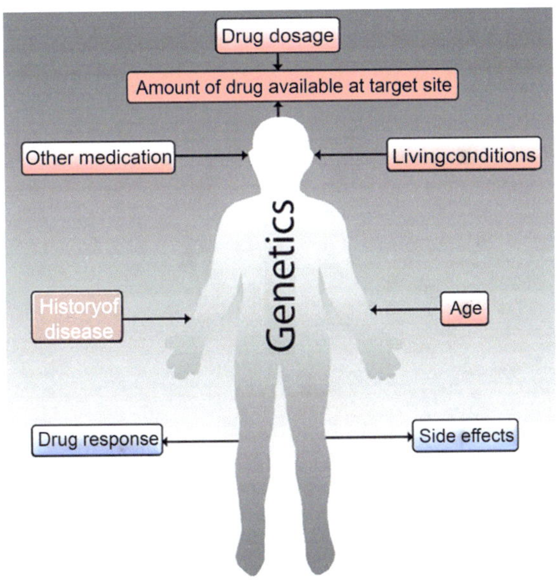

Figure 1.6. Genetic factors influencing adverse drug reaction.

Source: https://www.omicsonline.org/articles-images/2155-6156-4-248-g003.gif.

Further, the integration of pharmacogenetics into clinical practices can assist in enhanced patient outcomes through reduced hospitalization due to ADRs and overall healthcare expenditure. With the health sector slowly accepting pre-emptive pharmacogenetic testing, the potential to transform the practice of ADR management into an accurate and efficient process becomes evident, ultimately reaching the patients and the entire health system (Chenchula et al., 2024; Chiumia et al., 2024) (Figure 1.6).

1.2.3. Environmental and Drug Interactions

The intricate interaction between drug interactions and environmental determinants plays a significant role in the expression of ADRs. Environmental determinants such as climate, pollution, and exposure to diverse chemicals can modify drug action and metabolism. For instance, certain environmental toxins can compete at metabolizing sites in the liver with drugs and thus alter their therapeutic effect or toxicity. Apart from this, varying climatic factors can affect drug bioavailability, which may result in non-uniform treatment outcomes. This much complexity requires a consideration of a patient's exposure to the environment while administering drugs, since it may enhance the risk of ADRs. Such information becomes significant to personalize therapeutic regimens and adopt safer drug practices in diverse populations who encounter unique environmental barriers. Aside from external environmental factors, the construction of nanomedicines provides new opportunities and challenges for drug interactions. Nanotechnology aims to enhance drug delivery systems in a way that enables targeted therapy with minimal systemic exposure. As quoted, nanomedicine makes site-specific delivery possible with minimal influence of environmental factors on drug efficacy (Patra et al., 2018). However, such a novel approach will also potentially yield unforeseen interactions between nanoparticles and environmental materials, leading to various pharmacokinetic (PK) effects. The biocompatibility of engineered nanoparticles with organic and inorganic materials in various environments is yet to be explored. Therefore, careful observation and investigation are to fully comprehend how these new delivery systems interact with environmental conditions, so that therapeutic advancements do not unintentionally contribute to ADRs. Moreover, the interactive nature between drugs and the environment can impact cellular responses, and this could further render ADRs more complex. Environmentally induced cellular stress can impact drug potency and toxicity, modulating how drugs are metabolized in the body. For instance, varied levels of oxidative stress induced by environmental toxicants might activate cell death pathways that intersect with drug-induced responses (Galluzzi et al., 2018). Understanding the mechanistic pathways behind these interactions is crucial for developing safer pharmacotherapies. By integrating concepts in environmental science into pharmacology, researchers can better predict and prevent the risk of ADRs caused by such intricate interactions. This interdisciplinary approach may ultimately lead to more effective drug development and optimized therapeutic effects amidst a diverse array of environmental threats (Figure 1.7).

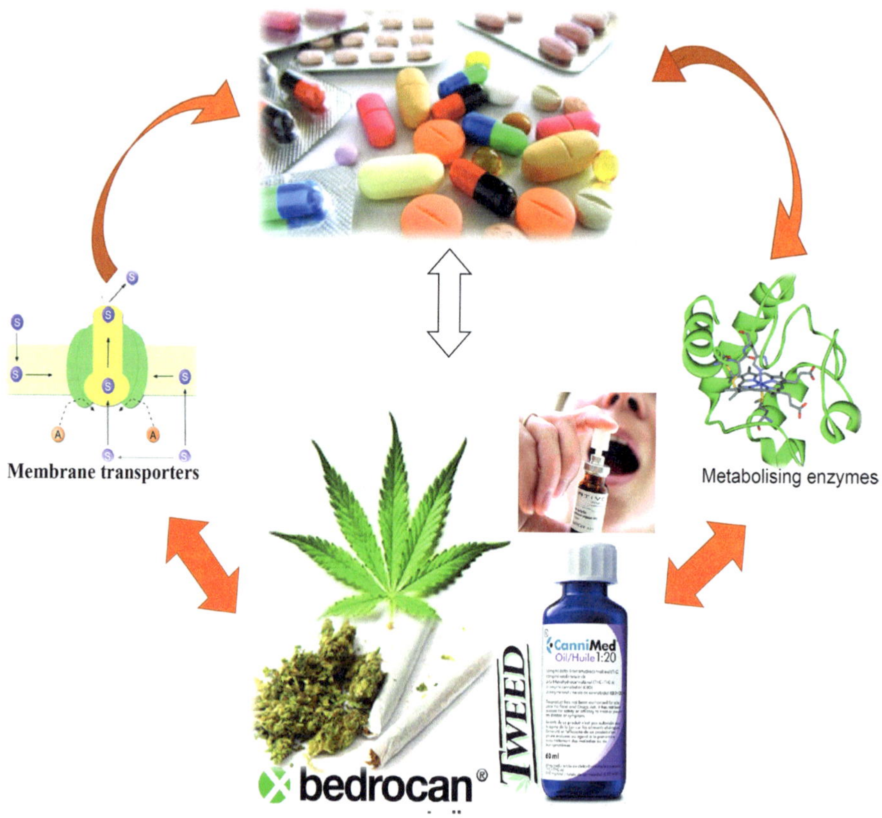

Figure 1.7. Environmental and drug interactions.

Source: https://pdhpe.net/wp-content/uploads/2016/08/environmental-factors.jpg.

1.3. Risk Factors for Adverse Drug Reactions

The occurrence of ADRs largely relies on the clinical and demographic characteristics of the patients, particularly among the elderly. The population is risk-prone because they tend to be on more than one medication at a time, and this can cause drug interactions. The body's physiological changes with advancing age also influence how drugs are absorbed, distributed in the body, metabolized in the liver, and excreted. As a result, ADRs may not exhibit the usual symptoms, making their detection and treatment challenging. Identification of vulnerable patients is essential, and tools like the GerontoNet ADR Risk Score have been developed to assist healthcare workers in identifying older patients at increased risk of developing adverse drug reactions (ADRs), ultimately resulting in targeted interventions aimed at reducing ADR occurrence (Onder et al., 2012). Considering the risks associated with ADRs, administering the wrong medicine to the elderly population is a significant concern. Misuse of medicines or in excessive amounts may result in serious problems, which is why each patient's regimen needs to be carefully examined. Visible as well as hidden criteria exist to allow efficient ways of prescribing medicines. Explicit criteria are used to determine the relevant dose and probable drug interaction, while implicit criteria rely on specialists' consensus and list the drugs to be avoided. Through systematic medication assessment tools, clinicians can perform important reviews that can address the individual needs of elderly patients, thus improving the quality of prescribing and reducing the incidence of ADRs (Corsonello et al., 2016). Moreover, when different experts collaborate, the detection and resolution of the risks of ADRs become easier. When doctors, pharmacists, and nursing staff work together in integrated pharmaceutical care, it enhances the safety and effectiveness of drug therapy for patients. Review of all medicines, taking pharmaceutical history, and the development of individual plans of care assist a better way of dealing with medications. If clinical professionals can visualize the entire medical record and clinical information, they can identify and manage potential drug-related risks. This combined approach underscores the importance of ongoing communication among medical professionals, fostering an environment in which ADR risks are effectively mitigated and patient safety is maximized (Corsonello et al., 2016).

1.3.1. Patient-Related Factors

Patient-related factors also play an important role in the cause and severity of ADRs. The age of the patients is also a deciding factor here, as elderly individuals are more prone to adverse drug effects. It has been seen that patients older than 65 years are more likely to have severe ADRs because of changes in their bodies, multiple drug therapy at a time, and the occurrence of more chronic diseases. This group was found to have severe ADRs at an odds ratio of 4.53, adjusted, meaning a fourfold increased risk compared to younger patients, and hence the implication of age in ADR development (Chiumia et al., 2024). That is why medical practitioners should give special attention to the group by cross-verifying medication risks to safeguard the patient against harmful impacts. ADRs are more likely to happen in persons with specific genders and different socioeconomic backgrounds. Women have been discovered, consistent with studies, to be apt to develop ADRs, and this is possibly due to their biological nature, hormonal changes, and individual susceptibility to drugs. Aside from gender, a person's level of income is a significant factor in their health conditions. In a study, a significant percentage of individuals with incomes below 2.5 lakh Indian rupees suffered moderately severe ADRs, illustrating the relationship between low socio-economic status and barriers in receiving optimal healthcare (Pavan et al., 2024). Once HCPs are aware of these correlations, they can develop improved treatments and provide beneficial information for every patient group. Additionally, how well patients understand their health and the medications they take can increase or decrease the risks of ADRs. If a patient does not know how to take medication prescribed to them, it might result in them not following directions and experiencing adverse effects. Being poorly educated about their medications can lead some patients to take incorrect doses, at an incorrect time, or with medication they should not be taking together. People who are health-educated can better manage their medications and prevent such risks. These are highly critical in situations where individuals will be taking more than one medication at the same time. If healthcare systems educate patients, they can achieve better treatment outcomes and diminish the effects of ADRs on individuals and the medical system, thereby making drug use safer (Figure 1.8).

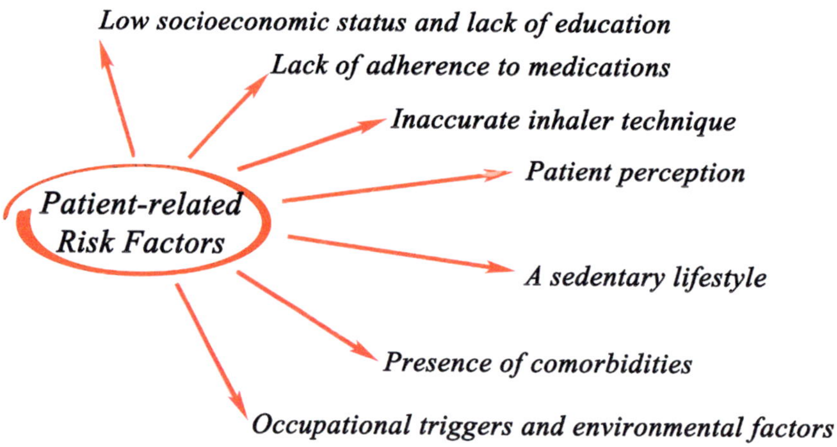

Figure 1.8. Patient-related factors.

Source: https://thumbs.dreamstime.com/z/seven-patient-related-risk-factors-239326571.jpg.

1.3.2. Drug-Related Factors

The process of drug-related factors in ADRs is mainly overseen by the drug's properties and the characteristics of the patient. The risk of ADRs is mainly affected by drug interactions, the correct dosage, and the way drugs are processed and used in the body. For example, using a combination of drugs at the same time can significantly raise the risk of serious ADRs. In a Malawian study, people using more than one antibiotic were shown by researchers to be 2.14 times more likely to experience serious ADRs than those using only one antibiotic. So, it is essential to manage and watch medications carefully, mainly when a person is taking multiple drugs. Patients' demographic factors are also significant in causing drug-related factors that lead to ADRs. Age, gender, and socioeconomic status play crucial roles in identifying a person's vulnerability to ADRs. In particular, older people had a 4.53 times greater chance of suffering severe ADRs compared to younger patients. Besides, poor patients may have difficulties getting the best care, which often makes it hard for them to follow complicated drug schedules. Such populations not only recognize at-risk groups but also highlight the necessity to administer drug treatment tailored to a patient's history, which can potentially counter the prevalence of ADRs. Furthermore, the severity of ADRs has the potential to impact a patient's health-related quality of life (HRQoL) severely, rendering identification of drug-related factors early in treatment vital. It was found in one study that many patients with ADRs suffered from moderately severe reactions that had a significant impact on their general well-being. It was found through multivariate analysis that the severity of the ADR, a person's income, and their age were the most important factors affecting HRQoL. As a result, clinicians are required to consider both the immediate and long-term effects of drugs on their patients' quality of life. Identifying these drug-related factors can ultimately enable patient-centered care and inform strategies to optimize therapeutic benefits, leading to a more preferable management of ADRs in clinical practice (Chiumia et al., 2024; Pavan et al., 2024) (Figure 1.9).

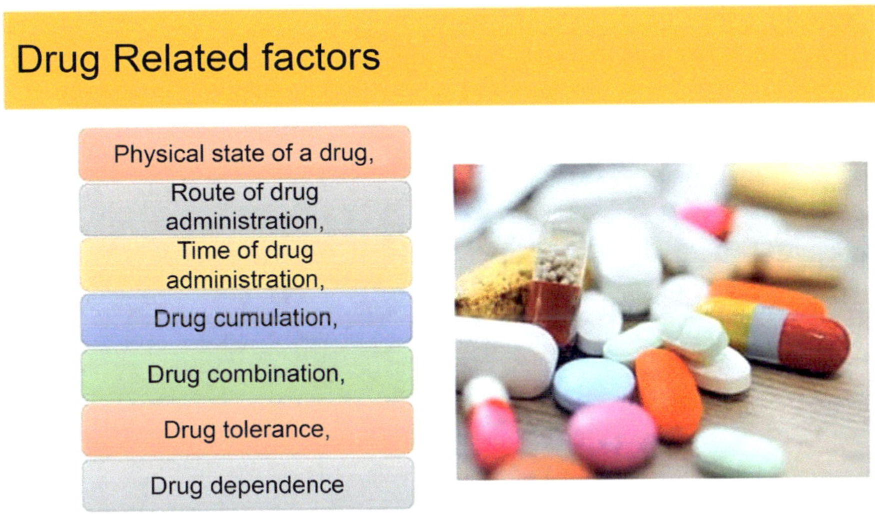

Figure 1.9. Drug-related factors.

Source: https://image.slidesharecdn.com/factorsaffectingdrugaction-200730092738/85/Factors-affecting-drug-action-in-Pharmacology-4-638.jpg.

1.3.3. Healthcare System-Related Factors

The health system has a decisive role in determining the incidence of ADRs, namely through its prescribing pattern and medication management policy. Different ways of prescribing and the fact that treatment schedules are complicated can lead to more ADRs. In particular, when patients are prescribed many drugs at the same time, the risk of adverse effects is much higher for older adults. The group usually deals with drug-related issues due to changes in their bodies and the existence of several other health conditions. Systematic review revealed that nearly 9% of hospital-discharged elderly patients have drug-related readmissions, of which a fraction is considered preventable, highlighting the systemic necessity of better medication management and education in healthcare environments (Moirana et al., 2023). Therefore, it is important to improve the way prescriptions are made and training to reduce the number of ADRs and make patients safer. Moreover, the quality and availability of healthcare services can either decrease or increase the chances of ADRs. In such areas, patients are not monitored regularly, so it is likely that drug reactions will not be found in time. The issue arises in nations where major public health problems exist. For instance, there was one systematic review that was characterized by an impressive 26.5% rate of hospitalization of ADRs in some African countries, primarily because of antiretroviral therapy (ART) complications (Moirana et al., 2023). More cases of ADR incidents suggest that the healthcare system does not have enough resources to handle treatment plans effectively. Therefore, addressing the problems in healthcare is crucial to prevent ADRs, so policy changes and additional investments should be made in this important area of public health. Besides setting rules and making drugs available, the way healthcare systems train professionals is important in avoiding ADRs. If health professionals can identify, deal with, and report ADRs, patient outcomes are better protected. Regularly teaching HCPs about medication safety is likely to encourage them to be careful in their work. For instance, a significant percentage of medication-related hospital readmissions for older adults were found to be preventable, indicating potential opportunities for clinicians to improve their information and communication regarding the complexity of treatment (Dai et al., 2024). As time passes, effective ways to avoid ADRs depend on pharmacists, physicians, and nurses collaborating in various areas. When healthcare workers are well-educated and work together, it may lower the risk of ADRs and help improve patient care (Figure 1.10).

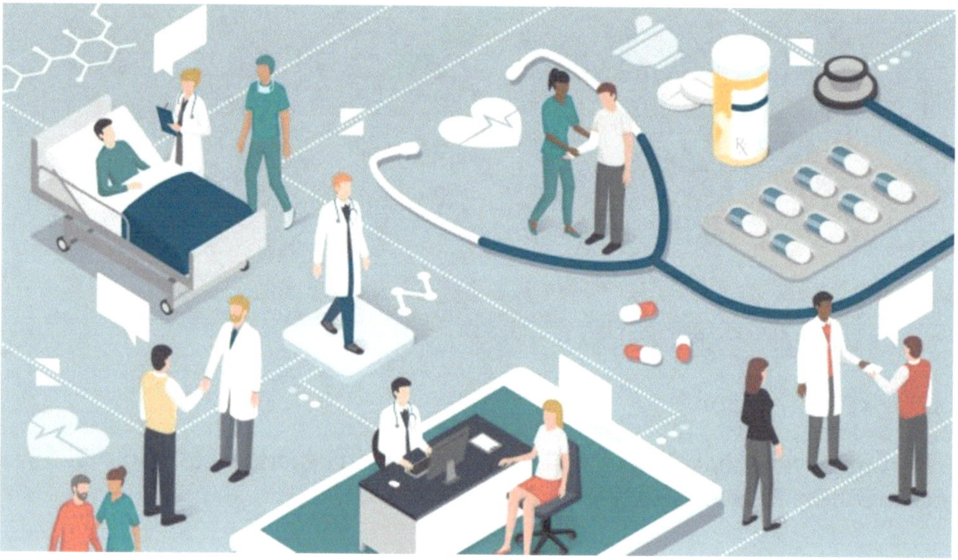

Figure 1.10. Healthcare system-related factors.

Source: https://online.stanford.edu/sites/default/files/styles/embedded_large/public/2020-08/%20 Introduction-to-Healthcare_SOM-XCHE0008.jpg?itok=ub93y0gH.

1.4. Detection and Reporting of Adverse Drug Reactions

Reporting and detection of ADRs is an important aspect of drug safety and pharmacovigilance. Because ADRs may endanger a patient's health, it is essential to regularly monitor and document them. Spontaneous reporting systems (SRS) play a crucial role in the process, as they allow healthcare providers and patients to report suspected ADRs, which helps in the broader understanding of a drug's safety profile. Analysis of data from these systems helps identify patterns and potential signals that inform regulators' practices and physicians' decisions. The primary challenge lies in the accurate identification of ADRs from vast amounts of data, indicating the need for rigorous methodologies for assessing the drug-ADR association (Gosho et al., 2024). All in all, improving the detection of adverse events is required to protect patients and pharmacovigilance. New ways of analyzing data are being recommended to help find more ADRs in SRS. While PRR and ROR are the main signals used in detecting ADRs, they may need detailed reviews for each ADR. A generalized mixed-effects model that has been proposed recommends a more effective approach to determining the relationships between several drugs and ADRs simultaneously, enhancing the detection process (Gosho et al., 2024). This method simplifies the analysis, making the results more accurate and correcting the false-positive results that are present in regular methods. Because of these methods, tracking drug safety is simpler, and fast action can be taken where needed. It is necessary to find alternative methods to identify ADRs, as they can sometimes be difficult to detect during pregnancy. Currently, the systems do not identify ADRs in specific groups and mix helpful signals with the rest of the background reports. EudraVigilance helps with finding ADRs in the European Economic Area, but it does not store data about exposure to medications during pregnancy. In this situation, a new algorithm has been developed to help identify ADRs by analyzing real cases in pregnant women. As the initial results suggest, this algorithm outperforms previous methods, providing an opportunity to make progress in pharmacovigilance and improve maternal health (Figure 1.11).

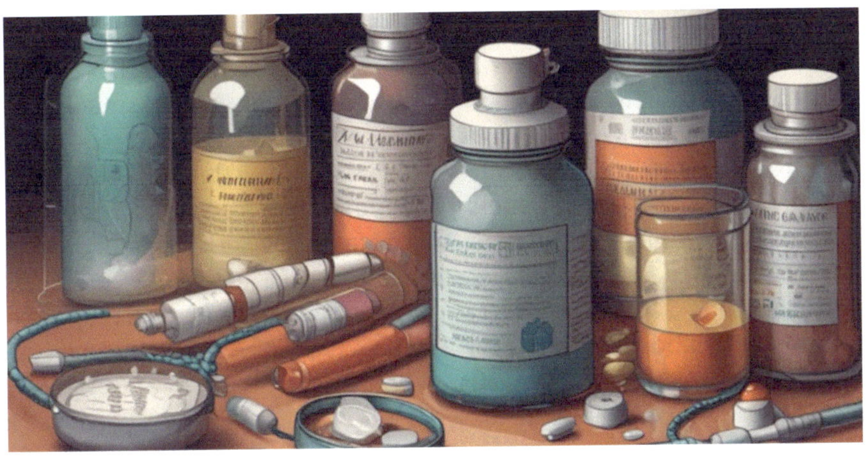

Figure 1.11. Detection and reporting of adverse drug reactions.

Source: https://assets.quizgecko.com/cdn-cgi/image/width=800,quality=90,format=webp/quiz/9d28f2446aaf5f1bb3ba128f16d20ade.jpg.

1.4.1. Methods for Detecting ADRs

ADR identification is critical for enhancing patient safety and optimizing drug therapy. Traditional methods, such as disproportionality analysis (DPA), have been conventionally used in pharmacovigilance to identify potential safety signals based on spontaneous event reports (SERs). However, based on a sparse data set, such methods may not be very skilled at ADR detection. Advances in technology in recent times have seen ML techniques introduced that enhance these detection methods by introducing more data. By integrating SER data with biological, chemical, and ADR data, scientists have demonstrated that ML algorithms outperform traditional DPA methods, yielding more accurate and comprehensive results. Therefore, the use of ML techniques could provide a more robust model of ADR detection and encourage improved practice in drug safety

(Schreier et al., 2024). In ADR detection, one of the new techniques is to use global trigger tools that flag possible ADRs from the patients' records. Retrospective reviews in healthcare have traditionally employed fixed tools to categorize ADRs according to how probable they were to occur, their severity, and their preventability. The tools typically employ the Naranjo scale as well as statistical methodology in determining how ADRs correlate with specific patient characteristics. Research into antibiotic-associated ADRs in Malawi has pointed out the prevalence of such occurrences and the efficacy of such methods. Approximately 24% of patients in a study had suspected ADRs, with severe incidences heavily affecting vulnerable populations, noting the necessity for good detection pathways within clinical facilities (Chiumia et al., 2024). Besides ML and global trigger tools, pharmacovigilance is also turning to real-time monitoring systems and electronic health records (EHRs) for the dynamic detection of ADRs. With these approaches, HCPs can monitor patient information on a regular basis and identify signals of potential harm from drugs. If various sources of data, such as treatment history, laboratory results, and patient information, are well-integrated into EHRs, it is fairly easy to identify ADRs. Furthermore, dashboards that indicate any abnormal trends can provide valuable insights to HCPs, motivating them to respond promptly. Thus, these advances suggest that an integrated approach—combining traditional practices, new advances in technology, and interdisciplinary examination of data—can significantly improve the monitoring of ADRs, ultimately enhancing patient safety (Schreier et al., 2024).

1.4.2. Importance of Reporting Systems

Effective reporting systems have an essential part in the surveillance and management of ADRs as the basis of pharmacovigilance. By enabling HCPs to document and report ADRs, these systems enable continuous monitoring of the safety and efficacy of drugs. This is critical in post-marketing surveillance, where the long-term effects of drugs are assessed among a larger population. Encouraging health care professionals' awareness of the significance of reporting systems enhances detection rates of ADRs. Following most research, e.g., (Eruaga et al., 2024) there is typically a large knowledge-practice gap regarding reporting guidelines and reporting practices among health care professionals. Hence, addressing this void through focused educational interventions (EIs) can tremendously improve drug regulation and overall patient safety, thereby instilling a culture of care and vigilance in healthcare institutions. Underreporting of ADRs remains a prevalent trend, reflecting the need for strong reporting systems that are easily accessible and easy to use. In environments like Nigeria, where issues such as limited resources and inadequate regulatory systems prevail, establishing robust reporting mechanisms is even more crucial. As propounded by Eruaga et al. (2024), the unique issues that confront countries with limited pharmacovigilance infrastructure underscore the necessity for effective reporting processes to enhance drug safety monitoring. By encouraging coordination among regulatory agencies, healthcare institutions, and drug producers, healthcare systems can create stronger and more effective reporting networks. This coordination not only increases the quantity of ADRs reported but also enhances the quality of data submitted for risk assessment, which improves public health outcomes and ensures that corrective action is implemented promptly. Moreover, the application of technology in reporting systems likewise offers viable alternatives to enhance the effectiveness and precision of ADR data collection. Internet-based platforms can facilitate real-time reporting, simplifying the process for healthcare practitioners. Healthcare practitioners can readily upload comprehensive reports through the use of mobile applications or online databases, thereby eliminating hurdles associated with conventional reporting systems. Moreover, as Hussain et al. (2021) found in their study, healthcare workers had positive attitudes towards ADR reporting, supported by simple protocols and readily accessible platforms. These results suggest that enhancing the technical infrastructure not only enhances the reporting rates but also facilitates the role of HCPs to become proactive in pharmacovigilance. Lastly, these advancements in reporting systems are most significant to reiterating the safety of therapeutic interventions, instilling an environment under which patient welfare is always accorded priority (Figure 1.12).

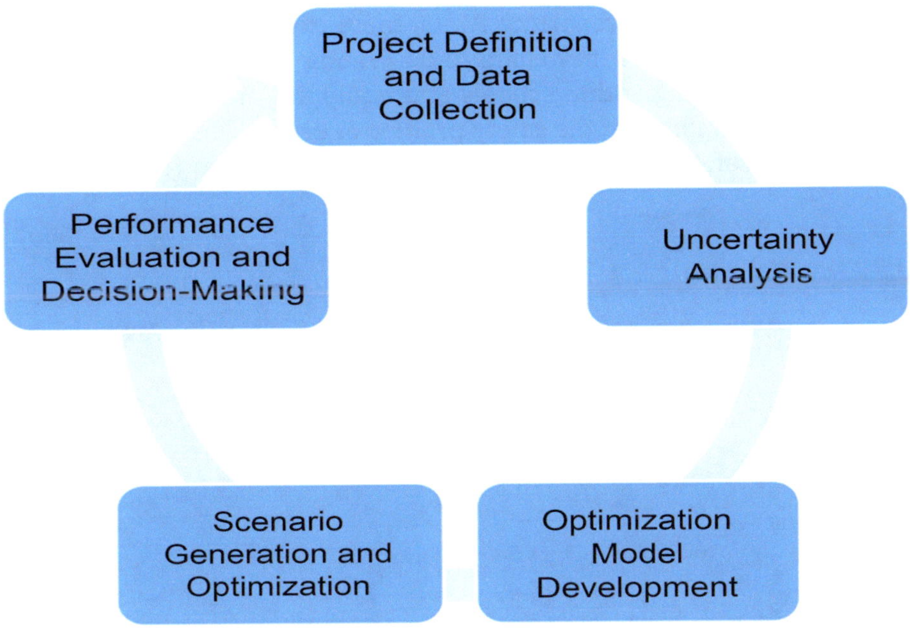

Figure 1.12. Importance of reporting systems.

Source: https://www.bplogix.com/hs-fs/hubfs/Adverse%20Event%20Reporting%20Challenges.png?width=1000&height=500&name=Adverse%20Event%20Reporting%20Challenges.png.

1.4.3. Role of Healthcare Professionals in Reporting

The role of the HCPs in the reporting of ADRs is key to advancing patient safety and enhancing pharmacovigilance. These practitioners are principal intermediaries responsible for the detection and reporting of ADR events, which feed back into providing data to regulatory agencies and facilitate continuing surveillance of drug safety. While their services are beneficial, the majority of studies demonstrate an alarming trend of underreporting among HCPs. Both ignorance about why reporting ADR is required and inadequate training are reasons why this trend exists. Interestingly, a survey within the primary healthcare setting revealed that the majority of HCPs, including nurses and pharmacists, were not knowledgeable enough about reporting, which was an enlightening gap to be addressed (Yuniar et al., 2024). EIs have emerged as the primary strategy to enhance the knowledge and attitudes of HCPs regarding the reporting of ADRs. Systematic reviews indicate that appropriately designed EIs, namely workshops, systematically improve rates of reporting ADRs as well as the overall awareness of pharmacovigilance among physicians. Studies indicate that participation in educational workshops can increase the odds of ADR reporting considerably, with outcomes reflecting an odds ratio of 6.26 for increased reporting after such interventions (Mónica et al., 2024). This heightened awareness not only educates healthcare professionals but also fosters a safety culture in healthcare settings. These measures are crucial in bridging the knowledge gap and in alerting HCPs to the fact that they can initiate the crucial action of ADR reporting and documentation. Ultimately, cultivating a proactive attitude towards ADR reporting among HCPs is essential for protecting patient health. The shared responsibility of HCPs for reporting and detection of ADRs cannot be overstressed, as effective reporting has the potential to lead to alterations in clinical practice as well as the development of safer drug regimens. From studies assessing attitudes towards reporting ADRs, there exists an enormous disparity between HCPs' intentions to report and what they claim to do (Yuniar et al., 2024). Therefore, focusing on the importance of ADR reporting within schools and equipping HCPs with proper resources and training will be essential in improving the safety profiles of drugs. This united effort can ultimately lead to improved patient safety and a more robust healthcare system (Figure 1.13).

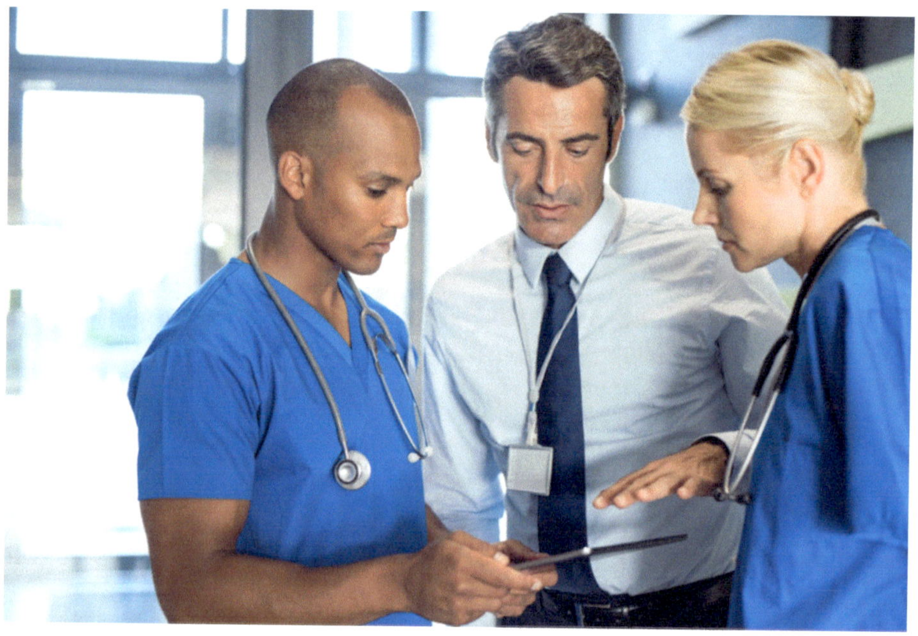

Figure 1.13. Role of healthcare professionals in reporting.

Source: https://s3.amazonaws.com/utep-uploads/wp-content/uploads/2017/09/07101640/need-healthcare-professionals.jpg.

1.5. Management of Adverse Drug Reactions

The management of ADRs is a critical aspect of pharmacovigilance and therapeutic intervention in clinical settings. The first step in good management is to spot and assess ADRs, which means that healthcare settings should have active monitoring and reporting systems. HCPs should be able to recognize the symptoms of ADRs so that they can take prompt action to prevent complications. In such cases, doctors may need to review the patient's medications, consider alternative treatments, or adjust the doses. When healthcare providers are alert and communicate well, the risk of adverse effects goes down and patient safety and results are improved. For ADR management to succeed, it is important to involve patients and educate them. Patients should be involved, since they can notice and report any possible side effects. Education programs can help patients recognize any unusual symptoms and report them promptly to their doctors. Besides, using mobile health applications can make it simpler to monitor medications and their side effects. Such real-time data gathering provides clinicians with information on ADRs, enabling them to select the most effective treatment options. Involving patients encourages them to take charge of ADR management and reminds them to adhere to their doctor's advice, thereby fostering a strong relationship between the patient and doctor. The management of ADRs plays a part in the bigger effort to enhance the quality of healthcare. Researching ADRs is important to learn about their causes and to develop new ways to manage them. New antibiotic therapies, for example, highlight the challenges posed by multidrug-resistant (MDR) organisms and the corresponding need for effective management strategies (Uddin et al., 2021). Furthermore, adherence to clinical guidelines, such as those proposed for the treatment of chronic conditions like psoriasis, can ensure a standardized approach to managing the adverse effects of medications (Nast et al., 2020). When professionals use research and best practices in daily healthcare, it helps them handle ADRs properly and protect patients' health while improving treatment results.

1.5.1. Strategies for Prevention

Practical strategies for preventing ADRs are essential to improve patient safety and healthcare outcomes. Structured reviews of medications are necessary, especially for older individuals who are likely to take multiple medications for various health conditions. Checking a patient's medications regularly may help find prescriptions that could be harmful and reduce the risk of drug interactions. Tools such as EHRs facilitate this process by providing HCPs with relevant patient information and medication histories, allowing for better clinical decision-making. Additionally, utilizing clinical guidelines developed for age-related pharmacotherapy can assist doctors in determining the most suitable treatment for each patient. By implementing such systematic reviews, healthcare providers can significantly reduce the incidence of ADRs and enhance the overall quality of care for at-risk populations, thereby addressing a substantial healthcare burden (Siobhán et al., 2024). Pharmacogenomics is a new way to prevent ADRs by adjusting drug treatment to each person's genetic makeup. With knowledge of how genes affect drug reactions, clinicians can prevent prescribing drugs that could harm patients due to their genetic makeup. Because of this approach, the chances of ADRs are reduced and the therapy is more effective. It is also important for healthcare providers to keep learning about pharmacogenomics, since this helps them take a proactive approach to avoiding ADRs. The integration of pharmacogenomic data into clinical practice can empower healthcare practitioners to make more informed prescribing decisions, thereby promoting safer medication use among patients (Tanwar et al., 2023). With the advancement of pharmacogenomics, healthcare systems may soon adopt a new approach to medication safety. Besides these approaches, having strong pharmacovigilance systems is important for spotting and monitoring ADRs. These systems, which utilize data mining and instant reporting, are crucial for identifying patterns of adverse reactions in many patients. When healthcare institutions systematically use and share data from EHRs, they can review the results of medications and identify potential risks associated with certain drugs. Additionally, providing educational materials on medications to patients helps them follow their treatment and discuss any concerns they may have with their doctors. By fostering a culture of patient engagement and vigilance, healthcare systems can enhance their capacity to prevent ADRs and thereby improve patient safety (Siobhán et al., 2024). If ADRs are handled together using these approaches, it will be easier to improve therapies and the quality of care in different medical settings (Figure 1.14).

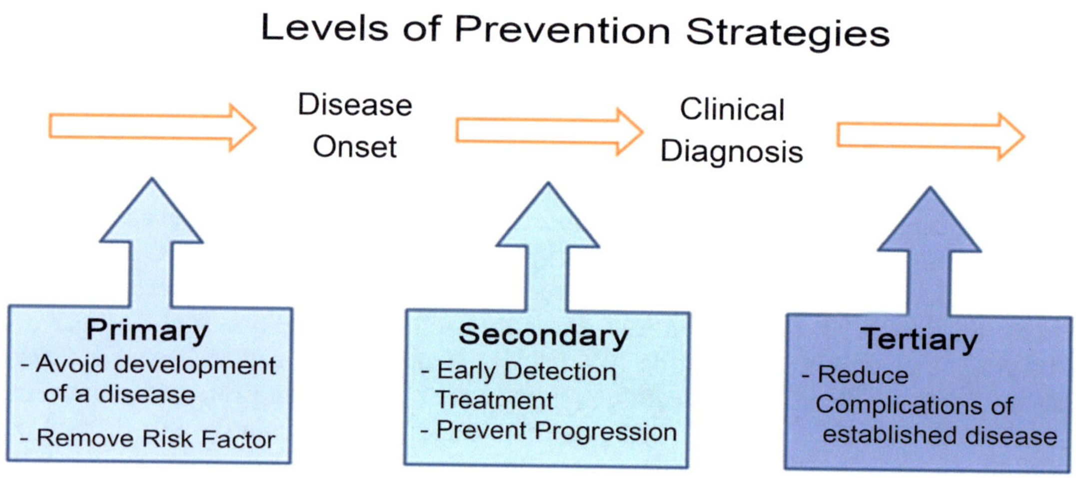

Figure 1.14. Strategies for prevention.

Source: https://bpb-us-w2.wpmucdn.com/edblogs.columbia.edu/dist/3/817/files/2017/04/prevention_strategy-1nr9qp0.jpg.

1.5.2. Treatment Options for ADRs

Management of ADRs must be multidimensional, not only to alleviate the symptoms but also to minimize the risk of recurrence in the future. The initial and most crucial step in managing ADRs is the identification and removal of the causative agent. The doctor must immediately analyze the relationship between the drug and the adverse effect. In situations where withdrawal is indicated, alternative therapy should be replaced. For example, individuals suffering from ADRs of pain-relief medications like acetaminophen, which are often prescribed and used, will have to switch over to alternative pain management protocols. These switches require consideration of the unique health profile of individual patients and cross-reactivity with substitute drugs, particularly considering that a few ADRs related to the use of acetaminophen are immune-mediated in nature, such as significant cutaneous reactions like SJS (Noah et al., 2023). Other than drug withdrawal, symptomatic management plays a key role in the treatment of ADRs. Symptomatic treatment can straightforwardly enhance the quality of life of a patient in dealing with the complexities of drug-induced complications. As an example, symptomatic treatment of ADRs caused by intranasal corticosteroids, such as epistaxis or headache, may include topical intervention or other analgesics that will not complicate existing conditions. A thorough analysis of safety data, as conducted by the Netherlands Pharmacovigilance Center, highlights the need for precaution in prescribing intranasal corticosteroids. Reporting of severe ADRs, including systemic complications like Cushing's syndrome, helps ensure constant surveillance of patients and makes them aware of potential side effects (Rollema et al., 2022). Ultimately, shared decision-making and patient education are essential components of ADR management. Health education about ADR signs and symptoms empowers patients to report the early occurrence of adverse effects, which initiates timely interventions.

Additionally, patients must be actively engaged in the treatment decision-making process, including discussions on the risks and benefits of recommended treatments. Such open communication enables healthcare providers to modify drug regimens to prevent ADRs while maximizing the efficacy of treatment regimens. This initiative can significantly enhance compliance and achieve optimal therapeutic outcomes, ultimately ensuring that patients receive safe and effective care for their health conditions through ADRs (Figure 1.15).

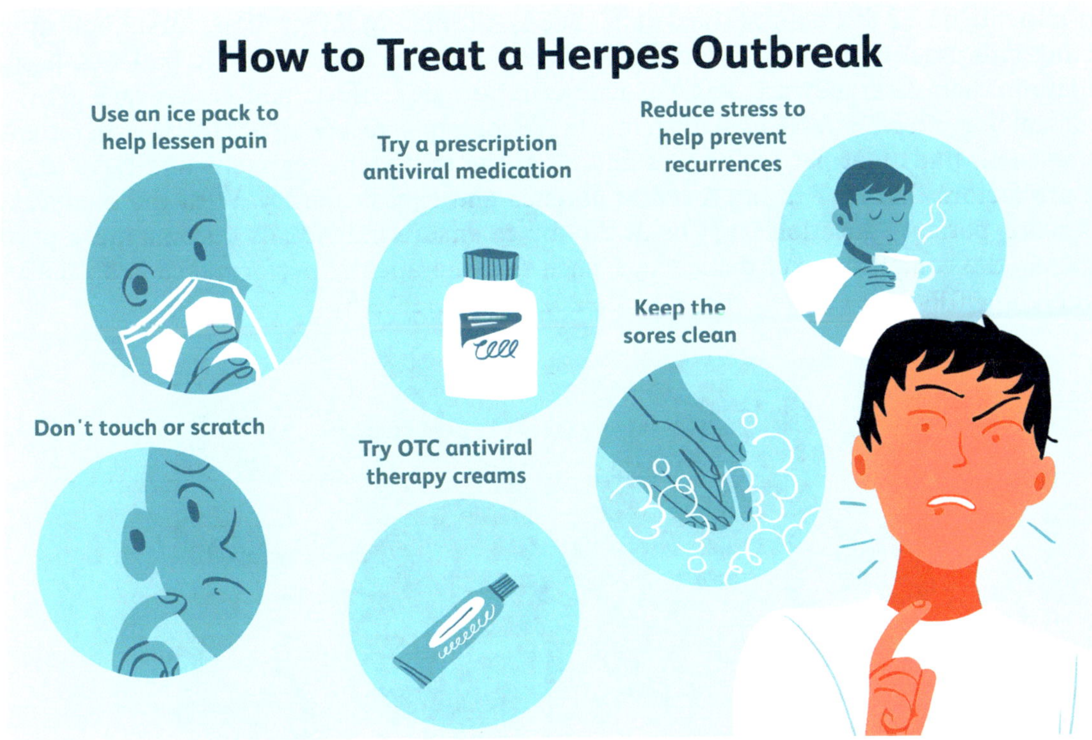

Figure 1.15. Treatment options for adverse drug reaction.

Source: https://www.verywellhealth.com/thmb/P148KQcgCt8w4WPmsNHd4VcphFQ=/1500x0/filters:no_upscale():max_bytes(150000):strip_icc()/herpes-treatment-3133020_color1-5b85557ac9e77c00576df991.png.

1.5.3. Patient Education and Counseling

Effective patient education and counseling are integral parts in the management of ADRs. By providing patients with comprehensive information about the medications being administered, including potential side effects, they can make informed decisions about their treatment. Practical counseling sessions help HCPs assess a patient's awareness of their treatment therapies given to them and provide precise counseling. Such interaction not only enhances medication adherence but also plays a vital role in the identification of early signs of ADR. For example, in tuberculosis (TB) patients undergoing anti-tubercular therapy, it has been found that patient counseling on the most common ADRs would significantly enhance their compliance with the treatment regimen, hence avoiding adverse effects in association with both ADRs and disease activity (Kaur et al., 2025). In addition, patient counseling regularly promotes an active approach of pharmacovigilance under which the HCPs can monitor and control ADRs more effectively. Organized interventions that entail training HCPs in recent studies have been shown to improve the efficiency of patient education programs. For instance, continuous education with occasional feedback greatly increased ADR reporting rates among HCPs, with evidence for the importance of an educated healthcare team in preventing ADRs. Such interventions are for developing a safety culture within medical facilities that enhances the capacity to recognize and act early on ADRs among patients, particularly vulnerable populations such as patients on TB treatment (Enazi et al., 2024). Ultimately, integrating patient education and counseling into practice not only favors better health but also empowers the patients. If patients participate in their care, they are better placed to report side effects and access care early, which is important for effective ADR management. In TB patients receiving anti-tubercular treatment (ATT), research finds that patient understanding of the treatment regimens and risks associated with it are factors that lead to improved adherence and health literacy. With the modernization of healthcare, patient education must be at the top to ensure individuals become more proficient in managing the complexities of their drugs, such that therapeutic performance is optimized and the trouble of ADRs is prevented (Kaur et al., 2025) (Figure 1.16).

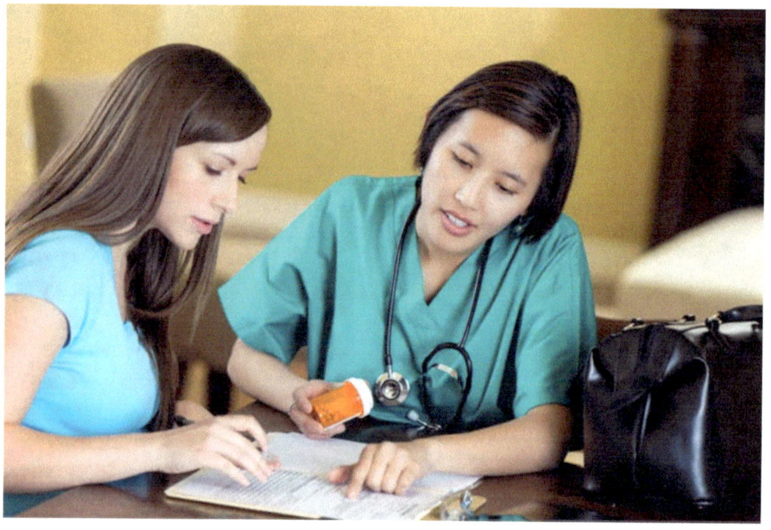

Figure 1.16. Patient education and counselling.

Source: https://www.amnhealthcare.com/siteassets/candidate-blog/nursing/contract/patient-education-in-nursing.jpg.

1.6. Regulatory Framework Surrounding Adverse Drug Reactions

The regulatory framework surrounding ADRs is crucial in ensuring patient safety and enhancing the efficacy of drugs. Regulatory bodies such as the U.S. Food and Drug Administration (FDA) and the European Medicines Agency (EMA) establish guidelines to monitor and manage ADRs throughout a drug's lifecycle. These agencies expect pharmaceutical companies to report any possible ADRs, whether they are noticed in clinical studies or after the drug is released. They are needed to spot and deal with any safety issues that could arise from the use of drugs by many people. Mandating detailed reporting enables these organizations to compile a comprehensive database that informs new laws and promotes safer practices, ultimately benefiting public health and reducing risks associated with drugs. In addition to the standard reporting methods, advancements in technology have enabled improvements in how ADR is detected and examined. For instance, automated systems like the Adverse Drug Reaction Detector (ADRD) utilize natural language processing (NLP) techniques to extract adverse drug events from free-text reports. Using these tools helps solve the problem of underreporting that has long affected ADR data collection, as proved by studies on SRS. With a more effective approach to analyzing and summarizing ADR cases, these systems may lead to faster actions and updates from regulators. Thus, integrating technological advancements within the regulatory framework is essential to bolster ADR monitoring and improve patient safety outcomes in healthcare environments (Naderian et al., 2024). Additionally, the study of ADRs highlights the importance for regulators to monitor and protect public health. A recent study conducted in Malawi highlighted the prevalence and characteristics of antibiotic-associated ADRs, indicating that approximately 24% of patients experienced suspected adverse reactions, with significant variations based on age and concurrent medications (Chiumia et al., 2024). This points out that regulatory bodies should use effective methods to assess the causes, severity, and preventability of ADRs. If ADR events are analyzed effectively, regulations can adapt to new issues and improve clinical practices. Keeping a close eye on these reactions guarantees patients are safe, which supports a healthcare system that responds and is trusted by the public.

1.6.1. Role of the FDA in ADR Monitoring

The FDA plays a pivotal role in the monitoring of ADRs, which are unintended and harmful effects associated with pharmaceutical products. It is the agency's primary task to check that drugs are safe and effective before they are approved for use. After thoroughly reviewing the results of clinical trials, the FDA continues to monitor drug safety by closely tracking its use after approval. By continuously monitoring, it is possible to identify ADRs that were not observed in the original trials, allowing healthcare providers to select the most effective treatment options. Furthermore, the FDA can enact regulatory measures, including issuing recalls or black box warnings, as necessary to protect public health from drugs that pose significant safety risks (Ahuja et al., 2015). HCPs and patients report adverse reactions after a drug is released, and this is how the FDA monitors these events. Although the system plays a crucial role in collecting information on drug safety, it also has certain limitations. In other words, the FDA admits that the data they receive cannot always prove a drug caused an adverse event, and cannot give a clear number of cases in the whole population. Consequently, the analysis of ADRs is often confounded by incomplete reports that lack detailed information on the adverse events experienced, leading to potential misinterpretations (Muñoz et al., 2014). For this reason, the FDA continues to seek better methods for monitoring ADRs and collecting data to ensure the accuracy of its findings. Due to the challenges in ADR reporting, the FDA is advocating for more data-driven methods to assess drug safety. It requires utilizing new technologies and large datasets to identify the connections between specific drugs and their side effects. The FDA aims to enhance its analytical capabilities to enable healthcare providers to utilize more detailed data in informed decision-making regarding drug therapies and mitigate associated risks. This progressive approach also serves to ensure that identified risks are communicated effectively to both HCPs and patients, fostering a culture of transparency and informed consent in pharmaceutical use (Ahuja et al., 2015). Because drug therapy is constantly changing, the FDA's efforts to manage ADRs will play a key role in keeping everyone healthy and using drugs safely (Figure 1.17).

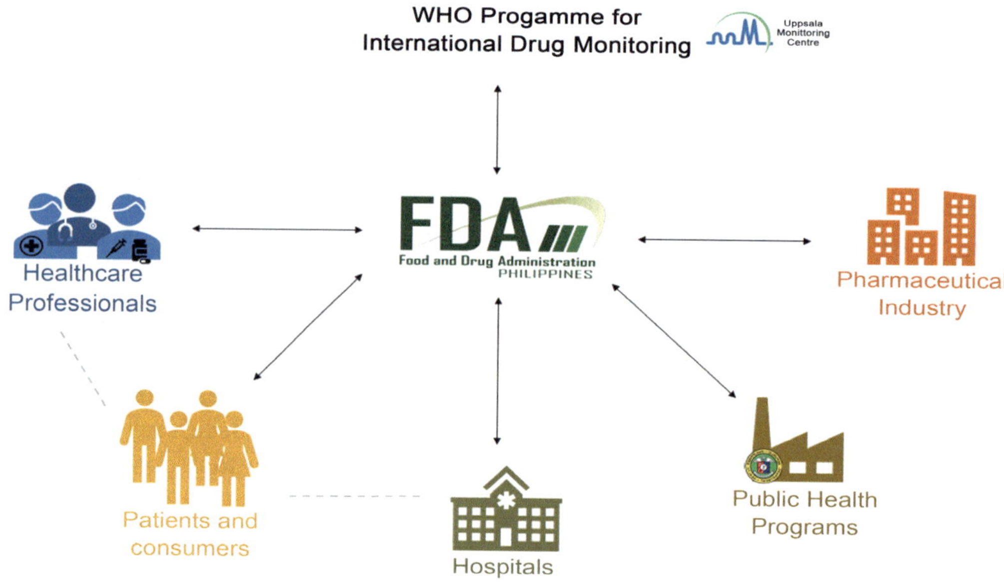

Figure 1.17. Role of the FDA in ADR monitoring.

Source: https://www.fda.gov.ph/wp-content/uploads/2022/08/PV-System.png.

1.6.2. International Guidelines and Regulations

The establishment of international regulations and guidelines on ADRs is crucial in upholding the safety of drugs globally. The International Council for Harmonization (ICH), among others, has established fundamental guidelines that govern pharmacovigilance operations across various nations. For example, the ICH E2B guideline emphasizes the importance of harmonized electronic communications that facilitate the effective collection and reporting of individual case safety reports (ICSRs). This framework enables Marketing Authorization Holders and National Regulatory Authorities (NRAs) to systematically evaluate ADRs, facilitating the easier identification of trends that may indicate safety problems. While countries work to harmonize their regulations, opportunities are lacking in instances where resources for robust pharmacovigilance systems are not available. Addressing such discrepancies through international collaboration is necessary to enhance the safety profile of medications (Lomeli-Silva et al., 2024). In addition to the harmonization efforts by ICH, other entities like the WHO play a key role in global surveillance of ADRs. Ever since the WHO Program for International Drug Monitoring came into being during the 1960s, countries have made greater use of pharmacovigilance systems to report and examine ADRs more effectively. Notably, the use of retrospective analysis through VigiBase, the WHO's international pharmacovigilance database, points towards the underlying necessity of continuous monitoring since extremely high numbers of ADRs are reported annually, some of them life-threatening (Kulkarni et al., 2022). These historical precedents demonstrate both the success of pharmacovigilance and the necessity of ongoing vigilance to adapt to new therapeutic developments. International vigilance for safety through enlightened regulation remains a dynamic process, demonstrating the sophistication of healthcare in the current era. With increasing therapeutic innovation, particularly in the development of biologics and next-generation therapeutics, international guidelines and regulations must also evolve to meet the growing challenges. The recent surge in emergency approvals of medicines, particularly during public health crises such as the COVID-19 pandemic, underscores the importance of agile pharmacovigilance procedures. To counter these rapid advances, the ICH and regulatory authorities must enhance their infrastructures not just to trace the approved medicines but also encompass real-world evidence that reflect broader patient populations. This entails incorporating patient experiences into ADR reporting work, which can lead to improved safety outcomes. Patient report inclusion in pharmacovigilance systems, as seen with initiatives like the UK's Yellow Card scheme, is an important aspect of how stakeholder engagement can reinforce regulatory action by prioritizing safety in innovation (Lomeli-Silva et al., 2024) (Figure 1.18).

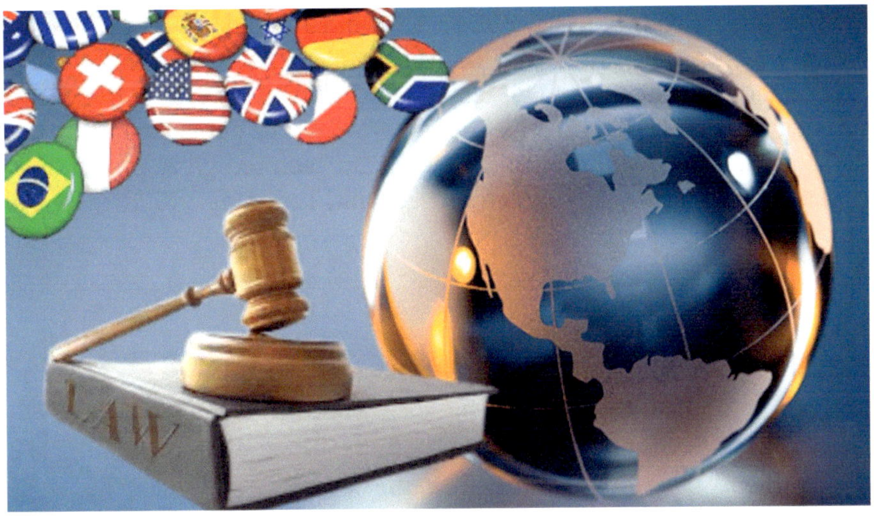

Figure 1.18. International guidelines and regulations.

Source: https://legalvidhiya.com/wp-content/uploads/2023/04/Screenshot-2023-04-10-at-12.48.56-AM.png.

1.6.3. Impact of Regulations on Drug Safety

Regulations play a vital role in ensuring drug safety, particularly in terms of ADRs. Organizations such as the FDA establish standards through rigorous tests and approvals, which pharmaceutical companies must comply with in order to have their products available on shelves. Characteristically, these regulations require thorough preclinical and clinical tests to assess the safety and efficacy of drugs before they are released to the public. This is to minimize the potential of ADRs by detecting danger earlier, thus protecting patients from adverse effects. Such systems are vital to creating a culture of accountability in the pharmaceutical industry, where compliance can ultimately determine a drug's success and its adoption in the medical community. By ensuring that safety procedures are implemented, regulation significantly minimizes the risk involved with ADRs. The climate around drug safety also shifts with advancing technology and techniques, creating drugs and tracking them.

The use of ML and artificial intelligence (AI) in the identification of ADR has become an essential component of existing regulatory processes. The technologies enable the prediction of potential drug toxicity and problems at high speed, even at preclinical stages, enhancing the overall drug safety profile. For instance, the employment of data mining and advanced modeling techniques enables the identification of complex interactions between drugs and patient populations. Such capabilities enable regulators and researchers to enhance their anticipation and response to safety issues. The integrated dynamic application of these technological developments into regulatory measures not only strengthens drug safety but also enables regulatory agencies to keep pace with the rapid development of drugs in the modern era's healthcare industry (Mohapatra et al., 2024). Despite such positive advancements made via regulatory actions, problems continue to exist, primarily regarding drug errors and their contribution to ADRs. A credible study noted that 35–45% of ADRs are caused by avoidable drug errors, highlighting the importance of continuous safety plan improvement. The studies show that while medication reconciliation and reviews are crucial, their effect on preventable ADR occurrence may be limited, such as in studies aiming at older patients with high-risk medications (Schmitz et al., 2024). Therefore, regulatory bodies must place greater emphasis on evidence-based guidelines that address these errors in a more holistic manner. By enhancing medication management practices, especially among vulnerable populations, regulations can lead to a decrease in the severity and frequency of ADRs. In general, a multi-faceted approach incorporating strict regulatory regulation with advanced technological innovation and education of drug safety is essential to encouraging drug safety and reducing the burden caused by ADRs.

Summary

As explained in this essay, ADRs may be mild or severe and can impact a patient's willingness to take medicines and their health outcomes. ADRs may occur due to patient-related factors and the manufacturing process of drugs. It is essential for healthcare providers to be vigilant and follow good pharmacovigilance practices to manage these reactions promptly. Informing patients about ADRs can help them report them, which makes the use of medicines safer. The acceptance of Ayurvedic medicine and similar treatments provides a new perspective on the discussion about ADRs. For instance, studies reveal that even widely accepted herbal treatments can lead to cutaneous ADRs, as evidenced by the observations regarding *Nagaradi lepa* (Kurikkal et al., 2024). As integrative medicine becomes more popular, it is essential to closely monitor and assess all types of medication, whether traditional or alternative. Being watchful in this way helps patients and also increases everyone's knowledge about the side effects of different drugs. In addition, recent research on medicines that help people with Alzheimer's sleep better shows that the results are not always precise. Although some medications show promise in improving outcomes, the potential for adverse reactions remains a significant concern (Bedward et al., 2024). From all the findings, it is obvious that continuous research and reporting are necessary to reduce the number of ADRs. If healthcare professionals, researchers, and patients join forces and share information, the healthcare community can develop safer and more effective treatments, which would enhance patient care and trust in medical treatments. ADRs cause significant problems in healthcare, making it essential to understand their full implications. Clinicians need to realize that ADRs can show different levels of severity and symptoms, which may affect how patients are treated and how safe they are. The creation of risk prediction models, including ADAPTiP, shows a significant step forward in this field. The model, which utilizes simple data, performed very well in identifying older individuals who might experience ADRs, with cross-validated area under the curve values of 0.75 and 0.83 in external validation. Such tools are essential for enabling HCPs to make informed decisions regarding medication reviews and potentially harmful prescribing practices, ultimately aiming to reduce the incidence of ADRs among vulnerable patient groups (Frydenlund et al., 2025). A significant focus within the realm of ADRs is the toxicological impact of specific medications, particularly poly (ADP-ribose) polymerase (PARP) inhibitors. They can result in several adverse reactions, for example, blood problems, stomach issues, and tiredness. To manage these reactions, regular blood tests are necessary to monitor the blood and refer patients to specialists when necessary. You can mitigate the effects of gastrointestinal toxicity by following a suitable diet and managing symptoms before they occur. In cases where fatigue is identified, a thorough assessment is critical, as its causes can vary widely, necessitating individualized management that may incorporate psychosocial interventions or pharmacotherapy (OZMASOOA et al., 2022). To reduce the chances of ADRs, HCPs should be proactive and always focus on the patient. It is essential to use strict monitoring methods, mainly for drugs that may interact with others. It is essential for clinicians to monitor patients' blood pressure and heart rate when using PARP inhibitors, as these medications can cause cardiovascular complications. If a patient presents with respiratory symptoms, it is essential to perform high-resolution CT scans to identify any underlying conditions, such as pneumonia. Overall, fostering a culture of vigilance that includes patient self-management education and multidisciplinary consultations can significantly enhance therapeutic outcomes while reducing the risk and severity of ADRs (OZMASOOA et al., 2022).

CLOSER LOOK

NATIONAL REGULATORY AUTHORITIES

National regulatory authorities (NRAs) are government-mandated agencies charged with designing, interpreting, and enforcing technical standards, licensing regimes, inspections, compliance actions, and adjudication across regulated sectors—ranging from pharmaceuticals and medical devices to finance, energy, telecommunications, food safety, and transport—acting as the primary institutional bridge between legal mandates and practical oversight in pursuit of public welfare, economic stability, or national security. Fully empowered under administrative-law frameworks, NRAs such as the U.S. Food and Drug Administration (FDA), European Medicines Agency (EMA), Japan's Pharmaceuticals and Medical Devices Agency (PMDA), India's CDSCO, Health Canada, Brazil's ANVISA, UK's MHRA, Australia's TGA, South Africa's SAHPRA, and others collectively represent national litigation-backed regulators with responsibilities including clinical-trial review, product licensing, post-market surveillance, labeling enforcement, recall authority, inspection of manufacturing sites, adverse-event monitoring, and establishing technical guidelines. In telecommunications, energy, and banking, analogous bodies like Ofcom (UK), India's CERC (Central Electricity Regulatory Commission), Kenya's Communications Authority, or Egypt's National Telecommunications

References

1. Padmaja, U., Adhikari, P., & Pereira, P. (2009). A prospective analysis of adverse drug reactions in a South Indian hospital. *Online Journal of Health and Allied Sciences*, *8*(3). http://cogprints.org/6959/Ahuja, V., Birge, J., Syverson, C., Huang, E., & Sohn, M. (2015). Quality management using data analytics: An application to pharmaceutical regulation. *Quality Management eJournal.* https://www.semanticscholar.org/paper/db0b88ad89cef3deda6ece5e512b3d544b8220d7 (accessed on 9 June 2025).

2. Al Enazi, H. H., Barnawi, Y., Omari, B. A., Al Fahad, W. A., & Al Onazi, M. (2024). Enhancing adverse drug reaction reporting in tertiary hospital in Saudi Arabia: An evaluation of methods and strategies. *Saudi Journal of Medical and Pharmaceutical Sciences.* https://www.semanticscholar.org/paper/19bf5799ea329848f46f58c83637dc6a49fd4462 (accessed on 9 June 2025).

3. Bedward, A., Kaur, J., Seedat, S., Donohue, H., Kow, C. S., Rasheed, M. K., Javed, A., et al. (2024). Pharmacological interventions to improve sleep in people with Alzheimer's disease: A meta-analysis of randomized controlled trials. *Expert Review of Neurotherapeutics, 24*, 527–539. https://www.semanticscholar.org/paper/57b7b388af626b5e0923ec2c7f2f3e68da143fb1 (accessed on 9 June 2025).

4. Bergenstal, R. M., Fleming, G. A., Heinemann, L., Holl, R., et al. (2017). Improving the clinical value and utility of CGM systems: Issues and recommendations: A joint statement of the European Association for the Study of Diabetes and the American Diabetes Association Diabetes Technology Working Group. https://core.ac.uk/download/132211400.pdf.

5. Burute, R. B., Burute, S. R., Karande, V. B., & Murthy, D. S. (2016). Awareness of adverse drug reactions in third M.B.B.S. students practicing self-medication. https://core.ac.uk/download/543134248.pdf (accessed on 9 June 2025).

6. Cervantes-Arellano, M. J., Castelán-Martínez, O., Marín-Campos, Y., Chávez-Pacheco, J., Morales-Ríos, O., & Ubaldo-Reyes, L. M. (2024). Educational interventions in pharmacovigilance to improve the knowledge, attitude and the report of adverse drug reactions in healthcare professionals: Systematic review and meta-analysis. *DARU Journal of Pharmaceutical Sciences, 32*, 421–434. https://www.semanticscholar.org/paper/d5f0be0eecb8ed6c4804dda601c721c1b5af9991 (accessed on 9 June 2025).

7. Chenchula, S., Atal, S., & Uppugunduri, C. (2024). A review of real-world evidence on preemptive pharmacogenomic testing for preventing adverse drug reactions: A reality for future health care. *The Pharmacogenomics Journal, 24.* https://www.semanticscholar.org/paper/10a7d2d5070c6fe8a61ceba870e527270107ee2c (accessed on 9 June 2025).

8. Chiumia, F., Chimimba, F., Nyirongo, H., Kampira, E., Muula, A., & Khuluza, F. (2024). Adverse drug reactions related with antibiotic medicines in Malawi: A retrospective analysis of prevalence and associated factors. *Drug, Healthcare and Patient Safety, 16*, 89–101. https://www.semanticscholar.org/paper/c9482d653330a829a8e018bacdc688054ef5de71 (accessed on 9 June 2025).

9. Corsonello, A., Jha, A., Leendertse, A., Somers, A., Spinewine, A., et al. (2016). *Geriatric Pharmacotherapy: Optimization Through Integrated Approach in The Hospital Setting.* https://core.ac.uk/download/55809733.pdf (accessed on 9 June 2025).

10. Dai, Z., Dai-Keller, Z., Lau, E. C. Y., Penm, J., et al. (2024). Prevalence of and risk factors for drug-related readmissions in older adults: A systematic review and meta-analysis. https://unsworks.unsw.edu.au/bitstreams/34ab9cf9-d3ef-4882-8953-4d1e10117428/download (accessed on 9 June 2025).
11. Danieletto, M., Dudley, J., Glicksberg, B., & Li, L. (2018). Processing of electronic health records using deep learning: A review. http://arxiv.org/abs/1804.01758 (accessed on 9 June 2025).
12. Eruaga, M. A., Bature, T., & Itua, E. O. (2024). Pharmacovigilance in Nigeria: Addressing challenges in ensuring drug safety and monitoring adverse effects. *GSC Advanced Research and Reviews, 18*, 78–82. https://doi.org/10.30574/gscarr.2024.18.3.0093.
13. Frydenlund, J., Cosgrave, N., Moriarty, F., Wallace, E., Kirke, C., Williams, D. J., Bennett, K., et al. (2025). Adverse drug reactions and events in an Ageing PopulaTion risk Prediction (ADAPTiP) tool: The development and validation of a model for predicting adverse drug reactions and events in older patients. *European Geriatric Medicine, 16*, 573–581. https://www.semanticscholar.org/paper/e8acb55ad11ecf7e409fdca198d6b564d19ec4b2 (accessed on 9 June 2025).
14. Galluzzi, L., Vitale, I., Aaronson, S. A., Abrams, J., Adam, D., Agostinis, P., Alnemri, E. S., et al. (2018). Molecular mechanisms of cell death: Recommendations of the Nomenclature Committee on Cell Death 2018. *Cell Death and Differentiation, 25*, 486–541. https://doi.org/10.1038/s41418-017-0012-4.
15. Garcia, G., Pacchini, V., Zamoner, W., Balbi, A., & Ponce, D. (2024). Drug-induced acute kidney injury: A cohort study on incidence, identification of pathophysiological mechanisms, and prognostic factors. *Frontiers in Medicine, 11.* https://www.semanticscholar.org/paper/d03104f2b21d27a38bc74c12fe941e7675db17fb (accessed on 9 June 2025).
16. Girgis, M. M. F., Farkasinszky, G., Fekete, K., Fekete, I., Vecsernyés, M., Bácskay, I., & Horváth, L. (2024). Seriousness and outcomes of reported adverse drug reactions in old and new antiseizure medications: A pharmacovigilance study using EudraVigilance database. *Frontiers in Pharmacology, 15.* https://www.semanticscholar.org/paper/5f5ce8cb4d05e61bb27bf55f826f633d8d86f353 (accessed on 9 June 2025).
17. Gosho, M., Ishii, R., Ohigashi, T., & Maruo, K. (2024). Multivariate generalized mixed-effects models for screening multiple adverse drug reactions in spontaneous reporting systems. *Frontiers in Pharmacology, 15.* https://www.semanticscholar.org/paper/c6554a14e04dc3bfbb8d02d2467d7dd1cf96dd01 (accessed on 9 June 2025).
18. Hussain, R., Hassali, M. A., Hashmi, F. K., & Akram, T. (2021). Exploring healthcare professionals' knowledge, attitude, and practices towards pharmacovigilance: A cross-sectional survey. *Journal of Pharmaceutical Policy and Practice, 14.* https://doi.org/10.1186/s40545-020-00287-3.
19. Jiang, H., Lin, Y., Ren, W., Lu, L., Tan, X., Lv, X., & Zhang, N. (2025). Potential inappropriate medications and drug–drug interactions in adverse drug reactions in the elderly: A retrospective study in a pharmacovigilance database. *Frontiers in Pharmacology, 16.* https://www.semanticscholar.org/paper/bfebce55c1c92f2eefeba65b1870e2f881df85eb (accessed on 9 June 2025).
20. Joaquim, J. J. M. (2023). *Assessment and Reporting of Adverse Drug Reactions to Iopromide: A Study of Risk Perception and Pharmacovigilance.* https://core.ac.uk/download/590219748.pdf (accessed on 9 June 2025).

21. Kamble, S. U., Bais, S. K., & Hugar, S. R. (2023). Review on adverse drug reactions. *International Journal of Advanced Research in Science, Communication and Technology.* https://www.semanticscholar.org/paper/b240d14c7b821b1dc1a42959265dff9ebf7cfba7 (accessed on 9 June 2025).

22. Kaur, J., Gupta, T., Saini, A., Khosla, P. P., Rani, N., & Verma, I. (2025). Adverse drug reaction of antitubercular drugs and impact of patient counselling on compliance in tuberculosis patients: A prospective study. *Current Drug Therapy.* https://www.semanticscholar.org/paper/97a1c6cefffe1f84c37915324a87d6e3deae54eb (accessed on 9 June 2025).

23. Khan, M., Hirsch, C., & Jones, A. M. (2024). Suspected adverse drug reactions associated with leukotriene receptor antagonists versus first-line asthma medications: A national registry-pharmacology approach. https://www.semanticscholar.org/paper/c6e8bbe576111911c7464bf6757db2ff780740b8 (accessed on 9 June 2025).

24. Kulkarni, S., Rieder, M., & Likić, R. (2022). Quo vadis (where are you going) pharmacovigilance? *British Journal of Clinical Pharmacology, 89.* https://www.semanticscholar.org/paper/cfbeb10ab2656d5d10022e1858182dc91a9e1d71 (accessed on 9 June 2025).

25. Kurikkal, H., Unnikrishnan, V., & Narayanan, M. (2024). Cutaneous adverse drug reactions on application of Nagaradi Lepa–A retrospective analysis. *International Journal of Ayurvedic Medicine.* https://www.semanticscholar.org/paper/346ab0593e28ebe6a9e49721fe07ff7e7fdad88c (accessed on 9 June 2025).

26. Lomeli-Silva, A., Contreras-Salinas, H., Barajas-Virgen, M. Y., Romero-López, M. S., & Rodríguez-Herrera, L. Y. (2024). Harmonization of individual case safety reports transmission requirements among PAHO reference authorities: A review of their current regulation. *Therapeutic Advances in Drug Safety, 15.* https://www.semanticscholar.org/paper/b48a538409797c38f67c5df4851a8bf1e562febb (accessed on 9 June 2025).

27. McGettigan, S., Curtin, D., & O'Mahony, D. (2024). Adverse drug reactions in multimorbid older people exposed to polypharmacy: Epidemiology and prevention. *Pharmacoepidemiology.* https://www.semanticscholar.org/paper/6931e8044f032e50049f4cdde5f3e77c484b9be1 (accessed on 9 June 2025).

28. Mohapatra, R., & Panda, P. (2024). Revolutionizing patient safety: Machine learning and AI for the early detection of adverse drug reactions and drug-induced toxicity. *Current Artificial Intelligence.* https://www.semanticscholar.org/paper/6cea6c1d52c10a5667b356a97e6e692dd7fd6d47 (accessed on 9 June 2025).

29. Moirana, E. L. (2023). *The Prevalence of Antiretroviral-Therapy-Related Adverse Reactions, Hospitalization, And Mortality Among People Living with HIV in Africa: A Systematic Review and Meta-Analysis.* https://core.ac.uk/download/590318230.pdf (accessed on 9 June 2025).

30. Montaño, D. (2022). Frequency and associations of adverse reactions of COVID-19 vaccines reported to pharmacovigilance systems in the European Union and the United States. *Frontiers in Public Health, 9.* https://doi.org/10.3389/fpubh.2021.756633.

31. Muñoz, M., Gómez-Ramírez, S., Liumbruno, G., & Grazzini, G. (2014). Intravenous iron and safety: Is the end of the debate on the horizon? *Blood Transfusion = Trasfusione del Sangue, 12*(3), 287–289. https://www.semanticscholar.org/paper/f12910cfd6514df0cdc4491a17db3a56613fca52 (accessed on 9 June 2025).

32. Naderian, S., Rahmani, R., & Samad-Soltani, T. (2024). A natural language processing

framework for detecting adverse drug reactions in clinical structured drug reviews. *International Journal of Drug Research in Clinics.* https://www.semanticscholar.org/paper/ac5cd0b576bb7b1ba766e7415ef0c5431e24f5d3 (accessed on 9 June 2025).

33. Nast, A., Smith, C., Spuls, P. I., Avila Valle, G., Bata-Csörgő, Z., Boonen, H., de Jong, E. M. G. J., et al. (2020). EuroGuiDerm guideline on the systemic treatment of psoriasis vulgaris–Part 1: Treatment and monitoring recommendations. *Journal of the European Academy of Dermatology and Venereology, 34*, 2461–2498. https://doi.org/10.1111/jdv.16915.

34. Ofori-Asenso, R., & Agyeman, A. A. (2016). Irrational use of medicines—A summary of key concepts. *Pharmacy, 4*, 35. https://doi.org/10.3390/pharmacy4040035.

35. Onder, G., Petrovic, M., & van der Cammen, T. (2012). *Adverse Drug Reactions in Older People: Detection and Prevention.* https://core.ac.uk/download/55848564.pdf (accessed on 9 June 2025).

36. Pandey, N., Kumar, S., Kumar, V. B., & Thakur, R. (2025). Study of drug utilization and adverse drug reaction pattern of anti-glaucoma drugs in patients with primary open angle glaucoma attending the glaucoma clinic at a tertiary care institute in Bihar, India: A cross-sectional study. *Journal of Clinical and Diagnostic Research.* https://www.semanticscholar.org/paper/b5c8883affeb6b1a07a1a27877ad4612468fd64a (accessed on 9 June 2025).

37. Panneerselvam, N., Kadhirvelu, P., Somasundaram, R., & Jayaprakash, S. (2019). A study on cutaneous adverse drug reactions reported in a tertiary care hospital, Kanchipuram. *Asian Journal of Pharmaceutical and Clinical Research.* https://www.semanticscholar.org/paper/6fdc3692936985d5209e64f7c922292188e25443 (accessed on 9 June 2025).

38. Patra, J. K., Das, G., Fraceto, L. F., Campos, E. V. R., Rodriguez-Torres, M. del P., Acosta-Torres, L. S., Díaz-Torres, L. A., et al. (2018). Nano based drug delivery systems: Recent developments and future prospects. *Journal of Nanobiotechnology, 16.* https://doi.org/10.1186/s12951-018-0392-8.

39. Pavan, G., Kumar, M., Murti, K., Dhingra, S., & Ravichandiran, V. (2024). Exploring the factors influencing the health-related quality of life in patients experiencing adverse drug reactions: A cross-sectional study. *Journal of Patient-Reported Outcomes, 8.* https://www.semanticscholar.org/paper/2702effc3658ddc78c3218e790730fe431466378 (accessed on 9 June 2025).

40. Rollema, C., van Roon, E. V., Ekhart, C., van Hunsel, F., & de Vries, T. D. (2022). Adverse drug reactions of intranasal corticosteroids in the Netherlands: An analysis from the Netherlands Pharmacovigilance Center. *Drugs–Real World Outcomes, 9*, 321–331. https://www.semanticscholar.org/paper/a090eec365fee9c9d88eef8195ba750d6b3c7436 (accessed on 9 June 2025).

41. Romoli, M., Mazzocchetti, P., D'Alonzo, R., Siliquini, S., Rinaldi, V. E., Verrotti, A., Calabresi, P., et al. (2018). Valproic acid and epilepsy: From molecular mechanisms to clinical evidences. *Current Neuropharmacology, 17*, 926–946. https://doi.org/10.2174/1570159x17666181227165722.

42. Schmitz, K., Lenssen, R., Wied, S., Laven, A., Berning, D., Thomeczek, C., Brokmann, J., et al. (2024). Impact of medication reconciliation and medication reviews on the incidence of preventable adverse drug reactions during hospitalization of elderly patients: A randomized controlled trial. *Die Pharmazie, 79*(9), 209–214. https://www.semanticscholar.org/paper/4366af28ea4b64abc48bfa32647a6ae098f4449a (accessed on 9 June 2025).

43. Schreier, T., Tropmann-Frick, M., & Böhm, R. (2024). Integration of FAERS, DrugBank and

SIDER data for machine learning-based detection of adverse drug reactions. *Datenbank-Spektrum, 24*, 233–242. https://www.semanticscholar.org/paper/46f3e8ff11d0e83aa3cc2abea32be72c8a8d2040 (accessed on 9 June 2025).

44. Sittiphan, S., Lim, A., Khurram, H., Dureh, N., & Dittakan, K. (2025). Epidemiology of reported serious adverse drug reactions due to anti-infectives using nationwide database of Thailand. *PLOS One, 20.* https://www.semanticscholar.org/paper/39dc8c352b6861393174ef74923d2657f9ff2cb7 (accessed on 9 June 2025).

45. Society of Obstetrics and Gynecology of Zhejiang Medical Association, Society of Urology of Zhejiang Medical Association, Committee of Breast Cancer of Zhejiang Anticancer Association, Committee of Clinical Pharmacy on Oncology of Zhejiang Anticancer Association (Preparation), & Committee of Urology of Zhejiang Society for Mathematical Medicine. (2022). Guidance on the management of adverse reactions induced by poly (ADP-ribose) polymerase inhibitors. *Journal of Zhejiang University. Medical Sciences, 51*(6), 765–774. https://www.semanticscholar.org/paper/784035e215c7773bf2c4521cc063cefd9f697b92 (accessed on 9 June 2025).

46. Spillers, N. J., Luther, P. M., Talbot, N. C., Ly, G. H., Downs, E., Lavespere, G., Pavlickova, D., et al. (2023). Association of acetaminophen with Stevens-Johnson syndrome and toxic epidermal necrolysis: Pharmacologic considerations and treatment options. *Cureus, 15.* https://www.semanticscholar.org/paper/43449904b1c4c789ea1ea12c2dc3f9c7d1e20bff (accessed on 9 June 2025).

47. Tanwar, D., Yadav, R. P., Saroha, A., & Sharma, P. (2023). Adverse drug reactions: Mechanisms, detection, and prevention strategies. *International Journal for Research Publication and Seminar.* https://www.semanticscholar.org/paper/0f2591658cafa9f3357b288116067415f94f2e62 (accessed on 9 June 2025).

48. Uddin, T. M., Chakraborty, A., Khusro, A., Zidan, B. M. R. M., Mitra, S., Emran, T. B., Dhama, K., et al. (2021). Antibiotic resistance in microbes: History, mechanisms, therapeutic strategies and future prospects. *Journal of Infection and Public Health, 14*, 1750–1766. https://doi.org/10.1016/j.jiph.2021.10.020.

49. Valdiserra, G., Mores, N., Rocchi, R. E., Sottosanti, L., Felicetti, P., Marchione, P., Laurenti, L., et al. (2023). Signal management and risk minimization strategy: A case study on Obinutuzumab and non-overt disseminated intravascular coagulation. *Frontiers in Drug Safety and Regulation.* https://www.semanticscholar.org/paper/64fb52b4c44591c92c603ebe8447ceefde4d792b (accessed on 9 June 2025).

50. Velasco Martín, A., & Velasco Sendra, M. (2018). *Reacciones adversas medicamentosas (RAM).* https://core.ac.uk/download/364251092.pdf (accessed on 9 June 2025).

51. Wanchoo, R., Karam, S., Uppal, N. N., Barta, V. S., Deray, G., Devoe, C., Launay-Vacher, V., et al. (2017). Adverse renal effects of immune checkpoint inhibitors: A narrative review. *American Journal of Nephrology, 45*, 160–169. https://doi.org/10.1159/000455014.

52. Yuniar, C. T., Fadhilah, R. Z., Anggadiredja, K., & Amalia, L. (2024). Healthcare professionals' attitudes towards adverse drug reactions reporting in primary healthcare settings: A cross-sectional survey. *Jurnal Manajemen dan Pelayanan Farmasi (Journal of Management and Pharmacy Practice).* https://www.semanticscholar.org/paper/c794f6e1350646ec7a5595373685f3f22bff37b8 (accessed on 9 June 2025).

53. Zaccaria, C., Piccolo, L., Gordillo-Marañón, M., Touraille, G., & de Vries, C. (2024). Identification of pregnancy adverse drug reactions in pharmacovigilance reporting systems: A novel algorithm developed in EudraVigilance. *Drug Safety, 47*, 1127–1136. https://www.semanticscholar.org/paper/4d27c886b642ac6e310fcbb44075be9ceb4fa57c (accessed on 9 June 2025).

54. Zhang, X., Chu, X., Wang, J., Gu, W., Fu, X., Zhang, J., Wang, C., et al. (2024). Retrospective analysis of survival and safety of bevacizumab biosimilar and original drug combination chemotherapy in non-small cell lung cancer. *Frontiers in Oncology, 14.* https://www.semanticscholar.org/paper/69a3c17a37cd1ea3d7f08bc9359ff9c742ed98b2 (accessed on 9 June 2025).

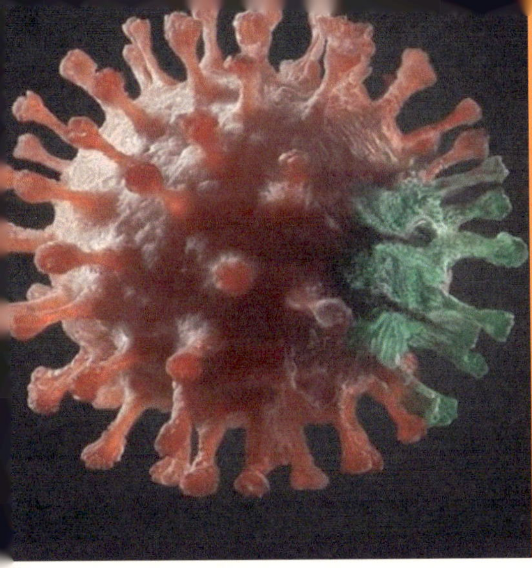

Chapter 2

EPIDEMIOLOGY AND RISK FACTORS FOR ADVERSE DRUG REACTIONS

Contents

Introduction

The phenomenon of adverse drug reactions (ADRs) is a highly complex issue within the field of healthcare that demands a complete understanding of their epidemiology and underlying risk factors. ADRs refer to the negative results of taking drugs that can cause serious health complications, including hospitalization for a long time and even death. Since drug use is becoming more complicated, doctors should be able to spot patients who might react badly and use methods to prevent it. The evidence base shows that genetic susceptibility, interaction between drugs, and patient-related factors play a significant role in determining whether patients develop ADRs, which calls for further predictive methods in clinical practice (He et al., 2025). Such studies are helpful in discovering the reasons that severe ADRs occur. Epidemiological studies rely on large datasets to identify patterns and relationships that inform clinical practice. It has been found through these studies that age, gender, and having a previous illness play a significant role in increasing the risk of adverse reactions. In addition, specific categories of drugs, mainly anti-infectives, are associated with a greater risk of serious ADRs, which means these patients should be watched closely. Careful analysis of these trends allows providers to design prevention strategies according to the patient profile, which can ultimately reduce the burden of ADRs in healthcare systems (Sittiphan et al., 2025). Pharmacogenomics' application to the clinic further enhances our capacity to predict and manage ADRs effectively. By understanding the genetic mechanisms of drug metabolism and the variability in an individual's response to a drug, clinicians can make more informed prescribing decisions that minimize the likelihood of adverse reactions. With the help of new ML and data analytics, it is now possible to create models that predict the start of ADRs from data that includes genetic, clinical, and demographic information. As a result, patients and treatment outcomes are made safer by addressing ADR risks proactively. With ongoing advancement in healthcare, the search for information in epidemiology and risk factors remains at the core of ensuring effective and safe drug therapy (He et al., 2025) (Figure 2.1).

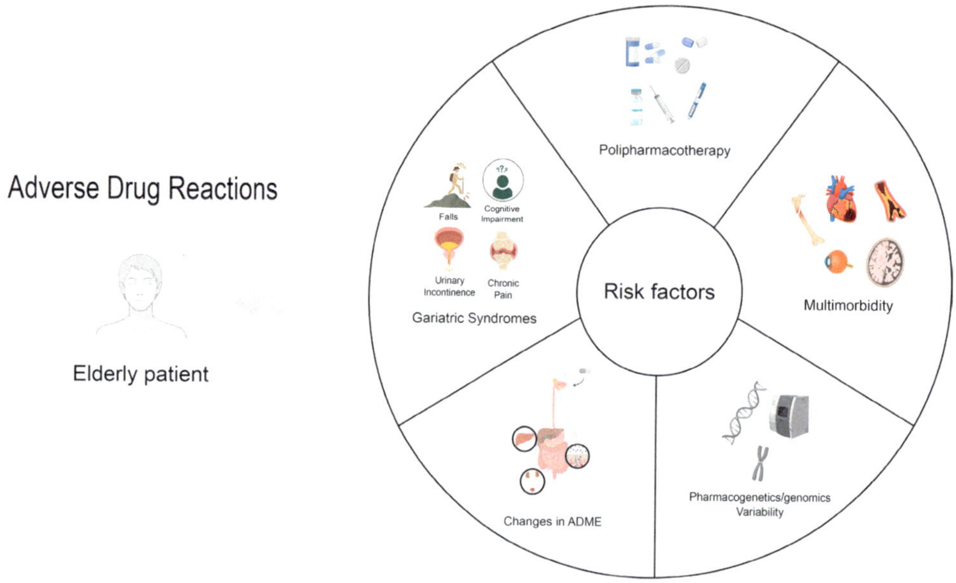

Figure 2.1. Epidemiology and risk factors for adverse drug reactions.

Source: https://www.mdpi.com/pharmaceuticals/pharmaceuticals-16-01542/article_deploy/html/images/pharmaceuticals-16-01542-g001.png.

Definition of Adverse Drug Reactions (ADRs)

The definition of ADRs encompasses a range of harmful responses that occur following the administration of pharmacological agents. ADRs are typically classified into two broad categories: Type A (predictable) and Type B (unpredictable) reactions. The majority of ADR cases are type A reactions, and they happen when a drug's pharmacological effects cause side effects that can usually be expected from its known profile. On the other hand, Type B reactions happen in unique ways and cannot be predicted by the drug's action so that they may cause significant and unexpected problems. Knowing about ADRs is important for healthcare professionals (HCPs) and for making patient safety better, as drug development keeps progressing and introducing more medicines in various treatment areas. Understanding how common ADRs are and what puts people at risk is possible through studying their epidemiology. It has been found in recent studies that ADRs are a key reason for hospitalizations and can seriously affect the health of people who are elderly or have several other health conditions. According to Christopher et al. (2022), the global burden of antimicrobial resistance (AMR) exemplifies a critical area where ADRs significantly influence mortality and morbidity rates, reinforcing the need for heightened awareness and vigilance in clinical settings. An examination of ADR epidemiology allows researchers to pinpoint the most dangerous drugs, factors related to patients' demographics, and health issues that increase the risk, so that HCPs can choose treatments more carefully. Additionally, it is crucial to identify the causes of ADRs so that their impact on public health can be minimized. Polypharmacy, age, genes, and existing health conditions play a big role in determining the chances of experiencing an ADR. Implementation of guidelines and risk management strategies informed by François et al. (2019) offers HCPs valuable frameworks for minimizing adverse effects while maximizing therapeutic benefits. Being aware of these risk factors encourages providers to discuss the safe use of medications with patients and helps them communicate more effectively. If these risk factors are recognized and addressed, the healthcare community can develop more effective prevention plans and help patients achieve better outcomes with their medications (Figure 2.2).

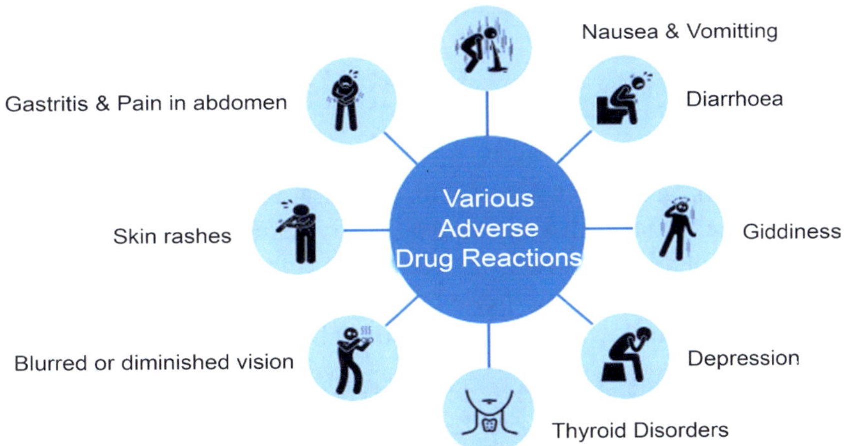

Figure 2.2. Adverse drug reactions.

Source: https://lh5.googleusercontent.com/LVRJw836Vrfl7mbmPUencGP6cUywtML4Cg3BK5ug1sxcafwk9KRILDR8lU1RVG3eKe3p91fqWq8Lqd4eVQcZGajPSC3pCMLV7oMSI7PaX0xPIfXaXXiJmdTSYac60Hd6ZgOavpdJ.

Importance of Studying ADRs in Public Health

Knowledge of ADRs is key to enhancing public health benefits, as their impact can be significant on patient safety and treatment outcomes. By studying ADRs, it is possible to detect what makes some people more likely to experience harmful drug effects, which helps in adjusting treatment plans for each person. In particular, elderly people, children, and patients with additional health issues are more likely to experience ADRs. A review of ADR reports helps healthcare providers identify the actions to take to avoid hazards, counsel patients more effectively, and revise their drug regimens. Noticing trends in ADRs allows regulatory bodies to provide rules that make drug use safer, which helps improve the health system. Studies on ADRs are important in the overall field of drug safety and pharmacovigilance. Although new drugs are thoroughly checked before being sold, it is still essential to continue monitoring them after they are approved. When more is known about ADRs, the process of developing drugs is improved, allowing scientists to identify and modify compounds with the most risks before they are widely distributed. For example, a study on the ChAdOx1 nCoV-19 vaccine highlighted the need for ongoing safety monitoring, as participants experienced adverse effects that informed subsequent research and public health guideline advisory recommendations (Voysey et al., 2020). Being careful like this gains the public's trust in drugs and also highlights why ADR studies should be part of everyday medical care to keep people healthy worldwide. In addition, ADRs can affect the cost of healthcare and the overall functioning of the system. As a result of ADRs, patients may need to stay in the hospital longer, receive treatment for a longer period, and incur additional healthcare expenses. Studies of these reactions enable public health agencies to calculate the total economic impact and provide guidance on actions that can reduce the number of ADRs. For instance, data from ADRs have played a crucial role in guiding health insurance policies that focus on strong, informed medication reviews before prescribing behavior, ultimately leading to a decrease in inappropriate healthcare spending (Zeppenfeld et al., 2022). Thus, studying ADRs in detail supports the creation of policies that prioritize public health and manage healthcare resources effectively in the long term.

2.1. Understanding Epidemiology

Epidemiology is a fundamental area in public health that examines how diseases affect the health and well-being of people in groups. It focuses on identifying risk factors associated with ADRs, which can lead to significant morbidity and mortality. By using different methods to count ADRs in various groups, epidemiologists can identify important links between individuals' backgrounds, the medications they take, and the outcomes observed in healthcare. With this data, health care providers can plan strategies to lower the dangers of using drugs.

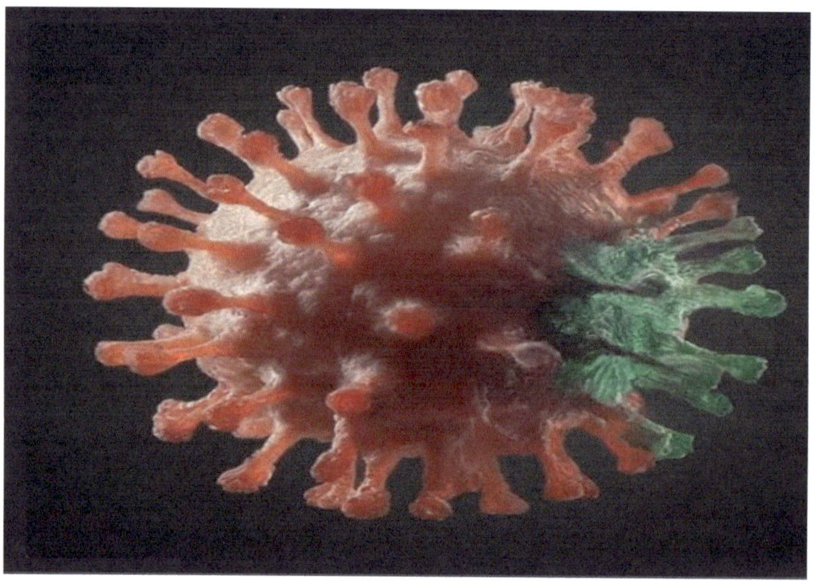

Figure 2.3. Understanding epidemiology.

Source: https://rectifymag.us/wp-content/uploads/2024/04/Gemini_Generated_Image_a17luga17luga17l-750x750.jpg.

Since some groups of people may react differently to certain medications, understanding the epidemiological situation helps doctors design the most effective treatment plans and ensure the safety of their patients. An in-depth study of skin problems caused by NSAIDs highlights the difficulties found in epidemiological studies of ADRs. Because these drugs are commonly used for their pain and inflammation-reducing properties, they often lead to side effects that vary from mild skin problems to severe reactions such as SJS. Many studies have highlighted that age, gender, and genetic background are among the factors that can contribute to these reactions. With a good understanding of these patterns, clinicians can identify individuals at risk and develop tailored treatment plans. This approach is necessary to enhance patient care and support public health efforts that inform patients about their medications and potential side effects, encouraging them to make informed decisions in collaboration with their doctors. Since drug-induced hypertension is an ADR, it is necessary to analyze the reasons behind it and the results for patients. Some medications, for example, glucocorticosteroids and nonsteroidal anti-inflammatory drugs (NSAIDs), can cause hypertension without showing any obvious signs, resulting in it being missed by doctors. According to studies, patients who have been diagnosed with well-controlled hypertension could have sudden rises in their blood pressure after taking these drugs. Since headaches and dizziness can be very subtle and different, it is important to watch patients who are given these drugs closely. When healthcare providers thoroughly study drug-induced hypertension, they can effectively prevent and manage it, ensuring that patients and healthcare professionals are prepared to deal with the condition (Figure 2.3).

2.1.1. Definition and Scope of Epidemiology

Epidemiology is essential in public health, as it studies how diseases affect different populations and what factors determine their spread. Epidemiology involves the number of cases and also the ways and reasons behind the health status of people in a population. To do this, one must study the complex interplay between the person, the environment, and genetic factors that contribute to the development of diseases, such as drug side effects. Epidemiologists conduct controlled trials and observational studies to identify the causes of specific health problems and associated risks. Epidemiological research helps to design effective actions and policies that lower the risk of ADRs, thus improving patient safety and the quality of treatments given to groups of people. The study of ADRs in epidemiology demonstrates how this field supports changes in medicine and drug monitoring. The goal of this field is to deal with the negative impacts of drug use, which can harm a patient and also influence the health of the general public. Epidemiologists can use the study of ADRs to discover patterns and possible reasons, such as drug-drug interactions, who the patients are, or their starting health conditions that result in these adverse effects. It is necessary to know about these factors to help HCPs create better preventive strategies and improve how they prescribe medications. As a result, epidemiology must ensure that the drugs used are not only effective but also safe for everyone to whom they are administered. When explaining risk factors for ADR, epidemiology points out that accurate design and reporting in clinical trials is very important. Randomized pilot and feasibility trials are a valuable way to check for possible ADRs before releasing a drug. Compliance with guidelines such as the Consolidated Standards of Reporting Trials (CONSORT) will make such studies more reliable and transparent, thereby ultimately increasing value to patient safety and informing regulatory agencies on the therapeutic applications of pharmaceuticals. Having many drugs available in the market makes it more challenging to know their risks. For this reason, an integrated epidemiological plan should employ rigorous study methods, utilize existing information, and regularly monitor the health outcomes of the population to address the causes of ADRs. As a result, epidemiology is leading the way in transforming public health and clinical care, enabling the more effective use of drugs among the general population.

2.1.2. Role of Epidemiology in Drug Safety

Epidemiology plays a critical role in enhancing drug safety by systematically studying the distribution and determinants of ADRs within populations. By closely studying patients, epidemiologists find out which groups of people are most likely to have ADRs. For example, changes in genetics, age, and other health issues can significantly impact a person's likelihood of experiencing adverse events. By analyzing large datasets and employing advanced statistical models, researchers can ascertain which drug-pathogen combinations present the most significant threat, as demonstrated in recent studies on AMR that reveal insights into the mortality rates associated with specific pathogen-drug interactions (Christopher et al., 2022). The use of data in healthcare helps doctors and also aids regulators in updating the way they approve drugs and monitor them after they are released. Additionally, the use of epidemiological methods in pharmacovigilance helps protect people from using unsafe drugs. After drugs are released, post-marketing surveillance gathers information on their safety, so their risks can be checked continuously. For example, during the recent COVID-19 pandemic, the deployment of vaccines necessitated extensive epidemiological rigor to systematically monitor side effects and adverse events, ensuring that public health decisions were informed by robust data regarding vaccine safety (Zhang et al., 2020).

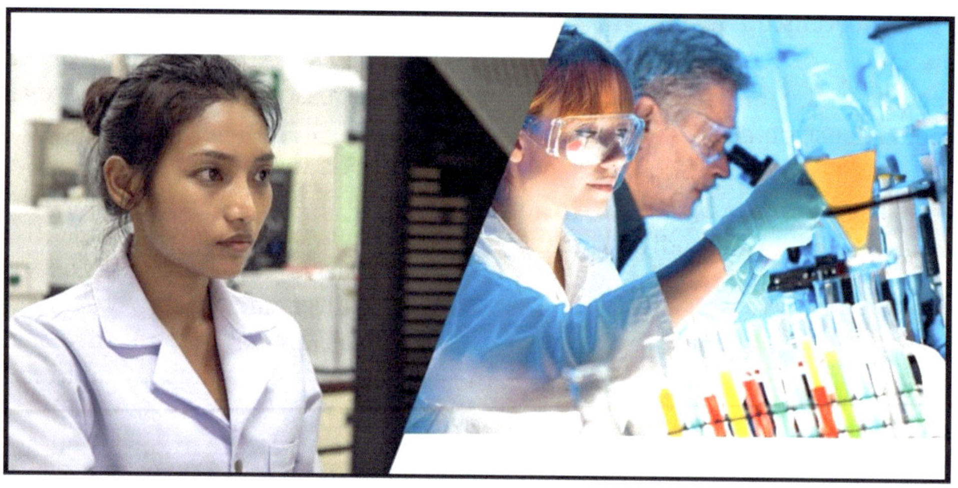

Figure 2.4. Role of epidemiology in drug safety.

Source: https://msc-epidemiology.online/wp-content/uploads/2015/11/Pharmacoepidemiology-Drug-Safety1.jpg.

Being vigilant is important to deal with the challenges brought by new drugs and therapies, since their safety may vary in different groups of people. Therefore, the epidemiological framework supports taking action to keep drugs safe by constantly monitoring and assessing them. Besides immediate safety, epidemiology also affects public health and policy in many ways. With the help of epidemiological studies, it is possible to direct healthcare policies and prioritize actions that improve drug safety. By understanding the seriousness and characteristics of ADRs, we can develop strategies to ensure safer prescribing, encourage patients to learn more, and enhance the regulations governing pharmaceutical products. In addition, these findings enable healthcare providers and patients to communicate effectively about risks, facilitating collaboration for patient safety. Without the help of epidemiology, it would be tough for healthcare to maintain the standards required to look after patient health in a complex medical environment (Figure 2.4).

2.1.3. Historical Context of ADR Studies

The historical context of ADR investigation has evolved significantly over the past century, driven by a series of milestone events and advances in pharmacovigilance. In the early years, ADR reporting primarily relied on the experiences and reports of doctors and patients. In the 1960s, the thalidomide tragedy made people realize that it was important to watch the safety of drugs closely. This incident resulted in the establishment of drug control bodies, such as the United States FDA and other organizations worldwide, that were given the mandate to verify drug safety and efficacy before approving them for the market. Due to these developments, formal methods for studying and monitoring ADRs were established, which ultimately led to changes in prescribing and safety guidelines for patients. At the same time, the scientific basis for ADRs was established by conducting epidemiological studies. Most of the early studies focused on just one group of drugs or a particular group of people. As research methods improved, researchers began to recognize that several factors contribute to ADR events. Experts realized that a person's genetic background, age, sex, and other medical problems could affect the chances and seriousness of ADRs. With the help of observational and experimental studies, epidemiologists can identify patterns and links that are crucial in assessing risks. This development enabled a better understanding of ADR risk factors, with the potential to inform more studies and improve patient care based on evidence-driven empirical findings, which reveal how different variables can impact drug safety outcomes, as noted by Brubaker et al. (2018). The development of technology has had a significant impact on the evolution of ADR research. The use of EHRs and big data analytics has dramatically changed the pharmacovigilance field in the last three decades. With access to big data, researchers can find ADRs that affect people in a population. Not only do these technologies enable the identification of adverse effects, but also the quantitative measurement of a drug's effectiveness in the real world through post-marketing surveillance. In addition, working together, pharmacologists, epidemiologists, and clinicians have provided a complete view of ADRs. This collaborative work is important in drug reaction complexities' management and the guarantee that patient safety should be of paramount importance in pharmacotherapy, as the understanding and implementation of guidelines set by institutions such as the European Society of Cardiology acknowledge that careful consideration of current recommendations is necessary for optimal medication use practices (Silvia et al., 2015).

2.2. Types of Adverse Drug Reactions

The categorization of ADRs is essential for understanding their implications in patient safety and public health. ADRs are primarily categorized into Type A and Type B reactions.

Type A reactions are caused by the direct effects of the drugs' properties. These reactions are often related to the drug dose and can include side effects such as sedation from antihistamines or gastrointestinal disturbances from NSAIDs. On the other hand, Type B reactions are unpredictable and happen without being caused by the drug's pharmacological effects. Sometimes, these reactions are allergic or very severe, and they are seen in a small number of patients, usually because of genetic or environmental causes, which makes it harder to treat patients with drugs. Knowing the epidemiology of ADRs helps us create preventive measures and improve the way treatments are given. Type A reactions occur frequently and are closely linked to factors such as a patient's age, sex, and other underlying health conditions. Sometimes, elderly individuals can be more sensitive to medications, which may lead to adverse side effects. Type B reactions are harder to deal with because they are unpredictable and may lead to hospitalization or death. It has been found through research that people with allergies or specific genetic traits are more likely to have Type B ADRs, which points to the importance of considering each patient's needs before prescribing. Healthcare providers should always watch for any signs of ADRs during the treatment of patients. In addition, the effects of both Type A and Type B reactions are felt in healthcare systems as well as in the health of patients.

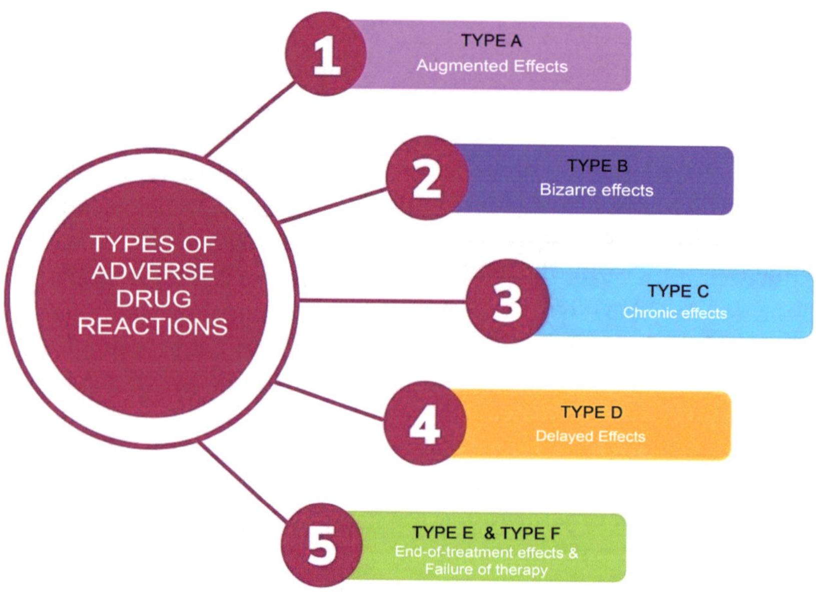

Figure 2.5. Types of adverse drug reactions.

Source: https://lh5.googleusercontent.com/u_xvKgpYqMmEyFb4Oi0T_13-mz-keUHVyVxpwKCvos4GU2Z71I6FsddZ8v73as--86rzjEuYKCzKtAAYJtpQyF0PMZUhxIhLmKnAn9J2gK5zn8yoxvRoW1gW0Jnn_9s1R2LB4j_8gGR9Ue0R-w=s1600.

For instance, ADRs lead to higher healthcare expenses, longer hospital stays for patients, and a lower quality of life, which puts a strain on the healthcare system. Recent analyses have quantified the burden of AMR, revealing significant mortality rates associated with drug-resistant infections, which are often consequences of suboptimal antibiotic use (Christopher et al., 2022).

Furthermore, during the COVID-19 pandemic, the emergence of various ADRs associated with new treatments and vaccines highlighted the importance of ongoing vigilance in pharmacovigilance efforts (Wiersinga et al., 2020). With proper monitoring and reporting, it becomes easier to manage the risks associated with ADRs, resulting in improved safety when using medications and better patient outcomes worldwide (Figure 2.5).

2.2.1. Type A (Augmented) Reactions

Type A (Augmented) reactions are the most prevalent form of ADRs, and they account for a high number of reported cases. The appearance of type A reactions is usually predictable because they occur as a natural part of using the drug within the proper dose. Rawlins and Thompson point out that Type A reactions are made up of overdosing, experiencing side effects, secondary effects, and interactions with other drugs. Noticing these reactions in pharmacology and epidemiology matters since they tell us how humans typically react to medication. Thus, management and monitoring of Type A reactions are imperative for achieving patient safety and therapeutic success, as their prevalence enables clinicians to be better prepared in advance for potential complications and modify treatment plans accordingly (Baldwin et al., 2018). Additionally, patients' individual features, such as changes in their genes, other health issues, and medications they are taking, influence the occurrence and severity of Type A reactions.

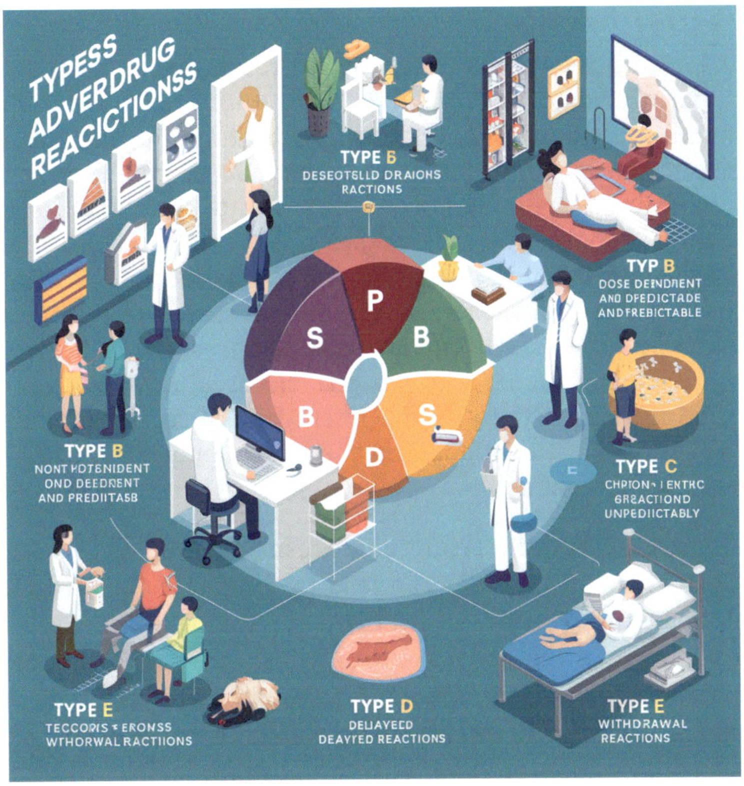

Figure 2.6. Type A (augmented) reactions.

Source: https://thepharmadaily.com/media/uploads/admin/2024/05/06/image-20240506133619-1.png.

The fact that patients are not the same means doctors should use personalized medicine when choosing drugs. For instance, elderly people are more likely to suffer from the harmful side effects of drugs. The older generation has been found to have impaired drug metabolizing capability and the ability to remove drugs, thus creating the accumulation of therapeutic agents and enhanced risk of toxicity (Bellanti et al., 2018). Moreover, when a patient has several health conditions, they are likely to take several drugs, which can result in Type A reactions because of possible drug-drug interactions. So, clinicians should be cautious when looking at patients' medical histories and drug use to avoid these anticipated side effects. To conclude, the occurrence of Type A reactions highlights the importance of having robust pharmacovigilance systems. It is important to improve monitoring to find out more about drug reactions and the people most at risk. Epidemiological studies tell healthcare providers which drugs often cause Type A reactions, which helps plan public health measures to reduce the risks of such reactions. Additionally, education interventions among healthcare providers are necessary, as greater awareness of the predictors and consequences of Type A responses will promote evidence-based prescribing behaviors (Baldwin et al., 2018). Overall, making an effort to identify and address Type A responses will enhance patient safety, increase the amount of care provided in pharmacotherapy, and benefit the overall health of the population (Figure 2.6).

2.2.2. Type B (Bizarre) Reactions

Type B (Bizarre) reactions, unlike Type A (Augmented) reactions, do not have a clear correlation with drug dosage or pharmacological effects. Sometimes, these reactions are unexpected and can happen in a limited number of patients, no matter how healthy they may be. Reactions of Type B may be caused by genetic factors or the immune system. Some people may have unique genetic variations that alter how drugs are metabolized, leading to unexpected side effects that were not identified during clinical trials. Since the causes of adverse reactions are unpredictable, it is challenging to identify the risk factors associated with them. Because of this, healthcare workers have few ways to prevent or control these events, which makes it necessary to study what leads to them. Type B reactions are also closely connected to the presence of previous conditions or the simultaneous use of other medications. Autoimmune diseases may increase the risk of unusual reactions, as the immune system's activity can be intensified by certain medications. Also, because many older people take several medications, the chances of unusual reactions are higher due to the increased risk of drug interactions.

It is essential to notice the link between antibiotic resistance and Type B reactions. For example, the misuse of antibiotics in clinical settings can lead to complications, as noted in recent studies highlighting the public health implications of antibiotic resistance (Christy et al., 2018). Such issues can alter the regular response of the body to drugs, which raises the chances of adverse effects. To understand the epidemiology of Type B reactions, we must examine their frequency in various groups. It is now believed that certain demographic elements, such as genetics or dietary habits, may influence a person's likelihood of experiencing unusual reactions. In particular, individuals consuming highly processed foods or those involved in intensive farming practices may face unique risks related to drug interactions, as seen with antibiotic residues (Christy et al., 2018). In addition, some foods can interact with drugs and cause unexpected results. Established conditions, such as the formation of bezoars, reveal intrinsic links between bizarre reactions and gastrointestinal health, adding another layer of complexity to this issue. For this reason, various methods, such as epidemiology, genetics, and lifestyle analysis, should be employed to better study and mitigate these adverse effects (Figure 2.7).

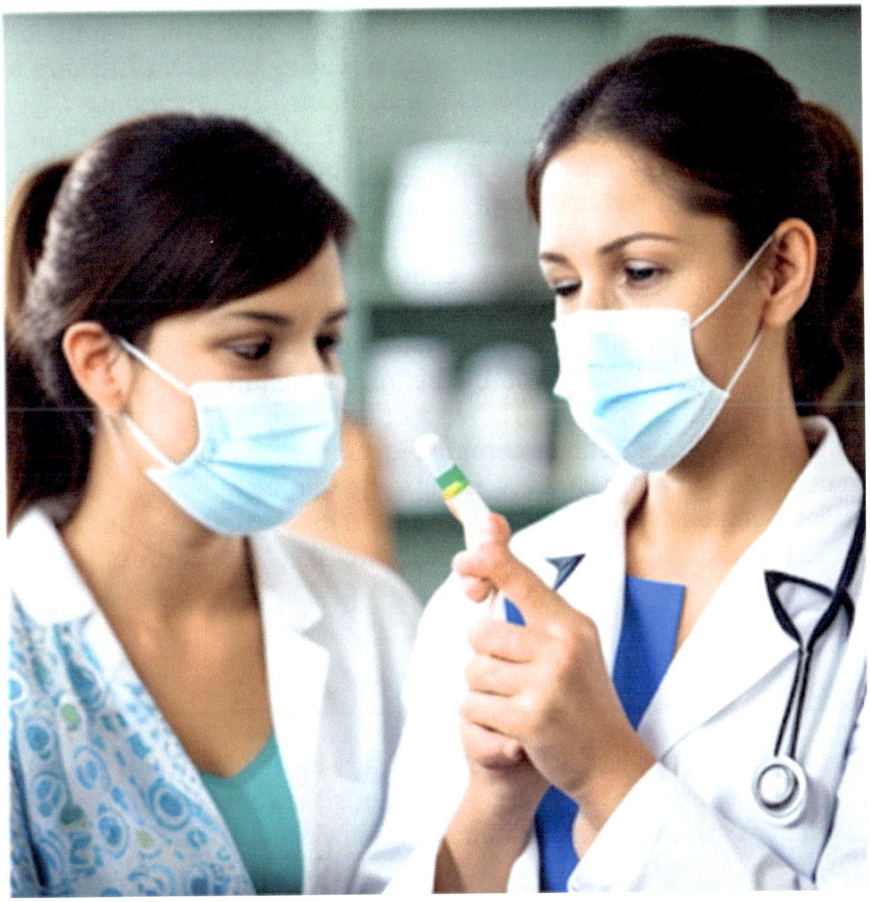

Figure 2.7. Type B (bizarre) reactions.

Source: https://blogger.googleusercontent.com/img/a/AVvXsEjzBmpcRVaBzLrnYxUEc_CUCUapPcz1fRscKxYkqwBjeBA_XaR5RumA2hOTDznDX032C7sqYZWSu7 j9A3RqBN1JGVmtCzj7Y5SH87wYWUMJBREcz2mdA0h37Dsm_327MR41TQasgLCjEK7c01jrlsIhmD_607MFQXsMJY4FViwuF7QIj2h8NJq5nCLhew=w521-h408.

2.2.3. Type C (Chronic) Reactions

Type C (Chronic) reactions are a significant category of ADRs characterized primarily by their chronic toxicity, additive effects, and delayed effects. Type C reactions have a propensity to emerge from the long-term use of individual pharmacologic agents, rather than from acute doses or brief courses of treatment. As an example, the risk of drug-induced liver injury (DILI) can rise with time for drugs such as acetaminophen, which are generally safe in standard therapeutic doses but can lead to full-thickness necrosis of the liver following long-term exposure to high doses. Additionally, their insidious nature of onset and non-specific clinical manifestations, which can mimic other liver conditions, complicate the identification of chronic reactions, making it difficult to diagnose and requiring extensive epidemiological information in order to devise effective management plans (Robert et al., 2022). The epidemiology of Type C reactions highlights their relatively low frequency of occurrence compared to immediate HSRs, but with great potential for severe consequences. Long-term ADRs tend to result in lasting health complications, including chronic liver disease, renal impairment, or endocrine disorders. The literature indicates that DILI, despite lower frequencies compared to acute reactions, remains a significant threat to public health due to its variability and complexity in presentation across different populations. Understanding Type C reaction risk factors, i.e., drug dose, duration of therapy, and patient factors like age and initial health status, allows for identifying high-risk groups. This approach emphasizes the importance of therapeutic interventions tailored to the individual to prevent long-term adverse reactions associated with certain drugs (Christopher et al., 2022). Besides, the investigation of chronic reactions is also critical in drug safety and pharmacovigilance. Continual monitoring of patient results connected with the long-term use of medication is critical in understanding the broader effect of Type C reactions. Long-term use of certain drugs, like antihypertensives and antimicrobials, has been proven to lead to the establishment of Type C reactions, which necessitates careful assessment in the process of standard clinical practice. The role of drug interactions in polypharmacy patients only adds to the obscurity of the arena of chronic reactions by emphasizing the cumulative effects of numerous agents. Health care providers navigating this complexity, though, call for greater coordination between clinicians, pharmacists, and epidemiologists to hone treatment protocols better so that these mitigate against the risk of chronic ADRs but address patients' multifaceted needs (Robert et al., 2022).

2.3. Prevalence of Adverse Drug Reactions

ADRs represent a significant challenge in contemporary healthcare, affecting patient safety and treatment outcomes. ADRs are more common in certain situations due to factors such as the type of medication, the patient's background, and the location where treatment is administered. In most cases, people who are older or have several health problems are more likely to have ADRs. A rise in the number of aging people and more chronic diseases is expected to result in a higher rate of ADRs and more healthcare pressure. Studies reveal that the chance of a serious ADR is higher for people who take several medicines at the same time. Understanding this variability is crucial for healthcare providers seeking to enhance patient care and utilize effective monitoring methods for those at the highest risk. ADRs occur due to both immune and non-immune responses within the body. Depending on a person's predispositions and the drug being used, these reactions can show in many different ways. For example, HSRs may cause serious consequences, so it is important to know how to manage and understand them as described in recent reviews of drug hypersensitivity. They mention the ways the immune system works and also list the various risk factors that can lead to more ADRs, such as genetic and environmental causes. Once these risk factors are spotted, HCPs can prepare for possible problems and design treatments to lower the risks. Thus, it is important to use this information in clinical settings to help patients and lower the number of ADRs. Moreover, progress in pharmacovigilance is designed to increase the identification and reporting of ADRs, which leads to improved safety of drugs. It is common in developing countries for adverse events to be underreported, as there are insufficient resources and awareness to address them effectively. It is crucial for healthcare systems to understand the epidemiology of ADRs so they can effectively address these issues. As cited, drug-induced liver injury (DILI) is a major concern due to both its prevalence and the seriousness of its consequences. Stronger monitoring and standardized reporting are crucial for identifying all ADRs and DILI, enabling medical staff to address them proactively. Thus, attention to ADR epidemiology will foster a safer medication landscape, ultimately enhancing patient outcomes and overall healthcare quality, potentially leading to better therapeutic decisions in clinical environments (Villarreal-González et al., 2023; Suzuki et al., 2024).

2.3.1. Statistics on ADR Occurrences

The prevalence and outcomes of drug adverse reactions (ADRs) highlight a significant public health concern at a global level. A study conducted in South Korea examined 44,122 cases of ADRs reported between 2009 and 2018, indicating that 56.2% were females and males accounted for 43.8% (Jeong et al., 2022). The data also indicated that individuals between the age group of 50–79 years made up 47% of the cases, showing the vulnerability of this age group to ADRs. This is a significant age since it might include individuals who are most likely to be on several medications and hence are at high risk of drug interaction and side effects. Disorders of the gastrointestinal system were the most common type of ADR, representing 25.8% of all reported cases, and this could suggest that certain classes of drugs pose an inherent risk to be monitored and prevented. The severity of the ADRs is also significant, with the research showing that 7.8% of the reported cases are of the severe type. The research also found some of the risk factors influencing the potential to develop severe ADRs, which are gender and age. For instance, males were also demonstrated to have a higher odds ratio (OR = 1.25) for developing severe ADR events compared to females, with particular ages like children and older people at greater risk (Jeong et al., 2022). These results mandate a thorough debate regarding the need for tailored pharmacovigilance approaches based on demographic factors. By determining the risk population profiles, the healthcare providers are well-positioned to implement more precise monitoring systems and, therefore, enhance the safety of patients as well as reduce the incidence of severe adverse reactions. In addition, the advent of drug safety methodologies, such as the combination of fault tree analysis and Petri net modeling, would be groundbreaking to avert ADR risks. These new approaches facilitate the qualitative and quantitative analysis of drug safety incidents, thereby exposing the underlying reasons for side effects. By using such models of analysis in healthcare settings, hospitals not only maximize medication error management but also optimize their risk management strategies. Emphasis on rational drug use and effective monitoring systems can eventually lead to improved medication safety levels, particularly for vulnerable groups, with a health system focused on patient well-being and ADR burden minimization. With ADR statistics development, the necessity of respective strategies and interventions to address them accordingly arises.

2.3.2. Variability in Prevalence Across Populations

The variability in the prevalence of ADRs among different populations is a significant concern in pharmacovigilance and clinical practice. Several factors can contribute to this, including genetic differences, environmental influences, and variations in lifestyle. Specific genetic changes, mainly in the genes responsible for drug breakdown, can make some people more prone to ADRs, but others may be protected from them. Some population-specific polymorphisms can cause drugs to be processed differently in the body, resulting in different reactions and more chances of harmful effects. Understanding these differences among populations is crucial for selecting the appropriate medications, ensuring patient safety, and developing personalized treatment plans tailored to each individual. Besides, factors such as a person's income, access to medical care, and public health rules are important reasons for the spread of ADRs among people. They may lead to a person being exposed to certain drugs and also to having side effects. People living in areas with limited resources are more likely to face risks because they often lack access to quality medicine, proper healthcare centers, or effective ways to treat diseases. For this reason, vulnerable groups suffer from ADRs more often than others. Therefore, it is evident that targeted actions are necessary to enhance healthcare quality and reduce risks, ensuring that everyone has equal health opportunities. Furthermore, the impact of AMR exemplifies the complexities of variability in drug reactions among populations. A number of recent studies have pointed out that AMR causes a great deal of death, mainly in lower-income regions, showing the significant difference in AMR between high and low-resource areas. AMR and ADRs are linked because bacteria become resistant and antibiotics cause specific reactions in the body. To develop effective strategies against AMR and ADRs, it is crucial to understand the relationship between AMR and ADRs. Improved understanding of the geographic and ethnogeographic variability, exemplified by the disparities in the prevalence of pathogenic variants influencing drug transport and metabolism, can ultimately contribute to more personalized medical approaches that enhance therapeutic efficacy and safety in diverse populations (Xiao et al., 2020; Christopher et al., 2022) (Figure 2.8).

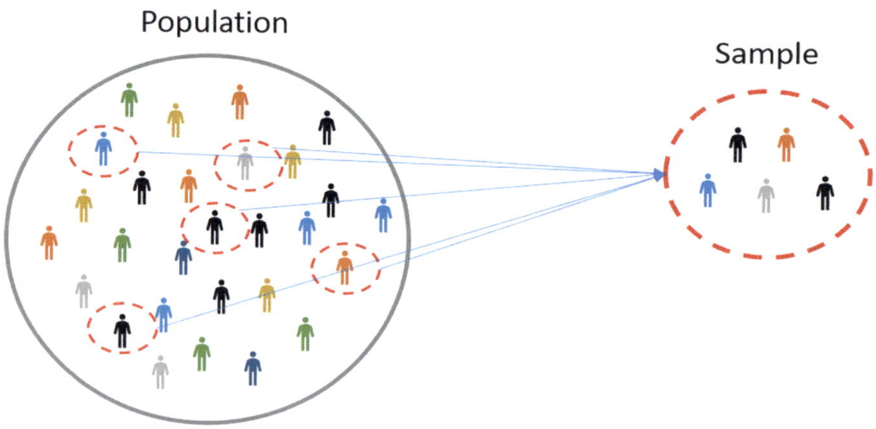

Figure 2.8. Variability in prevalence across populations.

Source: https://miro.medium.com/v2/resize:fit:1280/1*83WLnE2QTeOHSjbPJDVKfw.png.

2.3.3. Impact of ADRs on Healthcare Systems

ADRs are a global challenge to healthcare systems in that they have a direct bearing on patient outcomes and the use of healthcare resources. The commonality of ADRs makes it essential to adopt comprehensive approaches to pharmacovigilance, as they directly contribute to morbidity and mortality. To illustrate, it is estimated that millions of patients experience ADRs annually, which results in enhanced hospital admissions and longer stays in the health facility. Such side effects not only disrupt patient management plans but also overwhelm healthcare resources and call for additional medical treatment, which may increase healthcare spending. In many cases, ADRs can require alternative therapy, further entangle patient care, and increase drug interaction and treatment complication risks. Identifying the size and range of ADRs is essential to effectively organize and implement actions that neutralize their impact on patients and healthcare systems. The cost of ADRs is staggering, impacting both direct medical costs and indirect expenditures from lost productivity and extended healthcare needs. Studies have shown that ADRs are a significant determinant of healthcare expenditure, with hospitalizations accounting for a substantial share of those costs. The requirement for special treatment, additional diagnostic tests, and increased monitoring can account for increased spending and fiscal deficits on the providers' side. Additionally, the economic impacts of ADRs extend beyond immediate healthcare costs, with lost working time and reduced quality of life in affected patients, underscoring the need for health systems to adopt prevention measures. Investment in effective education, surveillance systems, and proactive patient care management methods can lead to a significant decrease in the prevalence of ADRs and their economic burden, ultimately benefiting patients and healthcare systems. A defining attribute of healthcare systems that are fighting the effect of ADRs is the increased requirement for training and better communication among HCPs. Effective drug handling and ADR prevention require HCPs to have the required knowledge and skills. An educated health workforce is crucial for ensuring the accurate identification of vulnerable populations and the effective implementation of preventive interventions. Furthermore, patient-professional communication needs to become paramount to enable decision-making alongside patients and enhance compliance with medication. Educational programs to improve provider education on risks associated with a multitude of drugs can enable better-educated prescribing practice. By creating a patient safety-oriented and sensitized culture, healthcare organizations can improve overall outcomes and reduce the occurrence of ADRs, finally leading to better patient care. The interdisciplinarity underscores the necessity for the central position of education, communication, and monitoring in countering the issue posed by ADRs in healthcare facilities.

2.4. Risk Factors for Adverse Drug Reactions

The landscape of ADRs is multifactorial, with several risk factors extending across demographic, genetic, and clinical parameters. Age is a significant factor here; elderly people are more likely to react badly to medicines because of their bodies, taking several medicines, and having other health problems. In addition, the rise in chronic diseases among older people increases the chances of bad reactions. In addition, taking certain medications may worsen arterial hypertension in the elderly, causing more health complications. Studies suggest that anticancer agents, in particular, may induce drug-induced hypertension, highlighting the importance of closely monitoring blood pressure and overall cardiovascular health in patients receiving such treatments (Ostroumova et al., 2022). As more people age and treatment plans become increasingly complex, it is essential to understand these interconnected risks to identify safer medications. A person's genetic background is an important factor in the risk of severe delayed drug hypersensitivity reactions (DHRs). More people agree that pharmacogenetics can help identify individuals who may be at risk of adverse reactions to certain drugs. For example, HLA-B*57:01 screening has proven successful in mitigating risks associated with abacavir use, underscoring the value of personalized medicine. Such advancements have illuminated how specific genetic markers can indicate vulnerability to severe cutaneous adverse reactions (SCAR) and drug-induced organ injuries, contributing to morbidity and mortality rates that can approach 40% in severe cases (Gomes et al., 2019). By using genetic screening in clinical care, it becomes easier to prevent ADRs, since healthcare providers can choose the right medicine for each patient and avoid dangerous reactions. Apart from age and genetics, other clinical factors, such as taking multiple medications and having underlying health issues, also play a significant role in causing ADRs. Those with several chronic illnesses usually take many medications, which raises the risk of drug interactions and more side effects. All these interactions can sometimes result in problems that are not immediately apparent. People who are treated with several drugs for conditions such as diabetes, hypertension, or heart disease may be more likely to suffer from adverse drug interactions since the drugs affect similar body processes. For this reason, it is crucial to monitor various medications and their potential side effects in clinical settings. Reviewing medications in detail and introducing protocols for managing many drugs at once can make patients safer and help reduce the chances of ADRs, leading to better treatment results (Figure 2.9).

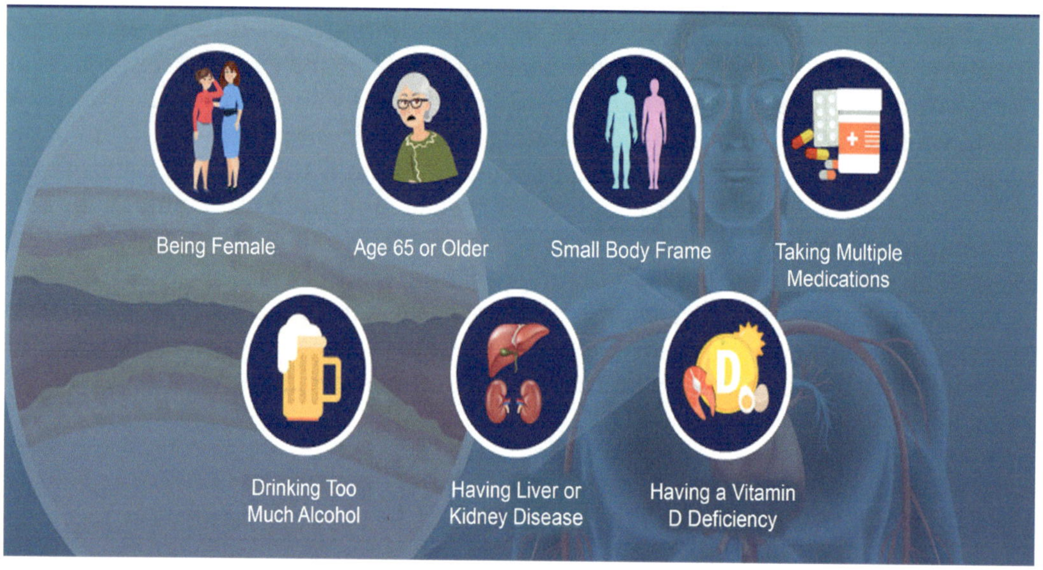
Being Female
Age 65 or Older
Small Body Frame
Taking Multiple Medications
Drinking Too Much Alcohol
Having Liver or Kidney Disease
Having a Vitamin D Deficiency

Figure 2.9. Risk factors for adverse drug reactions.

Source: https://drjockers.com/wp-content/uploads/2021/06/Statin-Drug-Side-Effects.jpg.

2.4.1. Patient-Related Factors (Age, Gender, Genetics)

Patient-specific factors such as age, gender, and genetics are relevant in the consideration during analysis of ADRs in clinical practice. Age significantly influences the PK and pharmacodynamics of medications. For instance, older individuals typically have physiological alterations that can alter drug metabolism as well as make them more vulnerable to ADRs. Such an age group is highly susceptible to polypharmacy, in which multiple drugs can interact negatively. Importantly, there is a model known as ADAPTiP that is employed to identify predictors of risk in older populations and that establishes a link between frailty, age, and hospitalization as a result of ADR. These results show the importance of age as a predictor in prescribing to minimize risk associated with ADR, which improves patient safety and therapeutic effectiveness (Frydenlund et al., 2024). Additionally, gender differences also play an important role in the occurrence of ADRs because of biological as well as sociocultural factors. Studies have indicated that females may be at greater risk owing to differences in body composition, hormonal changes, and the chance of polypharmacy, particularly in an aging population. Furthermore, cultural perceptions make women get higher doses or more medication than necessary, maximizing the risk of ADRs. Such imbalances require HCPs to consider gender-specific responses to treatment procedures. Through the integration of this knowledge into therapy planning and clinical judgment, the healthcare system can improve outcomes and minimize the incidence of side effects, demonstrating an indispensable component in the broader field of pharmacovigilance and patient safety (Pérez-Ingidua et al., 2024). A second patient-specific consideration, genetics, further complicates the ADR picture. Genetic differences among drug-metabolizing enzymes can lead to significant interindividual variability in drug response. Polymorphism among cytochrome P450 enzymes, for example, affects the metabolism of many drugs used in clinical practice, resulting in a small percentage of patients being ultra-rapid or poor metabolizers. This genetic diversity not only alters the efficacy of drugs but also the risk of ADRs, and pharmacotherapy should be more individualized. With the evolving pharmacogenomics, there are opportunities for tailoring drug therapy to suit a patient's genetic profile, potentially reducing the occurrence of ADRs and enhancing outcomes. Thus, the incorporation of genetic tests into clinical practice holds great potential to effectively mitigate risks from ADRs and provide safer drug usage (Frydenlund et al., 2024) (Figure 2.10).

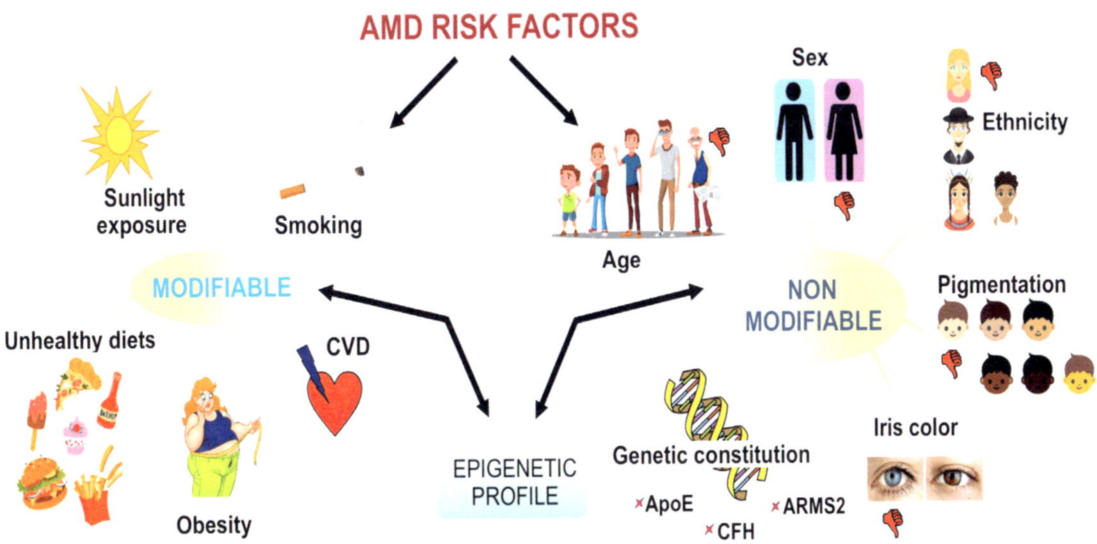

Figure 2.10. Patient-related factors (age, gender, genetics).

Source: https://pub.mdpi-res.com/ijms/ijms-24-02636/article_deploy/html/images/ijms-24-02636-g001.png?1675088908.

2.4.2. Drug-Related Factors (Dosage, Drug Interactions)

The incidence of ADRs can be significantly influenced by drug-related factors such as dosage and drug interactions. Proper dosage is necessary since changes in the amount could result in either too little or too much drug in the body. A drug's PK may vary depending on a person's age, sex, and organ function, so the usual dosage may need to be changed. If renal or hepatic function is not normal, lower doses should be used to avoid the drug from accumulating and becoming toxic. Therefore, the concept of therapeutic indices emphasizes that administering the correct dose is crucial for treating patients safely and effectively. Because of the rising number of drug overdoses, it is clear that managing doses according to each patient's needs is crucial and underlines the need for precise pharmacotherapy. Drug interactions are an important aspect of drug-related factors that may cause adverse reactions. When a person takes many drugs at the same time, it becomes more likely for pharmacodynamic and pharmacokinetic interactions to happen and cause unexpected ADRs. Since the elderly and those with chronic illnesses usually take several medications, there are concerns about possible interactions that could increase or reduce the effectiveness of drugs. Such interactions may alter how the body processes drugs, potentially leading to more challenging clinical outcomes. If HCPs are aware of possible interactions and follow clinical guidelines, they can help avoid such risks. Additionally, using dynamic drug monitoring may make it easier to identify potential interactions, thereby keeping patients safe and ensuring their treatments are optimized. Managing ADRs requires looking for both dosage-related and interaction-related factors that affect patients' outcomes. It is essential for healthcare providers to understand how drugs interact and why they must regularly monitor and adjust their patients' dosages. Moreover, open communication between healthcare workers and patients is essential, since patients often do not realize how important it is to report ADRs. Such systems help identify trends in ADRs and how drug safety has evolved over time. As indicated by recent studies, a proactive stance in understanding these drug-related factors is essential for improving patient outcomes, informing practice guidelines, and ultimately fostering safer medication use in clinical environments (Adithan et al., 2015; Brand et al., 2016).

2.4.3. Environmental Factors (Diet, Lifestyle)

Lifestyle and dietary habits are important environmental determinants that have a significant impact on the health consequences of an individual and potentially could affect the development of ADRs. Dietary habits, such as the consumption of processed foods, sugar, and trans fatty acids, can contribute to the development of chronic diseases, which in turn increase the risk factors associated with pharmacotherapy. For instance, obese or metabolic syndrome patients can have their PK and pharmacodynamics altered due to changes in organ function and body composition. All these alterations result in elevated drug levels and, therefore, the enhanced risk of ADRs. With this comes a realization of the inherent relationship between drug reaction and nutritional choice, making awareness essential in the epidemiological context, with calls for targeted nutritional intervention to limit risks associated with drug use. Lifestyle choices, including activity level and drug/alcohol intake, besides nutrition, also increase ADR risk profiles. Sedentary life and physical inactivity can exacerbate underlying illnesses such as hypertension and diabetes, which complicate drug therapy management. Secondly, the use of legal drugs such as tobacco has been reported to be linked with increased risk of negative outcomes among pharmacotherapy patients. For example, cigarette smoking is known to induce some of the drug-metabolizing enzymes, which can lead to reduced effectiveness or increased toxicity of drugs. These contacts emphasize the necessity for HCPs to consider a patient's lifestyle when creating treatment plans, promoting an interrelated strategy of drug therapy safety, incorporating both environmental and individual behaviors. Ultimately, the overlap between environmental influences—dietary and lifestyle—calls for an interrelated approach to assessing health risks associated with drug therapy. New findings bring to light non-traditional risk factors such as sleep health and psychological well-being, which are associated with adverse consequences following drug use. For instance, inadequate sleep has been found to have a detrimental effect on drug compliance, thus potentially increasing the level of drug interaction or drug side effects. In this regard, lifestyle and dietary interventions can not only act as preventive strategies against chronic diseases but also as methods to make drugs safer and more effective. Through the control of these determinants of environmental health, the incidence of ADRs can significantly be reduced and improved results for health in general may be promoted, as new studies on diet influences and lifestyle change assessments in drug therapy have indicated (Lu et al., 2024; Diancarlos et al., 2025) (Figure 2.11).

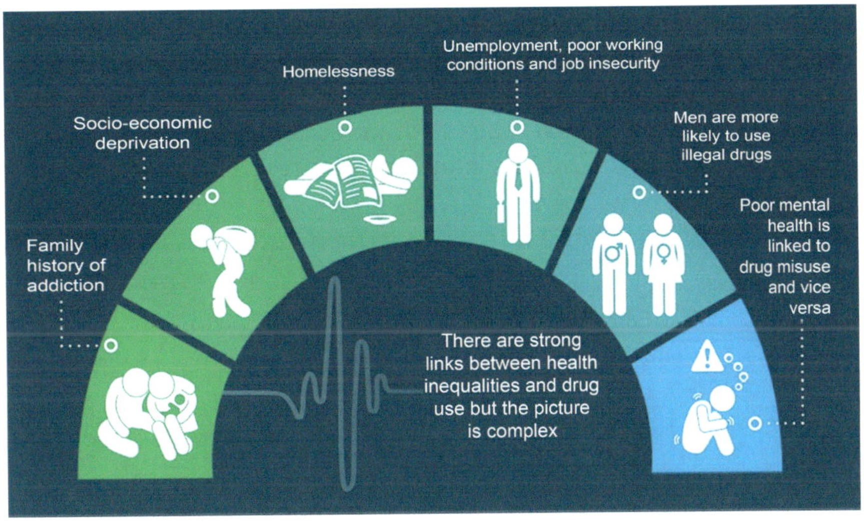

Figure 2.11. Environmental factors (diet, lifestyle).

Source: https://image1.slideserve.com/1603143/lifestyle-factors-affecting-health-l.jpg.

2.5. Methods of Identifying Adverse Drug Reactions

The identification of ADRs is a complex process that relies heavily on systematic methodologies to ascertain the relationship between drug exposure and resulting adverse effects. To start, clinicians investigate the patient's medication history, including the time, dose, and duration of use for every medication and any herbal or dietary supplements. This is very important, as ADRs usually develop within a specific time after taking the drug, so it is necessary to know the patient's medication plan. When comparing the frequency of liver injury to causes such as hepatitis and alcohol, doctors can focus more on possible drug-related causes. Moreover, the clinical patterns of liver injury and laboratory findings, including serum aminotransferases and bilirubin levels, help shape the diagnostic framework necessary for identifying specific ADRs and ruling out alternative etiologies (Robert et al., 2022). To make ADR identification more precise, new methods use both what doctors observe and laboratory tests. In cases of suspected DILI, healthcare providers utilize liver function tests (LFTs) to identify elevations in serum aminotransferases and alkaline phosphatase, which serve as indicators of hepatotoxicity. Additionally, using diagnostic algorithms enables doctors to distinguish between hepatocellular injury and cholestatic injury, thereby improving the diagnostic process. A study has found that careful monitoring after stopping the drug can prove if the adverse symptoms get better, suggesting that the drug may be responsible for the reaction. The necessity for detailed and careful diagnostic approaches underscores the challenges faced when attributing liver injury to specific medications, particularly in populations with multifactorial causes of liver disease (Robert et al., 2022). Using pharmacogenomic information in the process of identifying ADRs is a new area that shows a lot of promise. A person's genetic background can increase their chance of experiencing ADRs, mainly when they take certain medicines. For instance, specific human leukocyte antigen (HLA) alleles have been identified as risk factors for various drug reactions, suggesting the potential for personalized medicine in the realm of pharmacotherapy. By identifying genetic markers associated with adverse reactions, clinicians can prescribe drugs that are less likely to cause problems in those individuals. Although there is still much work to standardize genetic testing, the fact that genetic profiling can help with prescribing decisions is an exciting step that may significantly improve the way ADRs are handled (Figure 2.12).

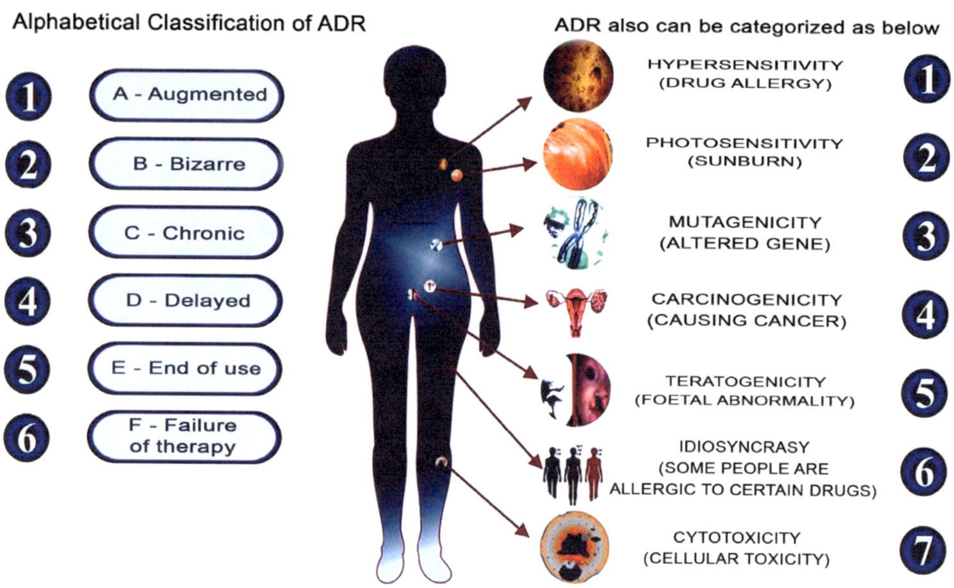

Figure 2.12. Methods of identifying adverse drug reactions.

Source: https://i.ytimg.com/vi/Qntov1vVS-4/maxresdefault.jpg.

2.5.1. Spontaneous Reporting Systems

Spontaneous reporting systems (SRS) play a significant role in the pharmacovigilance process, especially in the detection and assessment of ADRs. Unlike the randomized controlled trials, which are conducted under controlled circumstances, SRS employ real-world data (RWD) gathered post-marketing. The naturalistic approach allows the detection of rare and unexpected ADRs that may not have been evident in the pre-marketing phase. By using various statistical techniques, such as the reporting odds ratio (ROR) and the proportional reporting ratio (PRR), researchers can examine these spontaneous reports for safety signals. The ability to conduct these analyses on high volumes of data makes drug safety evaluations more valid and comprehensive, ultimately assisting public health programs aimed at minimizing drug adverse effects (Bondareva et al., 2024). The utility of SRS is evident in its application across different patient groups, such as hospital neonates undergoing intensive care. In a prospective observational study, the frequency of ADRs among admitted neonates was identified to be significantly high, with spontaneous reporting assuming a pivotal role in the identification of causative drugs and temporal profiles of these events. The SRS methodology allowed health professionals to actively query and browse spontaneous reports in institutional pharmacovigilance systems, collecting important data on the risk factors for ADRs in this vulnerable population (Leopoldino et al., 2023). Under the SRS viewpoint, this type of surveillance improves the understanding of how drug interactions and dosing influence neonatal health outcomes, thereby informing more specific pharmacotherapy. While they do have their utility, SRS are not without their limitations. They are prone to bias, such as underreporting and inconsistency in reporting activities, leading to missing data on drug safety. These limitations necessitate the use of robust statistical analysis to minimize bias and interpret the results accurately. In addition, while SRS help generate hypotheses regarding ADRs, findings must be substantiated by more rigorous studies before causality can be established. However, appropriately used, SRS remain a valuable component of the pharmacovigilance program, offering a low-cost means of monitoring drug safety post-marketing, especially in diverse clinical populations (Bondareva et al., 2024). To achieve this, they are a vital cinderblock in the ongoing struggle to safeguard public health from the threats posed by drugs.

2.5.2. Clinical Trials and Post-Marketing Surveillance

The way drug safety is managed depends largely on clinical trials and post-marketing surveillance, which are important for checking medication effectiveness and safety. Clinical trials, particularly those preceding a drug's approval, are meticulously designed to assess both the therapeutic benefits and potential ADRs among a controlled population. Although these trials provide important information about the drug's effectiveness, they often overlook rare and long-term side effects due to the small size of the groups and the short duration of the trials. When a medicine is used in practice, some risks may emerge that were not identified during trials. Therefore, it is essential to continue monitoring them through thorough post-marketing surveillance. Through vigilant monitoring, emerging patterns of drug utilization and adverse events can be systematically identified and addressed, thereby enhancing public health safety and contributing to a deeper understanding of medication effects in diverse populations (Frey, 2018). Clinical trials do not always reveal all the dangers of drugs, so post-marketing surveillance is needed to discover more about how safe they are. At this point, data is collected and regularly checked to identify any side effects that were not detected during the clinical trials. Some studies have shown that pharmacoepidemiology is necessary to spot links between medicines and rare side effects that doctors might miss. Sharing this information updates healthcare workers and government bodies. It also helps establish guidelines for patient care and safety. By employing diverse methodologies—including observational studies and the analysis of health records—researchers can elucidate the complex relationship between drug administration and potential adverse outcomes, thereby enhancing the accuracy of risk-benefit assessments in pharmacotherapy (Varanasi, 2012). Additionally, using data from post-marketing surveillance in clinical practice highlights concerns for patient safety and informs better prescription decisions. With the help of regulatory organizations, healthcare providers are able to closely watch the safety of the drugs they prescribe. Thanks to advisory alerts and updated guidelines, medical professionals can make the best decisions when prescribing treatments. As the epidemiological situation changes, researchers will continue to explore risk factors for ADRs, leading to the identification of those who are more likely to experience complications. Ultimately, the collaboration between clinical trial data and the insights gained from post-marketing surveillance fosters a comprehensive approach to drug safety, aimed at reducing the incidence of ADRs and improving patient outcomes (Frey, 2018) (Figure 2.13).

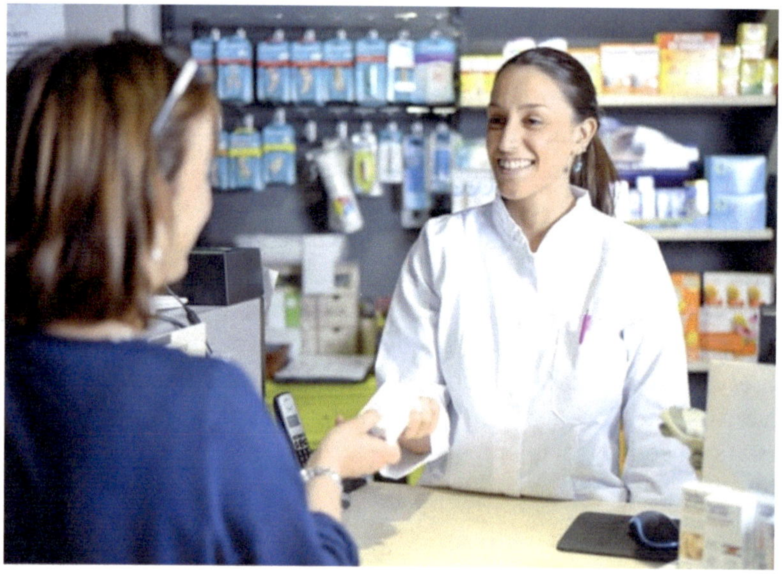

Figure 2.13. Clinical trials and post-marketing surveillance.

Source: https://www.aaps.ca/wp-content/uploads/Apr-7-clinical-research-program-600.jpg.

2.5.3. Electronic Health Records and Data Mining

The merging of EHRs and data mining methods has drastically transformed the field of pharmacovigilance, particularly in epidemiology and the identification of risk factors for ADRs. EHRs are detailed repositories of patient data, including demographic information, clinical histories, laboratory test results, and medication prescriptions. This large dataset is essential for successful data mining, enabling researchers to identify patterns and correlations that point to the development of ADRs. As indicated, the application of sophisticated computational algorithms to process EHR data would enable the identification of high-risk populations, where patients would be clustered into groups with similar profiles for increased targeted monitoring and intervention measures (Pretis et al., 2022). The trend of moving towards precision pharmacovigilance emphasizes the worth of such technologies as they can individualize drug safety assessments according to a patient's individual needs and condition. Data mining techniques applied in EHRs enable the provision of important information concerning ADRs and ADR risk factors through various approaches, including signal detection, temporal analysis, and prediction modeling. By such approaches, researchers can uncover seemingly subtle correlations between drug exposure and adverse outcomes that are otherwise not clearly visible in routine clinical trials. For instance, real-world evidence data analysis can identify rare ADRs encountered only after wider distribution of the drug, emphasizing the importance of surveillance that is supplementary to the extent of pre-approval studies (Yunn-Ho et al., 2019). Moreover, data mining facilitates researchers to understand the effect of patient factors such as age, gender, and comorbidities on drug response, which will result in high-risk population identification. This capability supports the need for integrating sophisticated analytical techniques with pharmacovigilance practice to ensure drug safety. Additionally, the application of EHRs and data mining can bring benefits to overall ADR management and patient safety in healthcare systems. By establishing more efficient pharmacovigilance systems, healthcare organizations can systematically get and analyze drug complication information, facilitating the detection of risks in a timely manner. This aligns with the aspiration to create intelligent hospitals where clinical decision-making will be informed by advanced systems for data gathering (Pretis et al., 2022). These technologies provide a gateway to more patient-centered therapy, whereby the prescriptions are tailored based on an individual's specific health environment and potential vulnerabilities to ADRs. The collaboration between healthcare providers, data analysts, and regulatory agencies will play a crucial role in utilizing these technologies to enhance drug safety and ultimately achieve better health outcomes for patients worldwide (Figure 2.14).

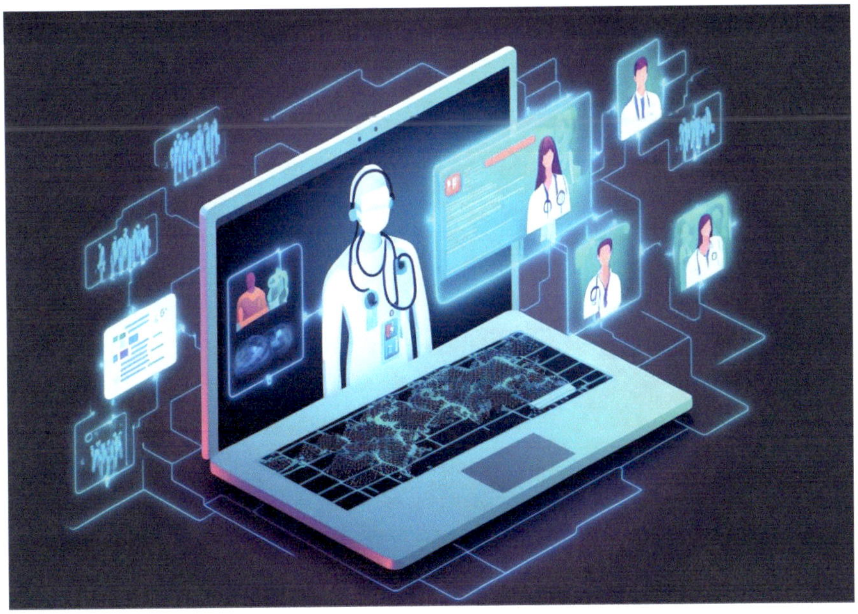

Figure 2.14. Electronic health records and data mining.

Source: https://datarundown.com/wp-content/uploads/2023/05/Data-Mining-Techniques-in-Healthcare.jpg.

2.6. Strategies for Minimizing Adverse Drug Reactions

Minimizing ADRs requires a multifaceted approach that begins with personalized medication management. When using this strategy, doctors take into account a patient's age, gender, ethnicity, and medical background since all of these can affect the chances of a serious ADR. For instance, a study highlighted the significant association between severe ADRs and variables such as age and a history of drug allergies, suggesting that HCPs should tailor prescriptions accordingly to mitigate risks (Sittiphan et al., 2025). If doctors carry out thorough assessments before prescribing, they can find patients who need special attention to avoid ADRs. This approach to patient care makes them safer and more likely to recover well, which highlights the importance of individualized care in preventing adverse reactions. Pharmacovigilance helps to keep an eye on drug safety and identify possible cases of ADRs.

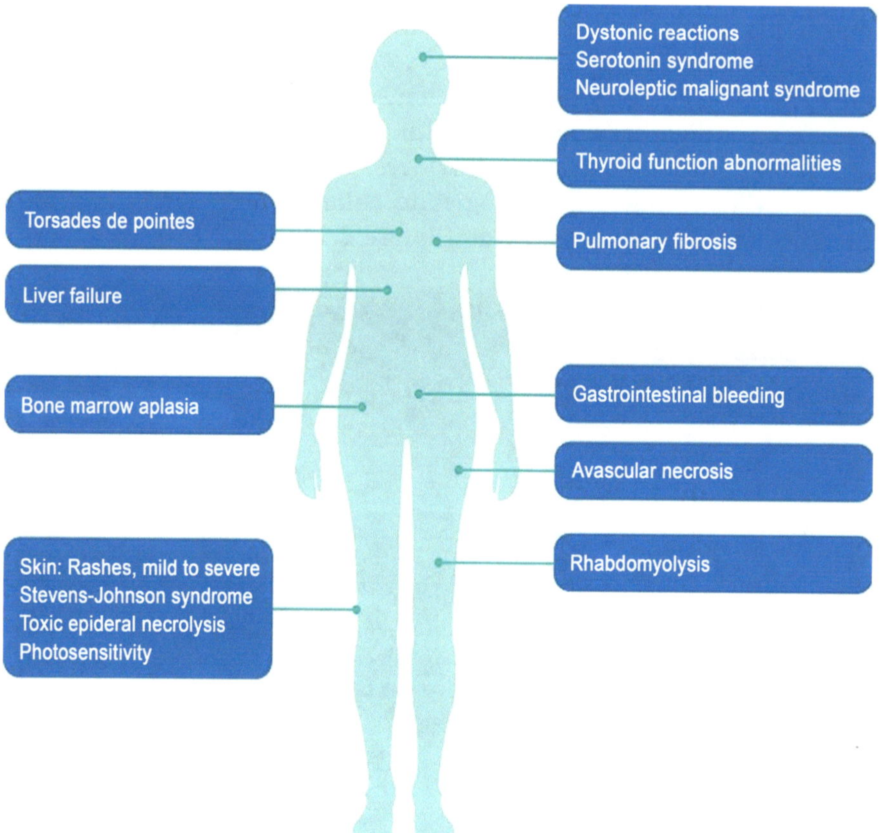

Figure 2.15. Strategies for minimizing adverse drug reactions.

Source: https://www.meded101.com/wp-content/uploads/2022/01/drugs-ge9ac8015b_640-scaled.jpg.

Effective reporting systems help identify ADR incidents and ensure that safety issues are addressed promptly as they arise. By employing tools such as EHRs and specialized software applications, healthcare providers can enhance the detection and reporting of ADRs in real-time, particularly in vulnerable populations, such as older adults who are often impacted by polypharmacy (Siobhán et al., 2024). They assist in keeping records and enable better data analysis, which results in safer ways to prescribe medications. A well-developed pharmacovigilance system helps HCPs spot signs of higher risks, which reduces ADRs and improves the quality of patient care. Moreover, having set medication review processes is important for avoiding ADRs in patients. Assessing medications regularly can uncover any inappropriate prescriptions, especially in older people who are likely to take many drugs together. Such reviews can utilize evidence-based guidelines and clinical decision support tools to optimize therapy and minimize the risk of adverse reactions (Siobhán et al., 2024). Having pharmacists, physicians, and nurses participate in these evaluations can bring diverse views and knowledge, ultimately improving care. If both healthcare workers and patients are educated about ADRs, individuals can be more involved in managing their medications and take care to avoid harm from drugs (Figure 2.15).

2.6.1. Risk Assessment and Management Protocols

Practical risk analysis and control measures are critical in minimizing the incidence of ADRs in the real world. The measures involve systematic protocols for identifying, analyzing, and regulating likely risks associated with pharmacological interventions. In populations being treated with highly active antiretroviral therapy (HAART), as reported by a study, a staggering 76% prevalence of ADRs occurred among the patients, pointing to the need for intervention.

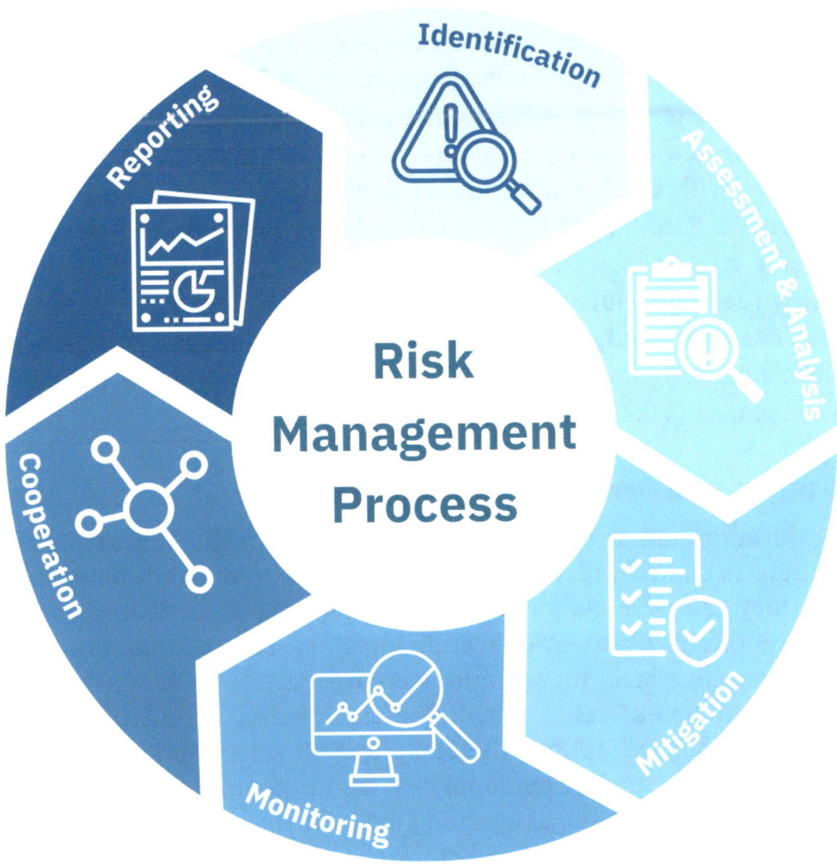
Identification
Assessment & Analysis
Mitigation
Monitoring
Cooperation
Reporting
Risk Management Process

Figure 2.16. Risk assessment and management protocols.

Source: https://assets-global.website-files.com/61ead44637176294fdd344ff/645bf3785d42518b7fb1437c_risk-management-process.png.

The study also noted major risk factors such as low CD4 counts and lower levels of education, emphasizing that communication and education measures that are appropriate could increase adherence to therapy as well as the detection of ADRs significantly. Ongoing risk assessment in HAART therapy necessitates the integration of patient education and surveillance of patients more frequently to recognize those who are at increased risk of developing adverse events, which will eventually result in better patient outcomes and protection against treating HIV infection (Moses et al., 2025). Along with the therapy monitoring, technology has been utilized to evaluate and control the risk, which improves the ability to detect ADRs more effectively. For instance, computerized drug interaction checkers allow for the detection of potential drug-drug interactions (DDIs), which are responsible for a significant proportion of the generation of ADRs. Studies have shown that patients with significant DDIs have 5.66 times higher opportunities of experiencing ADRs, pointing towards the importance of pharmacovigilance systems in healthcare settings. Moreover, training healthcare providers on how to use these technology devices can improve the effectiveness of medication management. By adopting an interdisciplinary model that merges human skills and technology-based assistance, caregivers can implement effective risk management policies that not only improve patient safety but also optimize therapeutic gains through knowledge-based decisions (Villanueva et al., 2025). Finally, encouraging a culture of responsibility and safety among medical staff is the key to ensuring effective risk management in ADRs. This involves creating an environment where HCPs are not afraid to report ADRs and learn from adverse events to avoid punishment. Including regular training and workshop sessions can propel a proactive risk assessment approach, empowering employees with the essential knowledge to detect early signs of ADRs and actively prevent complications. As exemplified in propofol sedation research, the occurrence of ADRs can be explained by some risk factors, i.e., the length of procedures and the ASA classification of patients. By regularly reading incident reports and integrating their findings into clinical practice, healthcare facilities can continually improve their risk management strategies, thereby ensuring patient safety and maintaining an assurance of excellence in care, even in the face of advanced pharmacological challenges (Villanueva et al., 2025) (Figure 2.16).

2.6.2. Patient Education and Informed Consent

Ensuring patient education and informed consent is critical in the context of ADRs, particularly given their implications in clinical practice. Patients should be told about the possible risks and side effects of the drugs they are given. As a result, people can take an active part in making decisions about their healthcare. Effective patient education encompasses clear communication of the risks associated with medications, which can be multifaceted, especially with substances known for their adverse reactions, such as non-steroidal anti-inflammatory drugs (NSAIDs). The epidemiology of NSAID-induced skin reactions exemplifies the complexity involved; patients must understand not only the general risks but also specific personal risk factors that might predispose them to severe reactions, as detailed in research findings regarding the incidence and characteristics of these events (Nurmala et al., 2024). Additionally, informed consent must be maintained after the initial use of a drug, as it necessitates ongoing communication between patients and healthcare providers. In many cases, nurses serve as the primary link between patients and their families. Understanding ADRs and reporting them accurately can significantly impact patient safety. Studies have shown that enhancing nursing staff's knowledge of ADRs can lead to improved patient education and ultimately better reporting practices (Bankar et al., 2023). If healthcare systems encourage nurses to share information with patients, the number of ADRs can be reduced and patients are more likely to have positive results from their treatments. Patient education and informed consent are even more important because medical care should be tailored to each patient. Understanding the patient's age, genetic background, and how they have responded to medications helps doctors and patients make informed decisions and discuss their treatment options. As illustrated in the analysis of ADRs associated with NSAIDs, different demographics exhibit varying susceptibilities due to factors like gender and comorbid conditions (Nurmala et al., 2024). When patients are educated, it helps them work with healthcare providers and also increases efforts to monitor the use of drugs in healthcare. All in all, educating patients effectively and obtaining their informed consent is crucial for reducing drug-related risks and making treatments safer (Figure 2.17).

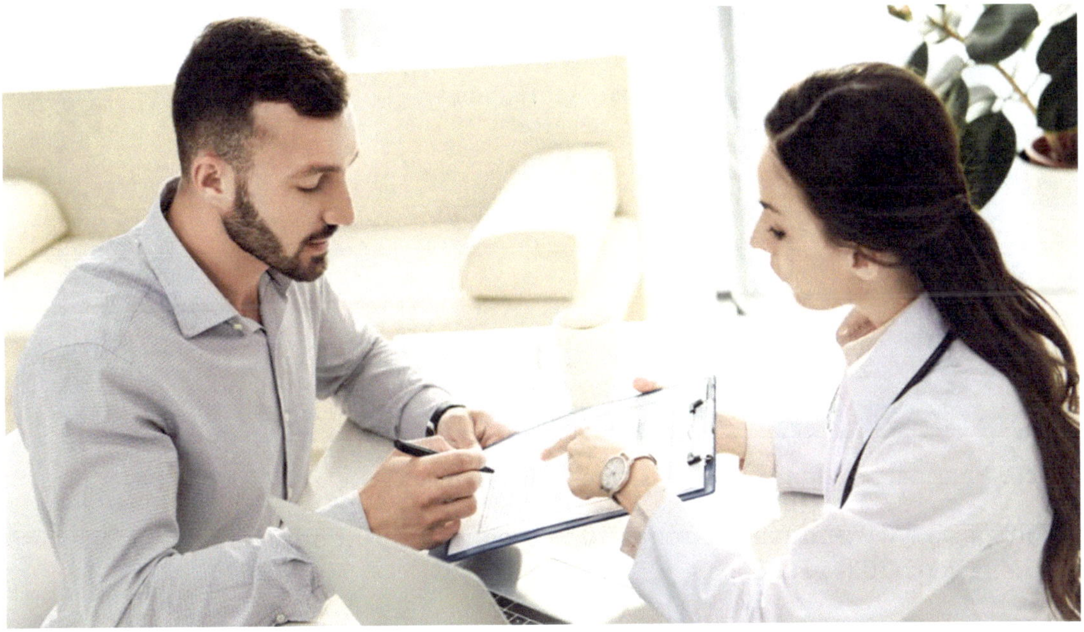

Figure 2.17. Patient education and informed consent.

Source: https://post.healthline.com/wp-content/uploads/2019/10/Patient_Doctor_Signing_1200x628-facebook.jpg.

2.6.3. Pharmacovigilance and Regulatory Measures

Pharmacovigilance is necessary for the efficacy and safety of drugs by systematic monitoring of ADRs that follow after the approval of drugs. Continuous surveillance reveals, analyzes, and interprets the risks of medicines to achieve patient safety. Pharmacovigilance operates through systems of reporting which include spontaneous reporting and more formal observational studies that aim at detecting possible ADRs in different populations. As ADRs can result in severe morbidity, healthcare workers and regulatory agencies have to cooperate to ensure the safety of medications on a daily basis. Studies have established that events related to medications are one of the primary causes of hospitalization. Specifically, between 1 in 10 hospital admissions in OECD countries can be attributed to such events, highlighting the immense importance of robust pharmacovigilance systems in mitigating risks and enhancing drug safety (Bienassis et al., 2022). Incorporation of regulatory elements in pharmacovigilance is crucial for the effective implementation of drug safety programs. Regulatory agencies such as the U.S.

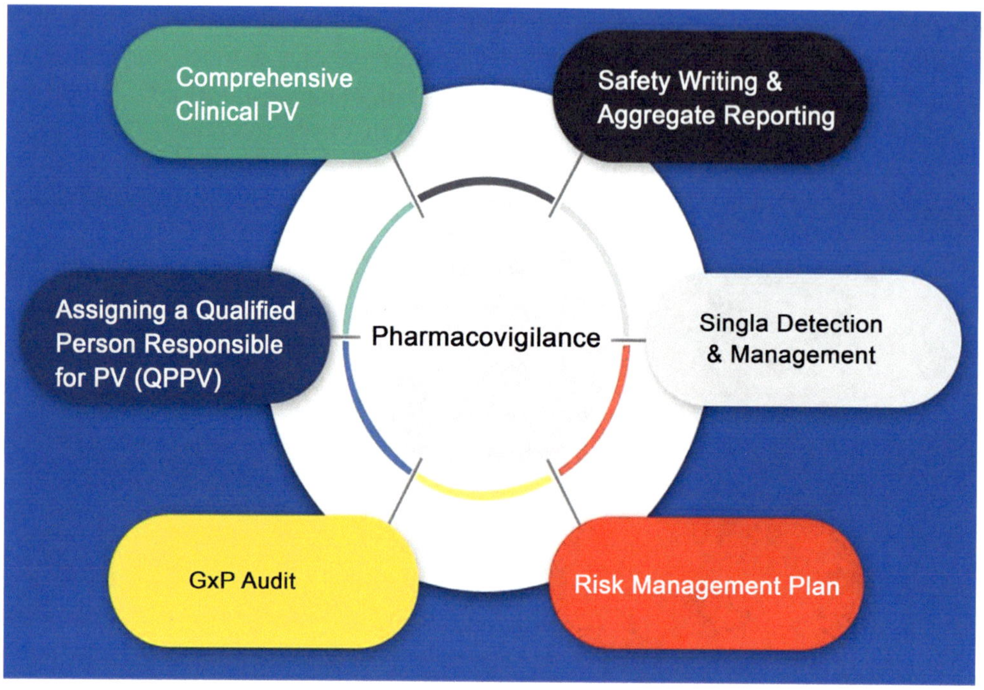

Figure 2.18. Pharmacovigilance and regulatory measures.

Source: https://www.indusnet.co.in/site/wp-content/uploads/2023/01/Future-Scope-Pharmacovigilance-1-1024x1024.jpg.

The FDA and the EMA mandate drug manufacturers to provide post-marketing adverse effects of their drugs to be accountable and transparent. These regulations help create a monitoring framework for the assessment of drugs even after the public approves them for use. In order to make these policies more effective, agencies encourage reporting of any unfavorable effects suffered by healthcare providers and patients, and developing a cumulative database of real-world evidence. This collaborative initiative is most essential in the administration of unique risks, which may vary based on demographic cohorts and comorbid medical illnesses. Thus, effective regulatory policies are essential for enabling the active administration of risks and informed decision-making in pharmacovigilance (Greenhawt et al., 2021). Additionally, ongoing education and training of healthcare practitioners in the field of pharmacovigilance should not be overstated. Empowering clinicians with the skill to identify and report ADRs can help healthcare systems develop an enhanced proactive system for ensuring drug safety. Training programs can help identify patients at high risk for adverse effects, allowing for individualized approaches to prescribing behavior. Considering the startling facts of medication-related harm, institutions must give top priority to these educational programs. Moreover, sensitization of the pharmacovigilance system can enable patients to become active participants in their care and assist in safety surveillance activities. Increased awareness among HCPs as well as among patients can more significantly impact overall pharmacovigilance and regulatory success, and that in turn can lead to safer prescribing practices and improved patient outcomes (Greenhawt et al., 2021; Bienassis et al., 2022) (Figure 2.18).

Summary

In conclusion, the increasing prevalence of ADRs presents significant public health challenges that require urgent attention. As we have seen in this essay, knowing the epidemiology of ADRs is important for making patients safer and improving their treatment results. It is essential to identify risk factors correctly in this process. It has been found that a patient's age, the amount of medicine they are taking, and their health issues play a significant role in the risk of ADRs. If healthcare providers pay attention to these variables, they can develop customized strategies to help patients and prevent risks. In addition, models used to predict anlotinib-related ADRs demonstrate the best approaches to clinical decision-making. Examining the past showed that diagnosis and the total dose of drugs were key reasons why ADRs happened among cancer patients. The use of advanced statistics to design effective models makes it easier for clinicians to predict and handle possible risks. In addition, addressing the issues with ADRs means being aware of how drugs interact with the body and the health of each patient. Studies, for example, the one on antibiotic-associated ADRs in Malawi, prove that reactions can be very different and can be quite severe in different populations. Since 24% of patients in these studies had ADRs, it is necessary to set up proper monitoring and assessment to lower the risks. As the medical community continues to evolve, enhancing our knowledge of ADR epidemiology and risk factors will be key in safeguarding patient health and ensuring the effective and rational use of medications (Chiumia et al., 2024; Qian et al., 2025).

The increased rate of ADRs has significant public health implications in the population and demands an exhaustive understanding of their epidemiology and risk factors. It is estimated that millions of people suffer from severe ADRs, which shows that strong evidence is needed to help doctors make decisions. Part of patient safety is to find out what kinds of reactions happen with drugs and who is most likely to experience them, such as the elderly or people taking many medications. When doctors consider each patient's risks and drug allergies, they can take better actions, which helps reduce the number of ADRs. As the case of AMR illustrates, complacency in controlling such risk factors is likely to exacerbate their effects on health, resulting in unnecessary morbidity and mortality in vulnerable populations (Christopher et al., 2022). Also, interactions between drugs, the environment, and genes make ADRs more challenging to deal with. As an example, variations in pharmacogenomics may cause people to react differently to drugs and face a higher risk of adverse side effects. It is now crucial for medical practitioners to employ a multidimensional approach when managing drug therapy. The use of predictive models that involve genetic testing helps doctors choose the best drugs and doses, thus lowering the chances of ADRs. At the same time, doctors are educated on the specifics of prescribing and closely watch patients who are taking risky drugs. Stakeholders are thus urged to incorporate such practices into regular care as part of a comprehensive approach to efficiently counter the occurrence of ADRs, thereby preventing high healthcare costs and adverse outcomes (François et al., 2019). Finally, addressing the epidemiology of ADRs requires not only addressing current problems but also promoting transparency and honest reporting in the healthcare sector. Setting up extensive surveillance networks can give valuable information needed for making clinical and policy decisions. They should make sure that healthcare providers, researchers, and regulatory agencies all cooperate. Healthcare organizations can utilize data analytics and real-time reports to identify patterns and potential safety issues with drug treatments. Along with efforts at bolstering reporting channels from patients, the ultimate goal is the creation of a safer pharmacological environment that prioritizes patients' health at the forefront but also decongests healthcare systems from ADRs (Christopher et al., 2022).

CLOSER LOOK

HEALTHCARE PROFESSIONALS (HCPS)

Healthcare professionals (HCPs) are formally trained and licensed individuals—including physicians, nurses, midwives, pharmacists, dentists, allied health professionals (e.g., physiotherapists, laboratory scientists, radiographers), community health workers and personal care assistants—whose core mission is to deliver, enable or support the provision of health services across prevention, curative, rehabilitative, and palliative care settings[1]. According to WHO, the global stock of health and care workers now exceeds approximately 70 million, yet a projected shortfall of 11 million is expected by 2030, contributing to huge disparities that leave nearly 60 percent of the world's population without access to basic services[2]. Physicians and advanced-practice providers (such as nurse practitioners, physician assistants and nurse anesthetists) typically diagnose, prescribe, and manage complex medical conditions—after many years of education, clinical placements, and licensure. Pharmacists advise on safe medication use, monitor regimens and in many jurisdictions prescribe under collaborative agreements[3], while nurses serve as essential coordinators of bedside care, patient advocacy and interprofessional communication[4]. Physiotherapists and other allied health professionals specialize in areas such as mobility, wound care, mental health, rehabilitation, public health, wound care or diagnostics[5]. Community health workers and health care assistants—classified by WHO as "associate professionals"—provide vital personal and preventive care under professional oversight, often bridging rural and underserved areas[6]. To ensure quality and patient safety, HCPs operate under regulated curricula, registration requirements, continued professional development mandates and clearly defined scopes of practice. Licensed handover tools such as SBAR and structured interprofessional rounds institutionalize clear communication among teams, reducing errors and improving outcomes[7],[8]. However, persistent funding gaps, ageing populations, COVID-related attrition, and inter-regional inequities exacerbate workforce shortages. Mid- and low-income countries face critical deficits (often more than 40 percent of trained staff intend to migrate), forcing widespread "task–shifting" to lesser-trained cadres and compounding burdens on health systems[9]. Despite these challenges, healthcare professionals remain the cornerstone of safe, equitable, resilient health systems, anchoring universal health coverage. Skilled, well-remunerated and supported HCPs not only restore health and dignity to individual patients, but also provide one of the most efficient returns on investment—potentially adding trillions of dollars to economies while averting millions of premature deaths by 2030[10].s

References

1. Adithan, C., & Sandhiya, S. (2015). Drug induced diseases (DID): Need for more awareness & research. *The Indian Journal of Medical Research*, *142*(1), 7. https://doi.org/10.4103/0971-5916.162086Baldwin, J., & Speck, A. (2018). *Drug Allergies*. DeckerMed Medicine. https://www.semanticscholar.org/paper/df4ee9e0bd52185d8679f039de043422ce23f8c0 (accessed on 9 June 2025).
2. Bankar, M., Tewari, S., & Kumar, S. (2023). Nursing professionals' awareness of adverse drug reactions and pharmacovigilance in an institute of national importance in India: A cross-sectional study. *Cureus*, *15*. https://www.semanticscholar.org/paper/78429b70627af462a05a045bf5f3db18df361793 (accessed on 9 June 2025).
3. Bellanti, J., & Settipane, R. (2018). The Floralia: A festive time for Romans and a demanding time for the allergist/immunologist. *Allergy and Asthma Proceedings*, *39*(3), 167–168. https://www.semanticscholar.org/paper/c815d1cf0d7961e6e6641f681224d9a8880c1a98 (accessed on 9 June 2025).
4. Bondareva, I. B., Zyryanov, S., Asetskaya, I., & Terekhina, E. (2024). Some features of statistical analysis of spontaneous adverse drug reporting data. *Kachestvennaya Klinicheskaya Praktika = Good Clinical Practice*. https://www.semanticscholar.org/paper/952fa299ffe6232eac2b16aea579acffb65a59b9 (accessed on 9 June 2025).
5. Brand, A., Evangelatos, N., & Satyamoorthy, K. (2016). Public health genomics: The essential part for good governance in public health. *International Journal of Public Health*, *61*, 401–403. https://www.semanticscholar.org/paper/1eba86dcad46128b60bed621f8a2e1b225454a45 (accessed on 9 June 2025).
6. Brubaker, L., Carberry, C., Nardos, R., Carter-Brooks, C. M., & Lowder, J. L. (2018). American Urogynecologic Society best-practice statement: Recurrent urinary tract infection in adult women. *Female Pelvic Medicine & Reconstructive Surgery*, *24*, 321–335. https://doi.org/10.1097/spv.0000000000000550.
7. Chiumia, F., Chimimba, F., Nyirongo, H., Kampira, E., Muula, A., & Khuluza, F. (2024). Adverse drug reactions related with antibiotic medicines in Malawi: A retrospective analysis of prevalence and associated factors. *Drug, Healthcare and Patient Safety*, *16*, 89–101. https://www.semanticscholar.org/paper/c9482d653330a829a8e018bacdc688054ef5de71 (accessed on 9 June 2025).
8. de Andrade, D. P., Marques, C. M., de Andrade, D. C. R., Lenzi, L., Oliveira, C. S., & de Figueiredo, B. C. (2025). Trends in tobacco smoking and bladder and lung-bronchial cancer rates among non-Hispanic white Americans (2000–2016). *Archives of Public Health*, *83*. https://www.semanticscholar.org/paper/7d5b72c3d7e30afd07d5711a1381e72cbc12baa6 (accessed on 9 June 2025).
9. De Bienassis, K., Esmail, L., Lopert, R., & Klazinga, N. (2022). The economics of medication safety. *OECD Health Working Papers*. https://doi.org/10.1787/9a933261-en.
10. De Pretis, F., van Gils, M., & Forsberg, M. (2022). A smart hospital-driven approach to precision pharmacovigilance. *Trends in Pharmacological Sciences*, *43*, 473–481. https://doi.org/10.1016/j.tips.2022.03.009.
11. Eldridge, S., Chan, C., Campbell, M. J., Bond, C., Hopewell, S., Thabane, L., & Lancaster, G.

(2016). CONSORT 2010 statement: Extension to randomized pilot and feasibility trials. *BMJ*. https://doi.org/10.1136/bmj.i5239.

12. Fontana, R. J., Liou, I., Reuben, A., Suzuki, A., Fiel, M. I., Lee, W. M., & Navarro, V. J. (2022). AASLD practice guidance on drug, herbal, and dietary supplement–induced liver injury. *Hepatology*, *77*, 1036–1065. https://doi.org/10.1002/hep.32689.
13. Frey, N. (2018). A study on the epidemiology of Stevens-Johnson syndrome and toxic epidermal necrolysis. https://www.semanticscholar.org/paper/d555617451d5e99e268831a7d76d9b0369ad3a04 (accessed on 9 June 2025).
14. Frydenlund, J., Cosgrave, N., Moriarty, F., Wallace, E., Kirke, C., Williams, D. J., Bennet, K., et al. (2024). Adverse Drug Reactions in an Ageing PopulaTion risk Prediction (ADAPTiP) tool: Development of a prediction model related to hospital admissions. *Age and Ageing*. https://www.semanticscholar.org/paper/1873c0d4baa02a626df14feca5657ac37b018826 (accessed on 9 June 2025).
15. Gomes, E., Marques, M., & Regateiro, F. (2019). Epidemiology and risk factors for severe delayed drug hypersensitivity reactions. *Current Pharmaceutical Design*. https://www.semanticscholar.org/paper/29d89b9d79936a3840bf90ef1cfb20ac74c06506 (accessed on 9 June 2025).
16. Greenhawt, M., Abrams, E. M., Shaker, M., Chu, D. K., Khan, D. A., Akin, C., Alqurashi, W., et al. (2021). The risk of allergic reaction to SARS-CoV-2 vaccines and recommended evaluation and management: A systematic review, meta-analysis, GRADE assessment, and international consensus approach. *The Journal of Allergy and Clinical Immunology: In Practice*, *9*, 3546–3567. https://doi.org/10.1016/j.jaip.2021.06.006.
17. He, M., Shi, Y., Han, F., & Cai, Y. (2025). Prediction of adverse drug reactions based on pharmacogenomics combination features: A preliminary study. *Frontiers in Pharmacology*, *16*. https://www.semanticscholar.org/paper/66c31d7018178cd393b67071c19e89003b9f804c (accessed on 9 June 2025).
18. Ho, Y. F., Hu, F. C., & Lee, P. I. (2019). The advantages and challenges of using real-world data for patient care. *Clinical and Translational Science, 13*(1), 4–7. https://doi.org/10.1111/cts.12683.
19. Huang, Z. (2016). The clinical medication safety based on Petri net monitoring. https://www.semanticscholar.org/paper/ae1ed3ac8d6d739e8fc8d7b0aa9b89fec5c414cf (accessed on 9 June 2025).
20. Iwamuro, M., Okada, H., Matsueda, K., Inaba, T., Kusumoto, C., Imagawa, A., & Yamamoto, K. (2015). Review of the diagnosis and management of gastrointestinal bezoars. *World Journal of Gastrointestinal Endoscopy*, *7*, 336. https://doi.org/10.4253/wjge.v7.i4.336.
21. Jeong, H., Chun, B., Kang, D., & Kang, H. (2022). Epidemiology and evaluation of adverse drug reactions in a Korean hospital database for spontaneous reports in the period 2009 to 2018. *International Journal of Clinical Pharmacology and Therapeutics*. https://www.semanticscholar.org/paper/3727dc623c714f9b6280916b10b658ec8d6d890c (accessed on 9 June 2025).
22. Lambertini, M., Toss, A., Passaro, A., Criscitiello, C., Cremolini, C., Cardone, C., Loupakis, F., et al. (2020). Cancer care during the spread of coronavirus disease 2019 (COVID-19) in Italy: Young oncologists' perspective. *ESMO Open*, *5*, e000759. https://doi.org/10.1136/esmoopen-2020-000759.

23. Leopoldino, R. W. D., Marques, D. P., Rocha, L. C. A., Fernandes, F. M., Oliveira, A., & Martins, R. (2023). Temporal profile of adverse drug reactions and associated clinical factors: A prospective observational study in a neonatal intensive care unit. *BMJ Open, 13*. https://www.semanticscholar.org/paper/d3c432bda821b4f7bce902ebdbe8c7ed07f20c00 (accessed on 9 June 2025).

24. Lu, Y., Sun, Y., Cai, L., Yu, B., Wang, Y., Tan, X., Wan, H., et al. (2024). Non-traditional risk factors for atrial fibrillation: Epidemiology, mechanisms, and strategies. *European Heart Journal*. https://www.semanticscholar.org/paper/f919905dac2b8529403495c3bc19c323052162d4 (accessed on 9 June 2025).

25. Mach, F., Baigent, C., Catapano, A. L., Koskinas, K. C., Casula, M., Badimón, L., Chapman, M. J., et al. (2019). 2019 ESC/EAS guidelines for the management of dyslipidemias: Lipid modification to reduce cardiovascular risk. *European Heart Journal, 41*, 111–188. https://doi.org/10.1093/eurheartj/ehz455.

26. Manyi-Loh, C. E., Mamphweli, S., Meyer, E. L., & Okoh, A. I. (2018). Antibiotic use in agriculture and its consequential resistance in environmental sources: Potential public health implications. *Molecules, 23*, 795. https://doi.org/10.3390/molecules23040795.

27. McGettigan, S., Curtin, D., & O'Mahony, D. (2024). Adverse drug reactions in multimorbid older people exposed to polypharmacy: Epidemiology and prevention. *Pharmacoepidemiology*. https://www.semanticscholar.org/paper/6931e8044f032e50049f4cdde5f3e77c484b9be1 (accessed on 9 June 2025).

28. Morice, A. H., Millqvist, E., Biekšienė, K., Birring, S. S., Dicpinigaitis, P. V., Domingo, C., Hilton Boon, M., et al. (2019). ERS guidelines on the diagnosis and treatment of chronic cough in adults and children. *European Respiratory Journal, 55*, 1901136. https://doi.org/10.1183/13993003.01136-2019.

29. Moses, N., Bukke, S. P. N., Goruntla, N., Mwandah, D. C., Abebe, B. A., Atwiine, F., Winnie, M., et al. (2025). Prevalence and factors associated with adverse drug reactions among patients on highly active antiretroviral therapy at a tertiary hospital in south western Uganda: A cross-sectional study. *PLOS One, 20*. https://www.semanticscholar.org/paper/5a178a9c1744d7cf32cb3607610f4d13cc395970 (accessed on 9 June 2025).

30. Murray, C. J. L., Ikuta, K. S., Sharara, F., Swetschinski, L. R., Robles Aguilar, G., Gray, A. P., Han, C., et al. (2022). Global burden of bacterial antimicrobial resistance in 2019: A systematic analysis. *The Lancet, 399*, 629–655. https://doi.org/10.1016/S0140-6736(21)02724-0.

31. Nurmala, S., Harrison, & Hasanah. (2024). Understanding NSAID-induced skin reactions: Implications for patient care. *International Journal on ObGyn and Health Sciences*. https://www.semanticscholar.org/paper/fa20cd2b3264b9cb27d43358dabe867a17c06f43 (accessed on 9 June 2025).

32. Ostroumova, O., Sychev, D., Kochetkov, A., Ostroumova, T., Kulikova, M. I., & De, V. A. (2022). Anti-cancer agents and drug-induced hypertension. *Medical Alphabet*. https://www.semanticscholar.org/paper/42a855eb1e45ff23dd225388008278803bb44394 (accessed on 9 June 2025).

33. Ostroumova, O., Sychev, D., Kochetkov, A., Ostroumova, T., Kulikova, M. I., & De, V. A. (2022). Drug-induced hypertension. *Medical Alphabet*. https://www.semanticscholar.org/paper/f5a4806c639fdec29a3965288134113aef1e304a (accessed on 9 June 2025).

34. Pérez-Ingidua, C., Rivas-Paterna, A. B., González-Perrino, C., Aleo-Luján, E., Ascaso-del-Rio,

A., Laredo-Velasco, L., Portolés-Pérez, A., et al. (2024). Adverse drug reactions in pediatric surgery: Prospective study on frequency and risk related factors. *BMC Pediatrics, 24*. https://www.semanticscholar.org/paper/50c3be737338e74d0cb483c636ae9387092eefd2 (accessed on 9 June 2025).

35. Priori, S. G., Blomström-Lundqvist, C., Mazzanti, A., Blom, N., Borggrefe, M., Camm, A. J., Elliott, P., et al. (2015). 2015 ESC Guidelines for the management of patients with ventricular arrhythmias and the prevention of sudden cardiac death. *European Heart Journal, 36*, 2793–2867. https://doi.org/10.1093/eurheartj/ehv316.

36. Qian, J., Ruan, C., Cai, Y., Yi, W., Liu, J., & Xu, R. (2025). Development and validation of a risk-prediction model for adverse drug reactions in real-world cancer patients treated with anlotinib. *Therapeutic Advances in Drug Safety, 16*. https://www.semanticscholar.org/paper/7f1e3413e834e3b8cc67f068158849dac7397272 (accessed on 9 June 2025).

37. Sittiphan, S., Lim, A., Khurram, H., Dureh, N., & Dittakan, K. (2025). Epidemiology of reported serious adverse drug reactions due to anti-infectives using nationwide database of Thailand. *PLOS One, 20*. https://www.semanticscholar.org/paper/39dc8c352b6861393174ef74923d2657f9ff2cb7 (accessed on 9 June 2025).

38. Suzuki, A., & Chen, M. (2024). Epidemiology and risk determinants of drug-induced liver injury: Current knowledge and future research needs. *Liver International, 45*. https://www.semanticscholar.org/paper/813ca6a0724c2688afbd323eb31af4054de11d4d (accessed on 9 June 2025).

39. Varanasi, V. (2012). Pharmacoepidemiology versus clinical pharmacology and epidemiology. *Advances in Pharmacoepidemiology and Drug Safety, 1*. https://www.semanticscholar.org/paper/4f2a7c937006b17f16f23015127d84d587ee0f4b (accessed on 9 June 2025).

40. Villanueva, R. I., Montero, C. B., Bulnes-Montánchez, M. E., Alva, L. S., Carrillo, J. S., Zevallos, A., & Salazar, F. (2025). Risk factors for adverse reactions to nurse-administered propofol during outpatient endoscopy: A cross-sectional study. *BMC Anesthesiology, 25*. https://www.semanticscholar.org/paper/97c235d37d39b7d7c19b32d1f9a6198fb563982b (accessed on 9 June 2025).

41. Villarreal-González, R., Canel-Paredes, A., Arias-Cruz, A., Fraga-Olvera, A., Delgado-Bañuelos, A., Rico-Solís, G. A., Ochoa-García, I. V., et al. (2023). Drug allergy: Fundamental aspects in diagnosis and treatment. *Revita Alegria Mexico, 69*(4), 195–213. https://www.semanticscholar.org/paper/40d50eebba43e4a250b03686d6aabf1e219488a5 (accessed on 9 June 2025).

42. Voysey, M., Costa Clemens, S. A., Madhi, S. A., Weckx, L. Y., Folegatti, P. M., Aley, P. K., Angus, B., et al. (2020). Safety and efficacy of the ChAdOx1 nCoV-19 vaccine (AZD1222) against SARS-CoV-2: An interim analysis of four randomized controlled trials in Brazil, South Africa, and the UK. *The Lancet, 397*, 99–111. https://doi.org/10.1016/s0140-6736(20)32661-1.

43. Wiersinga, W. J., Rhodes, A., Cheng, A. C., Peacock, S. J., & Prescott, H. C. (2020). Pathophysiology, transmission, diagnosis, and treatment of coronavirus disease 2019 (COVID-19). *JAMA, 324*(6), 782. https://doi.org/10.1001/jama.2020.12839.

44. Xiao, Q., Zhou, Y., & Lauschke, V. M. (2020). Ethnogeography and inter-individual variability of human ABC transporters. *Human Genetics, 139*, 623–646. https://doi.org/10.1007/s00439-020-02150-6.

45. Zeppenfeld, K., Tfelt-Hansen, J., Riva, M., Winkel, B. G., Behr, E. R., Blom, N. A., Charron, P., et al. (2022). 2022 ESC Guidelines for the management of patients with ventricular arrhythmias and the prevention of sudden cardiac death. *European Heart Journal, 43*, 3997–4126. https://doi.org/10.1093/eurheartj/ehac262.
46. Zhang, Y., Zeng, G., Pan, H., Li, C., Hu, Y., Chu, K., Han, W., et al. (2020). Safety, tolerability, and immunogenicity of an inactivated SARS-CoV-2 vaccine in healthy adults aged 18–59 years: A randomized, double-blind, placebo-controlled, phase 1/2 clinical trial. *The Lancet Infectious Diseases, 21*(2), 181–192. https://doi.org/10.1016/s1473-3099(20)30843-4.

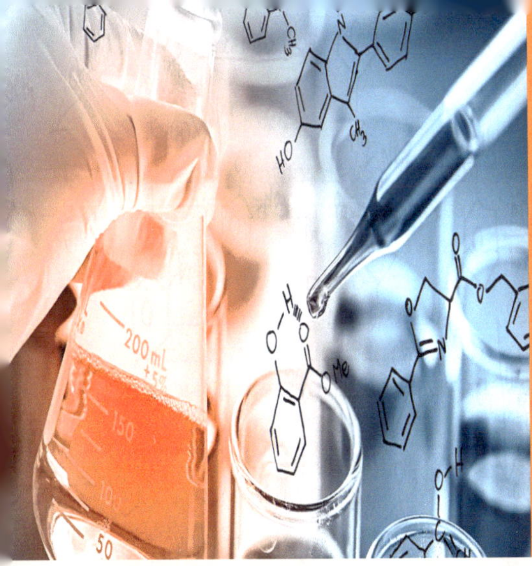

Chapter 3

MECHANISMS OF TYPE A REACTIONS

Contents

Introduction

In studies of the complexities of immune responses, understanding of the processes which control Type A reactions is pertinent. Such reactions, particularly related to oversteering hypersensitivity, offer valuable insight into the human immunological system. Induced by their acute and often severe nature, such reactions can be provoked by environmental allergens, such as pollen, as documented in various pathological studies. Interestingly, within a subgroup of atopic eczema patients, a distinct immunological reaction to type I allergy-inducing antigens has been reported, in which regulatory T cells and their cytokines are involved in mediating inflammation and eczematous responses. The analysis of such mechanisms not only explains the pathophysiology of allergic reactions but also highlights the necessity of personalized therapeutic interventions that recognize the specific cytokine patterns involved, such as in type A reactions and in therapeutic models, including patch testing with native pollen grains (Behrendt et al., 2008). In addition, the contrasting phenotypes of immunity to different allergens demonstrate the heterogeneity of Type A reactions. Recent research on platinum drugs, including oxaliplatin and carboplatin, emphasizes the immune mechanisms and clinical presentation. These drugs have been linked with diverse HSRs of varied severity and pathogenesis. For instance, data indicate that among reactive patients to oxaliplatin, high-frequency type I HSRs are common, and cytokine release reactions are seen in a significant proportion. The variability in immune response not only affects clinical outcome but also informs desensitization protocols, with implications for patient-directed management. The identification of unique biomarkers and endotypes for these reactions not only deepens understanding of individual patient responses but also illustrates the sophisticated interaction of immune mechanisms governing Type A reactions (Besz et al., 2023). The pathophysiologic information gained through the observation of such reactions is crucial to the design of effective treatment regimens and prevention strategies. As research continues to advance, it becomes increasingly evident that a knowledge of immunologic mechanisms directly impacts therapeutic modalities, such as desensitization protocols tailored to individual patients. The biphasic nature of Type A reactions, as illustrated in the case of allergic reaction to pollen, leads us to considering the immediate and the delayed phases of immune activation. A thorough analysis of these phases reveals the temporal patterns of cytokine release and cellular infiltration, which are crucial in forecasting potential complications during treatment. This collection of knowledge not only expands the scope of the science of allergology but also provides a foundation upon which to establish additional research endeavors aimed at reducing the adverse effects of Type A reactions and improving patient outcomes (Behrendt et al., 2008) (Figure 3.1).

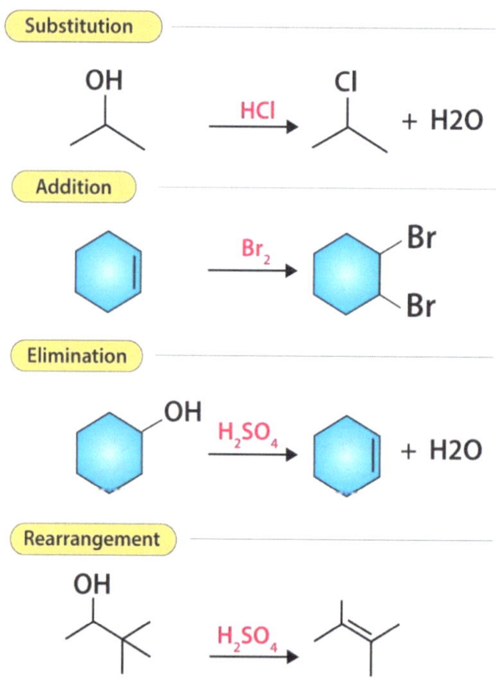

Figure 3.1. Mechanisms of type A reactions.

Source: https://edurev.gumlet.io/ApplicationImages/Temp/8743297_30fd1677-a6b0-4b26-a054-bb2c099e20ad_lg.png.

Definition of Type A Reactions

Looking into chemical reactions shows a variety of mechanisms that oversee their behavior. Of these, Type A reactions have a significant part because they are linear and can be reversed. Such reactions demonstrate that the reactants can revert to their original state, establishing a balance within the chemical system. The special thing about them is that they can react in both directions, helping to maintain a stable balance. Not only does reversibility influence the creation of products, but it also decides the speed of reactions, since the concentration of both reactants and products is important for the reaction's direction. A more detailed examination of Type A reactions reveals that advanced modeling approaches are necessary to accurately represent their behavior. The convergent reaction-diffusion master equation (CRDME)V2 is a notable advancement in this area, providing insights into the spatially continuous dynamics that underlie chemical interactions. When classical models are adapted to fit bimolecular interactions, the CRDME provides a useful way to understand the details of Type A reactions in living organisms. The implications of these interactions are vast, particularly in systems where diffusional processes and reaction rates are interconnected, which is often the case in cellular environments (Isaacson et al., 2018). In addition to the theory, Type A reactions also play a significant role in various practical areas, such as biochemistry and materials science. Exploring viscous, heat-conducting mixtures that react chemically requires an understanding of how chemical and thermodynamic forces interact. The use of partial mass and energy balances in these models demonstrates that thermodynamics is a crucial aspect of these processes. Understanding these interactions completely helps predict system behavior and reveals the details that make the system stable. By examining the interplay between reactions and the associated entropy production, researchers can gain critical insights into non-symmetric forces that emerge outside of equilibrium, thus enriching our grasp of Type A reaction dynamics (Bothe et al., 2013).

Importance in Organic Chemistry

The relationship between organic chemistry and other branches of science cannot be overstated, particularly in the aspect that complicated molecular interactions dictate numerous disparate reactions. The processes of Type A reactions are indicators of this complexity, demonstrating the importance of detailed mechanistic pathways in predicting chemical behavior and outcomes. Type A reactions are important to enable chemists to manage reaction conditions deliberately, maximizing yield and selectivity in synthesis. This versatility is based on a deep appreciation of the foundational mechanisms, ranging from nucleophilic substitutions to electrophilic additions, positioning organic chemistry at the keystone position in both theory and practice. In addition, when researchers attempt to uncover the intricacies of organic compounds, the important information developed through mechanistic studies facilitates improvements in medicinal chemistry, materials science, and environmental chemistry. One of the major fields within organic chemistry, which again underlines its significance, is the investigation of secondary organic aerosols (SOA). This subject is connected to Type A reaction mechanisms, as the atmospheric formation of SOA involves the reaction of many organic compounds under various conditions. The nature of these reactions requires a strong background understanding of the formation and transformation pathways that connect gaseous precursors and particulate material. This kind of research enhances our understanding of atmospheric quality and climate change, extending the relevance of organic chemistry beyond the laboratory and conventional settings. With environmental regulations tightening globally, it is increasingly important to understand the mechanisms of SOA formation, as emphasized by

Baltensperger et al. (2009), in the development of practical actions towards pollution control and sustainable approaches in atmospheric science and human well-being. Additionally, organic chemistry's relevance can also be observed in its root role in astrophysical investigations where organic compounds chemically drive molecular clouds. As explained by Blake et al. (1988), the dense molecular clouds theory not only leads theoretical research but also improves empirical studies of organic matter's contribution to the universe. This crossing illustrates how Type A reaction mechanisms function as analogs, allowing one to understand processes beyond Earth and broadening the scope of organic chemistry. By merging laboratory research with observational data from astronomical occurrences, scientists can begin making comparisons between Earthly organic reactions and those that exist throughout the universe. These discoveries can potentially complete gaps in our understanding and therefore shed light on the overall role of organic chemistry in revealing the fundamental mechanisms of terrestrial and extraterrestrial ecosystems (Figure 3.2).

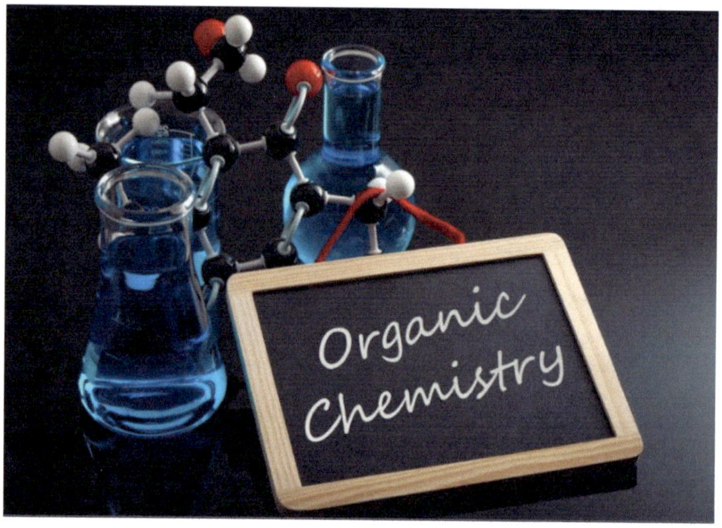

Figure 3.2. Organic chemistry.

Source: https://www.chemicals.co.uk/wp-content/uploads/2021/09/chalkboard-sign-saying-organic-chemistry-scaled-e1654607124262.jpg.

Overview of Mechanistic Pathways

In the intricate world of chemical kinetics, the ability to elaborate on mechanistic pathways is crucial in determining the dynamics of a reaction. Current advancements in formal modeling approaches suggest the use of directed multi-hypergraphs as chemical reaction networks, where molecules are represented as vertices and reactions are represented as hyperedges. Using integer-valued flows as a mechanism for representing pathways enables scientists to precisely comprehend the intricacies of such networks. It not only allows the investigation of reaction patterns but also enables the systematic enumeration of optimal and near-optimal paths. This procedure, in contrast to earlier methods such as Flux Balance Analysis, enhances the capability to formulate succinct mechanistic queries regarding the transformations occurring within Type A reactions, thereby paving the way for significant research contributions in metabolic engineering and synthetic chemistry (Andersen et al., 2017). Furthermore, the implementation of algorithms using computer automation has transformed the kinetic analysis process in chemical reaction networks. Advances like KiNetX simplify the examination of these networks that are derived from electronic structure calculations. The meta-algorithm determines the kinetic importance of species within a network, allowing researchers to focus their studies on the most important elements. By removal of kinetically irrelevant species, KiNetX simplifies complex reaction graphs to simpler, more interpretable forms, thereby illuminating the mechanisms at work. The sensitivity analysis incorporated into KiNetX ensures that the impact of rate constant variations on concentration changes is thoroughly understood, making mechanistic models more predictive. Thus, this computer-data-based approach underscores the value of kinetic analysis in expanding our understanding of Type A reaction pathways (Proppe et al., 2018). The ongoing advancement of mechanistic pathway analysis highlights the need for a synergy between theoretical modeling and computational methods. As model-construction techniques for the simulation of complex chemical networks improve, integration of frameworks that allow rigorous propagation of free-energy errors will be even more critical. These approaches provide the capability to probe varying reaction conditions and their impact on product distributions and reaction pathways, particularly in Type A reactions where specificity is crucial. The use of methodologies like KiNetX not only enhances the understanding of primary pathways but also directs the design of novel reactions through the prediction of the outcome of structural modifications in reactants. Mechanistic pathway investigation is, therefore, a cornerstone to the evolution of both scientific understanding and solution forms for chemical synthesis and reaction optimization (Figure 3.3).

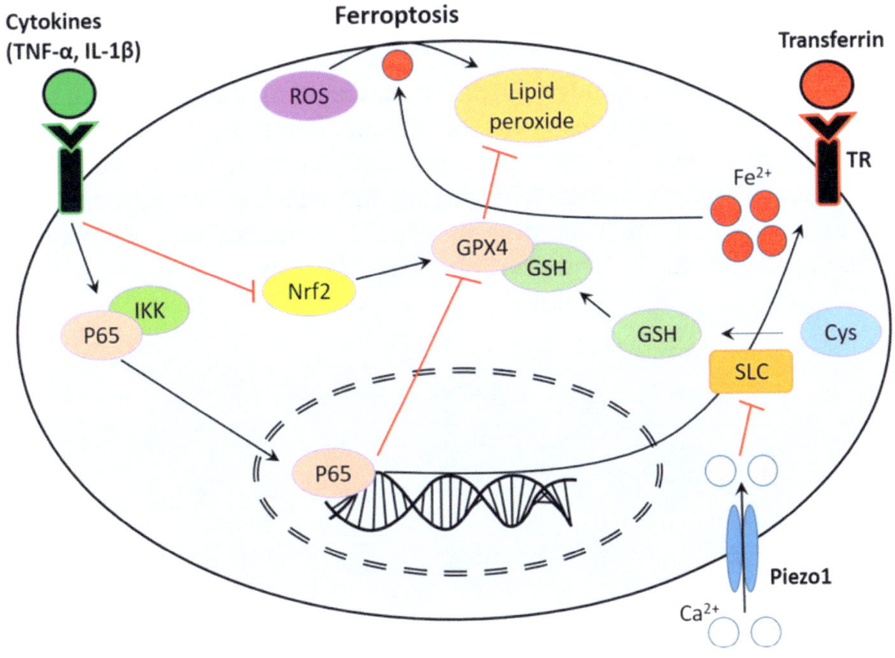

Figure 3.3. Overview of mechanistic pathways.

Source: https://www.researchgate.net/publication/369265896/figure/fig1/AS:11431281162145408@1685152219330/Overview-of-mechanistic-pathways-that-lead-to-ferroptosis-in-chondrocytes-While-TR.png.

3.1. Characteristics of Type A Reactions

Understanding the various factors that influence Type A reactions is crucial because they are highly complex. Such reactions depend on specific conditions and tend to manifest as distinct behaviors in various situations. One important trait is that they are affected by big variables such as temperature, pressure, and the amounts of reactants. They manage the speed and outcome of the reaction, proving why it is important to measure carefully in experiments. In particular, research on Type A reactions in explosive areas reveals that small changes in chemical reactions can lead to significant variations in the behavior of gases. The theoretical framework surrounding these reactions is bolstered by models that simulate conditions typical of deflagration and detonation, providing vital insights into the fundamental mechanisms at work (Kovalenko et al., 2018). Examining Type A reactions involves studying both their quantities and the ways they behave in various chemical environments. These reactions are often characterized by high reactivity and unpredictability, particularly during the combustion of hydrocarbons. Reaction viability and sustainability are judged mainly by the activation energy and pre-exponential factors, especially when there are changes in the conditions. In this case, gas-dynamical effects are particularly important, as they alter the reaction rates compared to steady-state combustion. The interplay between pressure fluctuations in gas streams and the resultant reaction velocity highlights the dynamic nature of Type A reactions, reinforcing the theory that minor alterations can yield nonlinear responses in chemical behavior (Kovalenko et al., 2018). The wider effects of Type A reactions can be explained by looking at their connection to entropy and thermodynamic stability. Every Type A reaction helps increase entropy, a fundamental concept in understanding biological and chemical processes. It demonstrates that reaction mechanisms are crucial in evolution, as they enable living things to reach more likely states, a fundamental principle of life. It is clear from this mechanism that, through random interactions, systems can form and contribute to important functions, such as the movement of energy and adaptation, in all types of environments. Recognizing the balance between reaction kinetics and thermodynamics enhances our understanding of Type A reactions and their significance in the process of natural selection and the organization of matter (Figure 3.4).

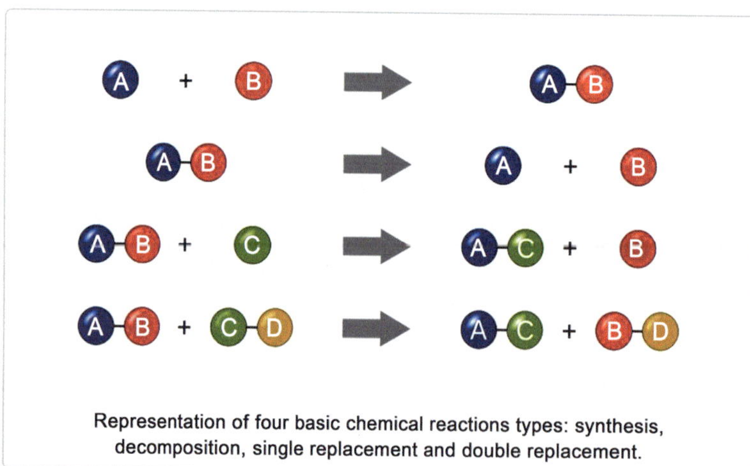

Figure 3.4. Characteristics of type A reactions.

Source: https://i.pinimg.com/originals/86/7a/10/867a10561de08bb10a0c364b85306a1f.jpg.

3.1.1. Reactant Structure and Properties

The molecular behavior of intricate chemical reactions, particularly those classified as Type A reactions, is significantly influenced by the complexity of the properties and structures of the reactants. Disposition of atoms in terms of geometry and electronic distributions within molecules has a primary role in determining how compounds react under collision. Molecular geometry, for instance, is directly responsible for dictating orientation and energy requirements for successful collisions of reactants, which is important in accounting for patterns of reactivity. In this, the correlation between structure and reactivity is demonstrated using various kinetic models, such as the Hill equation, which illustrates the nonlinear input-output relations frequently found in biological systems. These relationships highlight the importance not only of reactants themselves, but also of the way their structural features determine the topology of chemical processes within overall systems, thereby imposing fundamental limits on variation and adaptation in the living world (Frank et al., 2013). Reactant structure analysis is not just atomic construction; it is a systematic investigation of the influence of molecular properties on the mechanism of reaction. Properties such as steric hindrance, polarity, and electronegativity can be able to affect a reaction's speed and path significantly, showcasing the complexity of chemical dynamics. For example, very electronegative reactants can form stronger bonds with electrophiles, resulting in distinct reaction profiles. Additionally, steric influence may inhibit or enhance access into reactivity sites, therefore affecting overall kinetics. To observe these molecular attributes is to see with some refinement why some reactants are likely to preferentially experience Type A reactions compared with other reactants. In educational curricula, it becomes necessary to emphasize the interplay between structural chemistry and dynamics and to ensure students appreciate the underlying concepts that govern chemical reactivity and the extensive implications these concepts have on chemical education and practice (Dence et al., 1968). Furthermore, the integration of advanced structural information into reaction mechanism research fosters a deeper understanding of the relationship between molecular architecture and chemical behavior. The set of constituent molecular properties generally shapes the system-level interaction, highlighting the significance of collective behavior for understanding chemical processes.

The persistence of biological systems in following orderly patterns, as reflected by recurring input-output relations, suggests that structural conditions are secondary to an inherent order imposed on the dynamic randomness of chemical reactions (Frank et al., 2013). This magnificent synergy between structure and process deserves closer scrutiny of the way disparities in reactant properties can lead to different outcomes in Type A reactions in support of the contention that molecular design and intrinsic properties are centrally significant in reaction mechanism formation and pedagogic approach within the chemistry discipline (Dence et al., 1968) (Figure 3.5).

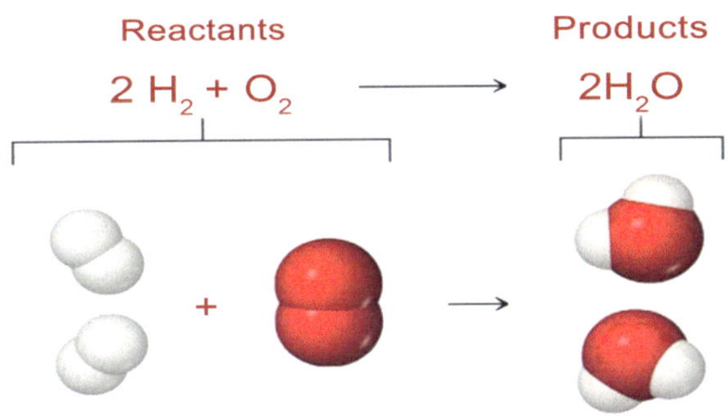

Figure 3.5. Reactant structure and properties.

Source: https://images.ctfassets.net/4yflszkpcwkt/2ujtH6BFhEgi330cbVM8aE/c7dc72d9b4f1404b6f13fde8b08eaa1a/Water.png.

3.1.2. Reaction Conditions and Environment

The way reactions are carried out and the environmental conditions are crucial for Type A reactions. Many things, including temperature, pH, and the existence of specific ions, can have a significant impact on how fast a reaction occurs and what is produced. For instance, the solubility and reactivity of vanadium depend a lot on the local environment. If vanadium compounds are added to water, reactions involving hydrolysis, changes in oxidation state, and ligand exchanges happen and are influenced by the pH and the concentration of the water. It is essential to understand these factors to explain reaction mechanisms, as the results may differ from those of the original vanadium compound.

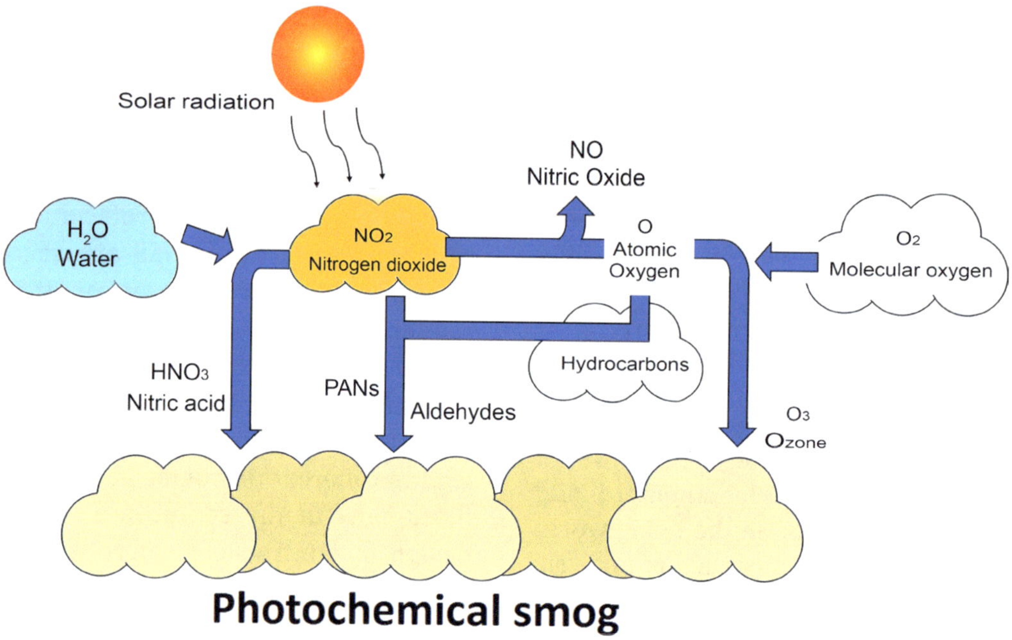

Figure 3.6. Reaction conditions and environment.

Source: https://energyeducation.ca/wiki/images/b/b6/Photochemsmog.png.

Such knowledge not only informs academic research but also provides keys to unlocking applications across environmental and biomedical domains, where the benefits or toxicity of vanadium species must be evaluated in diverse contexts (Dinda et al., 2025). Additionally, the organisms in these environments play a crucial role in controlling reaction conditions, as evidenced by research on diatoms. To deal with silica deficiency and pressure from algicidal bacteria, these unicellular eukaryotes change their metabolism. When genes are studied during stress, it is found that they activate proteins that help the body survive in challenging situations. This indicates that environmental conditions significantly influence how living things respond. The way metacaspases and similar enzymes express themselves reveals how diatoms adjust their biochemical processes in response to external conditions. These findings underscore that the outcome of Type Chemical compositions do not solely dictate a reactions but also by the ecological and physiological contexts in which these reactions occur (Bayramova et al., 2024). To sum up, understanding the conditions and environment helps us better comprehend Type A reactions. Different environments bring their problems and benefits, so chemical reactions there are always linked to their environment. Researchers can develop more accurate models of reactivity by examining how various factors affect the progression and outcome of reactions. It is imperative for this approach to be used in bioremediation as well as when making new types of drugs. Therefore, a comprehensive exploration of the mechanisms of Type A reactions should embed the complexities of environmental dynamics, thereby fostering innovative approaches that align with ecological principles and sustainability goals (Bayramova et al., 2024; Dinda et al., 2025) (Figure 3.6).

3.1.3. Kinetic and Thermodynamic Considerations

The interplay of kinetic and thermodynamic factors typifies the Type A reaction behavior across the board, particularly in complicated fluid systems with predominant chemical interactions. In attempts to understand the mechanics of viscous, heat-conducting mixtures, researchers have managed to explain how such chemical species engage in reactions as they conserve mass and momentum. A thorough understanding of the entropy of involved systems and interactions—more specifically, the non-symmetric nature of chemical interaction forces when chemical equilibrium is absent—strengthens our understanding of these reactions even further. Building an appropriate model requires a thorough understanding of both thermo-mechanical forces and chemical contributions, thereby enabling the development of generalized thermodynamic driving forces, which are essential mechanisms controlling the reaction path. This rigorous approach not only describes the dynamics of Type A responses but also illustrates the relevance of real-world applications in material science and chemical engineering (Bothe et al., 2013). Proceeding to thermodynamics, the application of the Clausius-Duhem inequality highlights the relevance of irreversible processes for Type A reactions. The transient network idea, advocated by original thermodynamic theorists such as Green and Tobolsky, encapsulates the complexity of strands and their interactions within a reaction network by considering them as chemical reactions. This perspective emphasizes the importance of defining thermodynamic values, both in and out of equilibrium, to gain optimal insight into reaction mechanisms. Finally, this theory encompasses not only the underlying theories of the work of earlier authors, such as Yamamoto and Tanaka-Edwards, but also narrows the gaps between kinetic theory and thermal equilibrium. Repeated consideration of mechanical history provides insights into the relationships between stress and heat generation, thereby enriching our understanding of how such reactions occur in a thermodynamic system (Palierne et al., 2000). Entering the realm of kinetic space, one sees that diffusion dynamics play a notable role in Type A reactions. The Maxwell-Stefan equations form a point of departure for understanding the diffusion velocities in such systems, referencing the influence of sound-speed on mass transfer processes. In particular, where diffusion velocities are smaller than the speed of sound, the model simplifies, and individual mass conservation is assigned to each component. These findings not only reveal the reduced complexity of diffusion processes but also shed light on the underlying thermodynamic unity present even in situations of simplification. The alliance between kinetic and thermodynamic interests ultimately decides the routes of Type A reactions, guiding their outcomes in a predictable as well as emergent manner. Hence, an overall strategy involving both kinetics and thermodynamics is required to further enhance our understanding of chemical reaction mechanisms under different environments.

3.2. Mechanistic Pathways

Understanding how Type A reactions work is crucial for comprehending the chemical interactions that regulate various biological processes. Typically, these pathways involve a series of reactions in which reactants are converted into products with the assistance of enzymes or catalysts. It is clear in Type A reactions that enzymes play a crucial role by facilitating the reaction and making it easier and faster. Thanks to this interaction, we can gain a deeper understanding of how reactions occur. For example, recent studies on the interplay between immune dysregulation and pathways in Type 2 diabetes mellitus (T2DM) highlight the complex regulatory networks that can influence reactions related to diseases such as non-Hodgkin lymphoma (NHL), thus emphasizing the significance of mechanistic pathways in health and disease contexts (Zhu et al., 2025).

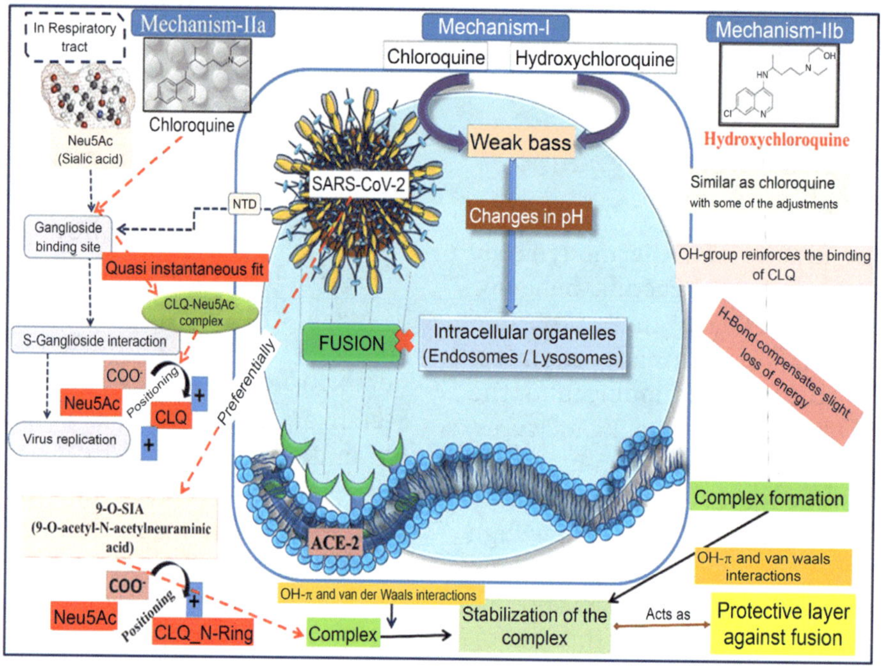

Figure 3.7. Mechanistic pathways.

Source: https://www.researchgate.net/profile/Kunal-Roy-3/publication/344064202/figure/fig10/AS:961898174496768@1606345804352/Schematic-representation-of-different-mechanistic-pathways-of-CLQ-and-HCQ-against.png.

Additionally, utilizing advanced computer methods in these pathways enables us to gain a deeper understanding of how chemicals interact with one another. Topological analysis aids in studying Type A reactions by illustrating the transformations from reactants to products. Using this approach, chemists can observe how electrons move and identify the various intermediates, thereby gaining a deeper understanding of the primary processes involved in these reactions. For example, using topological analysis, scientists have demonstrated the steps that bonds undergo as they form and break. In this context, the cyanide-type umpolung reaction exemplifies how such analyses can elucidate the complexity of reaction mechanisms, identify rate-determining steps, and delineate the sequence of events that define Type A reactions (Michalski et al., 2025). As scientists continue to study the mechanisms of Type A reactions, their discoveries are important for both medical and therapeutic fields. Understanding the key regulatory molecules and their connections to enzyme pathways may aid in the development of new drugs for metabolic disorders and cancers. Investigators can identify new biomarkers and treatment options by examining the shared molecular pathways between T2DM and NHL. Understanding these pathways in detail also helps explain the development and progression of diseases, highlighting the importance of detailed studies for public health and effective treatment. For this reason, further study of the mechanisms involved in diseases is very important for both basic and applied research (Figure 3.7).

3.2.1. Stepwise Mechanisms

The complexity involved in chemical reactions usually lies in the mechanisms by which they take place, and stepwise mechanisms have been amongst the current forefront research. They refer to a process that happens in individual steps, with the formation of intermediates along the way of the reaction. These intermediates can undergo significant changes, influencing the overall kinetics and thermodynamics of the reaction and thereby yielding alternative products. Stepwise processes permit stabilization at any intermediate stage, which is particularly important with multistep organic processes. This characteristic can lead to a deeper understanding of reaction kinetics and offers a path towards the design of selective catalysts. Finally, when considering Type A reactions in this model, the stepwise route typically allows subtleties that a concerted mechanism may suppress, revealing greater insight into the fundamental reactivity and selectivity evident in different systems. Within the realm of polymer chemistry, the use of stepwise mechanisms has received significant focus. The design and synthesis of polymers often involve deliberate control of intermediates in reactions to create properties of interest; hence, stepwise process knowledge is especially relevant. More generally, monomer structures and cross-linker development may be addressed according to this principle, highlighting how different mechanistic routes can control polymer material properties. The incorporation of dynamic covalent bonds in such materials opens up new opportunities for thermal response and processing, which are of great industrial interest. As explained in the literature, a better intrinsic understanding of such stepwise processes can inform the design of new polymer applications, enhancing functionality and recyclability of materials (Prez et al., 2019). Moreover, the subject of stepwise processes is also applied to catalysis, where zeolites serve as a traditional example of intricate chemical systems exhibiting such behavior. The study of methanol conversion into hydrocarbons reveals a competition between concerted and stepwise reaction mechanisms, resulting in different products. Advanced modeling techniques, particularly density functional theory (DFT)-based ones, allow researchers to mimic reaction conditions and unravel the interplay among reaction temperature, catalyst topography, and the presence of guest molecules. The stepwise nature of the mechanism, as illustrated in the synthesis of framework-bound methoxide intermediates, highlights the role played by individual factors in determining the kinetics and products of such zeolite-catalyzed processes. By allowing for control at the molecular level, such understanding is important in optimizing existing zeolite processes and driving novel technologies towards other feedstocks (Bailleul et al., 2016).

3.2.2. Concerted Mechanisms

Researching Type A reactions shows that there are detailed pathways that direct the change in molecular structures. They occur when bonds are simultaneously created and broken, all while passing through a single transition state without forming any intermediates. This approach is necessary to ensure that products are produced smoothly and without difficulty. The way these reactions happen together significantly affects their stereochemistry and regioselectivity, as is seen in many cycloaddition reactions. For instance, the 2 + 2 cycloaddition of tetrafluoroethylene and butadiene illustrates how the transition state configuration dictates product outcomes under kinetic and thermodynamic control, showcasing the delicate interplay of energy landscapes in concerted reactions (Houk et al., 2020). Such knowledge plays a crucial role in organic chemistry, where controlling the structure of molecules is often essential. Examining how concerted mechanisms function reveals that transition states are the most crucial part, as they possess the highest energy level during the reaction. By employing computational methods such as DFT, researchers have explored the potential energy surfaces of these reactions, allowing for predictions of reactivity and product distributions. The case of tetrafluoroethylene demonstrates that both steric and electronic factors can influence the course of a reaction. In particular, the preference for certain transition states often hinges upon the necessity for structural rearrangements that stabilize the transition state. This phenomenon can dictate whether a reaction pathway is favored (Houk et al., 2020). So, the way these mechanisms work is not only about bond reorganizations but is mainly controlled by energy and the structure of the molecules, which makes chemical reactions complex. Concerted mechanisms have a strong influence on the development of advanced polymers in materials science. Dynamic covalent linkages in polymer networks are gaining more attention, as they rely on concerted reactions to facilitate molecular rearrangements and enhance the properties of materials. As a result, these materials can react to heat and be recycled, aligning with today's environmental efforts. Using strong monomers and cross-linkers that take part in the same reaction, increases both the strength and the usefulness of materials. The latest research indicates that the reaction of vitrimers is closely tied to their physicochemical properties. Consequently, understanding how the various processes work in polymer chemistry enables the development of new ideas and improved performance in manufactured materials.

3.2.3. Role of Catalysts in Mechanisms

The intricate interplay of catalysts in chemical reactions, particularly in Type A reactions, ensures their central position in accelerating the rate of reaction without undergoing permanent change themselves. Catalysts can decrease the level of activation energy required to initiate a reaction, significantly reorienting the reaction path. Such a reorientation of energy profiles allows for reactants to be transformed into products more readily, pointing toward the catalysts role as facilitators rather than merely participants. They become more efficient in proportion to the complexity of reaction mechanisms involved, which is an observable situation when one sees modularity and hierarchical organization in metabolic pathways. These types of systems, which have preserved structures and functions, are strongly reliant on catalysts to maintain their sensitive balance as well as support adaptability to various conditions (Alberts et al., 2012). In this manner, catalysts do not simply influence direct reactions but also support broader biochemical networks through modulatory functionalities. Extending further into the unique role of cofactors, these simple constituents act as non-replaceable catalysts that optimize reaction mechanisms in Type A reactions. Cofactors add a unique level of regulation by being bound to enzymes, enabling more advanced interaction with small-molecule substrates. Based on their structural characteristics, cofactors are complex or straightforward; the latter can participate in extensive reactions, while the former can enable modular boundaries within more advanced pathways. This stratification adds to their importance, where some cofactors only occur at pivotal positions to regulate the fate of biochemical interactions. The control of chemical reactions through cofactors reveals a striking evolution of metabolic networks where even minor changes can lead to radical evolutionary advancement (Alberts et al., 2012). As such, knowledge of cofactor dynamics is necessary for achieving the complete set of catalytic activity in Type A reaction mechanisms. Technological and computational approaches have provided new strategies for analyzing chemical reaction networks, significantly advancing our understanding of the catalytic role. Intermediates and elementary steps are central to establishing such intricate networks, as catalysts are typically located at critical points along reaction pathways. Several methodologies exist, varying in effectiveness, scope, and completeness; some utilize chemical heuristics, while others require substantial human intervention. Future research can be anticipated to leverage these methodologies, combining stringent physical principles with insights from human intuition to design reaction pathways in an efficient manner. As catalyst research advances in innovative approaches, the likelihood of advancements in catalysis and reaction mechanisms increases, ultimately leading to improved applications in industrial and biological systems (Figure 3.8).

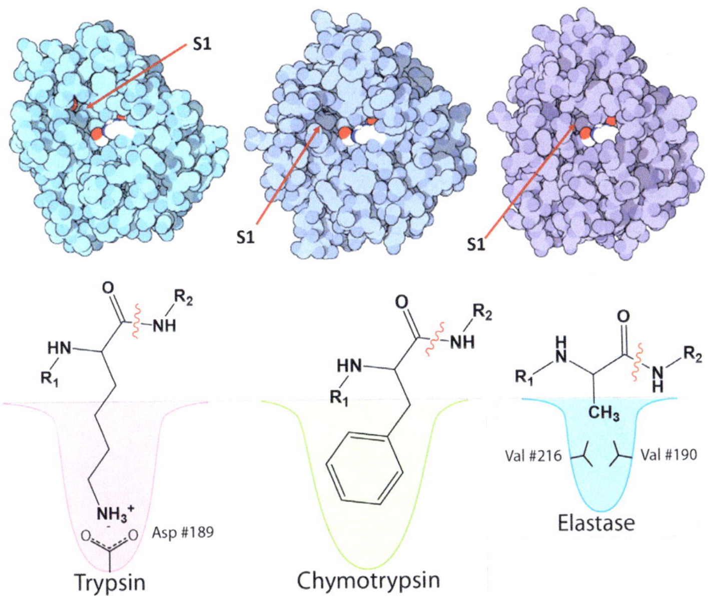

Figure 3.8. Role of catalysts in mechanisms.

Source: https://wou.edu/chemistry/files/2020/05/S1-binding-pocket-of-serine-proteases.png.

3.3. Types of Type A Reactions

Since biochemical reactions are highly complex, it is essential to comprehend the various mechanisms by which Type A reactions occur and their impact on the body. The most important aspect of these reactions is the presence of protein networks that are located in different areas of the cell. Unlike regular reactions that occur in the same environment, Type A reactions typically involve spatial changes that influence the way the reaction begins and concludes. Because of this variation, classical models might not be enough for metabolic control analysis. Innovations in understanding these interactions underscore how diffusion mechanics, combined with unique transport processes, significantly contribute to the control coefficients of Type A reactions, ultimately influencing cellular behavior in diverse environments (Kholodenko et al., 2002). Examining these various aspects reveals new insights into cellular signaling pathways and the biochemical mechanisms that govern them. The topic of Type A reactions encompasses more than biochemical reactions, as it also examines how cells adapt and interact with their environment. For example, some Type A reactions are capable of switching between active and inactive stages, allowing cells to respond quickly to environmental changes. Being able to adjust is key to homeostasis, as it allows the body to change its metabolic processes in response to changing conditions. Additionally, including diffusion in these reactions explains how cells manage their resources and maintain communication with one another. As highlighted in recent discussions surrounding metabolic control, the balance of fluxes within these heterogeneous networks underscores the significance of spatial factors, with diffusion acting as a crucial variable that contributes to the overall efficiency of Type A reactions (Pinto et al., 2017). Due to these numerous interactions, it is necessary to develop models that encompass all these elements. It is also clear from Type A reactions that their mechanisms and the environment in which they occur are closely connected. The way Type A reactions interact with cellular membranes is crucial, as it demonstrates that their outcomes depend on the environment's physical and chemical properties. These principles suggest that changes in membrane transport and the movement of signaling molecules can significantly influence both cell signaling and metabolic activity. According to these results, Type A reactions in a heterogeneous cell cannot be studied in isolation; they are interconnected with many other processes that control the cell's function. Understanding these mechanisms offers a holistic view of how cells navigate their environments, adapting to varying spatial constraints while maintaining essential biological processes (Kholodenko et al., 2002) (Figure 3.9).

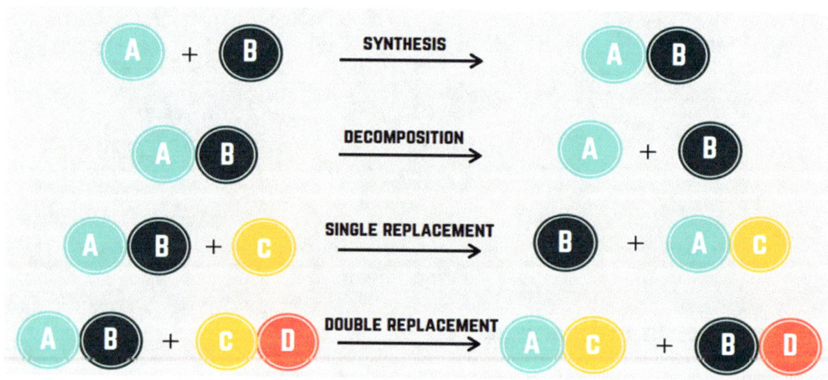

Figure 3.9. Types of type A reactions.

Source: https://chemistrytalk.org/wp-content/uploads/2023/03/Screen-Shot-2021-02-02-at-6.23.35-AM-1024x574-1.png.

3.3.1. Nucleophilic Substitution Reactions

Nucleophilic substitution reaction is revealed by the wealth of mechanistic pathways at the core of organic chemistry. Here, the encounter between nucleophiles and electrophiles plays a critical role in the loss of a leaving group and the formation of the new bond that ensues. The nature of the leaving group decisively controls the kinetics and mechanism employed in the reaction, affording either an SN1 or SN2 process. For instance, in SN1 reactions, leaving group departure leads to the formation of a carbocation that presents nucleophilic attack at any time, a feature firmly focused on in much mechanistic study. In SN2 reactions, the nucleophile instead attacks the electrophile directly, leading to a concerted process with a single transition state. Appreciation of these nuances not only sharpens the criticism of reaction kinetics but also enhances the predictive capability vis-à-vis product yield. A comparative examination of nucleophilic substitution reveals contrasting characteristics between aromatic and aliphatic systems. Specifically, aromatic nucleophilic substitution is different from uncomplicated paradigms and entails more complex mechanisms, such as the reaction of Meisenheimer complexes. In electrophile-nucleophile reactions with, say, phosphates, two channels were opened with direct attack on the phosphoryl center and secondary routes at aromatic carbons. HPLC and NMR are essential analytical tools in this instance for unraveling the mechanisms. Notably, variation of kinetic parameters like the nucleophilic rate constants (kN) reflects the intricacy of the electrophilic center. The ensuing Bronsted-type plots also confirm mechanistic differences, demonstrating consistent slopes that represent varying reaction mechanisms, thus contributing to the overall debate of nucleophilic reactivity in substitution reactions (Aguayo et al., 2013). As mechanistic insights continue to develop, the role of photocatalysts in facilitating nucleophilic substitution reactions becomes more significant. Recent research into photoinitiated radical processes has highlighted the role played by various photocatalysts in controlling the efficiency and product selectivity of such reactions. By subjecting experiments to varying photocatalytic conditions, scientists can control the initial radical formation and propagation steps, resulting in unique quantum yields and chain lengths. For example, n-C4F9I-based research highlights the regioselectivity diversity and mechanistic proposals based on the use of various photocatalysts, thereby offering a multifaceted understanding of the processes involved in nucleophilic substitutions. This study has profound implications for organic synthesis in general, supporting the importance of controlled conditions in observing and understanding the intricate mechanisms of nucleophilic substitution reactions (Damian et al., 2020).

3.3.2. Electrophilic Addition Reactions

Electrophilic addition reactions demonstrate the detailed nature of molecular interactions and highlight a range of reactivity and selectivity that is key in organic chemistry. As the reactions occur, an electrophilic species combines with a nucleophile to form a reactive intermediate. This is very important since it determines the ways the reaction can proceed, which in turn affects the outcome and how the product is formed. The theoretical frameworks, particularly those grounded in DFT, provide valuable insights into these mechanisms. Scholars have underscored the importance of indices like the electrophilicity ω and nucleophilicity N, which serve as pivotal markers to predict and rationalize the behavior of reactants in electrophilic addition scenarios (Contreras et al., 2004). They help us learn more about reaction kinetics and also clarify how specific sites in functional groups become active. Further analysis of the structure reveals that the electronic properties of the reactants play a significant role in determining the outcome of electrophilic addition reactions. The way molecules react at different points can be explained with the help of electronic density response functions. The position of electrons on the double bond indicates how the substituents will react to incoming electrophiles, typically resulting in regioselectivity and stereoselectivity, both of which are important in synthetic organic chemistry. Using global and local reactivity indices, chemists can predict where reactions will occur, which helps them determine how to conduct experiments. Additionally, the presence of solvents can alter the reactivity of certain areas and result in various outcomes. These dynamics exemplify the interplay between theoretical predictions and practical applications in the realm of organic synthesis (Contreras et al., 2004). The study of electrophilic addition reactions ultimately helps explain basic chemical reactions and contributes to the creation of complex organic molecules. As research in the field advances, studying reactions with empirical data helps improve and explain their details. Thanks to empirical analysis and DFT-based indices, chemists can effectively deal with electrophilic species and determine the optimal conditions for producing the desired products. Because both theories and experiments are combined, synthetic methodologies will continue to develop and can be applied in new ways to pharmaceuticals and materials. In conclusion, embracing the diverse avenues afforded by these reactions is essential for harnessing their full potential in ongoing and future research within organic chemistry (Domingo et al., 2016).

3.3.3. Elimination Reactions

Elimination reactions exemplify a significant field of organic chemistry that requires a thorough understanding of mechanistic pathways. More specifically, elimination reactions involve the removal of one hydrogen atom and one leaving group to create a π-bond at the end. The rules governing elimination reactions can be remarkably complex and require students to be able to distinguish between multiple mechanisms, such as E1 and E2.

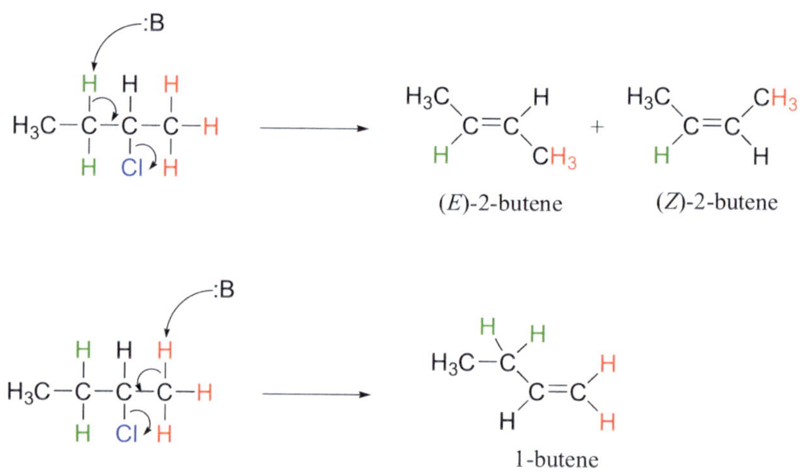

Figure 3.10. Elimination reactions.

Source: https://external-content.duckduckgo.com/iu/?u=https%3A%2F%2Fchem.libretexts.org%2F%40api%2Fdeki%2Ffiles%2F281219%2Fimage082.png%3Frevision%3D1&f=1&nofb=1&ipt=96331cb5b317282bcf98730cdd55f263137c489a3bbdfe79df4126494808a366.

In schools, differentiation is critical here because uncertainty might be caused when students are unable to predict reaction outcomes. Recent studies have shown that students assign enormous significance to the nature of starting substrates when predicting products, a phenomenon that highlights the importance of conceptual clarity in such reactions. As they progress, the students must not just memorize the mechanistic steps but also explain why these steps correspond to the reactivity of various substrates, as presented in a study on students' understanding in organic chemistry (Kevin et al., 2025). A significant characteristic of elimination reactions is the role of the base involved, overshadowed by the property of the substrates. The pathway by which elimination occurs—whether through a bimolecular (E2) or unimolecular (E1) reaction—is highly influenced by the strength of the base. Strong bases in E2 assist in removing a β-hydrogen and the leaving group as a concerted operation to form a double bond. However, E1 reactions consist of a two-step mechanism with intermediate carbocation formation before the removal of the proton. This contrast among the mechanisms is reflected in the synthetic methods employed in organic chemistry and highlights the rich perspectives that students must maintain in equilibrium. Correspondingly, teachers are encouraged to support learners in understanding these complex interactions by developing a comprehensive understanding that integrates the properties of the substrates and the bases within elimination conditions (Kevin et al., 2025). Moreover, the implications of elimination reactions extend beyond intellectual curiosity, as they are of actual importance to synthetic organic chemistry. Rational predictability of the elimination paths is an effective tool that can be applied to create novel compounds with specific functional groups. For instance, systematic investigation of lipid A derivatives, as revealed by research involving mass spectrometry, points towards the importance of understanding the organic components' cleavage mechanisms. These findings encourage a comprehensive exploration of elimination pathways, describing the fragmentation pattern and potential for discrimination between isomers due to structural differences. With students well-trained to distinguish between these processes, the applicability of their knowledge could significantly encourage advancements in drug discovery and molecular synthesis. Understanding, therefore, the nuances of elimination reactions plays a fundamental role in shaping the future of organic chemistry as a discipline (Figure 3.10).

3.4. Factors Influencing Type A Reactions

The occurrence of Type A reactions is largely influenced by the combination of environmental and genetic factors. Scientific studies indicate that changes in nature and those caused by humans can alter ecological systems, which in turn affect biological responses throughout a person's lifetime. This illustrates why it is essential to comprehend all the factors involved in Type A reactions. The distribution of essential nutrients among the atmospheric, biospheric, and oceanic systems is crucial. Changes in the supply of nutrients due to human actions alter the factors that lead to Type A reactions, necessitating species adaptation accordingly. This dynamic relationship accentuates the need to assess current states of planetary systems to predict potential shifts in biological responses, thereby elucidating the broader implications for ecosystem resilience and habitability as discussed by Mcelroy et al. (2025) Besides environmental causes, the way an organism's genes are structured is significant for Type A reactions. Genes, together with epigenetic and exogenous factors, form the information necessary for development and for the similarity between parents and their children. Because these systems are connected, they are important for understanding biological reactions. Even though genetic information is important for development, the way these hereditary systems interact lets organisms adjust to different environments. In Type A reactions, the quick responses to stimuli from biology play a big role in shaping the course of evolution. The evolutionary significance of these mechanisms highlights a complex framework in which proximate and ultimate information converge to influence how organisms navigate their environments, as elaborated by Griffiths et al. (2017). Additionally, changes in the environment and internal bodily processes can introduce further challenges to the factors that influence Type A reactions. Changes in the climate, loss of habitat, and less availability of resources cause different pressures on organisms, which makes them respond in various ways. Being able to adapt is crucial; organisms rely on both their genetic makeup and environmental changes to survive. In addition, studying these processes enables us to anticipate future responses in various situations, highlighting the importance of integrating multiple disciplines in conservation biology and ecology. Because the causes of Type A reactions keep changing, it is still necessary to study how genes and the environment work together. As a result, these studies will increase our knowledge about resilience and resource management, which is very important for dealing with today's global ecological and climate issues.

3.4.1. Solvent Effects

The influence of solvents on kinetics and mechanisms of Type A reactions is extremely profound in that solvents possess the ability to change radically reaction pathways and activation energies. It is exceedingly evident for enzymatic processes where solvent dynamics are coupled with substrate transformations. For instance, differentiation in reaction rates and selectivity can often be traced to solvent attributes such as dielectric constant, viscosity, and hydrogen bonding capability. The enzymatic activity may also change significantly in a transition between different solvents, causing changes in the transition states and intermediates' stability.

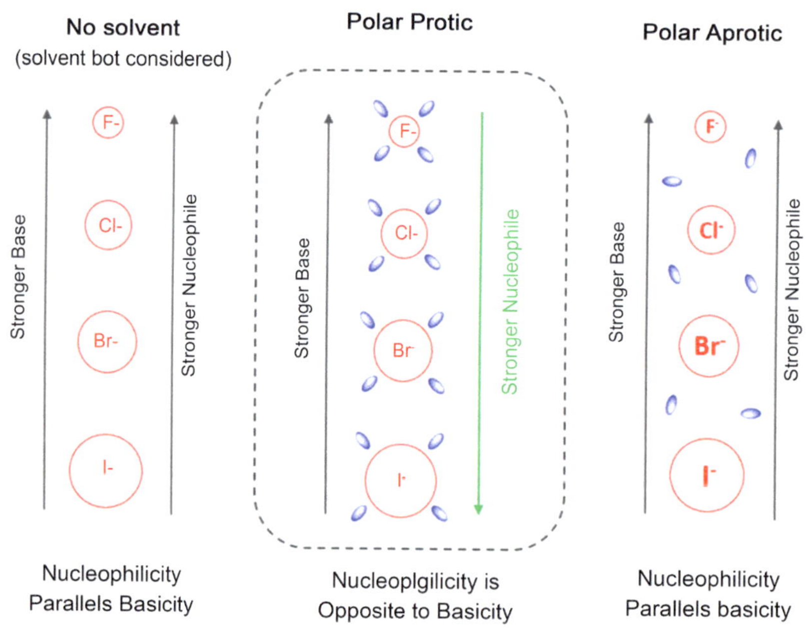

Figure 3.11. Solvent effects.

Source: https://www.chemistrysteps.com/wp-content/uploads/2019/11/The-Effect-of-Polar-Protic-and-Aprotic-Solvents-on-Nucleophilicity-and-Basicity-768x608.png.

These effects play a significant role in understanding the mechanisms at work, as they have the ability to modulate the reactant conversion process and product formation in a desirable manner, thereby highlighting the solvent's role as an active participant in the reaction process. Quantitative solvent effect studies of enzymatic reactions often employ techniques such as isotope labeling and pH-rate profiles to unravel the intricacies of enzymatic catalysis. For example, in carbapenem synthetase, solvent deuterium isotope effects provide valuable insights into substrate adenylation and ring formation, which are rate-limiting steps. Here, isotopic solvent composition can probe the hydrogen transfer pathways, in effect proving that solvent changes can make a substantial difference in enzyme conformation and function. The experiment shows that the interaction of solvents with the enzyme-substrate complex is not only efficient in modifying the binding affinities but also in influencing the mechanistic pathways that the reactions follow. These results enable a more vivid realization of the manner in which solvents can regulate efficiency and product of reactions and play their pivotal role in Type A mechanisms. Studies concerning the hydrolytic deamination of cytidine offer further evidence of the effect of solvents on enzyme action, illustrating the complex interplay between solvent properties and the products of reactions. 15N and deuterium isotope effect measurements demonstrate that isotopic solvent composition can significantly influence reaction rates, modulating substrate commitment to bond breakage. Notably, alterations within the solvent environment, such as the transition from H2O to D2O, reveal significant differences in enzymatic competence, demonstrating that solvent interactions play a crucial role in determining biochemical process rates. These findings illustrate the delicate balance in enzymic systems wherein solvent molecules possess the ability to stabilize certain transition states or intermediates, thus modifying the reaction landscape. This polyvalent solvent effect is crucial in determining the mechanisms of Type A reactions and provides insight into controlling conditions for biochemical reactions and designing catalytic strategies (Figure 3.11).

3.4.2. Temperature and Pressure

The relationship between temperature and pressure is crucial for understanding Type A reactions, particularly in catalysis. When temperatures rise, reactions occur more quickly because the heat helps molecules collide and break their bonds, which is necessary to overcome the activation energy barrier. At the same time, pressure affects the concentrations of the reactants and the way particles are organized, both of which can decide how the reaction proceeds. RuO_2 demonstrates that altering the temperature or pressure can significantly impact the course of a reaction. Specifically, the findings of a recent density-functional theory based kinetic Monte Carlo study highlight that while surface structure variations between different crystal facets of RuO_2 affect binding energetics, the overall catalytic activity remains comparable under certain elevated temperature and pressure conditions, challenging traditional notions of catalytic sensitivity and performance (Reuter et al., 2015). Type A reactions allow us to examine how temperature and pressure work together using rate-controlling mechanisms. Identifying the degree of rate control (DRC) offers a robust framework for determining which steps limit overall reaction rates. Researchers analyze kinetic parameters in simulated conditions to determine how changes in temperature and pressure affect the rates and mechanisms of chemical reactions. Observing how these forces affect reactants provides a clearer understanding of their behavior in various situations. Particularly, DRC approaches utilized in kinetic Monte Carlo simulations showcase that small modifications in environmental factors lead to significant changes in the rate-limiting steps, revealing kinetic sensitivities that are critical in the design and optimization of catalytic systems (Baranski et al., 2008). Both temperature and pressure play a significant role in determining the stability and reactivity of the chemicals involved in Type A reactions. When temperature goes up, there are more high-energy molecules, which may result in more undesired byproducts. Changes in pressure can also influence the position of equilibrium and, therefore, the amount and type of products formed. The idea that temperature and pressure are important in catalysis promotes a viewpoint that looks at both the speed of reactions and their stability. Having this detailed view is crucial for developing catalysts and processes, especially in industries where achieving the right results is paramount. By examining these connections more closely, chemistry can make progress in both fundamental and applied fields, and generate new ideas for catalysis and other areas (Figure 3.12).

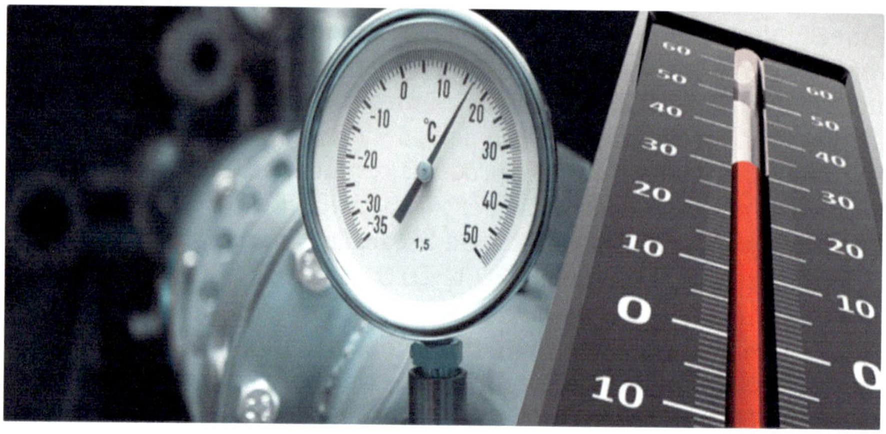

Figure 3.12. Temperature and pressure.

Source: https://www.carelusa.com/pressure-and-temperature.

3.4.3. Concentration of Reactants

In chemical reactions, the concentration of reactants plays a crucial role in determining both the reaction rate and the overall efficiency of the process. While examining the mechanism in Type A reactions, one must note that concentration changes do not only influence the reaction rate but also the kinetics involved in the reaction between the reactants. For instance, raising the concentration of reactants is likely to enhance the likelihood of molecule collisions, thereby accelerating the formation rate of the products. The relationship constitutes a fundamental concept in reaction kinetics, where higher concentrations are likely to enhance reaction development and completion conditions. On the other hand, as described in recent research, reactant concentration dynamics can become complicated, particularly when issues such as catalyst poisoning arise, potentially modifying anticipated outcomes and resulting in significant changes in the reaction's effectiveness, as noted by Froment et al. (2009). Additionally, the importance of reactant concentration is further demonstrated by its influence on catalytic efficiency and reactor design. Particularly, microreactor reactions coated on walls involve complex mass transfer-reaction regimes that are closely linked with reactant concentration profiles. Experiments indicate that the different orders of the reaction and varying levels of concentration may result in different conversion rates, thereby ruling out assumptions in reduced models. The dependence of the resistance to mass transfer on the concentration of reactants underscores the need for a high-level knowledge of catalyst activity, where the best conditions can yield improved flow efficiency and transform reactant more effectively.

Chemists are in a position to optimize reaction conditions more effectively with these variables, thereby making catalytic systems more practical and economical, as evidenced by Rodrigues et al. (2013). Besides, concentration crossovers in reactants not only affect reaction kinetics but also lead to novel phase behaviors in chemical systems. A finding by various studies indicates that under certain conditions, reactions may exhibit nonlinear behavior and anomalous scaling effects, particularly when reactants are close to critical concentrations. In some cases, such as unimolecular reactions, steep crossovers to asymptotic scaling can be realized even with minimal departures from critical parameters. The significance of such events emphasizes the intricate dynamics between reactant concentration and general Type A reaction dynamics. As scientists continue to investigate the effects of varying reactant amounts, a deeper understanding emerges, revealing the driving processes that govern reaction mechanisms. This insight can be used to inform the formulation of future advances in chemical engineering and applied science.

3.5. Applications of Type A Reactions

In many areas of chemistry, Type A reactions have played a key role in advancing approaches, particularly in catalysis and synthesis. Such reactions, which involve the transfer of a functional group from one molecule to another, demonstrate crucial aspects of how complex reactions occur. For example, Type A reactions can produce important intermediates used in pharmaceuticals and agrochemicals. The importance of catalysts is proven by the continuous research on ways to boost reaction efficiency and selectivity. This matters significantly for the environment, as better catalysts help reduce both waste and resource consumption, which aligns with the principles of green chemistry. As a result, Type A reactions are now used in industrial processes because they are flexible and useful in today's synthetic chemistry. Type A catalysis is especially important, mainly because it helps ceria-supported metal catalysts in oxidation reactions. The special redox abilities of ceria create a beneficial support system that enhances the performance of catalysts, underscoring the practical relevance of Type A reaction mechanisms in real-world applications. As an illustration, ceria-supported transition metal nanoparticles are highly effective in converting carbon monoxide (CO) into carbon dioxide, which is necessary for reducing toxic emissions in various industries. In these cases, the active oxygen species formed at the metal-support interface help the reaction and also make the whole process more efficient. Furthermore, studies have shown that the selectivity and reactivity of these catalysts can be enhanced by adjusting the dispersion of the metal and the structure of the ceria support, highlighting the importance of Type A reactions in detail and their practical applications. In addition, Type A reactions are important for making new energy conversion and storage technologies. For example, preferential oxidation of carbon monoxide (PROX) is a critical reaction in hydrogen fuel cells, where the efficient conversion of hydrogen and minimization of CO impurities is essential for performance. Thanks to new insights into Type A reaction mechanisms, catalysts can now selectively oxidize CO in the presence of H2, thereby preventing catalyst poisoning and increasing efficiency. It has been found that the surfaces of ceria and the kind of catalytic metals involved can both shape the results of these reactions, leading to some configurations being more selective and active. For this reason, Type A reactions are significant in modern chemistry because they help achieve sustainable and efficient chemical reactions.

3.5.1. Synthesis of Pharmaceuticals

The intricate process of drug synthesis is at the heart of creating effective medicines, particularly those with targeted action on specific biochemical pathways. Among the various synthetic methods employed, Type A reactions are pivotal to drug biosynthesis, offering paths that are both selective and efficient. This selectivity is especially valuable, as it allows for the synthesis of compounds that exhibit great specificity to their biological targets, thereby minimizing unintended side effects. Recent developments in synthetic methodology have enabled the construction of more complex molecules, significantly enhancing the pharmacological profiles of novel drug entities. The continuous development of such synthetic pathways not only streamlines the manufacturing process but also increases the overall yield of the target drug reagents, highlighting the importance of being aware of the underlying mechanism in Type A reactions. In the broader context of pharmaceutical synthesis, the introduction of sophisticated analytical methods can prove revolutionary. These methods can be used to shed light on the complex structures and drug-target interactions, which is needed to develop safer and more effective drugs. For instance, the application of high-performance liquid chromatography (HPLC) and mass spectrometry in drug synthesis has enhanced the ability to track reaction progress and product purity. Furthermore, studies such as the one on HXLPP-WCX sorbents demonstrate the importance of developing sophisticated separation techniques that efficiently extract drugs from complex matrices, as they significantly contribute to the recovery and analysis of active compounds under various environmental conditions.

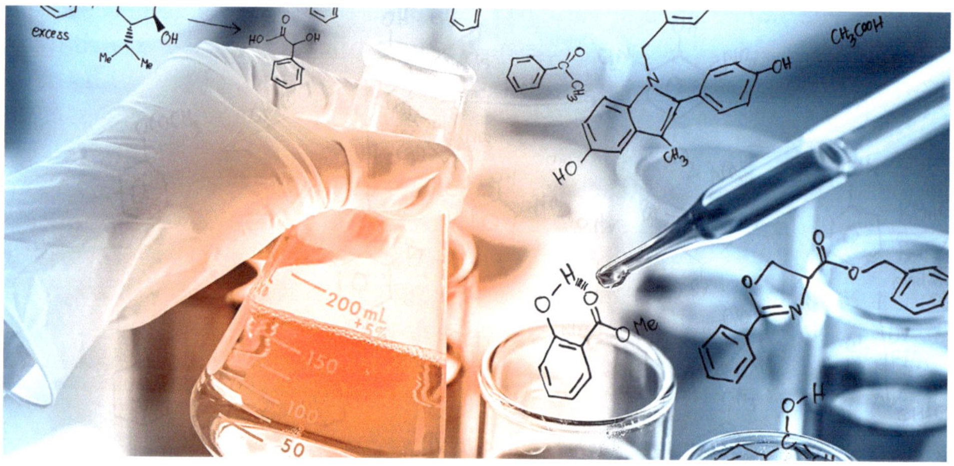

Figure 3.13. Synthesis of pharmaceuticals.

Source: https://master-chimie.univ-grenoble-alpes.fr/medias/photo/master-2-organic-synthesis-for-pharmaceutical-and-agronomical-industries_1494863642244-jpg?ID_FICHE=116993.

By enhancing such techniques, researchers can keep the synthesis of drugs not only efficient but also adhere to Environmental Protection Agency (EPA) regulations and guidelines. Furthermore, computer-based approaches are increasingly being recognized for their contribution to pharmaceutical development through the modeling of drug action and synthetic route in silico. Such approaches provide critical insight into the kinetics and mechanisms of drug action, as well as how drug efficacy changes under varying environmental conditions. This trend is best exemplified by the study on prostaglandin H synthase-1 (PGHS-1), which showed how computational modeling could be used to forecast the pharmacological actions of NSAIDs in different environments. Researchers can use this predictive model to foresee resistance mechanisms and design combination therapies that could be optimized. The synthesis of drugs, therefore, not only calls upon traditional chemical means but also increasingly on these advanced computational tools, a testament to the multi-dimensional character of drug discovery in Type A reaction settings (Figure 3.13).

3.5.2. Industrial Chemical Processes

Industrial processes are central in the chemistry field for making the compounds that form modern materials and technologies. This is well illustrated by the synthesis of arene-ruthenium-sulfur clusters, where new techniques help to improve catalysts and their use. Specifically, the comprehensive work detailed in Chapter Two of the pertinent thesis elucidates the synthesis of various higher nuclearity clusters, such as $[Ru_5S_4(cymene)_4](PF_6)_2$ and $[Ru_4(S_2; SO; cymene)_4](PF_6)_2$. Through X-ray crystallography, these clusters are grouped, and it is found that their valence electrons play a crucial role in shaping their structure, thereby enhancing our understanding of their applications in catalysis and materials. Such insights are invaluable as they pave the way for more efficient and tailored chemical processes in industrial settings that require precision and reliability (Guo et al., 1999).

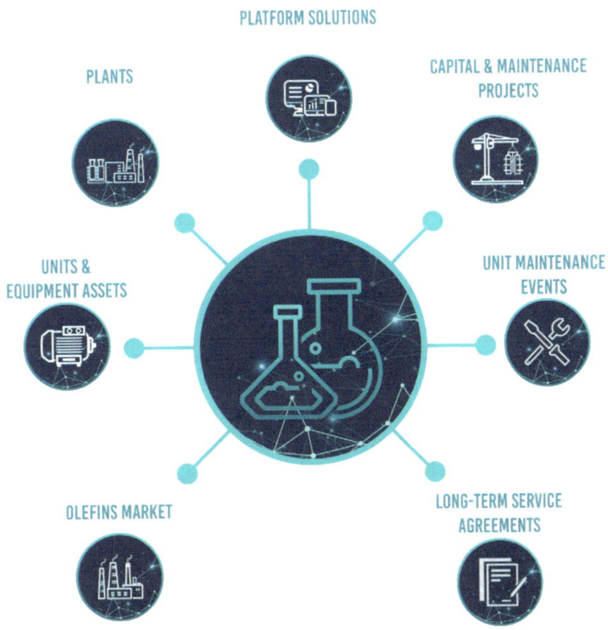

Figure 3.14. Industrial chemical processes.

Source: https://media.industrialinfo.com/database/chemical_processing/images/chemicalProcessing_lowPoly_diagram.png.

As technology improves, industrial chemical processes continue to evolve, making the details of reactions increasingly important. Important information is provided on the ways arene-ruthenium-sulfur clusters are formed and handled in controlled experiments. The study demonstrates that the structure of a cluster depends on the structure of its molecules and the conditions used in its synthesis. Besides, examining unusual signals in NMR spectra helps to determine and confirm the structure and activity of these complexes. This intricate understanding of the mechanisms not only supports academic inquiry but also has practical implications for optimizing industrial applications, whereby the efficiency of Type A reactions can be maximized (Guo et al., 1999). Additionally, the intricacies of industrial chemistry involve examining arene-ruthenium-nitrogen complexes, which is another important field of study. In Chapter Three of the thesis, the synthesis and characterization of relevant complexes, such as [$RuCl_2(NH_3$; cymene)] and [$Ru(NH_3)_3$(cymene)] $(PF_6)_2$, are thoroughly discussed. The process of these reactions illustrates the complex pathways associated with Type A reactions. Learning about these pathways supports the development of new catalysts and also helps increase the quantity and quality of products produced in industries. The systematic approach to investigating the formation mechanisms of these complexes offers insights into optimizing processes that are foundational to many industrial applications, further supporting the ongoing evolution of chemical manufacturing methods (Guo et al., 1999) (Figure 3.14).

3.5.3. Environmental Chemistry

The intricate interplay between Type A reactions and environmental chemistry is crucial in understanding the biochemical transformations that occur within ecosystems. Type A reactions, characterized by their intrinsic mechanistic patterns, can significantly influence the equilibrium of several chemical compounds in the environment. For instance, the reactions generally involve redox reactions where electron exchange defines the chemical landscape. When analyzing pollutants, such as heavy metals or organics, Type A reaction mechanisms help determine their reactivity and modes of degradation. The change in form can either alleviate or aggravate environmental problems, depending on the individual reactants and conditions.

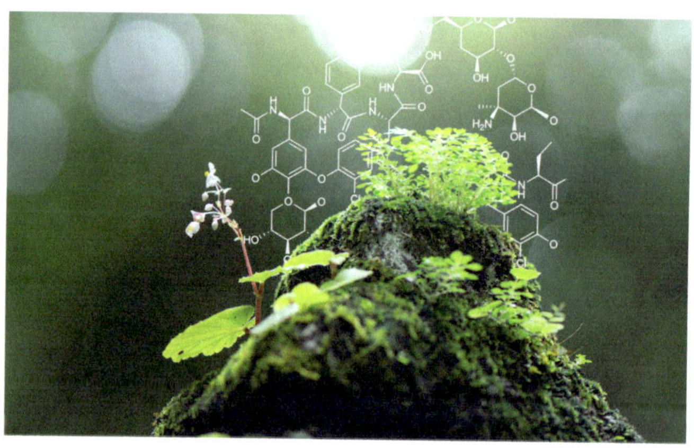

Figure 3.15. Environmental chemistry.

Source: https://www.agro-chemistry.com/wp-content/uploads/2020/07/cefic-launches-bio-based-chemicals-sector-group.jpg.

Therefore, demystifying the intricacies of Type A reactions is essential for developing effective remediation measures. By applying findings from recent studies, we can enhance our understanding of the mechanisms and their impact on environmental health (Ebenhoeh et al.,

2013). In addition to pollution, the impacts of Type A reactions also encompass nutrient cycling in various ecosystems. For example, such reactions make it simple for compounds of nitrogen and phosphorus to be transformed, which is critically essential in plant growth and ecosystem productivity. With nitrification and denitrification reactions, Type A reactions play a crucial role in regulating nutrient levels in soil and water ecosystems. Biogeochemical cycling is critical in maintaining ecological stability, particularly in areas where natural resources are disrupted by human activities such as agricultural production and urbanization. By knowing the mechanistic elements of these reactions, we can have better approaches for sustainable land use management and water management. These tactics are crucial in mitigating the effects of nutrient overloading, which often leads to adverse processes such as eutrophication within aquatic ecosystems (Pinto et al., 2017). Additionally, awareness of Type A reactions helps quantify the dynamics of greenhouse gases, particularly in the context of climate change. Reactions of carbon compounds are central in atmospheric chemistry and directly contribute to global warming potential. The interaction between Type A reaction mechanisms and the decomposition of organic matter yields the production of greenhouse gases, such as methane and carbon dioxide. Carbon cycling is not merely a theoretical process, but an urgent global issue, as the emission of these gases has a dramatic influence on the composition of the atmosphere and climate models. Through the study of reaction mechanisms, researchers can establish the potential for carbon sequestration and explore possibilities for lessening the effects of climate change. Ultimately, an interdisciplinary approach to studying Type A reactions in environmental chemistry can lead to innovative solutions to global environmental issues (Ebenhoeh et al., 2013) (Figure 3.15).

3.6. Challenges in Studying Type A Reactions

Exploring Type A reactions raises numerous issues that hinder scientists' progress in this field. The reactions are often very complex because they depend on many factors that can impact the outcomes. For example, it is crucial to observe how structures evolve during these reactions, although it is challenging to measure. According to recent studies, the changes in shape and strength of black phosphorus-based composites indicate that significant volume expansions during lithiation can lead to a decrease in the battery's capacity. It suggests that observing these subtle details would be very difficult without using electrochemical atomic force microscopy, which reveals a vital gap between theory and experiment in studying Type A reactions. Moreover, how Type A reactions cause damage are very challenging. In particular, the role of interfaces and solid electrolyte interphase (SEI) formation is critical yet underexplored. It is clear from studies of black phosphorus-based anodes that the way the materials are held together in composites may not be strong enough to deal with the stresses caused by electrochemical reactions. Also, it is not always easy to link the way operations are conducted with the performance outcomes, which makes the study more complicated. It is crucial to have comprehensive frameworks that can identify and explain how materials degrade, particularly when we aim to understand how certain material properties interact in use. Exploring these materials is crucial to establishing reliable performance measures and identifying more suitable materials for actual use. Another important issue is the combination of new electrochemical systems and determining their operational limits. In studying reactions involving proton exchange membrane (PEM) water electrolyzers, for instance, researchers grapple with understanding the degradation mechanisms that accompany reduced platinum group metal (PGM) loadings. While researchers strive to enhance performance and reduce costs, it remains crucial to understand how factors such as catalyst order and the interaction between layers impact the system's efficiency and lifespan. The way Type A reactions behave under different conditions highlights the importance of collaboration among materials science, chemistry, and engineering. Handling these challenges requires developing improved experimental methods and rapid tests that assess the impact of new materials and designs on Type A reactors, which enables them to perform better and last longer (Figure 3.16).

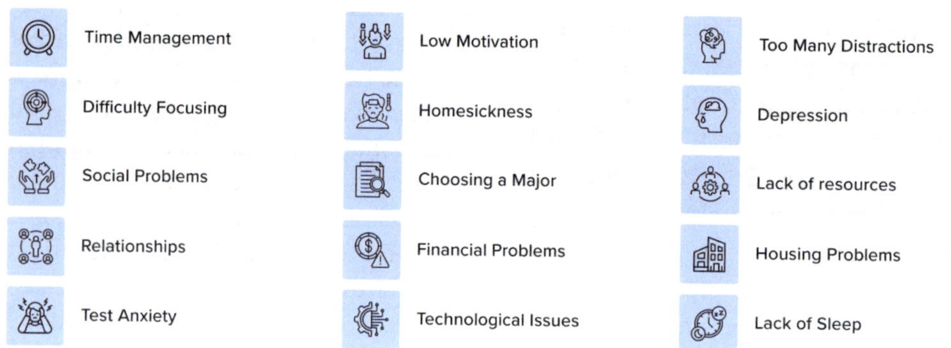

Figure 3.16. Challenges in studying type A reactions.

Source: https://assets-global.website-files.com/620e4101b2ce12a1a6bff0e8/6491879f0e42bb135f29cd1d_Infographics_15%20Most%20Common%20Student%20Problems%20And%20Their%20Solutions_APRIL2023.webp.

3.6.1. Complexity of Reaction Mechanisms

Investigation into the intricacies of reaction mechanisms reveals the complex nature of Type A reactions, in which numerous factors influence the direction of chemical conversions. The understanding of the mechanisms is highly complicated by the existence of many possible intermediates and transition states that can appear in a chemical reaction. Because these intermediates are likely to involve numerous molecular conformations and kinetic barriers, they give rise to a dynamic situation that defies classical reaction kinetic models. This is particularly relevant when attempting to observe how different conditions, such as temperature and pressure, are able to stabilize or destabilize specific intermediates and cause the preferred reaction pathway to alter. Therefore, the comprehension of the full scope of a Type A reaction mechanism includes an understanding of not only the reactants and the products but also the subtleties of each step of the reaction mechanism. When considering specific instances of Type A reactions, it is found that the complexity can be compounded by the reaction environment, which may include catalytic surfaces or solvating influences. For example, solid catalysts can create new routes that are possibly not available in solution-phase reactions and introduce fresh levels of complexity. The reactions in the solid state are likely to occur in a series of steps, involving diffusion processes, surface interactions, and adsorption phenomena, all of which are likely to alter the effective mechanism. Moreover, advanced materials like zeolitic imidazolate frameworks (ZIFs) present compelling examples wherein reaction mechanisms are characterized by their porous nature. The interplay of the structural properties of ZIFs and molecular interactions not only facilitates catalyzed reactions within them but also instills a degree of architectural stability, allowing for complex reaction pathways (Wang et al., 2022). Simulation of such complex reaction mechanisms requires sophisticated computational techniques that can account for the multicomponent nature of the processes. PALM model system and other similar models that can simulate chemical kinetics in reactive environments have brought about a new era of studying chemical reactions, particularly in urban areas. By concatenating various gas-phase chemistry mechanisms, these models can simulate the influence of environmental conditions on reaction routes and thereby enhance their understanding of the resulting complexity. Of particular significance is the application of structured models, such as the Carbon Bond Mechanism 4, which illustrates the substantial differences in prediction capability between alternative reaction mechanisms and highlights the necessity of a sophisticated strategy for Type A reaction investigation. Studying these mechanisms enables scientists to combat the challenges of chemical reactivity complexity in different environments more effectively, thereby contributing to wiser applications in fields such as catalysis and environmental chemistry (Khan et al., 2021) (Figure 3.17).

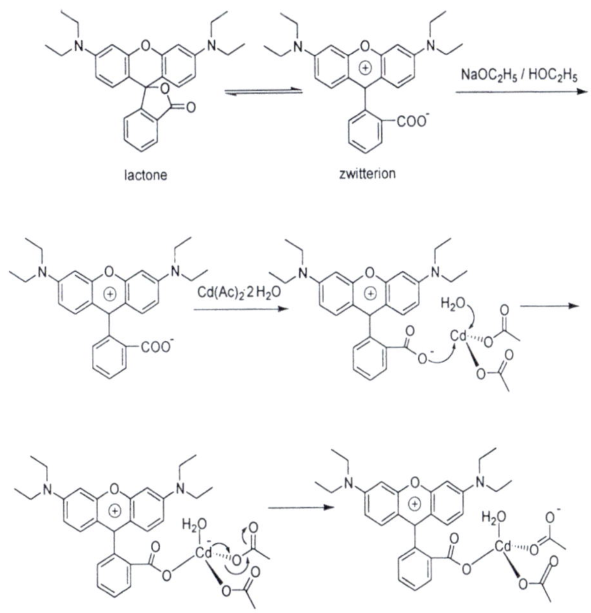

Figure 3.17. Complexity of reaction mechanisms.

Source: https://www.priyamstudycenter.com/wp-content/uploads/2021/09/enzymes-function-and-catalysis-reaction.png.

3.6.2. Limitations of Experimental Techniques

For Type A reactions, being precise in the way experiments are performed is important. Still, the approaches used in research can sometimes lead to results that are not accurate. Methods such as kinetic studies and mechanistic trapping can be influenced by factors like temperature fluctuations and environmental impurities. These reasons may lead to unreliable data or incorrect interpretations of the pathways involved. Additionally, RWD can differ from what is expected, which further complicates the process of obtaining accurate results. Such differences highlight the need for researchers to exercise caution, as issues in the experiment setup may not accurately reveal the true details of reaction mechanisms; therefore, they should analyze the data more thoroughly. A further problem is that chemical databases are the primary sources of information for carrying out experiments. The way Type A reaction mechanisms are understood depends on how accurate and complete the data is. A study on this topic highlights that although existing systems are beneficial, they often fail to consider all possible outcomes, thereby overlooking alternative ways to understand reaction pathways. Showing only part of a chemical reaction may cause scientists to prefer some routes over others that could be equally valid. Thus, the findings from experiments might only cover a limited part of the real range of processes involved in Type A reactions. In addition, computational models predict results well, but they still have some restrictions. For example, new studies in machine learning (ML) present a novel approach to predicting retrosynthetic reactions using information from patents. It can overcome some of the usual problems found in rule-based and other ML models. Still, it reveals that relying solely on data has its own problems, mainly due to the limitations of how well the datasets represent the situation. With many types of chemical reactions included in Type A reactions, the limited scope of the training data may obscure important aspects or mechanisms, indicating that additional development and improvement of experimental methods are necessary for a thorough understanding (Figure 3.18).

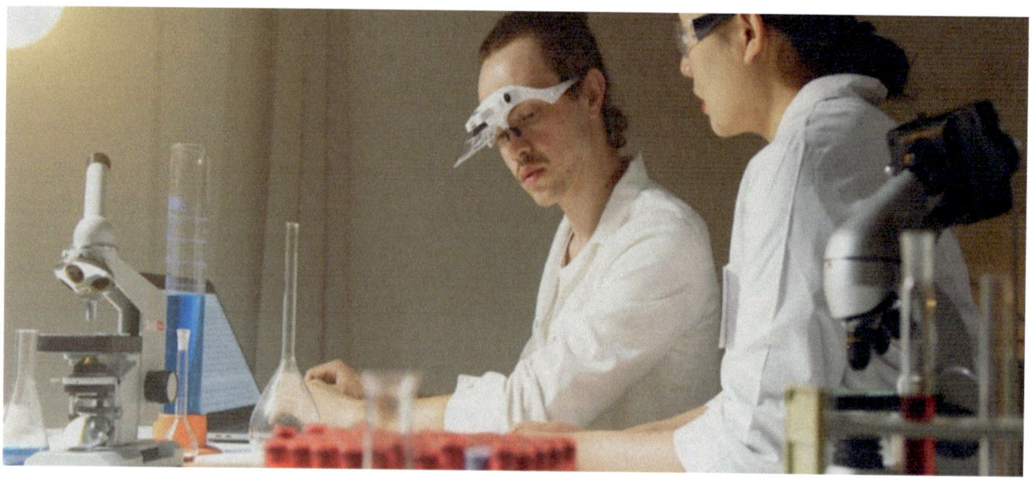

Figure 3.18. Limitations of experimental techniques.

Source: https://www.enago.com/academy/wp-content/uploads/2022/11/ResearchDesign_Global.jpg.

3.6.3. Computational Modeling Approaches

Advances in computational modeling approaches have significantly transformed the study and analysis of reaction mechanisms, particularly for Type A reactions. The application of algorithmic strategies allows researchers to efficiently screen and identify relevant intermediates and elementary steps crucial to developing valid prediction models. Various methodologies exist, each with a varying range of applications, level of screening thoroughness, and reliance on heuristics and human involvement. These computational approaches not only surpass the ability to model chemical reaction networks but also facilitate systematic investigation of multi-interaction schemes. By leveraging both computational rapidity and chemical awareness, researchers can gain a more advanced understanding of Type A reactions, positioning such methodologies at the forefront of current chemical science (Reiher et al., 2018). The application of theoretical modeling frameworks is a convenient way to manage the complexity of biological systems and Type A reaction dynamics.

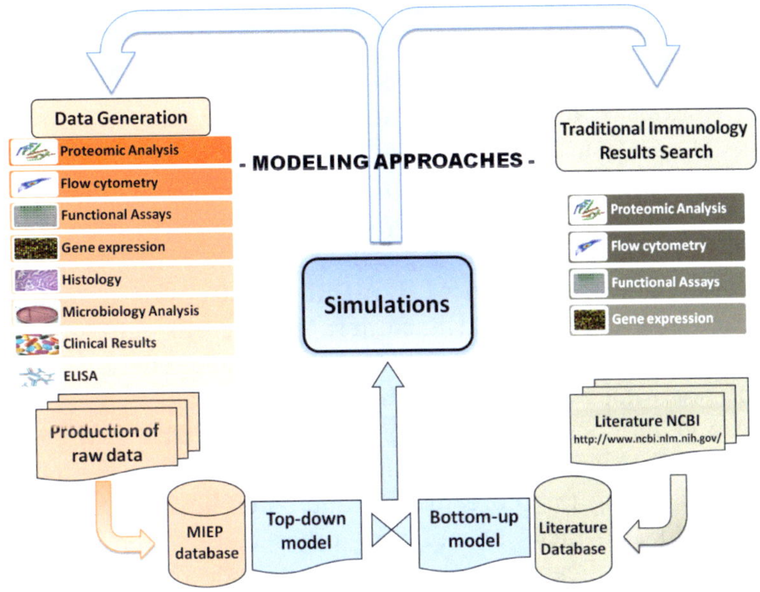

Figure 3.19. Computational modeling approaches.

Source: https://www.nibib.nih.gov/sites/default/files/inline-images/ISB.3.2.jpg.

Models can distill the intricate behavior and numerous interactions in biological networks into more manageable forms, enabling insights that are difficult to access by experimental approaches alone. The disconnected boundary between computational modeling and biology is evident through the use of computer programming languages like BlenX, which effectively translates high-level descriptions of biological networks into practical applications. Through the breakdown of complex reaction mechanisms into basic elementary reactions, Gillespie's stochastic approach can be effectively utilized, thereby changing our approach to Type A reaction modeling (Priami et al., 2010). This pioneering use of a computational approach illustrates the growing importance of multidisciplinary approaches in developing our understanding of reaction mechanisms. Moreover, with the ongoing escalation of the complexity of reaction mechanisms, the emphasis on compositional modeling approaches is all the more imperative. Compositionality enables researchers to deal with the combinatorial explosion of potential interactions by systematically decomposing complex systems into their functional components. This methodology not only facilitates analysis but also yields more robust model construction, as demonstrated in numerous applications across biological systems. By exploring the relationship between elementary reactions, computational modeling techniques can provide greater insight to Type A reaction kinetics, enabling further study and empirical verification. The interplay between theoretical advancements and computational advancements, therefore, has a lot of potential for the development of reaction mechanism research, showcasing the marriage of systematic modeling with computational practice (Priami et al., 2010; Reiher et al., 2018) (Figure 3.19).

Summary

The study of Type A reactions has revealed the detailed processes involved in these immune reactions, mainly when using β-lactam antibiotics. Immediate HSRs often happen because of genetic predispositions. Research has identified specific genetic markers, notably the HLA-DRB1*10:01 allele, as significant risk factors for these reactions, with findings indicating an increased likelihood of immune-mediated responses among individuals who carry this genetic variant. Because of this, patients who are at risk can be appropriately recognized and cared for, resulting in fewer bad reactions to medications. As highlighted in contemporary studies, this understanding is paramount for enhancing patient safety and optimizing therapeutic strategies (Barrett et al., 2020). Considering these findings further, it is possible to make better decisions about the risk of using β-lactam antibiotics. The association of HLA-DRB1*10:01 with immediate HSRs advocates for a more personalized approach in pharmacotherapy, wherein genetic screening can inform treatment decisions. Due to these advancements, it is evident that genetic testing should be utilized in clinics, as it has the potential to significantly impact the management of allergies. In addition, information from these genetic studies can help create treatments that reduce the chances of HSRs and improve patient outcomes. This evolution in understanding aligns with broader trends in personalized medicine, aiming for more precise and safer healthcare delivery (Bianchi et al., 2015). Experts in this field also focus on studying other factors that may increase the risk of Type A reactions. Although significant progress has been made in identifying HLA-related risks, it remains necessary to explore other parts of the genome that may affect immune responses and enhance our understanding of hypersensitivity. Researchers should also utilize genome-wide association studies to identify additional genetic factors that contribute to adverse drug reactions. When investigators examine more than HLA markers, they may uncover new information that can significantly enhance the management and care of Type A reactions in hospitals. Hence, the future of immunological research and its applications hinges upon sustained inquiry into the mechanisms driving these reactions (Barrett et al., 2020).

Exploring the details of Type A reactions provides us with important insights into biochemical reactions. These reactions are primarily based on the way substrates bind to enzymes, which is crucial for metabolic pathways and cellular function. Being aware of the regulations involved in these interactions reveals more about the ways biological systems keep their functions stable. Due to factors such as concentration and environment, these processes may yield different outcomes. For this reason, this variation shows that biological systems are constantly changing yet can still create patterns of order. For instance, while an initial expectation might align with conventional biochemical theories, real-world observations frequently deviate, pointing toward the complexities of living systems and their operational frameworks, as illustrated in foundational research on enzyme kinetics and interaction models (Ebenhoeh et al., 2013). Another important point to note is that sometimes a system's response to inputs does not match what is expected. Often, these systems exhibit S-shaped outcomes that deviate from the Michaelis-Menten model. The fact that this happens in biology is a sign that there is a detailed organization of processes inside cells. The Hill equation explains how enzymes behave in different conditions. Such insights not only enhance our comprehension of enzymatic function but also provide a scaffold for exploring the regularities that biology imposes in the face of disorder, as discussed in several contemporary analyses of biochemical processes (Frank et al., 2013). Also, the combination of various biological elements is crucial for this type of input-output relationship. As subsystems work together, they help form the main characteristics of the system and decide how well and what happens in Type A reactions. Such aggregation often results in a structure that maintains stable outcomes, despite changes, by exhibiting an order that helps dissipate information as it moves through the components of a biochemical system. Examining measurement and precision is crucial for understanding how different patterns of scaling occur, and for highlighting the role of structure in biology. Ultimately, recognizing the interplay between aggregation, measurement, and input-output relationships is crucial for elucidating the mechanisms of Type A reactions and their functional significance in living organisms (Frank et al., 2013).

CLOSER LOOK

FLUX BALANCE ANALYSIS

Flux Balance Analysis (FBA) is a constraintbased computational framework that predicts steadystate flows—"fluxes"—through a reconstructed metabolic network by solving a linear optimization problem under massbalance and enzymeactivity constraints. The heart of FBA is a stoichiometric matrix S that encodes all intracellular reactions (rows = metabolites, columns = reactions): it enforces $S \cdot v = 0$, ensuring mass inputs and outputs are balanced at steady state, and thus no accumulation occurs in any metabolite pool. The system is inherently underdetermined (more reactions than metabolites), so FBA introduces lower and upper bounds on each flux—based on reaction reversibility, measured uptake rates, thermodynamic directionality, or enzyme capacity—and defines a linear objective function $Z = c^T v$, where c reflects a biological goal such as maximum growth, ATP yield, or product formation. Solving this linear program selects one flux vector among many feasible solutions, providing a biologically plausible metabolic phenotype without requiring kinetic parameters or rate laws.

FBA's power lies in its scalability and its ability to explore genome-scale models in silico—thousands of metabolites and reactions—facilitating applications across metabolic engineering, synthetic biology, systems medicine, and antibiotic or cancer drug target discovery. For instance, FBA has helped optimize microbial hosts for enhanced ethanol, succinate or lycopene production, and predict gene essentiality in pathogens or hostpathogen interactions. FBA can also be extended via techniques like flux variability analysis (FVA) to characterize alternate optima, loopless or thermodynamic FBA (tFBA/TFA) to eliminate infeasible cycles, and dynamic FBA to simulate temporal changes from environmental perturbations.

Despite limitations—such as dependence on the assumed objective function, sensitivity to missing reactions in reconstructions, and static steadystate assumption—FBA remains the most widely adopted constraintbased modeling approach in systems biology, prized for its minimal data requirements, computational efficiency, and ability to generate testable hypotheses linking genotype to metabolic phenotype.

References

1. Aguayo, R., Arias, F., Cañete, A., Zuñiga, C., Castro, E. A., Pavez, P., & Santos, J. G. (2013). Dual nucleophilic substitution reactions of O,O-Diethyl 2,4-dinitrophenyl phosphate and thionophosphate triesters. *International Journal of Chemical Kinetics*, *45*(3), 202–211. https://doi.org/10.1002/kin.20756Aissa, I., Kilár, A., & Dörnyei, Á. (2021). Study on the CID fragmentation pathways of deprotonated 4′-monophosphoryl lipid A. *Molecules, 26*. https://www.semanticscholar.org/paper/3f7393a74553b4118363dad6710e799cf1be0788 (accessed on 9 June 2025).
2. Alberts, B., Andreini, C., Balche, W. E., Barker, H. A., Benner, S. A., Berge, C., Braakman, R., et al. (2012). *The Compositional and Evolutionary Logic of Metabolism*. http://arxiv.org/abs/1207.5532 (accessed on 9 June 2025).
3. Alia, S., Padgett, E., Chan, A. L., Blair, S. J., Medina, S., Reeves, K., Yu, H., et al. (2024). (Invited) Degradation mechanisms, diagnostics, and mitigation in proton exchange membrane water electrolyzes. *ECS Meeting Abstracts*. https://www.semanticscholar.org/paper/37df83e182cdb960268a02051c4c4f44540a9286 (accessed on 9 June 2025).
4. Andersen, J. L., Flamm, C., Merkle, D., Stadler, P. F., et al. (2017). *Chemical Transformation Motifs–Modelling Pathways as Integer Hyper Flows*. http://arxiv.org/abs/1712.02594 (accessed on 9 June 2025).
5. Annila, A. (2007). *Natural Process–Natural Selection*. https://core.ac.uk/download/186331453.pdf (accessed on 9 June 2025).
6. Arnett, S. O., Gerratana, B., & Townsend, C. (2007). Rate-limiting steps and role of active site Lys443 in the mechanism of carbapenem synthetase. *Biochemistry, 46*(32), 9337–9345. https://www.semanticscholar.org/paper/e15540568539f404bfbeb5000bae57becd315573 (accessed on 9 June 2025).
7. Bailleul, S., De Wispelaere, K., & Van Speybroeck, V. (2016). *Towards Molecular Control of Elementary Reactions in Zeolite Catalysis by Advanced Molecular Simulations Mimicking Operating Conditions*. https://core.ac.uk/download/55855326.pdf (accessed on 9 June 2025).
8. Baltensperger, U., Claeys, M., Dommen, J., Donahue, N. M., et al. (2009). *The Formation, Properties and Impact of Secondary Organic Aerosol: Current and Emerging Issues*. https://core.ac.uk/download/4882143.pdf.
9. Baranski, A. S., Boudard, C., Campbell, C. T., Chorkendorff, I., Dumesic, J. A., et al. (2008). *Examination of the Concept of Degree of Rate Control by First-Principles Kinetic Monte Carlo Simulations*. https://core.ac.uk/download/267951742.pdf.
10. Barrett, S., Blanca, M., Blanca-López, N., Carr, D. F., et al. (2020). *Beta-Lactam-Induced Immediate Hypersensitivity Reactions: A Genome-Wide Association Study of a Deeply Phenotyped Cohort*. https://core.ac.uk/download/334954369.pdf (accessed on 9 June 2025).
11. Bayramova, E., Petrova, D. P., Marchenkov, A., Morozov, A., Galachyants, Y. P., Zakharova, Y., Bedoshvili, Y., et al. (2024). Differential expression of stress adaptation genes in a diatom *Ulnaria acus* under different culture conditions. *International Journal of Molecular Sciences, 25*. https://www.semanticscholar.org/paper/d57723e224d18220edb4469b3bccfa74f45c2dc8 (accessed on 9 June 2025).

12. Behrendt, H., Darsow, U., Eyerich, K., Foerster, J., et al. (2008). *Pollen Grains Induce a Rapid and Biphasic Eczematous Immune Response in Atopic Eczema Patients.* https://core.ac.uk/download/16432577.pdf (accessed on 9 June 2025).
13. Besz, K. M., Burgos, A., Castells, M., de las Vecillas, L., et al. (2023). *Differential Presentation of Hypersensitivity Reactions to Carboplatin and Oxaliplatin: Phenotypes, Endotypes, And Management with Desensitization.* https://core.ac.uk/download/599239048.pdf (accessed on 9 June 2025).
14. Bianchi, M., Facco, G., Grazzini, G., Liumbruno, G. M., et al. (2015). *Leukoreduction of Blood Components: An Effective Way to Increase Blood Safety?* https://core.ac.uk/download/54532479.pdf (accessed on 9 June 2025).
15. Blake, G. A. (1988). *Chemistry in Dense Molecular Clouds: Theory and Observational Constraints.* https://core.ac.uk/download/10211213.pdf.
16. Borrull, F., Bratkowska, D., Cormack, P. A. G., Fontanals, A., et al. (2010). Synthesis and application of hyper crosslinked polymers with weak cation-exchange character for the selective extraction of basic pharmaceuticals from complex environmental water samples. https://core.ac.uk/download/9029849.pdf (accessed on 9 June 2025).
17. Bothe, D., & Dreyer, W. (2013). *Continuum Thermodynamics of Chemically Reacting Fluid Mixtures.* https://core.ac.uk/download/289298815.pdf (accessed on 9 June 2025).
18. Branco Pinto, D., Constales, D., Marin, G., & Yablonsky, G. S. (2017). *Kinetic Intersections as A Source of Information on Rate Coefficients.* https://core.ac.uk/download/91288153.pdf (accessed on 9 June 2025).
19. Contreras, R. R., Parra-Mouche, J., & Pérez, P. (2004). Quantitative representation of reactivity, selectivity and site activation concepts in organic chemistry. https://core.ac.uk/download/288897646.pdf (accessed on 9 June 2025).
20. Demin, O., Goltsov, A., Goltsov, G., & Goryanin, I. (2010). *In silico* screening of nonsteroidal anti-inflammatory drugs and their combined action on Prostaglandin H Synthase-1. https://core.ac.uk/download/228176861.pdf (accessed on 9 June 2025).
21. Dence, J. B., Gray, H. B., & Hammond, G. S. (1968). *Chemical Dynamics.* https://core.ac.uk/download/4890307.pdf.
22. Deo, S., Dooley, K., Janik, M. J., & Rioux, R. M. (2020). *Influence of Metal Nuclearity and Physicochemical Properties of Ceria on The Oxidation of Carbon Monoxide.* https://core.ac.uk/download/650640332.pdf (accessed on 9 June 2025).
23. Dinda, R., Garribba, E., Sanna, D., Crans, D. C., & Costa Pessoa, J. (2025). Hydrolysis, ligand exchange, and redox properties of vanadium compounds: Implications of solution transformation on biological, therapeutic, and environmental applications. *Chemical Reviews.* https://www.semanticscholar.org/paper/8956deb6bc45bcb5316ec1abbe17af3a937a4c47 (accessed on 9 June 2025).
24. Domingo, L. R., Pérez, P., & Ríos-Gutiérrez, M. (2016). *Applications of the Conceptual Density Functional Theory Indices to Organic Chemistry Reactivity.* https://core.ac.uk/download/288909223.pdf.
25. Du Prez, F., Leibler, L., & Winne, J. (2019). *Dynamic Covalent Chemistry in Polymer Networks: A Mechanistic Perspective.* https://core.ac.uk/download/299792670.pdf (accessed on 9 June 2025).

26. Ebenhöh, O., Flis, A., Pokhilko, A., & Stitt, M. (2013). Adjustment of carbon fluxes to light conditions regulates the daily turnover of starch in plants: A computational model. https://core.ac.uk/download/29151105.pdf (accessed on 9 June 2025).

27. Frank, S. A. (2013). Input-output relations in biological systems: Measurement, information and the Hill equation. https://core.ac.uk/download/pdf/81921706.pdf (accessed on 9 June 2025).

28. Froment, G. F., Reis, F. D. A. A., Rice, S. A., & Mattos, T. G. (2009). Phase transitions and crossovers in reaction-diffusion models with catalyst deactivation. http://arxiv.org/abs/0906.3150 (accessed on 9 June 2025).

29. Gomes, J., Ho, S., Kawthekar, P., Liu, X., et al. (2017). Retrosynthetic reaction prediction using neural sequence-to-sequence models. http://arxiv.org/abs/1706.01643 (accessed on 9 June 2025).

30. Griffiths, P. E., & Stotz, K. (2017). Genetic, epigenetic and exogenetic information. https://core.ac.uk/download/131214859.pdf (accessed on 9 June 2025).

31. Guo, L. (1999). The synthesis and characterization of new higher unclarity arene-ruthenium-sulfur clusters (Master's thesis, Massey University, New Zealand). https://core.ac.uk/download/162617233.pdf (accessed on 9 June 2025).

32. Houk, K. N., Liu, P., Mackey, J. L., Pemberton, A., et al. (2020). Concerted [4 + 2] and stepwise (2 + 2) cycloadditions of tetrafluoroethylene with butadiene: DFT and DLPNO-UCCSD(T) explorations. https://core.ac.uk/download/323078702.pdf.

33. Hunter, K. H., Groenenboom, L. A., Farheen, A., & Becker, N. M. (2025). Student conceptualizations and predictions of substitution and elimination reactions: What are they seeing on the page? *Chemistry Education Research and Practice*. https://www.semanticscholar.org/paper/e16520665fef63b6990aa5a4052674fbbe4047a8 (accessed on 9 June 2025).

34. Isaacson, S. A., & Zhang, Y. (2018). An unstructured mesh convergent reaction-diffusion master equation for reversible reactions. http://arxiv.org/abs/1711.04220 (accessed on 9 June 2025).

35. Khan, B., Banzhaf, S., Chan, E. C., Forkel, R., Kanani-Sühring, F., Ketelsen, K., Kurppa, M., et al. (2021). Development of an atmospheric chemistry model coupled to the PALM model system 6.0: Implementation and first applications. *Geoscientific Model Development, 14*, 1171–1193. https://doi.org/10.5194/gmd-14-1171-2021.

36. Kholodenko, B. N., Peletier, M. A., & Westerhoff, H. V. (2002). Control of spatially heterogeneous and time-varying cellular reaction networks: A new summation law. https://core.ac.uk/download/301661846.pdf (accessed on 9 June 2025).

37. Kovalenko, I. L., Nalisko, M. M., Sobolev, V. V., Ustimenko, A., et al. (2018). The macro kinetics parameters of the hydrocarbon's combustion in the numerical calculation of accidental explosions in mines. https://core.ac.uk/download/288815745.pdf (accessed on 9 June 2025).

38. McElroy, M. (2025). Global change: A biogeochemical perspective. https://core.ac.uk/download/pdf/42850184.pdf.

39. Michalski, M., & Berski, S. (2025). Mechanistic pathways in cyanide-mediated benzoin condensation: A comprehensive electron localization function (ELF) and catastrophe theory

analysis of the umpolung reaction. *Molecules, 30*. https://www.semanticscholar.org/paper/a3ebf7daca74fda52f3485161fff0a2d414f226c (accessed on 9 June 2025).

40. Palierne, J. F. (2000). Rheothermodynamics of transient networks. http://arxiv.org/abs/cond-mat/0007368 (accessed on 9 June 2025).

41. Priami, C., & Zámborszky, J. (2010). BlenX-based compositional modeling of complex reaction mechanisms. http://arxiv.org/abs/1002.4065 (accessed on 9 June 2025).

42. Proppe, J., & Reiher, M. (2018). Mechanism deduction from noisy chemical reaction networks. http://arxiv.org/abs/1803.09346 (accessed on 9 June 2025).

43. Reiher, M., Simm, G. N., & Vaucher, A. C. (2018). Exploration of reaction pathways and chemical transformation networks. http://arxiv.org/abs/1810.07490 (accessed on 9 June 2025).

44. Reuter, K., & Wang, T. (2015). Structure sensitivity in oxide catalysis: First-principles kinetic Monte Carlo simulations for CO oxidation at RuO_2(111). https://core.ac.uk/download/532709023.pdf (accessed on 9 June 2025).

45. Rodrigues, A. E., Al-Rawashdeh, A., Alfieri, A., Berger, R., Berger, R., Cao, R., Damköhler, G., et al. (2013). *Regime Mapping and The Role of The Intermediate Region in Wall-Coated Microreactors*. https://core.ac.uk/download/9843918.pdf (accessed on 9 June 2025).

46. Said, S., Shutt, R. R. C., Zhang, Z., Lovett, A. J., Howard, C. A., & Miller, T. (2024). Electrochemical atomic force microscopy of black phosphorus composite anodes: Electrode destabilization and degradation mechanisms in alkali-ion batteries. *ACS Applied Materials & Interfaces, 16*, 43512–43525. https://www.semanticscholar.org/paper/93fc065aa29cfe6eeab8c08e9823ebd1cfd7b423 (accessed on 9 June 2025).

47. Snider, M., Reinhardt, L., Wolfenden, R., & Cleland, W. (2002). 15N kinetic isotope effects on uncatalyzed and enzymatic deamination of cytidine. *Biochemistry, 41*(1), 415–421. https://www.semanticscholar.org/paper/ce0069f6df24bae975b3a682724b4477598ddbdc (accessed on 9 June 2025).

48. Wang, H., Pei, X., Kalmutzki, M. J., Yang, J., & Yaghi, O. M. (2022). Large cages of zeolitic imidazolate frameworks. *Accounts of Chemical Research, 55*, 707–721. https://doi.org/10.1021/acs.accounts.1c00740.

49. Whittaker, A. G., Taflove, A. S. C. H., Abramovitch, R. A., Adam, D., Agostino, A., Agostino, A., Agostino, A., et al. (2013). *Modern Microwave Methods in Solid State Inorganic Materials Chemistry: From Fundamentals to Manufacturing*. https://core.ac.uk/download/16462397.pdf.

50. Yerien, D. E., Barata-Vallejo, S., Mora Flores, E. W., & Postigo, A. (2020). The role of photocatalysts in radical chains in homolytic aromatic substitution, radical addition to olefins, and nucleophilic radical substitution mechanisms. *Catalysis Science & Technology, 10*, 5113–5128. https://www.semanticscholar.org/paper/972c8cf771dfdced4dedf903fc1ce5744440d5e4 (accessed on 9 June 2025).

51. Zhu, Y., Liu, J., & Wang, B. (2025). Integrated approach for biomarker discovery and mechanistic insights into the co-pathogenesis of type 2 diabetes mellitus and non-Hodgkin lymphoma. *Diabetes, Metabolic Syndrome and Obesity, 18*, 267–282. https://www.semanticscholar.org/paper/302386608f989e99fa9f6be74acce02d1c378c75 (accessed on 9 June 2025).

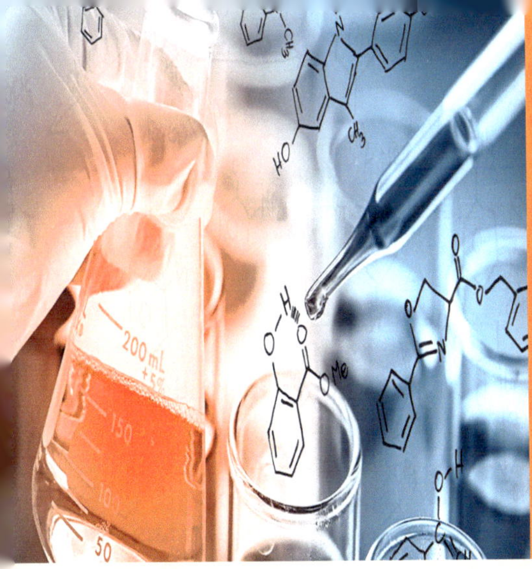

Chapter 4

MECHANISMS OF TYPE B REACTIONS

Contents

Introduction

The drug substances and bodily processes interaction will typically result in complex, pre-emptive responses, the most significant being adverse drug reactions (ADRs). This is especially so with Type B reactions, which are defined by their idiosyncratic pattern and unpredictability, compared to the predictable Type A reactions. Type B reactions occur regardless of dose and are not easily explained by the pharmacological effects of the drugs; hence, they are very challenging both clinically and research-wise. Drug-induced acute kidney injury (DI-AKI) is a typical example of such reactions wherein renal function is impacted to a significant degree by the combined effect of more than one nephrotoxic drug. Investigating such mechanisms has the potential to provide informative details concerning patient treatment and treatment regimens, as well as understanding the implications of patient outcomes, thus emphasizing the need to expand our understanding towards Type B reactions in the clinic (Garcia et al., 2024). Perhaps the most potent aspect of Type B reactions is their correlation with innate genetic and environmental factors that may predispose individuals to such reactions. Unlike Type A reactions, which are often preventable through dose reduction or careful medication management, Type B reactions require a more detailed examination of patient-specific factors. These include genetic polymorphisms that can interfere with the metabolism of certain drugs and leave patients susceptible to renal damage after exposure to environmental nephrotoxins. The multifaceted nature of these reactions underscores the importance of patient-specific treatment approaches that consider genetic determinants, enabling clinicians to better predict and manage the risks associated with specific drugs. This personalized medicine model is fundamental in avoiding the adverse impact of drugs responsible for DI-AKI and ultimately translates into patient survival and quality of life (Garcia et al., 2024). Moreover, the intrinsic complexity of Type B reactions also pertains to the variability in injury mechanisms that can occur, exhibiting a spectrum of phenomena worthy of close examination. These mechanisms can vary from immune-mediated responses or interactions that trigger inflammatory processes, illustrating how some patients develop a heightened susceptibility and react especially to specific drugs. For instance, the variability in response to drugs like Vancomycin is indicative of the stealthiness of DI-AKI, with certain patients facing significant problems others do not. Mapping these different tracks makes the multifactorial pathophysiology of Type B reactions understandable and emphasizes the urgency for further research and clinical observation. It enables the healthcare community to develop models that more accurately identify populations at risk and optimize therapeutic strategies, ultimately leading to improved patient outcomes in the care of acute kidney injuries (Figure 4.1).

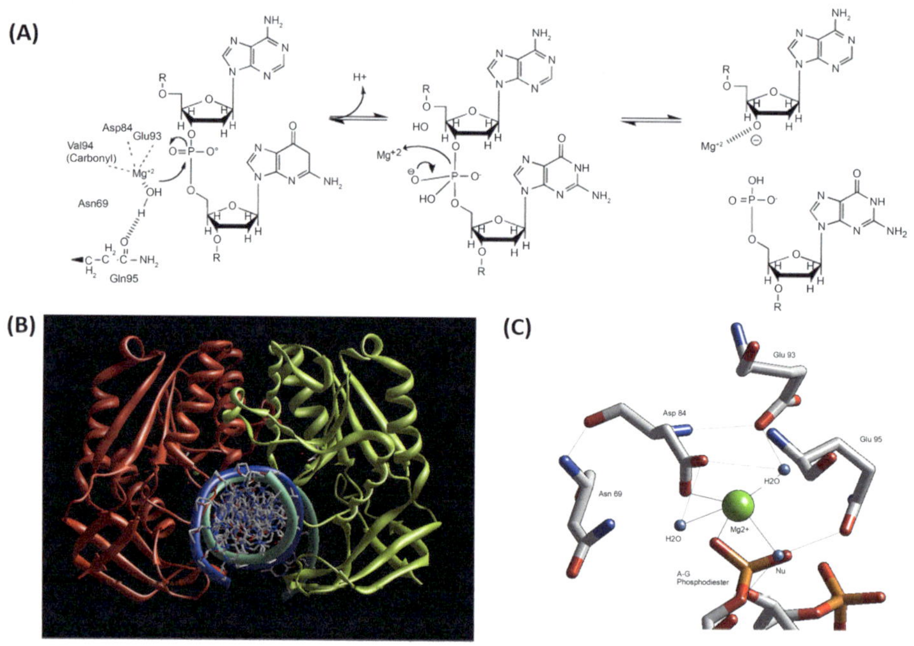

Figure 4.1. Mechanisms reactions.

Source: https://wou.edu/chemistry/files/2020/05/BglII.png.

Definition of Type B Reactions

Often, the detailed nature of biochemical reactions helps us understand how cellular functions are controlled. Type B Reactions are particularly notable for their specificity and efficiency, especially during heterocyclization reactions. The process involves constructing a cyclic structure from a linear building block, which is crucial for producing various natural products. Type B Reactions are used to point out how enzymes assist in creating a wide range of cyanobactin structures. Thus, to understand Type B Reactions, you must recognize their reaction type and also appreciate the important roles they play in the body. Type B Reactions can only be understood by considering their chemical process and biological importance. The reactions are usually carried out by enzymes that help convert substrate molecules in particular ways. For example, cyanobactin demonstrates how Type B Reactions handle amino acid residues, ultimately forming complex heterocycles. With this framework, enzymes like TruD can keep the substrate and catalyze different reactions one after another. Thanks to this specificity, the compounds are stable and active, allowing for more studies on their possible use in pharmaceuticals and biotechnology.

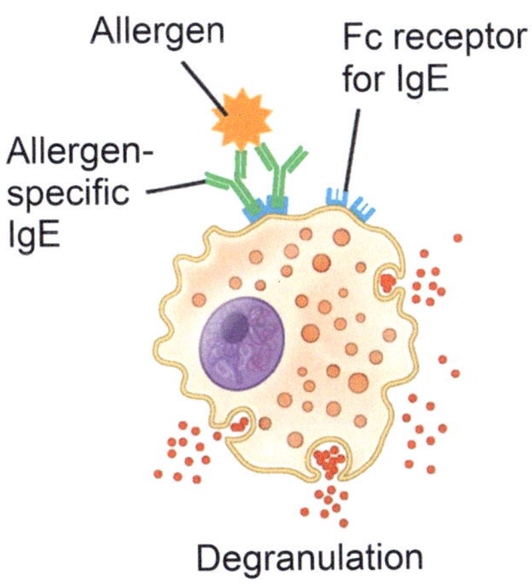

Figure 4.2. Hypersensitivity reactions.

Source: https://encrypted-tbn0.gstatic.com/images?q=tbn:ANd9GcR79S1SfWc7-jJxg1qraRYRYh4rmQwMi9IdIA&s.

Type B Reactions are significant in both synthetic biology and medicinal chemistry, not just in the field of science for its own sake. Experts are utilizing their understanding of these reactions to develop new drugs for medical use. Because Type B Reactions are both processive and specific, they facilitate the development of efficient methods for synthesizing complex molecules. Moreover, since these reactions do not cause harmful side effects, they increase the amount of product and are helpful in making new drugs and natural products. Now that scientists are constantly researching and revising our understanding of enzymatic reactions, Type B Reactions will likely make significant contributions to future discoveries and strengthen the connections between biochemical processes (Figure 4.2).

Importance in Chemical Reactions

In the intricate web of chemical reactions, the mechanisms of Type B reactions provide insight into the broader context of science. Type B reaction phenomena, which are predominantly classified according to their need for specific immunological pathways, demonstrate the intersection of biochemistry and pharmacology. This is notably the case in chronic rhinosinusitis (CRS), where crossing of the immune responses leads to diverse clinical manifestations. Endotype differentiation, for example, T2, T1, and T3, provides a fundamental understanding of how these reaction mechanisms induce physiological and therapeutic responses. Systematically exploring the pathways activated during Type B reactions enables scientists to devise targeted approaches that address the underlying causes of disease, rather than just its symptoms. Therefore, the importance of understanding these reactions extends beyond the academic arena and plays a crucial role in optimizing patient care and developing effective medical therapies in conditions like CRS (Klimek et al., 2025). Additionally, the use of chemical reactions in biocatalysis emphasizes their function in promoting environmental sustainability and the production of renewable resources. Investigating

Type B reaction mechanisms involves not only examining enzyme interactions but also the intricate webs that direct these interactions. An illustration of the degree to which complex biochemical pathways could be used to address pivotal global concerns, such as climate change, is the synergy of action of bacterial enzymes in lignin breakdown. Identification of the cooperative mechanism between enzymes, such as ligninases and their supportive counterparts, is a paradigm shift in biochemical studies. Understanding these processes enables scientists to develop more effective biomass conversion methods, thereby supporting an improved carbon economy (Liang et al., 2025). The ramifications of such processes are far-reaching beyond the laboratory setting to impact bioprocessing-dependent industries and environmental stewardship. Ultimately, the identification of Type B reactions represents a crucial area for advancing scientific research and treatment approaches. While research continues in the field of immunology, particularly about diseases with defective immune function, the possibility of precision medicine increases. The establishment of specific endotypes in disorders like CRS not only enhances personalized therapeutic approaches but also fosters an understanding of disease heterogeneity. Additionally, recognizing the mechanisms that support Type B reactions has implications for interdisciplinary cooperation and practice, thereby bridging the gaps between practice and theory. Interestingly, being in control of these chemical reactions has far-reaching implications, enabling scientists and clinicians to engineer new strategies towards optimizing patient outcomes. With the further growth of this field, the significance of Type B reactions will undoubtedly be a part of the advancement of both health and ecological conservation (Klimek et al., 2025; Liang et al., 2025) (Figure 4.3).

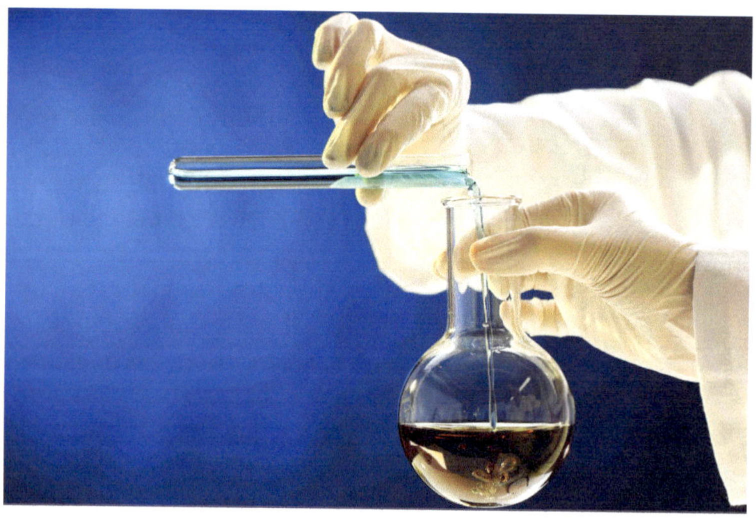

Figure 4.3. Chemical reactions.

Source: https://www.thoughtco.com/thmb/UeH0yjOI18KZ6K3EubTPIvlrISs=/3867x2578/filters:no_upscale():max_bytes(150000):strip_icc()/155006089-56a1327b3df78cf7726851bf.jpg.

Overview of Mechanisms

To understand how Type B reactions work in chemistry, one should examine their mechanisms, which highlight the detailed interactions among molecules and the transfer of energy. The way these reactions unfold is affected by many factors, including reaction kinetics and thermodynamics, which control the speed and extent of each process. Because there are many aspects to chemical systems, they can use different methods to produce products. Such studies demonstrate that many of these reactions involve specific transitional states, illustrating how molecules are rearranged as the reaction progresses. In addition, examining these transitional states helps us understand the reasons behind certain reaction pathways and their outcomes, which enhances our knowledge of reaction mechanisms.

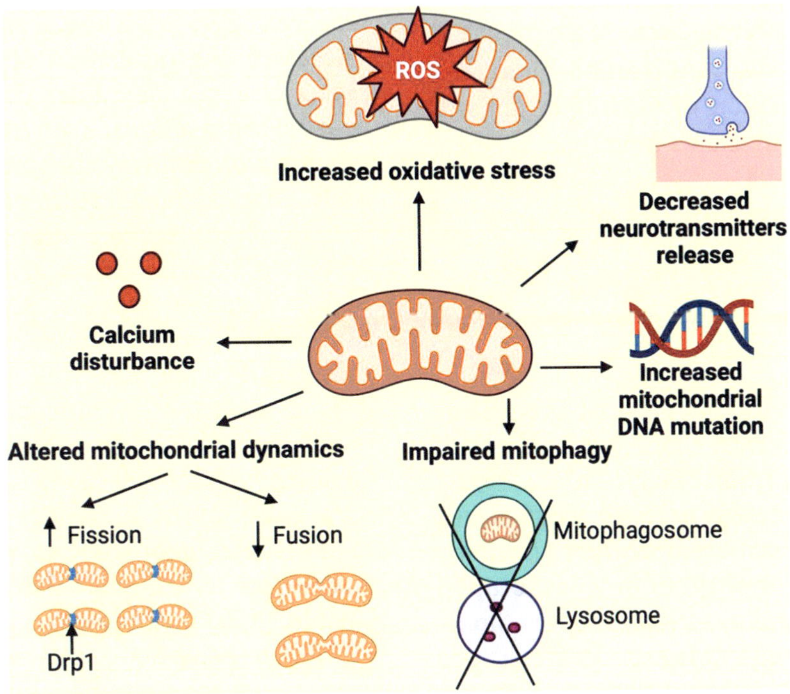

Figure 4.4. Overview of mechanisms.

Source: https://www.researchgate.net/publication/370180380/figure/fig1/AS:11431281249960573@1717735254405/Simplified-overview-of-mechanisms-associated-with-mitochondrial-dysfunction.tif.

An important thing to note about Type B reactions is that some happen directly, while others take a concerted pathway. Direct mechanisms involve reactants colliding and undergoing changes one after another, whereas concerted mechanisms involve several bonds changing simultaneously, facilitating the reaction's rapid progression towards the product. For instance, Oberhummer et al. (1994) discuss nuclear reactions proceeding through a direct mechanism and their implications for solar hydrogen burning, a vital process in stellar chemistry, ultimately contributing to our understanding of supernovae and the stellar lifecycle. In the same way, these rules apply to complicated organic reactions, where different intermediates, bond formations, and breakages occur simultaneously, resulting in a wide variety of end products in chemistry. Considering the structures involved and their effects on the reaction process adds more to our knowledge of Type B reactions. Recent experimental evidence highlights the significance of specific chemical structures, such as aliphatically substituted and bridged polycyclic aromatic hydrocarbons (PAHs), in the context of combustion environments. Using advanced techniques such as mass spectrometry, researchers have identified which small aromatic compounds are crucial for forming soot, thereby helping to explain combustion chemistry. As outlined by Adamson et al. (2018), these findings suggest that alkylated aromatics serve a dual purpose: not only as reactants in PAH growth but also as crucial intermediates in a network of reactions that govern soot nucleation. Therefore, a thorough examination of these mechanisms highlights their significance in various areas of chemistry (Figure 4.4).

4.1. Characteristics of Type B Reactions

The identification of Type B reactions involves considering their typical characteristics, which differentiate them from other reaction types. These reactions commonly exhibit a compounded interaction of factors, like temperature sensitivity and concentration-dependent reactants. Furthermore, Type B reactions are commonly dominated by their kinetics, exhibiting a complex interaction between activation energy and molecular dynamics. This is supplemented by difficulties of direct experimentation; it is tough to obtain macrokinetic parameters by trustworthy means due to the microscopic character of reaction zones, as quoted in by Kovalenko et al. (2018). Numerical experiments are hence applied in modeling such reactions to successfully review the complexity of explosive combustion, illustrating the velocity, pressure, and temperature gradients throughout the reaction. In Type B reactions, the rate-controlling mechanisms of the reaction often involve a distinct set of energy barriers to be crossed before product formation is feasible. Effective activation energy is a significant principle of learning about how reactions will proceed under varying conditions. For instance, where stationary-state reactions occasionally exhibit characterizable activation energy profiles, Type B reactions often demonstrate a high degree of sensitivity to external stimuli, such as shock waves and temperature changes. This is where dynamic modeling, based on the non-linear characteristics of gas dynamics typical in combustion phenomena, sets in, having been prioritized and pursued through research aggregated by Kovalenko et al. (2018). Therefore, the prediction of Type B reactions requires a robust model that allows for the proper representation of kinetic parameters and reaction pathways in practical applications. Another important feature of Type B reactions is their ability to take multiple pathways, out of which intermediates are created as part of the reaction process. Such intermediates can exert dramatic influences upon resultant products formed, and this is the reason why it is of essential significance to understand reaction networks as well as intrinsic kinetics. Such complexity will likely demand systematic investigations of reactivity patterns related to molecular geometry as well as electronic structures, as suggested in consideration of chemical dynamics. Besides, with better modeling techniques being sought by researchers, the goal is to construct simplified kinetic mechanisms that can be applied for real-world usage, such as predicting outcomes under emergency explosions in confined spaces, thus taking us closer to an understanding of the mechanisms of Type B reactions.

4.1.1. Reaction Conditions

The pathways of Type B reactions depend significantly on the reaction conditions that are set in place. Factors such as temperature, pressure, and concentration influence both the rate and the type of products formed during a reaction. For example, higher temperatures typically cause reactant species to become more active, which in turn accelerates reactions. Nevertheless, when these conditions are used, side products can form, which may reduce the efficiency and the final amount of the product. Having a good grasp of these conditions is crucial, particularly when conducting complex reactions that require accurate and predictable results, demonstrating their value in various industries and laboratories.

Besides the laws of thermodynamics, the stability of biological systems when conditions change can reveal important information about Type B reactions. The metabolic pathways of Escherichia coli and other organisms are highly resilient to changes in genes or environmental conditions. As noted by Almaas et al. (2007), these pathways can maintain functionality even in the presence of perturbations, a feature strongly tied to the maintenance of a balanced flux sum around key metabolites.

Thanks to this stability, it is clear that changes in reaction conditions can alter the distribution of fluxes and may have a bigger impact on the cell's ability to adapt than just the rate of the reaction. This aspect highlights the importance of maintaining balanced reaction conditions to achieve the desired metabolic results and prevent any harmful effects. The role of structure in catalysis adds complexity to understanding the conditions required for a reaction. Different facets of catalysts, exemplified in the kinetic Monte Carlo study of RuO_2 by Reuter et al. (2015), demonstrate how variations in surface structure can lead to differing reaction pathways, even under similar operational conditions.

As a result, the traditional belief that the structure of metals matters most is challenged, because specific features are now seen to play a bigger role than the metal's general structure. This research highlights that both the primary properties of catalysts and their surface activity should be considered when designing reactions, which helps advance our understanding of Type B reactions and their mechanisms (Figure 4.5).

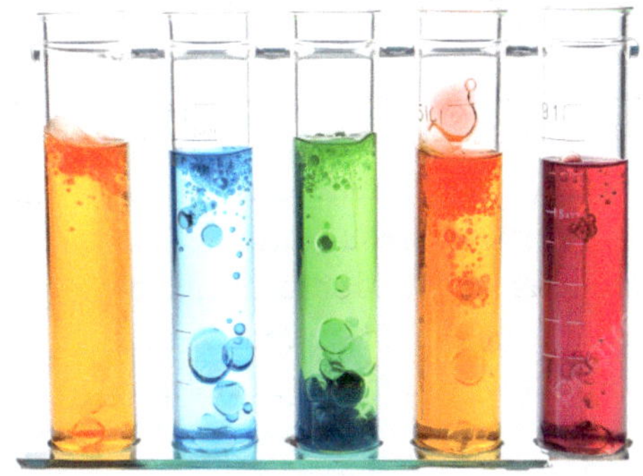

Figure 4.5. Chemical reaction.

Source: https://png.pngtree.com/png-clipart/20231016/original/pngtree-the-chemical-reaction-in-test-tube-png-image_13321931.png.

4.1.2. Reactants Involved

Understanding the intricate nature of Type B reactions requires an in-depth examination of the reactants involved in the process. For the case where specific hydrocarbons are under analysis, the combination of iso-octane and 1-hexene can serve as a sufficient illustration. Laboratory results determine that mixtures with 82% content of iso-octane and 18% composition of 1-hexene exhibit unusual patterns of reactivity, showing that the addition of 1-hexene leads to higher reactivity compared to the pure iso-octane. This deviation from anticipated behavior is crucial for understanding the low-temperature reaction mechanisms common to Type B reactions, as evidenced by the presence of cool flame effects and negative temperature coefficient zones. The ability to identify and study the dominant reactants, along with their corresponding interactions, thereby provides access to insightful interpretations of the intrinsic chemical mechanisms behind such processes and the energy profiles of these reactions (Barbé et al., 2006). As researchers explore the chemistry of Type B reactions further, the significance of reactant structure and reactivity cannot be overstated. The molecular structure of the reactants, such as naphthyl radical and vinylacetylene, at low temperatures can control reaction pathways and product formation. Laboratory experiments, as well as theory, have established that naphthyl radicals can create barrierless reactions to yield complex PAHs such as anthracene and phenanthrene. This highlights the reality that PAHs, being commonly associated with high-temperature environments, can be synthesized under milder conditions, hence opposing current presumptions in the area. Overcoming perceived constraints in this scenario not only deepens our understanding of Type B reactions but also highlights the importance of the multifaceted interactions that reactants can experience, thereby predicting the distribution of the final product's outcomes (Ablikim et al., 2018).

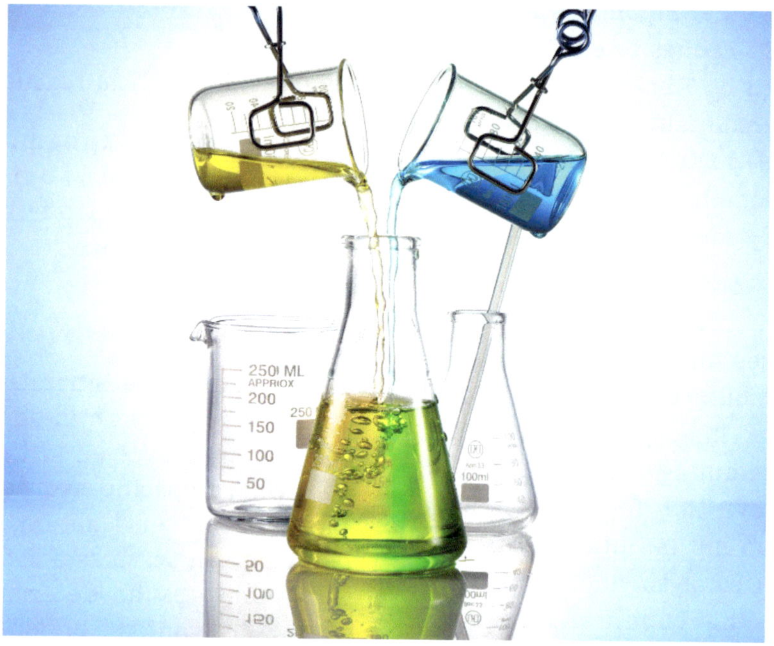

Figure 4.6. Limiting reactant of a chemical reaction.

Source: https://www.thoughtco.com/thmb/id_f2lgphtT4_IE0EwKePYdyvHY=/6572x5250/filters:fill(auto,1)/simple-experiment-58b5b3325f9b586046bbfa7f.jpg.

The knowledge obtained through the study of reactants that participate in Type B reactions has deep-reaching implications both theoretically and practically for chemical science applications. Through the disclosure of the roles of certain reactants and their interactivity, researchers can develop predictive models to account for reactivity under various conditions, ultimately informing synthetic strategies and optimizing industrial processes. In addition, understanding the processes involved in product formation from mixtures of different hydrocarbons enables the optimization of performance in fields such as fuel technology and environmental chemistry. An understanding of reactants, therefore, transcends mere scholarly interest; it is foundational to technological advancements in energy efficiency and environmental sustainability. The acquisition of information from such findings creates a clearer context for chemical reactions and widens the line of investigation into Type B reactions with new avenues for new developments that are scientifically and practically applicable (Figure 4.6).

4.1.3. Energy Changes

During chemical reactions, the way energy changes can give us interesting insights into the properties of matter. The changes mainly influence the way Type B reactions work in energy they cause. Such reactions typically exhibit significant changes in enthalpy and entropy, and the way energy is utilized during the reaction depends on whether it is input or released. The use of theoretical frameworks for energy transformations helps predict how quickly reactions will occur and what their equilibrium will be, which guides the development of more efficient industrial processes. A prime example is the role of hydrogen, an energy carrier characterized by high energy density, which impacts numerous applications from transportation to agriculture (Alia et al., 2024).

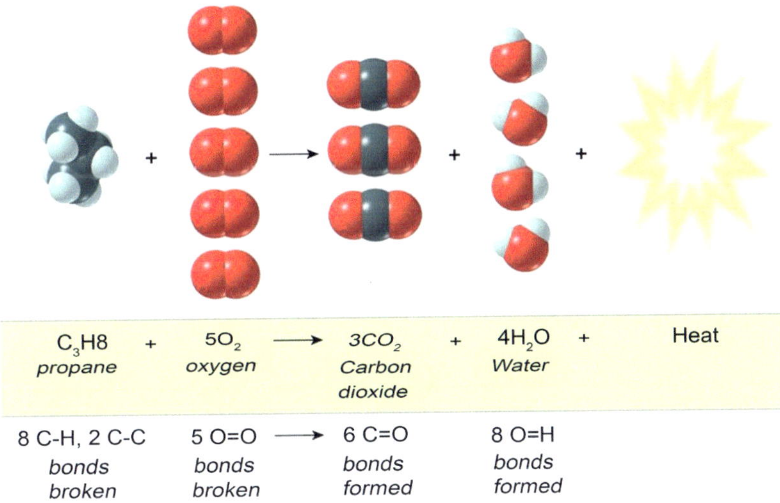

Figure 4.7. Energy changes.

Source: https://image1.slideserve.com/1563673/chemical-bonds-and-energy3-l.jpg.

Therefore, understanding energy changes in Type B reactions can help identify opportunities for improved and innovative approaches in reaction engineering. The processes involved in Type B reactions also have various changes in energy, especially when they cross from one state of matter to another. For instance, when exploring the catalytic degradation and efficiency of PEM water electrolyzers, it becomes evident that the choice of catalysts significantly influences the energy landscape of the reactions. The oxidation processes occurring at the anode and cathode, moderated by the presence of metal catalysts like iridium, affect both reaction kinetics and energy consumption (Alia et al., 2024). Additionally, the structure of catalysts can alter energy barriers, thereby influencing the pathways of chemical reactions. The performance of catalysts demonstrates both the challenges of chemical reactions and the vital role of materials science in enhancing a reaction's efficiency and lifespan. Furthermore, the close connection between the structure of materials and their energy indicates that any defects in crystalline materials are of great importance. An examination of how cavity defects in compounds such as 3-nitro-1,2,4-triazol-5-one (NTO) influence thermal decomposition illustrates this relationship vividly. By analyzing molecular dynamics, it is clear that the energy levels of intermediates and products are influenced by the amount of defects, providing a clearer picture of how degradation occurs under heat. The reaction rate can either decrease or increase at certain defect levels because the crystal structure plays a significant role in energy changes during Type B reactions. They help us better understand energy changes, which form the base for new strategies to boost material performance in reactive conditions (Figure 4.7).

4.2. Types of Type B Reactions

The intricate topography of Type B reactions is characterized by the diversity of mechanisms that facilitate the substitution and conversion of ligands in coordination complexes. This is underlined by the ligand substitution, which is central to the definition of the stability and reactivity of metal ion complexes. The process not only influences the kinetic character of the reaction but also the thermodynamic process. For instance, in a ligand replacement within an inner sphere complex, the accompanying changes might significantly affect the electronic nature of the coordination sphere. This type of change is representative of the dynamic character of coordination chemistry, where the stability of alternative configurations is constantly being questioned by external factors, i.e., the availability of alternative ligands and solvent effects, thus enabling various reaction routes to be manifested. Moreover, one of the most distinguishing properties of Type B reactions is the distinction between associative and dissociative mechanisms, wherein two distinct pathways regulate the ligand substitution process.

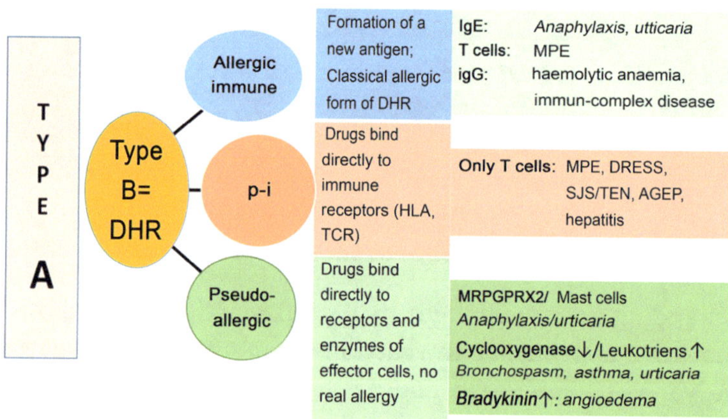

Figure 4.8. Types of type B reactions.

Source: https://www.researchgate.net/publication/331565445/figure/fig4/AS:11431281246357093@1716345674893/Classification-of-type-B-reactions-modified-from-10-Adverse-drug-reaction-are.png.

Associative processes commonly entail a concerted transition state wherein a more complex intermediate is developed prior to attaining the ultimate product. In contrast, dissociative mechanisms enable the release of the ligand before it can coordinate with a new ligand. The choice among these mechanisms is dictated by various parameters such as the electronic character of the metal center, the steric demand of the involved ligands, and solvent interactions. This binary aspect not only emphasizes the intricacy of ligand dynamics but further enhances our understanding of how metal ions are involved in intricate interactions on various substrates. Regarding Type B reactions, the role of the immediate environment in ligand substitution reactions becomes essential. For instance, changes in temperature, pressure, or solvent polarity will likely have a remarkable influence on the rate and efficiency of reactions. In addition, the presence of catalysts can facilitate such transformation by enabling lower activation energy options. The interaction between metal ions and ligands remains a dynamic subject of interest for scientists, particularly in areas such as catalysis and materials science. The investigation of Type B reactions, therefore, yields important information regarding the ensuing processes which dictate ligand action in polymeric systems, enhancing their applicability in both theoretical and practical research in coordination chemistry (Figure 4.8).

4.2.1. Substitution Reactions

Substitution reactions have a significant impact in organic chemistry. They include different methods where one part of a compound is replaced by another. Their importance is clear, as they are widely used in the production of essential substances, such as pharmaceuticals and agrochemicals, in synthetic chemistry. For instance, the Lewis acid-catalyzed Pudovik reaction exemplifies a robust substitution mechanism that facilitates the effective construction of phosphoric esters, compounds crucial for a myriad of applications, including their role in biological systems and clinical treatments (Keglevich, 2023).

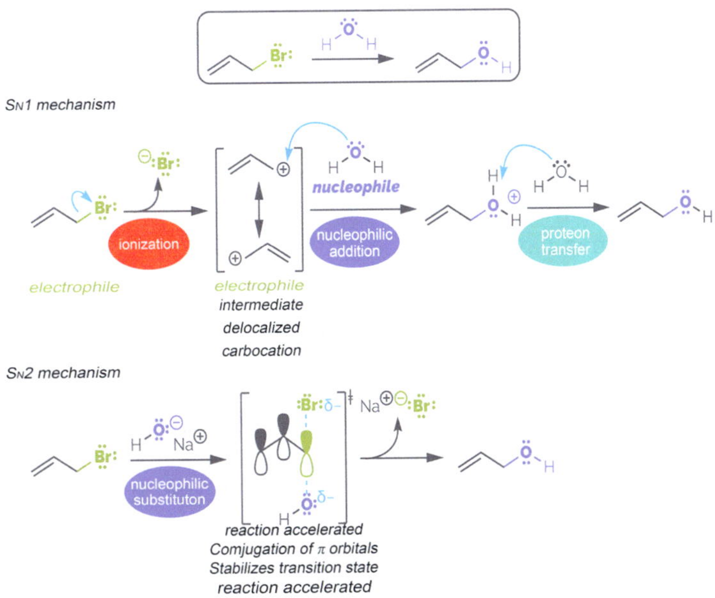

Figure 4.9. Substitution reactions.

Source: https://images.squarespace-cdn.com/content/v1/62185f3b81809a6fd03ddbb5/408007 7a-4516-4b43-ba9e-c56baa5325d7/Example5.png?format=1500w.

They demonstrate the significance of substitution in chemical science, as it helps both in learning and in practical chemistry. Moreover, these reactions are flexible and can be used to introduce various groups into molecules under different conditions. A special type of these reactions is ion-pair-assisted nucleophilic substitution, in which alkynyl trifluoroborates react rapidly with sp^3-carbon electrophiles. This approach can utilize inactivated alkyl triflates and propargyl methane sulfonates to produce products typically observed in Sonogashira-type reactions. The underlying mechanism reveals not only the necessity of a careful approach to electrophilic reactivity but also emphasizes the role of ion-pair organic complexes, as explored through computational chemistry and real-time NMR experiments, which elucidate the nature of the interaction during the substitution process (Liu et al., 2022). These findings demonstrate that nucleophiles play a crucial role in facilitating reactions to proceed efficiently. Additionally, the manner in which a reaction is carried out can significantly impact the products and their quality. Substitution will work well if the solvent, temperature, and the use of a catalyst are all set correctly. The Pudovik reaction demonstrates this point, as a Lewis acid catalyst significantly influences the reaction, enabling it to be applied to a wide range of substrates while mitigating the difficulties caused by sensitive functional groups. Better ways to adjust these parameters help produce more products and also lead to discoveries in synthetic organic chemistry. With knowledge of substitution reactions, chemists can utilize them to develop more complex and important substances, which aid in the progress of many scientific areas (Figure 4.9).

4.2.2. Elimination Reactions

In organic chemistry, the complexities of elimination reactions provide valuable insights into molecular behavior and transformation pathways. Various types of elimination, primarily categorized by whether they are of the unimolecular or bimolecular type, emphasize different mechanistic approaches to bond breakage and product formation. Unimolecular eliminations (E1) are typically a two-stage process in which the leaving group departs first, creating an intermediate carbocation. This entails a heavy reliance on the stabilization of the product cation, emphasizing the significance of factors such as substrate shape and solvent polarity in influencing reaction rates and product ratios. Conversely, bimolecular eliminations (E2) are concerted reactions that entail the breaking and making of bonds simultaneously and hence are susceptible to steric hindrance and the base employed. These mechanistic differences eventually determine the selection of conditions for desired outcomes in synthetic chemistry. Elimination reactions are not only theoretical but also have practical applications in various synthetic procedures. For instance, polyfluorinated aryl compounds tend to undergo elimination reactions, leading to useful intermediates in organic synthesis. Investigations into such reactions illustrate the versatility of polyfluorinated aryl alkynes and alcohols, which can be converted into crucial structural motifs of drugs and agrochemicals. Such transformations through elimination reactions provide a hint of their pivotal role in synthesizing intricate organic molecules. Additionally, the intricate mechanisms of these reactions can be elucidated by the necessity for chemoselective and regioselective outcomes, which necessitates an understanding of the underlying principles that control elimination reactions in developing efficient synthetic protocols. Furthermore, studies have enlightened new modes and conditions under which elimination reactions can be optimized for laboratory and industrial utility. Chapter analyses in more recent work indicate there are situations where noncovalent interactions are highly significant in dictating the direction of such reactions. For example, when a thermally activated monoprotonated species is contained within a macrocyclic cavity, drastic deviations from normal gas-phase behavior were reported, giving rise to competitive elimination processes. Such observations suggest that the environmental context, e.g., molecular encapsulation or solvent complexation, can significantly influence the elimination processes involved. Therefore, a critical understanding of elimination reactions supplemented with theoretical estimates and experimental evidence emphasizes the intricate interdependence of structural factors governing chemical reactions and encourages the design of synthetic methods (Liu, 2021; Moorthy et al., 2023) (Figure 4.10).

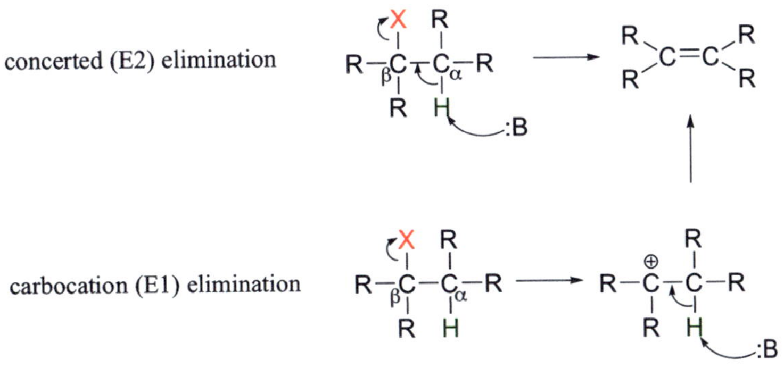

Figure 4.10. Elimination reactions.

Source: https://files.mtstatic.com/site_4334/3246/0?Expires=1747890420&Signature=GmoyFryEBTC-1ZUT17jLsqp~7bSL5FJNEHsfP-G~HGl1WWlrAlMxE2IiO0dtLf~WYKW9p51Z6vaq55GqlKgiBfGNu3mNK4KAZeUzld3v8Bn48ZI6ZkHJ0oTwY8FZ8wt2O5u5XKE2ymc7BYxAAKq06pesIlB6O6nmCKZlgYAD2yU_&Key-Pair-Id=APKAJ5Y6AV4GI7A555NA.

4.2.3. Rearrangement Reactions

Rearrangement reactions exhibit an interesting aspect of organic chemistry, particularly when examining the mechanisms of Type B reactions. These reactions usually turn a substrate into an isomer by moving atoms or groups inside the molecule, forming a new and stable structure. Epoxides are very flexible in rearranging reactions. For example, recent studies have revealed that PenF and AsqO enzymes help convert epoxides under biological conditions, changing the way complex organic transformations are performed. By promoting a cationic rearrangement that yields quaternary carbon centers, these enzymes provide insightful models for understanding rearrangement mechanisms, illustrating both nature's ingenuity and the potential for synthesizing complex structures from simpler precursors (Garcia-Borràs et al., 2017). Using this approach, studying the transformations of carbon systems gives more insight into rearrangement reactions. Molecular dynamics simulations have shown the way carbon clusters develop into fullerene structures. Simulations show that there are two steps: the first involves a transition to a hollow sp^2 shell, marked by a significant drop in potential energy. This change in structure highlights the role of temperature and energy, as well as the specific molecular interactions that drive these changes. During the critical moments leading to fullerene formation, the insertion of remaining carbon chains illustrates the complexity inherent in rearrangement reactions, providing a clear picture of the structural evolution involved in these processes (Knizhnik et al., 2017). Besides simply rearranging structures, these reactions are often crucial in creating new chemical compounds and devising innovative methods for their synthesis. Understanding the principles of rearrangement mechanisms, chemists can devise innovative methods to construct complex molecules with numerous useful functions. It is most noticeable in natural products and pharmaceuticals, since rearrangement reactions can help create a wide range of bioactive compounds from basic starting materials. Consequently, the interplay of enzymatic catalysis and synthetic chemistry in the study of rearrangement reactions not only elucidates the underlying principles of Type B reactions but also paves the way for advancements in synthetic methodologies, demonstrating the relevance and utility of these mechanisms in contemporary organic synthesis (Garcia-Borràs et al., 2017; Knizhnik et al., 2017) (Figure 4.11).

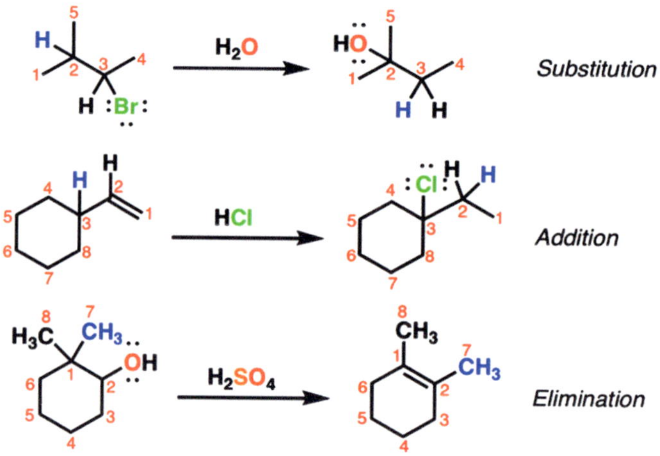

Figure 4.11. Rearrangement reactions.

Source: https://s11452.pcdn.co/wp-content/uploads/2019/12/5-three-examples-of-rearrangement-reactions-in-substitution-alkene-addition-and-elimination-reactions.gif.

4.3. Kinetics of Type B Reactions

The kinetic behavior analysis of Type B reactions reveals a complex interplay of reaction rates and concentration variations that are usually at odds with the accepted chemical rules. These reactions can exhibit nonlinear response properties that are better described using the Hill equation than the traditional Michaelis-Menten method, which is well-known in enzyme kinetics. This disparity can be attributed to taking into consideration the intricate dynamics of the biological systems, which tend to exemplify nonconstant input-output relations in the interactions between the subsystems, as highlighted in the application of biological input-output relations (Frank et al., 2013). For Type B responses, reactant and product agglomeration serve to impose order on the apparent disorder and eventually govern the observed kinetic behavior in these systems. Additionally, component aggregation plays a crucial role in understanding how Type B reactions evolve over time. The associated processes are not standalone, as they interact dynamically with other biochemical pathways, affecting the global efficiency and regulation of metabolic processes. Structural constraints surrounding such interactions play a significant role in determining the effect that a change in substrate concentration has on reaction velocities. Therefore, emergent order in the kinetics of Type B reactions can be accounted for through the systemic nature of these biological inputs and outputs, which integrate data from across subsystems to characterize their aggregate behavior. All of these features are at the heart of understanding how enzymes function under various environmental conditions, significantly influencing reaction performance and efficiency. The implications of these kinematic patterns extend far beyond scholarly interest; they are critical to our understanding of evolutionary fitness and flexibility. Because biological shape generally adheres to the shape established by fundamental kinetics, natural selection tends to favor organisms that can manage their enzymatic processes successfully within these firm limits. Since responses tend to follow detectable scaling patterns of reaction, the identification of such dynamics provides a foundation for inferring how evolutionary pressures shape biochemical pathways over time. The marriage of kinetic analysis and the theory of evolution thus yields a coherent mechanistic framework for describing the mechanisms of Type B reactions, demonstrating the influence of structure and process in determining biological function and diversity (Frank et al., 2013). Further studies of these responses hold the promise of yielding significant advances in biotechnology and medicine, thereby expanding our knowledge of the intricacies of life (Figure 4.12).

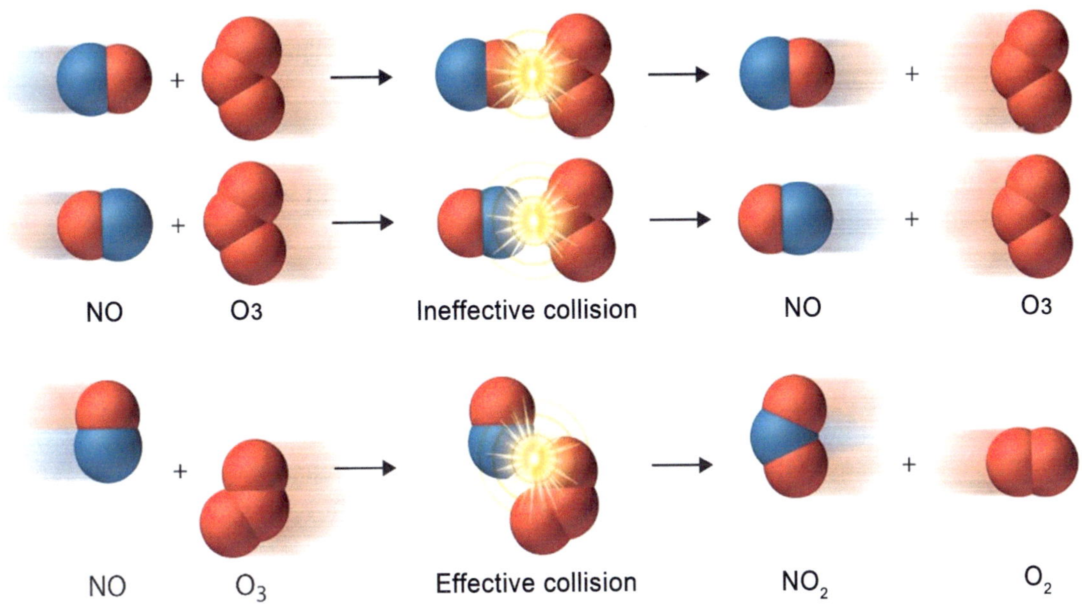

Figure 4.12. Chemical kinetics.

Source: https://files.mtstatic.com/site_4334/49924/0?Expires=1747892084&Signature=W3I007dIu7BY5Z8T3AXDCUSMl1sIYSooM71HgSUsmaeaCLTdVGTXjTX98MhJZvlojANIyYHJL6A5rpdUuYEkCc83AH-mY--RxUhCh7xQ7vMZ9j3mWx0bjguIInQVxe8Nc505KImsxVnRyZEhcSkULJ-Fciif1SpLinfPlr1qipU_&Key-Pair-Id=APKAJ5Y6AV4GI7A555NA.

4.3.1. Rate Laws

Since Type B reactions are complex, it is essential to understand rate laws thoroughly, as they are the primary descriptors of their kinetics. They explain how the levels of reactants in a system influence the rate at which a reaction occurs, providing important insights into biological processes. In Type B reactions, rate laws can vary significantly due to the presence of enzymes, the concentrations of each substance, and environmental conditions. Importantly, scientists use Michaelis-Menten kinetics to discuss enzymatic reactions and determine how changes in substrate amounts influence the speed of the reaction. This ability to forecast events demonstrates the importance of having accurate rate laws for modeling dynamic processes in both biochemistry and physiology. Upon closer examination, the selection of a rate law can have a significant impact on modeling metabolic pathways. Michaelis-Menten and similar laws give a convenient and effective way to understand how enzymes react in Type B reactions. It has been found in recent studies that the accuracy of these models depends on the accuracy of their parameters, which represent biological facts. The study demonstrated that using enzyme parameters in the rate law yielded results comparable to those of the actual process, highlighting the importance of accurate parameterization in developing kinetic models. Conversely, ignoring important biochemical details often leads to incorrect predictions, so it is crucial to identify rate laws that are easy to use yet capture the complexity of biochemical networks. Additionally, examining various rate laws helps us gain a deeper understanding of how metabolic processes are regulated. Some studies have found that using rough rate laws can still give helpful information about Type B reactions, primarily when the amount of substrate is well controlled. In some cases, when there is sufficient substrate, simpler models may be sufficient to predict the reaction, eliminating the need for complex explanations. The ability to adapt demonstrates that using rate law approximations is effective, especially in large-scale modeling, where efficiency is crucial. Nevertheless, the findings highlight a more nuanced perspective, suggesting that detailed mechanistic approaches often enhance prediction accuracy when adequate data are available, thereby providing a comprehensive framework for future research in enzyme kinetics and metabolic pathways (Bordbar et al., 2016; Pinto et al., 2017).

4.3.2. Factors Affecting Reaction Rates

In the intricate world of chemical reactions, several critical factors significantly dictate the rates of these reactions, largely influencing Type B reaction mechanisms. Temperature is one of those key factors that play an important role in reaction dynamics. As temperature increases, the kinetic energy of molecules also rises, leading to more frequent and intense collisions between reactant particles. This elevated activity increases the likelihood of overcoming the activation energy barrier required for reactions to occur, thereby accelerating the overall reaction rate. Lower temperatures tend to slow reaction rates as molecular motion is slow, with reduced frequency of collisions and lower accessible energies for successful interactions among reactants. Hence, temperature control can be an economically viable step in optimizing reaction kinetics in Type B mechanisms, indicating its inherent importance in chemical reactions. The reactant concentration also turns out to be a crucial step that affects the rate of reaction, particularly in Type B reactions where the interaction among species is of utmost relevance. Higher concentrations of reactants tend to lead to higher frequencies of collisions, which subsequently increase the likelihood of reactions taking place. This is elucidated by collision theory, which stipulates that the rate of reaction goes up with increased concentration of reactants because the greater the number of particles in a volume, the greater the chances of colliding with one another. Furthermore, for electrochemical devices such as electrochemiluminescence devices (ECLDs), electrolyte concentrations have been observed to influence both electron transfer kinetics and reactant mass transfer, which are also at the core of the mechanisms powering these models. Thus, control of reactant concentrations is a method of effective regulation of reaction rates. The second important factor in calculating reaction rates is how catalysts affect them. Catalysts are chemicals that significantly enhance the rate of reaction without being consumed in the reaction process. Catalysts provide an alternative pathway for reactions, where the activation energy threshold is lower than that of the reaction without a catalyst. Such an alteration ensures a higher number of effective collisions within a given time span, thereby accelerating the rate of reaction. In Type B reactions, the presence of a suitable catalyst can have dramatic consequences, such as enabling complex biochemical pathways that otherwise would be too slow to be viable. The application of catalysts offers a route to more efficient processes for reactions, underlining the intrinsic significance of catalysts to the kinetics of chemical reactions. Thus, it is of utmost importance that anyone learning about the mechanisms of Type B reactions and their uses learn about catalyst behavior (Figure 4.13).

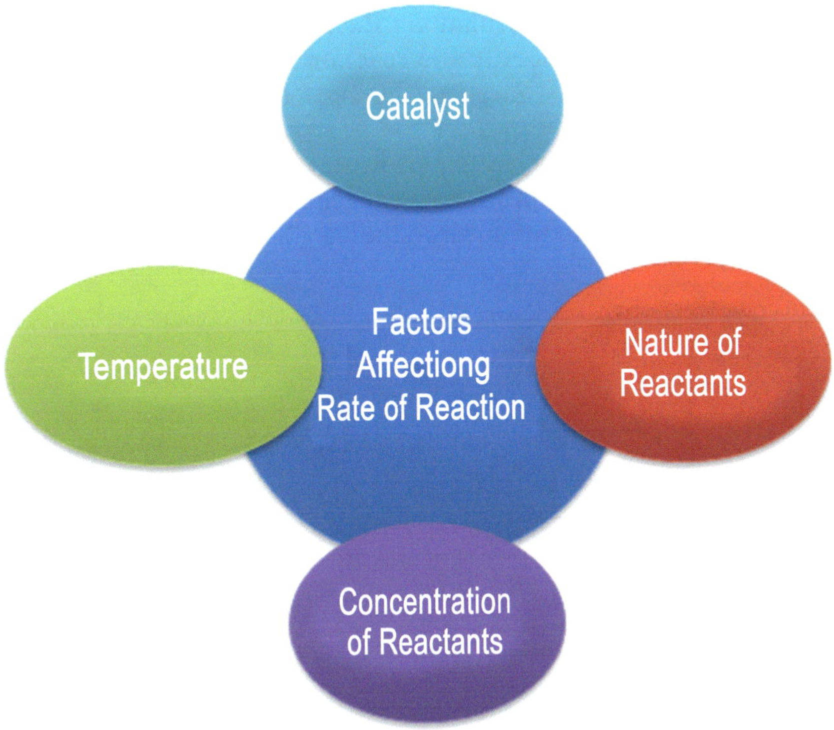

Figure 4.13. Factors affecting reaction rates.

Source: https://images.saymedia-content.com/.image/t_share/MTc0NjM5MTYzODk4MDEzNjg2/chemical-reactions-and-chemical-equations.png.

4.3.3. Experimental Methods for Kinetic Studies

To explore Type B reactions, scientists must employ robust techniques that are capable of revealing the details of how reactions occur. Many studies utilize well-stirred reactors because they maintain a uniform reaction environment, allowing researchers to accurately set the temperature and concentrations. Scientists can use experiments to determine how chemical kinetics influences the course of reactions by varying the equivalence ratios and inlet temperatures. It is necessary to use this controlled setting to separate each reaction, so their impact on the whole process can be thoroughly examined. In addition, combining computational simulations with experimental findings helps to explain reaction mechanisms in greater detail than can be seen solely through experimentation. During recent investigations, monitoring changes in reactant and product concentrations is crucial for analyzing kinetics. According to studies on methane oxidation at different dilution levels, measuring the mole fraction shows the connection between reaction rates and how stable the system is. Examining these states by analyzing production rates and sensitivity reveals the importance of specific recombination reactions. When researchers determine which reactions are responsible for ignition and extinction, they can design more accurate kinetic models. Thorough investigations are necessary to understand Type B reactions and to determine how temperature and concentration impact the entire reaction process. More progress in understanding Type B reactions has been made through bifurcation analysis, which explains how the system can become unstable and exhibit oscillations. By studying the temperatures at which unstable solutions occur, scientists can determine the conditions that encourage oscillations during hydrocarbon combustion. The technique enables the observation of multiple states in the reaction system, as demonstrated in studies on the oxidation of heavier hydrocarbons. Altering the strength of recombination can significantly impact the system's stability, and this can alter the occurrence of oscillations. Importantly, such investigations into the kinetic behaviors in experimental settings significantly contribute to the broader understanding of combustion processes and chemical kinetics, shedding light on their complexities and providing directions for future studies (Pinto et al., 2017; Battin-Leclerc et al., 2020) (Figure 4.14).

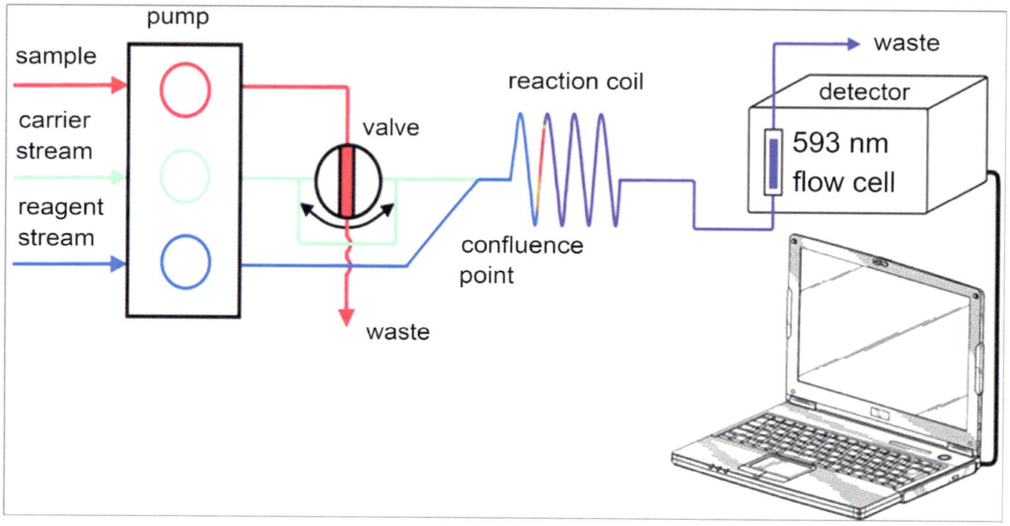

Figure 4.14. Experimental methods for kinetic studies.

Source: https://cdnintech.com/media/chapter/40717/1512345123/media/image64.jpeg.

4.4. Mechanistic Pathways

The intricate nature of biochemical interactions necessitates a deep understanding of mechanistic paths, particularly in Type B reactions. The study of molecular interactions illustrates how these paths control the activity of biological systems under varying conditions. For instance, Type B reactions typically involve enzymatic activity that regulates metabolic pathways, illustrating the responsive nature of cell behavior. As such responses continue, they can establish a cascade of events that influence not only metabolic rate but also the organism's generalized physiological state. The interconnectedness of these pathways underscores the need for identifying key regulatory points that can serve as therapeutic targets in disease controlled by metabolic dysregulation. A critical examination of Type B reactions reveals a correlation between certain mechanistic pathways and disease states, such as Type 2 diabetes mellitus (T2DM). Existing evidence suggests that immune-mediated pathways significantly contribute to the co-pathogenesis of type 2 diabetes mellitus (T2DM) and non-Hodgkin lymphoma (NHL) (Zhu et al., 2025).

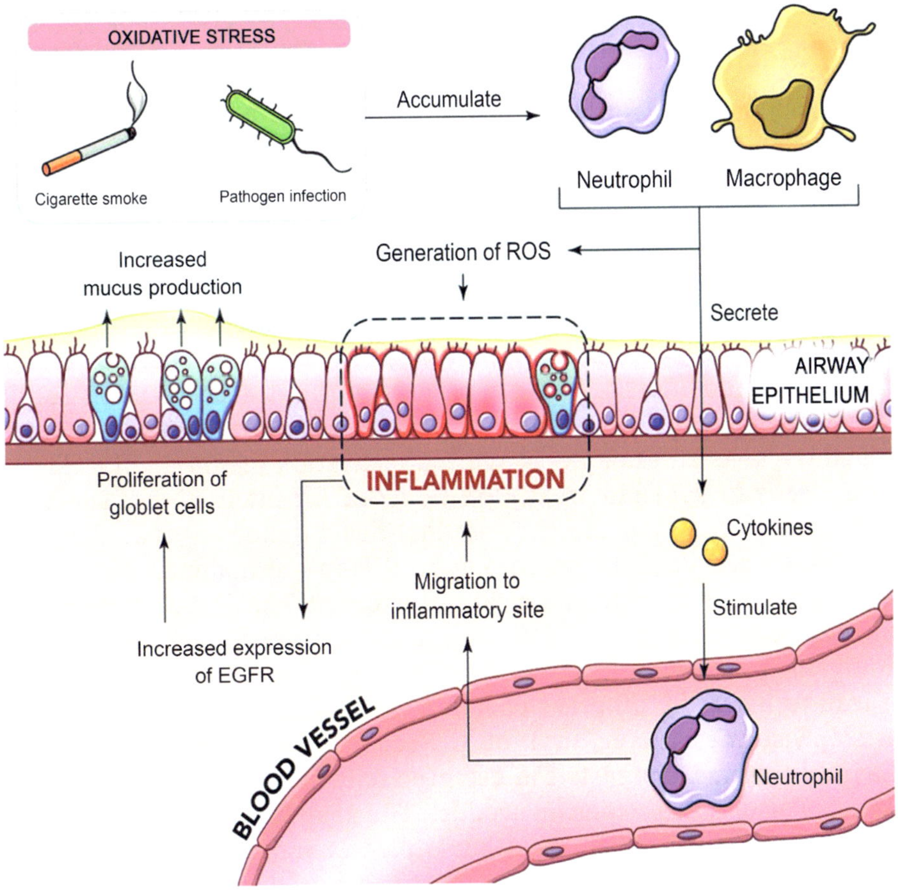

Figure 4.15. Mechanistic pathways.

Source: https://www.mdpi.com/biomolecules/biomolecules-10-00144/article_deploy/html/images/biomolecules-10-00144-g003.png.

Analyzing overlapping biomarkers of the two diseases enables scientists to define the manner through which disrupted metabolic processes result in multiple health outcomes. This intersectional approach enables the identification of hub genes that can illuminate the mechanistic pathways underlying the simultaneous onset of these diseases. The identification of mechanistic pathways provides us with essential information about how metabolic disorders are interconnected and with ramifications for clinical intervention. The evolution of chemical processes, such as the cyanide-type umpolung reaction, provides a clear example of mechanistic pathways at work. A detailed analysis reveals that benzoin condensation proceeds through various transition state geometries, with the reaction dynamics involving the formation of large intermediates (Michalski et al., 2025). The evolution of electron density in the reactions reflects the complex nature of bond formation and molecular stability. Scientists can determine dynamic electron framework changes through topological analysis to gain a comprehensive understanding of reaction mechanisms. These findings not only enhance our understanding of individual response profiles but also contribute to our overall understanding of how mechanistic pathways direct the development of new chemical methods and therapeutic regimens (Figure 4.15).

4.4.1. Stepwise Mechanisms

It is clear from studying Stepwise Mechanisms in Type B Reactions that the process typically occurs in separate stages, allowing for the control of the reaction's progression. Thanks to this, chemists are able to make reactions that can be adjusted to achieve particular results. One intriguing manifestation of stepwise mechanisms is evident in the synthesis of cerium oxide nanoparticles (CeNPs). The synthesis of antioxidants and prooxidants depends on the conditions used, which can lead to significant variations in their activities. Adding polyvinylpyrrolidone in steps yields nanoparticles with different oxidation states. This variability influences their catalytic properties, as evidenced by the enhanced peroxidase-mimicking activity of PVP-CeNPs-Pts, highlighting the importance of structural modifications that evolve throughout each reaction step (Nadiia et al., 2025). Based on the compounds that participate in these reactions, they can either promote or hinder specific pathways. As an example, in thermal activation of supramolecular assemblies, the outcome's chemoselectivity depends greatly on noncovalent interactions. The DBOA complexed with b-cyclodextrin study clearly demonstrates this idea by showing that the protonated DBOA undergoes collision-induced dissociation in a typical stepwise manner. However, when similar interactions occur within the macrocyclic cavity of cucurbit[7]uril, the pathway shifts to involve a stepwise homolytic bond cleavage. Here, the reaction mechanism not only reflects the influence of the surrounding environment on reaction dynamics but also illustrates how subtle changes at each stage can lead to markedly different chemical behaviors (Moorthy et al., 2023). Going into more detail on stepwise mechanisms in Type B Reactions shows how they work effectively in complicated chemical systems. Chemists can use precise control at every stage to create reactions that yield better rates or produce a specific product. The analysis of CeNPs and their catalytic roles demonstrates that stepwise mechanisms can be applied in various fields, including biochemistry and material production. The various actions and features of each intermediate in a pathway enable scientists to develop new ideas in nanotechnology and biochemistry. Such investigations not only expand the understanding of reaction dynamics but also open avenues for future research into more efficient catalytic systems, exemplifying the profound significance of stepwise mechanisms in advancing chemical sciences (Nadiia et al., 2025).

4.4.2. Concerted Mechanisms

The complexity of concerted mechanisms is at the core of the structure of Type B reactions, where bonding and bond-breaking take place in a single transition state. This aspect of concerted mechanisms diverges strongly from stepwise mechanisms, which may yield intermediates that can stabilize or destabilize the overall reaction course. In particular, concerted mechanisms are characterized by increased reaction efficiency, resulting in cooperative transition-state stabilization. For instance, zeolite catalysis exhibits the stabilization effects of the zeolite framework, demonstrating how local environments prefer concerted pathways. Based on studies, the transition state stabilization, facilitated by zeolite confinement of the reaction intermediates, results in lowered activation energies and consequently improved reaction kinetics (Cabral et al., 2018). This is a particularly significant effect to examine in light of structural variability between different zeolites. Exploring the mechanistic details of concerted processes provides additional insight into electron density distributions that are crucial in determining reactivity and selectivity. The concurrent interactions in concerted processes are described by the quantum theory of atoms in molecules, whereby electron density analysis provides a transparent operational background. By mapping electron distribution and interaction, researchers can differentiate between confinement and interaction energies that contribute comparatively to catalysis. Notably, the concerted bonds that are formed in zeolite reaction sequences provide a classic example of how cooperation can result in desirable reaction outcomes. In this case, the synergy between interacting species, such as the multicoordinated methyl cation—is indicative of the role played by concerted interactions in facilitating the efficient overcoming of activation barriers within catalytic landscapes (Cabral et al., 2018). Unlike solely concerted processes, Type B reactions illustrate the delicate balance between transition state stabilization and reaction selectivity in acid-catalyzed processes. The acid catalysis observed in transformations, including the conversion of sugars to furans, demonstrates how the reaction routes can be influenced by both Brønsted and Lewis acid activation. Since high-efficient yields of key intermediates are most critical, the combined processes that follow in these context-rich reactions must be studied as a whole. Studies confirm that understanding how reactants and solvents behave in different catalytic conditions can significantly contribute to simplifying such processes. Through studies of such interactions, chemists can harness concerted mechanisms in a manner that minimizes byproducts and maximizes desired reaction products, recalling the profound effects of catalytic environments on Type B reaction behavior (Figure 4.16).

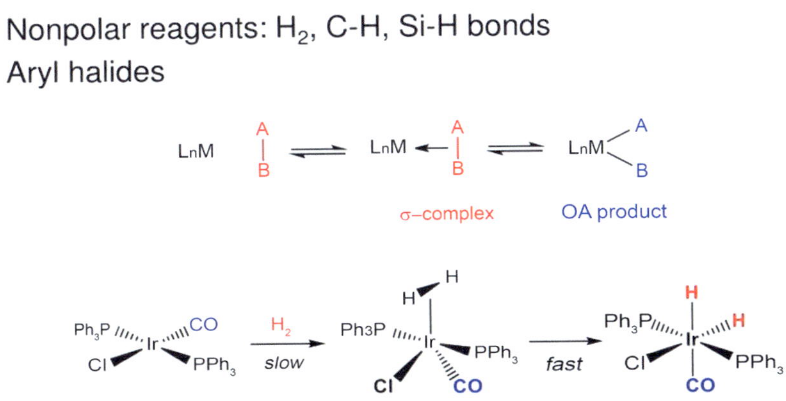

Figure 4.16. Concerted mechanisms.

Source: https://image2.slideserve.com/4751306/concerted-mechanism-l.jpg.

4.4.3. Role of Catalysts

The presence of catalysts significantly affects the details of how reactions happen, mainly in Type B reactions. Many times, catalysts enable reactions to occur at mild temperatures or pressures that would be required otherwise. They do more than increase speed; they target specific processes to make the desired products more efficiently. For instance, alumina surfaces exemplify this phenomenon, serving as support materials that contribute to the synthesis of environmentally persistent free radicals (EPFRs) through their active Lewis acid–base sites. These sites interact with substrates to create different reaction pathways leading to EPFR formation, which contrasts starkly with the pathways that would dominate in the absence of a catalyst (Altarawneh et al., 2023). The structure of the catalyst's surface plays a significant role in determining the reactions, underscoring the key role of catalysts in influencing the outcomes of chemical reactions. Organic synthesis using new methods often depends on the important role of transition metal catalysts. A good example is found in the synthesis of complex polycyclic compounds, which typically involves numerous different reactions. Recent research has highlighted the effectiveness of homogeneous gold(I) catalysis in facilitating cascade reactions that synthesize multiple bonds in a single step. They demonstrate how a catalyst is vital since it helps create complex structures from basic building blocks. Mechanistically, the gold(I)-catalyzed processes rely on the formation of Novas bonds through strategic rearrangements and interactions with substrate molecules (Semleit et al., 2020). This demonstrates that catalysts play a crucial role in organic chemistry reactions, as they affect both the rate and the mechanism of the reaction. Besides making processes more efficient, catalysts also have an effect on the environment. Especially, EPFRs that develop on surfaces, such as alumina used in catalysts, show their catalytic effects and also raise concerns about environmental pollution. When chemists know how radicals are formed, they can come up with ways to reduce the creation of pollutants. Using catalysts wisely, researchers can ensure that harmful by-products are minimized and the main chemical products are increased. The ongoing exploration in this area promises to yield further insights into how catalyst-enhanced pathways can lead to sustainable methodologies in chemistry, ultimately contributing to both academic scholarship and practical applications in environmental science (Altarawneh et al., 2023). Because catalysts play a key part in reactions and society, they are essential to current chemical research (Figure 4.17).

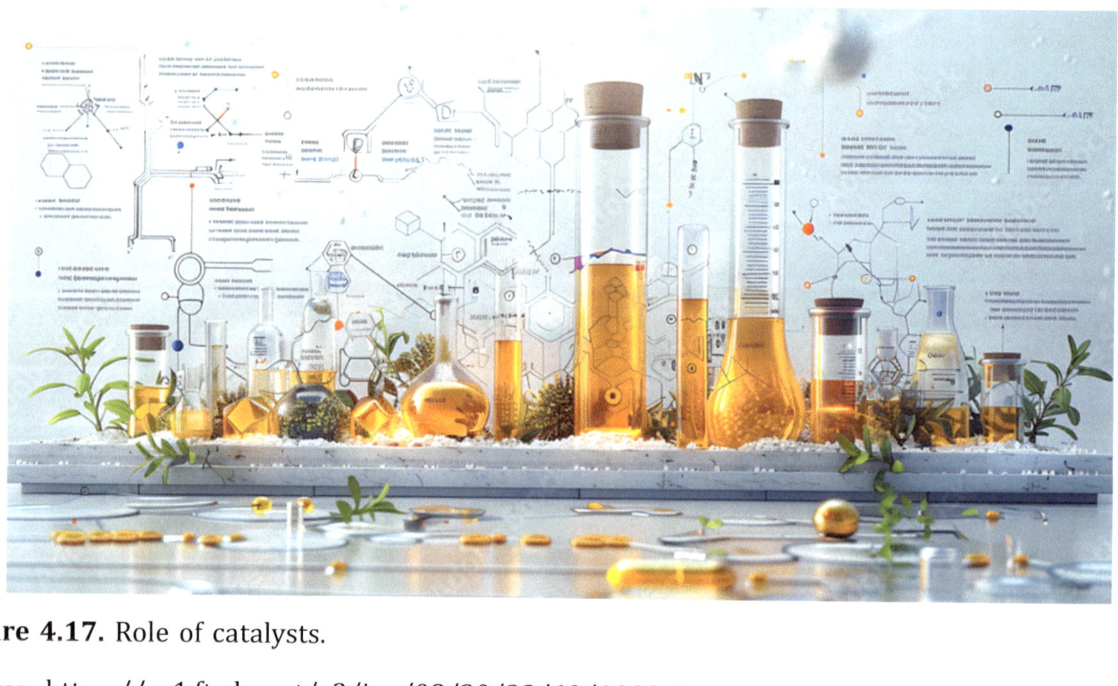

Figure 4.17. Role of catalysts.

Source: https://as1.ftcdn.net/v2/jpg/08/30/33/60/1000_F_830336044_3OaXGfTBAaEKQzrtt2fhHEcNBO3Nfoyo.jpg.

4.5. Applications of Type B Reactions

In exploring the broad applications of Type B reactions, a range of key chemical reactions of importance to various domains of synthetic chemistry and materials science is identified. The reactions typically involve the transformation of substrates through mechanisms that facilitate the rearrangement of bonds, enabling the creation of new compounds with defined properties. For instance, in the chemical industry, Type B reactions allow chemists to design and synthesize complex molecules that serve as active pharmaceutical ingredients in medication. The ability to control molecular structures via such reactions makes such reactions highly important in drug development, where accuracy and efficiency are paramount. As the demand for new materials and therapeutic agents becomes increasingly pressing, Type B reactions remain invaluable as part of producing cutting-edge solutions in the chemical sciences. Among the numerous advances that have resulted from Type B reaction knowledge, the integration of computational tools has revolutionized applications in industrial chemistry. Use of algorithms in searching reaction networks enables intermediates to be recognized as well as prediction of reaction paths, with the ultimate optimization of reaction conditions. Such computational techniques vary in heuristic dependency as well as completeness, according to recent research that discusses numerous algorithmic strategies for searching chemical networks (Reiher et al., 2018). By combining the capabilities of technology with the mechanisms of Type B reactions, scientists can make a dramatic improvement in production rates and resource utilization in the industry. This integration of computer and chemical science represents a paradigm shift toward increasing the economic feasibility and sustainability of chemical processes, and aptly demonstrates the practical applications of Type B reactions in modern science. The existing research on Type B reactions offers opportunities for cutting-edge research and innovation in various fields. In environmental chemistry, for example, understanding the mechanistic models of Type B reactions can be applied to develop effective remediation techniques for pollutants. By uncovering the route and intermediates in biodegradation, chemists can engineer systems to catalyze the breakdown of poisonous compounds (Pinto et al., 2017). Similarly, advances in Type B reactions guide the development of green chemistry principles, which seek to minimize environmental impact while maximizing security and efficiency in chemical production. Encouragement for incorporating Type B reaction mechanisms into holistic approaches to study enhances their potential as driving forces not only of chemical research but also of sustainable practices aligned with global environmental goals.

4.5.1. Synthesis of Organic Compounds

Examining the various ways organic compounds are synthesized in Type B reactions highlights the complexity of biochemical reactions and the role of environmental factors involved. Glycine and methylamine, found in meteorites, are good examples of organic molecules that prompt us to question how they formed outside of Earth. The production of these compounds depends on the number of precursor molecules and the level of processing they undergo in their host bodies. Researchers can use isotopic analysis to understand how they were formed and to spot the effects of processes from outside the solar system, suggesting that many of these routes happen in places and conditions unlike those in laboratories. Therefore, understanding these varied conditions is essential for developing a comprehensive understanding of organic compound synthesis in diverse environments (Aponte et al., 2025). In Type B reactions, metabolic pathways can give important clues about how organic compounds are made. Metabolism is structured in a way that allows us to understand better how chemicals are changed in the body. Research on metabolism explains that the use of recurring substances in cellular structures results in a wide range of reactions in organisms. They work together to facilitate the complexity of organic reactions by utilizing conserved enzymes and cofactors to aid in these reactions. The belief that core metabolic functions are modular suggests that these pathways are significant for the whole process of biosynthesis. Consequently, exploring the modular aspects of metabolism not only elucidates organic synthesis but also hints at the evolutionary trajectories that influence biochemical organization (Alberts et al., 2012). Type B reactions in organic chemistry also enable us to discuss the effects that various environmental factors can have on the course of reactions. Observations of meteoritic compounds demonstrate that changes in temperature, pressure, and chemical composition can yield significantly different outcomes in organic reactions. It shows that the environment in which a reaction takes place can limit organic synthesis and affect the amount and kinds of products produced. By understanding these influences, chemists can develop new approaches to synthesizing organic chemicals and gain a deeper understanding of how organic molecules form and persist in the environment. Through elucidating these dynamic interactions between environment and synthesis pathways, researchers can refine their approaches to chemical innovation (Aponte et al., 2025) (Figure 4.18).

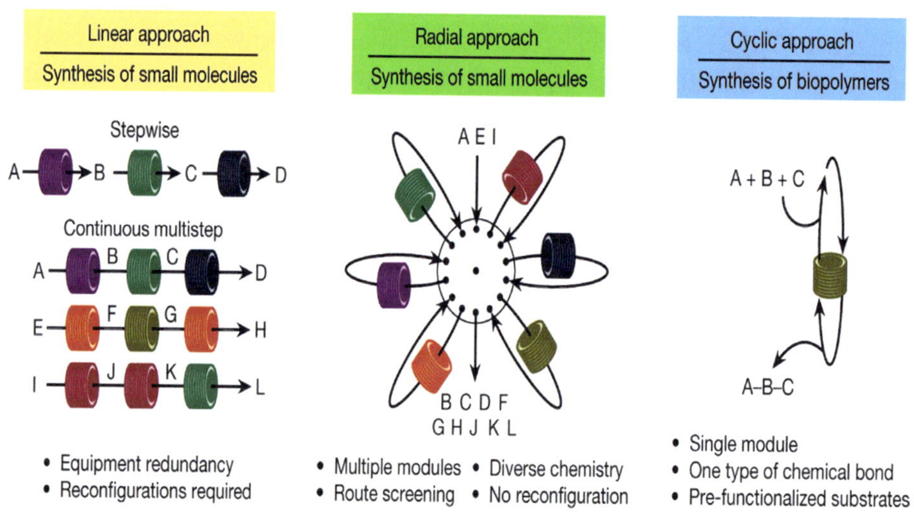

Figure 4.18. Synthesis of organic compounds.

Source: https://media.springernature.com/full/springer-static/image/art%3A10.1038%2Fs41586-020-2083-5/MediaObjects/41586_2020_2083_Fig1_HTML.png.

4.5.2. Industrial Applications

The search for efficient and sustainable industrial applications is increasingly governed by the advancement of chemical reactions, particularly Type B reactions. Type B reactions, which are commonly found with their unique mechanisms and conversions, present cogent opportunities for innovation in materials science, particularly in the development of luminescent materials. A thrilling demonstration of this is in the application of boron-nitrogen (B-N) compounds, with their phenomenal electronic structures that are perfectly suited for application to organic light-emitting diodes (OLEDs) and other electroluminescence technology. The synthetic pathways leading to these compounds tend to depend on Friedel-Crafts-type reactions, highlighting the forefront position of Type B mechanisms in the creation of light technology. Due to ongoing efforts committed to enhancing synthesis techniques and enhancing luminescent efficiency, B-N compounds are an indispensable component in the present evolution of optoelectronic applications and possess the groundbreaking ability in Type B reactions (Lin et al., 2024). Another significant route for industrial applications involves the reduction of greenhouse gases to valuable chemicals, and Type B reactions provide new avenues for carbon utilization. The electrolysis of CO_2 to carbon monoxide (CO) is a prime example, as it is the convergence of sustainability and chemical engineering. Toshibas work on developing low-temperature zero-gap type CO_2 electrolysis cells demonstrates the practical applications of these Type B reactions. With proper design, scientists have overcome efficiency and stability challenges by ensuring that bulk electrolysis cells can perform as well as their miniaturized counterparts. Such development not only facilitates conversion of CO_2 to valuable chemical feedstocks but also provides the gateway to a circular economy, closing the gap between industry operations and carbon neutrality as well as sustainability goals (Fujiwara et al., 2023). The controllability of parameters for Type B reactions has direct implications for the operational stability of industrial processes, which is crucial for commercialization. For instance, in the case of CO2 electrolysis, the pressure and humidity of the cathode are among the parameters of highest significance in addressing common stability issues, such as flooding and salt deposition. A mechanistic strategy toward managing these conditions can lead to extended lifetimes of operation, as proof of the validity of mechanistic understanding in real environments. Moreover, the research validating a consistent performance over extended periods demonstrates the sustainability of employing such electrolysis systems on a large scale. As industries place greater importance on green practices, the judicious application of Type B reactions is likely to continue delivering revolutionary outcomes, maximizing efficiency and ecology in various industries (Fujiwara et al., 2023).

4.5.3. Biological Significance

Because radiation affects the body in many ways, it is essential to understand how Type B reactions are regulated. High linear energy transfer (LET) radiation, for instance, exhibits markedly different biological effects compared to low LET radiation, leading to significant implications for cellular integrity and organismal health. The difference is very clear in the damage to biochemical structures in cells, which can become severe and sometimes irreparable after exposure to high-LET radiation. The variations observed in biochemistry are significant because they ultimately lead to damage to cells and organs. Such nuances are necessary for comprehending not only the immediate impacts of radiation but also the long-term consequences of exposure, particularly in contexts such as cancer therapy and radiobiological assessments (Wiley et al., 1972). Further study of biology reveals that Type B reactions involve multiple layers of information processing for growth and the transmission of traits from one generation to the next. In this situation, genetic inheritance helps send information that is important for cellular functions. Still, the role of epigenetics brings a new element to the study of biology. The latest discussions in evolutionary biology indicate that both epigenetic and exogenetic inheritance play important roles in development. These mechanisms function in tandem with traditional genetic inheritance, providing deeper insight into how traits are expressed and how organisms adapt to their environments, thereby highlighting the multifaceted nature of biological information, which is essential in assessing Type B reactions (Griffiths et al., 2017). Studies of biological significance also include the ways in which evolution is affected, primarily through the use of proximate and ultimate biology. Proximate biology examines the immediate causes of development and heredity, and information is crucial in these areas. On the other hand, ultimate biology examines the evolutionary reasons behind these mechanisms, serving as a link between rapid biological changes and the slow process of evolution. It clarifies how genetic, epigenetic, and exogenetic systems interact to explain Type B reactions. Therefore, grasping these concepts becomes essential not only in the study of radiobiological phenomena but also in appreciating the broader implications of biological inheritance and adaptation in evolving organisms (Griffiths et al., 2017).

4.6. Challenges in Studying Type B Reactions

In exploring the complexity of Type B reactions, a range of problems emerges that may hinder overall comprehension. The primary challenge is identifying all intermediates and elementary steps involved in these reactions. The complexity of such reactions, typically involving multiple channels and a potential for numerous side reactions, renders mechanistic investigation challenging. Since the researchers are trying to map such networks, the demand for definite identification can lead to issues, particularly in trying to identify key intermediates that are short-lived or unstable. Without sufficient certainty regarding the full spectrum of intermediates, any inferences made about reaction mechanisms may end up being deficient or misleading. Thus, a robust methodology is needed to accurately capture these aspects for the advancement of the Type B reaction field and to render findings credible and actionable. Algorithmic approaches have been proven to be significant tools in exploring reaction network complexity, yet with possible detriments. Whereas these methods can carry out investigations and yield data systematically well, their variation in scope of application and exhaustiveness creates complexities for researchers. For instance, some chemical approaches may involve great use of heuristics and excessive use of human input, leading to incomparable outcomes. Additionally, the performance of such algorithms can be variable, which has an impact on the overall investigation rate for Type B reactions. As such, the application of automated techniques must be closely scrutinized, so that a well-balanced mix of human knowledge and chemical heuristics can be established to enhance knowledge. These factors underscore the need for future studies to leverage the expertise of both computational approaches and human intuition in reaction mechanism studies (Reiher et al., 2018). Furthermore, physical sophistication in designing experiments is crucial to understanding the mechanisms of Type B reactions. The experimental complexities that arise from performing experiments with the same accuracy as these reactions can complicate data interpretation and introduce possible sources of error. In an attempt to replicate conditions likely to induce Type B responses, investigators face the challenge of regulating external variables, such as temperature, pressure, and concentration. Thus, inconsistency in experimental outcomes can conceal embedded patterns and interrelations fundamental to the understanding of reaction mechanisms. Overcoming physical constraints of this nature through careful experimental design, coupled with advances in technology, can provide more tangible insight into Type B reaction dynamics. With progress in the discipline, it will become essential to give high importance to the coordination of sound experimental techniques with computational approaches in solving these questions and unraveling the mechanisms of Type B reactions (Pinto et al., 2017).

4.6.1. Complexity of Reaction Mechanisms

The complexity in reaction mechanisms stems from the numerous reactants and the intricate ways in which they transform into products. In Type B reactions, the complexity is evident, as several pathways can occur, and slight changes in the environment can lead to different outcomes. The way observed products appear can be misleading, as many intermediate species and dynamic balances may be involved. For instance, research indicating the significance of aliphatically substituted and bridged PAHs provides a case in point; the structural intricacies revealed through advanced mass spectrometry elucidate a web of interactions facilitating PAH growth and soot formation in combustion environments (Adamson et al., 2018). The fact that these compounds react at so many points to the main idea that chemical complexity depends on molecular structure, which determines how they react and what they form. Going further into biochemistry, signal transduction in cells is a good example of how reaction mechanisms can be more complicated. Cells react to many outside signals through complex signaling systems, which use different receptors to cause different effects in the body. Different receptor activations can lead to various intracellular signaling pathways, showing how complex biochemical reactions can be. Because molecular interactions are not fixed, the environment and the amount of reactants can change the course of the reaction. With BioNetGen, rule-based modeling enables the study and understanding of how different signals interact within a cell. By systematically addressing such complexities, researchers can gain a deeper understanding of the specific pathways activated and their implications for cellular behavior (Faeder et al., 2017). Additionally, because Type B reactions are complex, it is necessary to employ various analytical methods to fully comprehend their processes. Such complexity is often understood by using advanced modeling to visualize and predict the results of reactions in various situations. With these techniques, it is possible to uncover pathways that are difficult to detect in regular experiments. The interactions leading to the formation of larger, bridged aromatic hydrocarbons, as highlighted by studies in combustion contexts, illustrate just one example of how modeling can claw back the layers of abstraction surrounding complex reactions (Adamson et al., 2018). With the help of both theory and experiments, researchers are able to understand the steps in chemical reactions better and relate them to the observed facts (Figure 4.19).

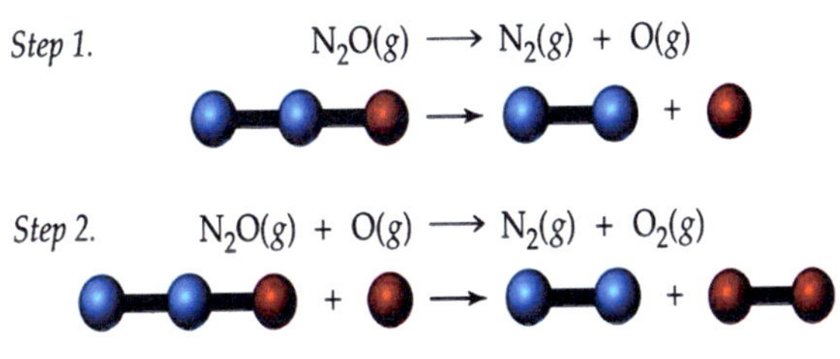

Figure 4.19. Reaction mechanisms.

Source: https://slideplayer.com/slide/13794232/85/images/6/Reaction+Mechanisms+Determine+the+overall+reaction%2C+the+reaction+intermediates%2C+and+the+molecularity+of+each+individual+elementary+step.jpg.

4.6.2. Limitations of Current Models

The inherent complexity of Type B reactions generates a critical need to discuss our current models and understanding, particularly in relation to their implications for the development of sustainable processes. Recent advances highlight several key areas where current paradigms are lacking, particularly in regard to electrochemical reactions. Despite the long history of scientists employing electrochemical pathways to split water into hydrogen and oxygen, the inefficiencies of such reactions constrain their application. Current models fail to account for the complexities of catalysts explicitly designed to stabilize reaction intermediates, thereby preventing optimization for effective water-splitting reactions, which in turn impact the effectiveness of subsequent reactions, such as CO_2 reduction (Seh et al., 2017). This implies that existing theories must evolve to accommodate for the advanced dynamics in multi-electron and proton transfer reactions across Type B mechanisms. In the field of photocatalytic CO_2 reduction, the limitations of current models are gratefully apparent. For example, considerable progress has been made in identifying materials suitable for CO2 conversion; however, the dominant focus remains on a limited list of semiconductor nanoparticles. This narrow focus misses the multidimensional character of materials like indium oxide, which possess unique surface properties conducive to photocatalysis. Furthermore, the oversimplification of reaction mechanisms hinders our understanding of the complexity of interactions between CO2, the catalyst surface, and light absorption (Laura et al., 2014). Therefore, failure to incorporate such complexity leads to a misestimation of photocatalytic performance and an inaccurate realization of the active sites needed for the efficient production of solar fuel. This gap thus calls for revolutionary approaches in model development that can address the intricate nature of Type B reactions. Additionally, current theoretical models tend to overlook the environmental factors under which the photocatalytic reaction occurs. For effective use of Type B reactions, conditions such as temperature fluctuation and efficacy in CO_2 capture must be factored into current models. Research shows moderate temperature variations can significantly enhance the activity of photocatalysts, but existing models assume constant conditions that rarely happen in real life (Laura et al., 2014). Such environmental variations are not accounted for, and thus predictions regarding the viability and scale-up of solar fuel technology are inaccurate. Thus, an overarching paradigm shift to more adaptable and holistic modeling is required to transcend our current constraints of knowledge regarding Type B reaction mechanisms and pave the way towards sustainable chemical solutions.

4.6.3. Need for Advanced Techniques

New findings about Type B reactions have demonstrated the need for advanced methods in both research and clinical work. Typically, traditional approaches to studying biochemical processes do not adequately explain the details of intermediates and the kinetics of reactions. The growth of nanomedicine demonstrates that modern technologies enable doctors to control drug delivery with greater precision, thereby enhancing the effectiveness of therapeutic agents. When nanotechnology is used, therapies can be designed to target specific cells or tissues, thereby enhancing the success of treating chronic diseases. By integrating these methodologies, researchers and clinicians can better elucidate the nuances of Type B reactions, ultimately leading to more reliable and successful patient outcomes through enhanced diagnostic and therapeutic strategies (Patra et al., 2018). Moreover, the advent of sophisticated data management tools such as the Cambridge Structural Database (CSD) has revolutionized the accessibility of structural information crucial for understanding reaction mechanisms. The repository collects a vast amount of data on crystallography, which helps scientists study the interactions and pathways of reactions in Type B reactions. With this database, it is easier to find connections between the structure of molecules and their reactions, which helps predict the results of chemical reactions. With the help of detailed structural data and experimental findings, researchers can predict how a reaction will occur. As the CSD continues to evolve, its role in bridging gaps in our understanding of complex reactions will become increasingly vital, highlighting the necessity for advanced techniques in chemical research (Colin et al., 2016). The importance of such new approaches is very high, especially as biochemical research starts to focus on more detailed systems. Since Type B reactions are difficult to predict, it is essential to employ advanced methods to gain a deeper understanding. With the aid of new imaging and modeling technologies, scientists can observe and manipulate reactions at the molecular level. They support our understanding of Type B reactions and also facilitate the discovery of new drugs and personalized treatments. By fostering a multi-disciplinary approach that encompasses both advanced biophysical techniques and cutting-edge materials science, the scientific community will be better positioned to tackle the complexities inherent in biochemical mechanisms (Colin et al., 2016; Patra et al., 2018).

Summary

While studying Type B reactions, it has become clear that the way reactants and conditions affect the outcome is very complex. These reactions depend on realizing that temperature, pressure, and certain catalysts can have a significant impact on the way and speed at which reactions occur. This understanding affects many areas, including both industrial chemistry and environmental science. Investigations have shown, for instance, that the composition of reactive mixtures can significantly impact their reactivity and efficiency, as demonstrated by studies examining iso-octane and 1-hexene mixtures, which showcased distinctive low-temperature behavior in their reaction profiles (Barbé et al., 2006). Therefore, the lessons learned from Type B reactions play a crucial role in facilitating the progression of chemical reactions. In addition, the classification of indications for leucoreduction reveals three main categories for evaluating the success of these treatments. The categorization distinguishes between evidence-based indications, those substantiated by robust data, and those supported by observational studies, as well as those of undetermined efficacy (Barbé et al., 2006). By using this approach, it is clear that using evidence is vital in both hospitals and research labs when dealing with possible adverse reactions to blood transfusions. Making the link between theories and real-world applications enhances the safety and effectiveness of transfusion medicine. Additionally, these classifications are useful in directing future studies, allowing new research to build upon existing knowledge and also address unresolved issues. To sum up, looking at the mechanisms of Type B reactions points out how complicated they are and also how important they are in different fields. As people continue to explore the fundamental elements of these reactions, the opportunities for new applications increase significantly. For example, gaining insight into how temperature and pressure interact in certain reactions can enhance the design of synthetic pathways in organic chemistry. Similarly, clarifying the mechanisms underlying leukocyte reduction can lead to improved transfusion practices and patient outcomes (Bianchi et al., 2015). Ultimately, enhancing our understanding of Type B reactions is crucial for advancing both theoretical models and practical applications, thereby facilitating the field's progression toward one centered on science and medicine.

The detailed structure of biological systems gives us helpful information about Type B reactions. Such reactions typically contradict the standard models that biochemistry has established. Although it is often assumed that processes follow Michaelis-Menten kinetics, numerous studies have found that the Hill equation provides a better description. This difference in findings suggests that more complex processes are at work than those described by the Michaelis-Menten theory. By examining these discrepancies, we can gain a deeper understanding of how biological systems function and adapt, revealing a tapestry of interactions, regulations, and feedback loops that govern Type B reactions and their contributions to broader biological phenomena (Ebenhoeh et al., 2013). Understanding how Type B reactions work mainly depends on studying the aggregation processes in biological systems. Even though there is disorder at the molecular level, the interaction of these components usually produces outputs that have regular patterns. The process of aggregation helps unite different parts of the body to give consistent reactions to the environment. It is worth noting that the Hill equation pattern, unlike traditional kinetics, can be explained through the principles of aggregation, measurement, and scaling. It becomes clear from this how the structure of a cell helps control the processes in the body. Thus, the dynamics of Type B reactions can be better appreciated when viewed within this framework, illustrating the intricate balance between order and disorder in biological design (Frank et al., 2013). All in all, a comprehensive study of Type B reactions requires an understanding of the primary rules that govern biological input-output connections. The combination of aggregation, exact measurement, and different views on scale explains the factors that control these reactions. While evolving, biological systems are influenced by both the biochemical processes occurring within them and the broader structures established through their interactions with the environment and various components. With this knowledge, we see that Type B reactions are crucial and that biological systems can adjust and thrive in various conditions. Hence, a complete analysis of these mechanisms provides valuable insights into natural selection and the evolution of complex life forms (Ebenhoeh et al., 2013; Frank et al., 2013).

CLOSER LOOK

LOW-TEMPERATURE REACTION MECHANISMS

At temperatures well below ambient (from a few hundred down to ~10 K), chemical reactivity enters a fundamentally different mechanistic regime: instead of the familiar Arrheniustype slowdown with falling temperature, many radicaldriven reactions proceed with little or no temperature dependence—or in some cases, they even speed up—because they occur over **barrierless** or gently sloping potentialenergy surfaces, becoming effectively **collisional complexes** that react as soon as they form; for instance, both laboratory CRESU experiments (using Laval nozzles to reach T ≈ 10 K) and theoretical masterequation analysis show that **$OH + O_2$, CN + NO**, and similar radical–neutral processes often retain high bimolecular rate constants even down to tens of kelvins. In particular astrochemical kinetics of **$O + OH \rightarrow H + O_2$** have been simulated using hyperspherical quantum dynamics, predicting a nearly constant rate coefficient from 10–39 K—matching highresolution measurements—underlining the role of **quantum mechanical tunneling** and longrange attraction in cold environments. Similarly, studies of **$OH + H_2$** on cold ice surfaces (~ 60–80 K) reveal reaction rate constants that plateau at low T consistent with an **atomtunneling pathway**, along with large kinetic isotope effects that illuminate reaction bifurcations even when classical energy barriers would otherwise halt reactivity. In oxygenated volatile organic compound oxidation—central to polar tropospheric and nighttime chemistry—the mechanistic web includes unimolecular **RO_2 (peroxyradical) hydrogen shifts**, **Criegeeintermediate rearrangements**, and pressuredependent branching that emerge only at low T or low NO_x regimes; the **automated Reaction Mechanism Generator (RMG)** has played a vital role in identifying such pathways across large compound libraries, although uncertainties in barrier heights produce large rate uncertainties at < 250 K. Theoretical methods have had to adapt too: standard Arrhenius extrapolation often fails in the lowT regime, and alternative approaches using **loweigenvalue expansions**, full **masterequation simulations**, **variational transitionstate theory**, and explicitly **nonBorn–Oppenheimer dynamics** are required to capture pressure and energytransfer effects that dominate at cold temperature. In sum, lowtemperature reaction mechanisms—whether in cold planetary atmospheres, interstellar clouds, or nocturnal boundary layers—are enabled by barrierless or tunneling pathways, pressuredependent stabilization, unimolecular branching, and the delicate interplay between collisionless quantum dynamics and collisional energy transfer, demanding tightly integrated experimental and computational models to decode their behavior.

References

1. Zhao, L., Kaiser, R. I., Xu, B., Ablikim, U., Ahmed, M., Evseev, M. M., Bashkirov, E. K., Azyazov, V. N., & Mebel, A. M. (2018). Low-temperature formation of polycyclic aromatic hydrocarbons in Titan's atmosphere. *Nature Astronomy*, *2*(12), 973–979. https://doi.org/10.1038/s41550-018-0585-yAdamson, B. D., Ahmed, M., Hansen, N., et al. (2018). Detection of aliphatically bridged multi-core polycyclic aromatic hydrocarbons in shooting flames with atmospheric-sampling high-resolution tandem mass spectrometry. https://core.ac.uk/download/294625769.pdf.
2. Alberts, B., Andreini, C., Balche, W. E., Barker, H. A., Benner, S. A., Berge, C., Braakman, R., et al. (2012). The compositional and evolutionary logic of metabolism. http://arxiv.org/abs/1207.5532 (accessed on 9 June 2025).
3. Alia, S., Padgett, E., Chan, A. L., Blair, S. J., Medina, S., Reeves, K., Yu, H., et al. (2024). (Invited) Degradation mechanisms, diagnostics, and mitigation in proton exchange membrane water electrolyzes. *ECS Meeting Abstracts*. https://www.semanticscholar.org/paper/37df83e182cdb960268a02051c4c4f44540a9286 (accessed on 9 June 2025).
4. Almaas, E., Covert, D. Y., Lee, D., Gerdes, G., Ghim, C., Goebl, M., et al. (2007). Metabolite essentiality elucidates robustness of *Escherichia coli* metabolism. http://arxiv.org/abs/0708.1865 (accessed on 9 June 2025).
5. Altarawneh, M., Assaf, N. W., Hussain, H. M., & Dlugogorski, B. (2023). Structural properties of alumina surfaces and their roles in the synthesis of environmentally persistent free radicals (EPFRs). *Nanotechnology Reviews, 12*. https://www.semanticscholar.org/paper/51b5623c90d3495b8133856a535aa8c7428053f8 (accessed on 9 June 2025).
6. Aponte, J. C., Charnley, S. B., Dworkin, J. P., et al. (2025). Pathways to meteoritic glycine and methylamine. https://core.ac.uk/download/pdf/323104146.pdf (accessed on 9 June 2025).
7. Barbé, A., Battin-Leclerc, F., Benson, S. W., Buda, F., Callahan, C., Ciajolo, A., al. (2006). Experimental and modeling study of the autoignition of 1-hexene/iso-octane mixtures at low temperatures. http://arxiv.org/abs/physics/0603236 (accessed on 9 June 2025).
8. Battin-Leclerc, F., Faravelli, T., Herbinet, O., Marin, G., et al. (2020). The role of chemistry in the oscillating combustion of hydrocarbons: An experimental and theoretical study. https://core.ac.uk/download/286549690.pdf (accessed on 9 June 2025).
9. Bianchi, M., Facco, G., Grazzini, G., et al. (2015). Leukoreduction of blood components: An effective way to increase blood safety? https://core.ac.uk/download/54532479.pdf (accessed on 9 June 2025).
10. Bordbar, A., Dräger, A., Flamholz, A., Joshi, A., Kinoshita, A. B. C., Canelas, A. B., Dräger, A., et al. (2016). Evaluation of rate law approximations in bottom-up kinetic models of metabolism. https://core.ac.uk/download/323065299.pdf.
11. Branco Pinto, D., Constales, D., Marin, G., et al. (2017). Kinetic intersections as a source of information on rate coefficients. https://core.ac.uk/download/91288153.pdf (accessed on 9 June 2025).
12. Cabral, N. D., Paredes, E. N., Peruchena, N. M., et al. (2018). Study of confinement and catalysis effects of the reaction of methylation of benzene by methanol in H-Beta and H-ZSM-5 zeolites by topological analysis of electron density. https://core.ac.uk/download/287882610.pdf (accessed on 9 June 2025).

13. Caratzoulas, S., Davis, M. E., Gorte, R. J., et al. (2014). Challenges of and insights into acid-catalyzed transformations of sugars. https://core.ac.uk/download/33115410.pdf.

14. Dence, J. B., Gray, H. B., & Hammond, G. S. (1968). Chemical dynamics. https://core.ac.uk/download/4890307.pdf.

15. Ebenhoeh, O., Flis, A., Pokhilko, A., et al. (2013). Adjustment of carbon fluxes to light conditions regulates the daily turnover of starch in plants: A computational model. https://core.ac.uk/download/29151105.pdf (accessed on 9 June 2025).

16. Faeder, J. R., & Sekar, J. A. P. (2017). An introduction to rule-based modeling of immune receptor signaling. http://arxiv.org/abs/1709.06658 (accessed on 9 June 2025).

17. Frank, S. A. (2013). Input-output relations in biological systems: Measurement, information and the Hill equation. https://core.ac.uk/download/pdf/81921706.pdf (accessed on 9 June 2025).

18. Fujiwara, N., Kofuji, Y., Mikoshiba, S., Kitagawa, R., Matsunaga, A., Kikuchi, I., & Shimotori, S. (2023). Development of durable large-sized CO_2 electrolysis cells for industrial applications. *ECS Meeting Abstracts*. https://www.semanticscholar.org/paper/f81e421e1f410a589b58700a4ba7100b4c424d22 (accessed on 9 June 2025).

19. Garcia, G., Pacchini, V., Zamoner, W., Balbi, A., & Ponce, D. (2024). Drug-induced acute kidney injury: A cohort study on incidence, identification of pathophysiological mechanisms, and prognostic factors. *Frontiers in Medicine, 11*. https://www.semanticscholar.org/paper/d03104f2b21d27a38bc74c12fe941e7675db17fb (accessed on 9 June 2025).

20. Garcia-Borràs, M., Hirayama, Y., Houk, K. N., et al. (2017). Enzyme-catalyzed cationic epoxide rearrangements in quinolone alkaloid biosynthesis. https://core.ac.uk/download/323080002.pdf.

21. Grady, C., Daigger, G., Love, N., & Filipe, C. (2011). Biological wastewater treatment. https://www.semanticscholar.org/paper/9f74aab3fed3459fecbdc8046d61da743ab0703e (accessed on 9 June 2025).

22. Gray, H. B., & Langford, C. H. (1968). *Ligand Substitution Dynamics*. https://core.ac.uk/download/4886900.pdf.

23. Griffiths, P. E., & Stotz, K. (2017). Genetic, epigenetic and exogenetic information. https://core.ac.uk/download/131214859.pdf (accessed on 9 June 2025).

24. Groom, C. R., Bruno, I., Lightfoot, M. P., & Ward, S. C. (2016). The Cambridge Structural Database. *Acta Crystallographic Section B: Structural Science, Crystal Engineering and Materials, 72*, 171–179. https://doi.org/10.1107/s2052520616003954.

25. Guan, W. J., Ni, Z., Hu, Y., Liang, W., Ou, C. Q., He, J., Liu, L., et al. (2020). Clinical characteristics of coronavirus disease 2019 in China. *New England Journal of Medicine, 382*, 1708–1720. https://doi.org/10.1056/nejmoa2002032.

26. Hoch, L. B., Wood, T. E., O'Brien, P. G., Liao, K., Reyes, L. M., Mims, C. A., & Ozin, G. A. (2014). The rational design of a single-component photocatalyst for gas-phase CO_2 reduction using both UV and visible light. *Advanced Science, 1*. https://doi.org/10.1002/advs.201400013.

27. Keglevich, G. (2023). Organophosphorus chemistry: From model to application. *Beilstein Journal of Organic Chemistry, 19*, 89–90. https://www.semanticscholar.org/paper/3d5133718529a950ad0375b9f95319f1e33c99f5 (accessed on 9 June 2025).

28. Klimek, L., Becker, S., Haxel, B., Cuevas, M., Huber, P., Chaker, A., Pfaar, O., et al. (2025). [Different immunological types of CRSwNP in the context of the new European EAACI nomenclature: Part 1: Hypersensitivity reactions of type IVa-c as a correlate to T1, T2, and T3 endotypes]. *HNO*. https://www.semanticscholar.org/paper/c6fe3d72fa213028ec0c711c289be447a37c74f1 (accessed on 9 June 2025).

29. Knizhnik, A. A., Lebedeva, I. V., Popov, A. M., et al. (2017). Transformation of amorphous carbon clusters to fullerenes. http://arxiv.org/abs/1708.01557 (accessed on 9 June 2025).

30. Koehnke, J., Bent, A. F., Zollman, D., Smith, K., Houssen, W. E., Zhu, X., Mann, G., et al. (2013). The cyanobactin heterocycles' enzyme: A processive adenylase that operates with a defined order of reaction. *Angewandte Chemie International Edition, 52*, 13991–13996. https://doi.org/10.1002/anie.201306302.

31. Kovalenko, I. L., Nalisko, M. M., Sobolev, V. V., et al. (2018). The macro kinetics parameters of the hydrocarbon's combustion in the numerical calculation of accidental explosions in mines. https://core.ac.uk/download/288815745.pdf (accessed on 9 June 2025).

32. Liang, C., Lin, L., Xu, T., Kang, G., Liu, Z., & Li, B. (2025). The *Pseudomonas* ligninolytic catalytic network reveals the importance of auxiliary enzymes in lignin biocatalysts. *Proceedings of the National Academy of Sciences of the United States of America, 122*(4), e2417343122. https://www.semanticscholar.org/paper/4c0de5861f3b503ba194059721b335f1aa36b53a (accessed on 9 June 2025).

33. Lim, H., Park, J., Hong, J. I., & Shin, I. S. (2020). Diffusion and kinetic-controlled electrochemical reactions for improving the performance of solution-based electrochemiluminescence devices. *Bulletin of the Korean Chemical Society, 41*, 362–365. https://www.semanticscholar.org/paper/af02257f18f1eb729e75586c76e5829f2fc86f09 (accessed on 9 June 2025).

34. Lin, M., & Liang, J. (2024). Boron-nitrogen compounds in luminescent materials: A review of applications and synthesis methods. *Highlights in Science, Engineering and Technology*. https://www.semanticscholar.org/paper/9fe25c253bd1aff6643e2250fad95222523c9ac3 (accessed on 9 June 2025).

35. Liu, S., Tormena, C., Hammond, G., & Xu, B. (2022). Broadly applicable ion pair-assisted nucleophilic substitution of sp^3-carbon electrophiles with alkynyl trifluoroborates. *Organic Letters*. https://www.semanticscholar.org/paper/357fd80346417756e726978927bcd812433e9aef (accessed on 9 June 2025).

36. Liu, Z. (2021). Fluorinated aryl boronates as units in organic synthesis. https://www.semanticscholar.org/paper/cd3096f714f469d581c12de5fdabd0d9571547f9 (accessed on 9 June 2025).

37. Michalski, M., & Berski, S. (2025). Mechanistic pathways in cyanide-mediated benzoin condensation: A comprehensive electron localization function (ELF) and catastrophe theory analysis of the umpolung reaction. *Molecules, 30*. https://www.semanticscholar.org/paper/a3ebf7daca74fda52f3485161fff0a2d414f226c (accessed on 9 June 2025).

38. Moorthy, S., Lambert, H., Mohan, N., Schwarzlose, T., Nau, W., Kalenius, E., & Lee, T. C. (2023). Noncovalent modulation of chemo selectivity in the gas phase leads to a switchover in reaction type from heterolytic to homolytic to electrocyclic cleavage. *Angewandte Chemie*. https://www.semanticscholar.org/paper/0b1e240fb7d995adb75e0c2854032d666a84fbda (accessed on 9 June 2025).

39. Oberhummer, H., & Staudt, G. (1994). Direct mechanism in solar nuclear reactions. https://core.ac.uk/download/25165879.pdf.

40. Patra, J. K., Das, G., Fraceto, L. F., Campos, E. V. R., Rodriguez-Torres, M. P., Acosta-Torres, L. S., Díaz-Torres, L. A., et al. (2018). Nano based drug delivery systems: Recent developments and future prospects. *Journal of Nanobiotechnology, 16*. https://doi.org/10.1186/s12951-018-0392-8.

41. Reiher, M., Simm, G. N., & Vaucher, A. C. (2018). Exploration of reaction pathways and chemical transformation networks. http://arxiv.org/abs/1810.07490 (accessed on 9 June 2025).

42. Reuter, K., & Wang, T. (2015). Structure sensitivity in oxide catalysis: First-principles kinetic Monte Carlo simulations for CO oxidation at RuO_2(111). https://core.ac.uk/download/532709023.pdf (accessed on 9 June 2025).

43. Seh, Z. W., Kibsgaard, J., Dickens, C. F., Chorkendorff, I., Nørskov, J. K., & Jaramillo, T. F. (2017). Combining theory and experiment in electrocatalysis: Insights into materials design. *Science, 355*. https://doi.org/10.1126/science.aad4998.

44. Semleit, N., Kreuzahler, M., & Haberhauer, G. (2020). Gold(I)-catalyzed allene–diene–alkyne coupling reaction to polycycles. *European Journal of Organic Chemistry, 2020*, 6629–6634. https://www.semanticscholar.org/paper/8a8fd8b94b74ce2118d44b7b6cd4225ca88d2dfe (accessed on 9 June 2025).

45. Wang, T. B., Li, L. J., Tao, Y. T., Ning, L., Jin, S. H., Cen, K., & Lu, Z. Y. (2024). Influence of cavity crystal defects on the thermal decomposition mechanism of NTO. *Journal of Physics: Conference Series, 2891*. https://www.semanticscholar.org/paper/f5cc856aaaf90986b9f8286aa3ad7d54c34729ea (accessed on 9 June 2025).

46. Wiley, A., Jr. (1972). A review: Some biological effects of high LET radiations. https://core.ac.uk/download/pdf/10297185.pdf (accessed on 9 June 2025).

47. Yang, M., Zhang, S. B., Zhang, M., Li, Z. H., Liu, Y. F., Liao, X., Lu, M., et al. (2024). Three-motif molecular junction type covalent organic frameworks for efficient photocatalytic aerobic oxidation. *Journal of the American Chemical Society*. https://www.semanticscholar.org/paper/5bb96dbccd9997f2e86bc275615e345386eb399c (accessed on 9 June 2025).

48. Zholobak, N. M., Dubova, I., Deineko, A., Kalinovych, V., Nováková, J., Matolínová, I., Prince, K. C., et al. (2025). A PVP-stabilized cerium oxide–platinum nanocomposite synthesized in TEG: Pro-/antioxidant activities. *Nanoscale Advances, 7*, 1686–1697. https://www.semanticscholar.org/paper/6bfc339940886125bdb156986d164555c5a5266f (accessed on 9 June 2025).

49. Zhu, Y., Liu, J., & Wang, B. (2025). Integrated approach for biomarker discovery and mechanistic insights into the co-pathogenesis of type 2 diabetes mellitus and non-Hodgkin lymphoma. *Diabetes, Metabolic Syndrome and Obesity, 18*, 267–282. https://www.semanticscholar.org/paper/302386608f989e99fa9f6be74acce02d1c378c75 (accessed on 9 June 2025).

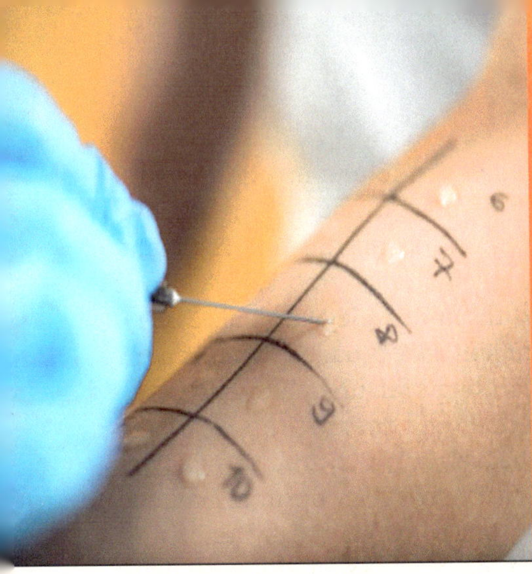

Chapter 5

DRUG HYPERSENSITIVITY REACTIONS

Contents

Introduction

Drug hypersensitivity reactions (DHRs) are a significant issue in clinical medicine, characterized by ADRs due to immunologically mediated effects. The responses range from mild cutaneous manifestations to fatal anaphylaxis, for which the correct diagnosis and treatment are necessary to prevent harm to the patient. Recent evidence indicates that beta-lactam antibiotics are prevalent in causing HSRs, particularly in children, where misdiagnosis is the norm due to overlapping presentations with viral infections. Such characterization and discrimination of these reactions into non-immediate and immediate forms is essential to clarify their mechanistic underpinnings as well as managerial implications. Furthermore, the high negative predictive value (NPV) of single-day drug provocation tests (sdDPT) makes precise evaluation necessary before attributing a drug as a putative allergen and thus enabling clinical decisions in drug prescribing (Genis et al., 2024). Meanwhile, drug hypersensitivity is not limited to antibiotics but encompasses many therapeutic classes, prompting a demand for accelerated research into individualized treatment methods. Intravenous (IV) iron replacement, for instance, is typically employed when rapid restitution of iron reserves is imperative; however, bouts of HSRs may mar its application. Desensitization regimens, such as the one involving ferric carboxymaltose, have emerged as vital modalities in the therapy of established hypersensitive patients to prevent depriving necessary therapies unnecessarily. Systematic desensitization regimens establish the protocol wherein practitioners can address drug hypersensitivity problems without provoking adverse results, thus maintaining the efficacy of essential therapies (Şeyma et al., 2024). The adoption of such desensitization regimens into practice is testament to a broader commitment to patient safety and personalized medicine. With growing understanding of drug hypersensitivity, an urgent need arises to create more advanced diagnostic approaches and therapeutic regimens attuned to the specific needs of the individual patient. Continued research into DHRs holds promise for improving outcomes for patients, highlighting the pressing need to strike an optimal balance between therapeutic efficacy and safety. With the introduction of advanced diagnostic systems and treatment protocols, healthcare practitioners are now able to reduce the risks associated with drug hypersensitivity and enhance the provision of more effective and safer drug management among multicultural patient populations. The combination of rigorous assessment and innovative treatment modalities will indeed shape the dynamic future of DHR in the clinical setting (Figure 5.1).

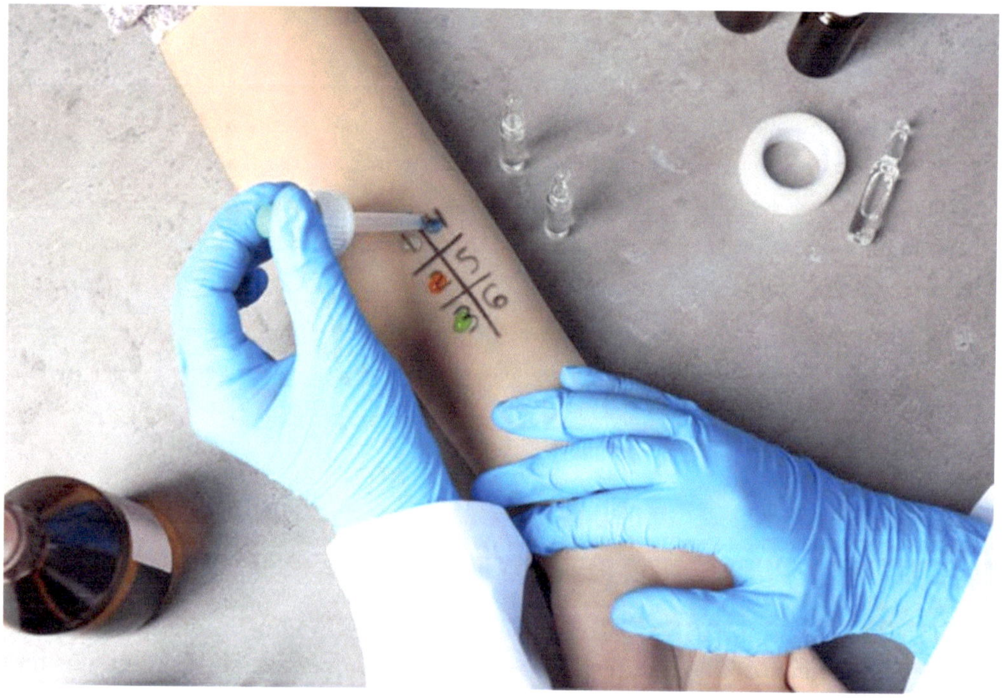

Figure 5.1. Drug hypersensitivity reactions.

Source: https://images.medindia.net/patientinfo/950_400/allergy-tests-are-used-to-diagnose-drug-hypersensitivity-reactions.jpg.

Definition of Drug Hypersensitivity Reactions

A comprehensive understanding of DHR is essential for healthcare practitioners, as these reactions represent a significant clinical challenge. When someone is drug hypersensitive, their immune system responds strongly to a particular drug, which may result in anything from minor skin rashes to very dangerous anaphylaxis. It is possible to divide this immune reaction into immediate and delayed types, with immediate reactions mainly involving IgE antibodies and delayed reactions involving T cells. Evidence indicates that drug-related allergies account for a notable portion of emergency department visits, with studies revealing that 14.4% of drug-related cases resulted in such visits, highlighting the profound implications of DHR on patient safety and public health (Pagani et al., 2022). Examining these reactions can lead to improved methods for preventing and treating DHR in various patient populations. The role of T cells, particularly T regulatory cells (Tregs), in DHR provides insight into the underlying mechanisms of these responses. Research has demonstrated that some patients may develop multiple drug hypersensitivities (MDH), characterized by clinical and immunological reactivity to various drugs. In cases of MDH, Tregs generally exhibit heightened activity, allowing them to modulate immune responses effectively (Daubner et al., 2011). As an illustration, these cells can stop T-cells from multiplying, which could prevent bad drug reactions in people with monoallergy, but not in patients with MDH. Since T-cell activation differs in monoallergic and MDH patients, it is essential to employ specific approaches to diagnose and treat each patient to achieve better outcomes. The effects of DHRs are not limited to treating the patient and also involve safety aspects of drugs. As more people develop allergies to medications, it is essential for healthcare practitioners to be aware of common triggers, including antibacterials, analgesics, and radiocontrast agents. Elevated reporting of drug allergies and associated anaphylaxis underlines the importance of thorough patient histories and proactive therapeutic management (Pagani et al., 2022). Besides, the review found that there is variability in ED visits related to drug-related hypersensitivity, so healthcare providers are now developing better screening methods for people who are at risk. If healthcare providers can identify people who are more likely to have drug hypersensitivity, then they can monitor them better and apply preventive measures, and choose the appropriate treatments, which may reduce the occurrence of such reactions (Figure 5.2).

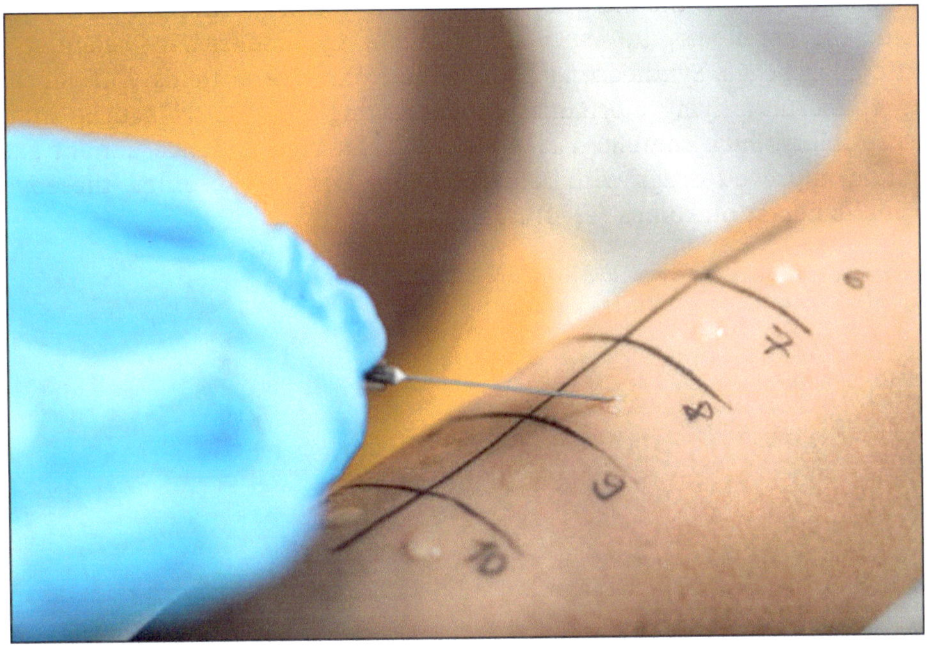

Figure 5.2. Skin prick allergy testing.

Source: https://media.istockphoto.com/id/1167052053/photo/skin-prick-allergy-testing.jpg?s=612x612&w=0&k=20&c=JU6zT7NZmOn_vGRF8dMbkC03eUoxDHDn3SwFghV76vw=.

Importance of Understanding Drug Hypersensitivity

Drug hypersensitivity is crucial for both patient safety and the overall efficacy of pharmacotherapy. Because ADRs affect a significant proportion of hospitalized patients, with rates estimated at over 6% and at over 100,000 deaths per year in the United States alone, the severity of the problem is considerable. These ADRs may be Type A or Type B, the former being very unreliable and mostly of an immunoallergic type. Thus, being aware of the potential for hypersensitivity can direct clinicians and patients toward the necessity for careful drug selection, monitoring, and potential alternative therapy. Clinicians' recognition of drug hypersensitivity can enable improved diagnosis and appropriate management schemes, ultimately translating into improved patient outcomes and reduced healthcare expenditure in association with ADRs. Genetic susceptibility has also emerged as a fundamental factor to consider in drug hypersensitivity. Recent evidence has suggested that certain genetic variations, primarily those in the HLA genes, are associated with allergic cross-reactivity to drugs such as penicillin. Such discoveries necessitate a personalized medicine strategy that takes into account genetic backgrounds when prescribing medications. Some correlations between specific genetic markers and drug reactions were demonstrated in studies involving over 600,000 participants, highlighting the complex nature of drug hypersensitivity and the need for ongoing pharmacogenomics research. As genetic testing becomes increasingly prevalent in the clinic, familiarity with these associations will enable healthcare providers to identify patients at heightened risk and modify pharmacologic treatment accordingly, mitigating the risk of severe HSRs. Furthermore, an interdisciplinary collaboration among scientists researching drug hypersensitivity is essential to further our understanding of its mechanisms and risk factors. Forming a collaborative network of clinicians, researchers, and geneticists can yield a more unified approach to identifying risk populations and designing effective preventive measures. By designing solutions to challenges such as the intricacy of metabolic pathways involved in drug-induced liver injury (DILI) and the immunological aspects of inducing hypersensitivity, scientists can develop new therapeutic approaches. Synthesizing knowledge from several fields will aid in augmenting understanding of the underlying mechanism and drawing insights from drug metabolism and individual susceptibility. Such combined feedback will not only enhance patient safety but also aid in formulating improved drugs with reduced hypersensitivity profiles, thereby significantly transforming public health outcomes (Figure 5.3).

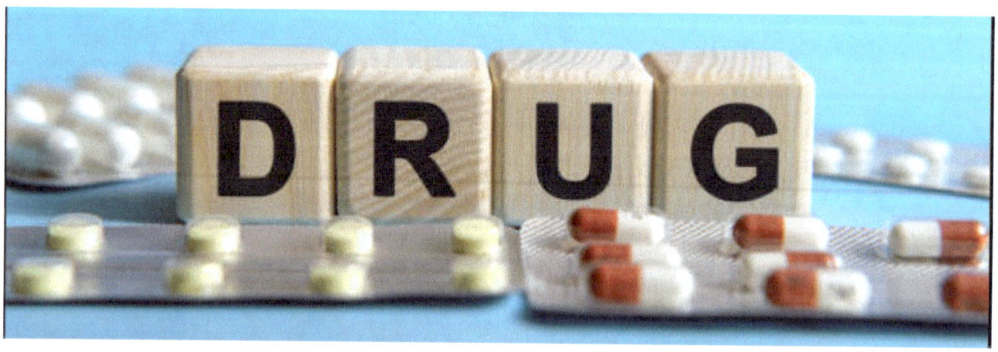

Figure 5.3. Drug.

Source: https://media.istockphoto.com/id/1214400864/photo/drug-text-on-cubes-drug-tablets-in-blisters-to-reduce-disease-symptoms.jpg?s=612x612&w=0&k=20&c=C9CjVCS-xShi6J4m4J5xwWEhW1YgCBY_zwUm6qjFArU=.

5.1. Types of Drug Hypersensitivity Reactions

It is essential to be aware of the various drug hypersensitivity reactions (DHRs) to effectively manage patients and ensure their safety. Gell and Coombs have grouped these reactions into four main categories. Type I HSRs, also known as immediate hypersensitivity, are mediated by immunoglobulin E (IgE) and can result in anaphylaxis, which is life-threatening. This kind of reaction can appear within a few minutes after contact with the drug and is marked by urticaria, angioedema, and difficulty breathing. In contrast, Type II HSRs happen when antibodies against drug-modified cells cause cytotoxicity, which may result in hemolytic anemia or thrombocytopenia. If clinicians are aware of these mechanisms, they can anticipate potential allergic reactions in certain patients and ensure the most effective treatment with the lowest risk. In paragraph 5, it is explained that Type III and Type IV reactions have different ways they develop and different symptoms than each other.

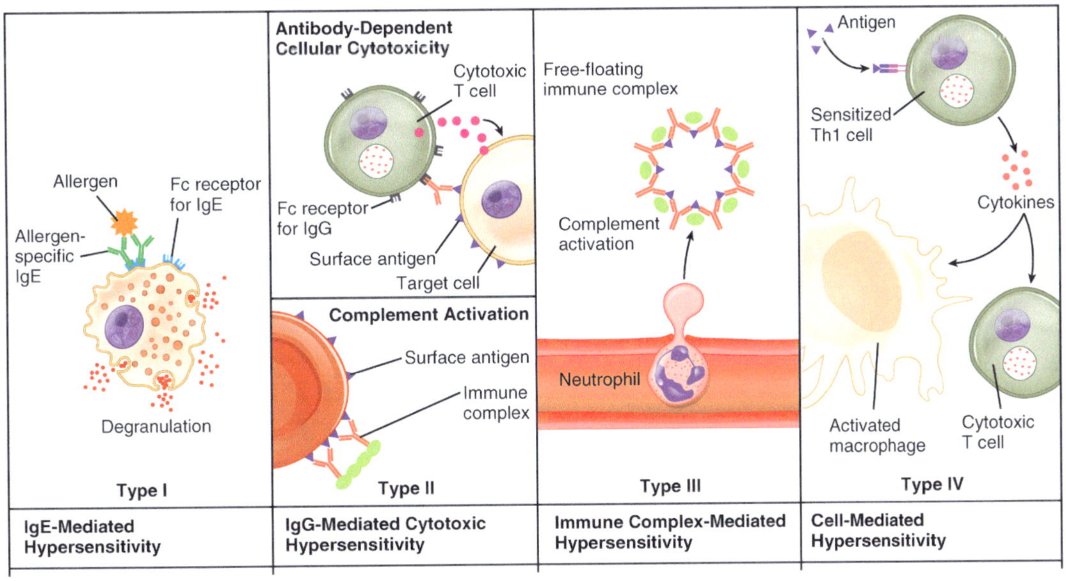

Figure 5.4. Types of drug hypersensitivity reactions.

Source: https://philschatz.com/anatomy-book/resources/2228_Immune_Hypersensitivity_new.jpg.

In Type III hypersensitivity, immune complexes form and accumulate in tissues, causing inflammation and tissue damage. Such reactions may show up as general symptoms, for example serum sickness, or as local problems, such as vasculitis. Instead, Type IV hypersensitivity, also known as delayed-type hypersensitivity, is primarily controlled by T cells rather than antibodies. Reactions often occur 48–72 hours after drug exposure and include conditions such as contact dermatitis or drug-induced Stevens-Johnson syndrome (SJS). For instance, hypersensitivity to antiepileptic drugs (AEDs), as assessed in a clinical cohort, often results in severe cutaneous adverse reactions (SCAR) linked to specific genetic markers like HLA-B*1502, emphasizing the importance of personalized medicine in managing these complex reactions (Cohen et al., 2011). The frequent occurrence of DHRs shows that it is imperative to watch and report in clinical settings carefully. It has been found that chemotherapy drugs such as paclitaxel and docetaxel are responsible for inducing HSRs in cancer patients. Notably, ADRs associated with these agents can manifest as respiratory distress or severe anaphylaxis, potentially leading to fatal outcomes. A recent study found that out of 258 recorded ADRs, 30 cases were classified as HSRs with paclitaxel being a significant contributor (Begum et al., 2022). By using scales such as the WHO-UMC causality assessment scale, it becomes easier to assess the frequency and severity of these reactions. It is essential for healthcare providers to monitor ADRs to improve patient care, introduce preventive actions, and create safer treatment settings (Figure 5.4).

5.1.1. Immediate Hypersensitivity Reactions

Immediate HSRs are a dangerous subgroup of DHRs, characterized by acute onset of reactions typically within minutes after exposure to an offending agent, e.g., a drug. They are primarily mediated by IgE antibodies produced on first exposure to an allergen and cause mast cell degranulation on subsequent exposures. Common presentations include urticaria, angioedema, bronchospasm, and, in the most dangerous scenarios, anaphylaxis.

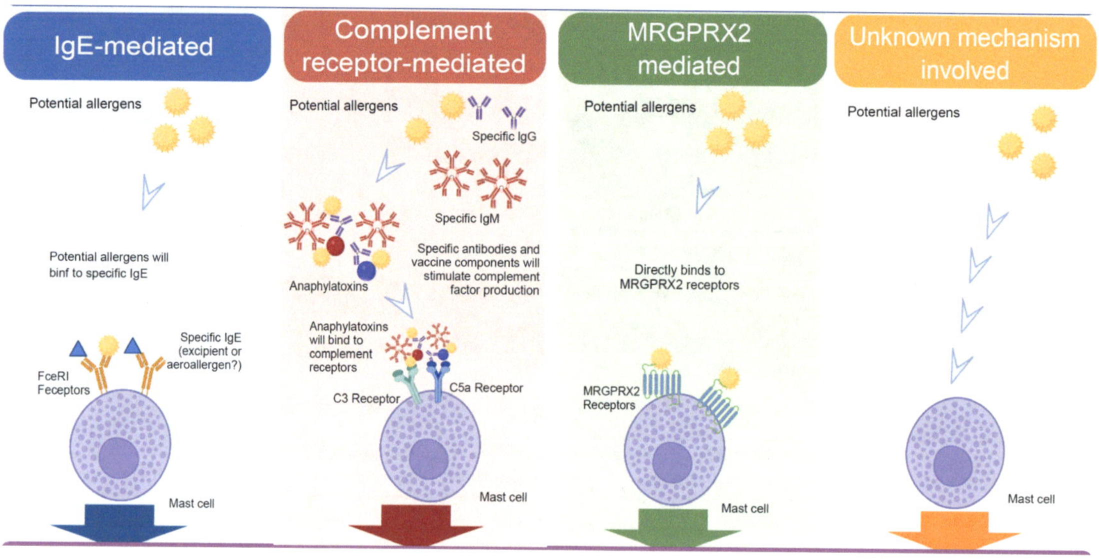

Figure 5.5. Immediate hypersensitivity reactions.

Source: https://www.mdpi.com/biomedicines/biomedicines-10-01260/article_deploy/html/images/biomedicines-10-01260-g001.png.

The clinical significance of such reactions is that they can be potentially life-threatening, and hence, early diagnosis and treatment are required. An understanding of the immunologic processes underlying them is important because it enables clinicians to treat and prevent recurrent attacks in sensitized patients accordingly, thereby ensuring patient safety through effective drug therapy. The immediate hypersensitivity reaction can be diagnosed by a multidisciplinary approach with routine use of patient history, physical examination, and cutaneous testing. When it comes to beta-lactam antibiotics, the most common culprits for immediate reactions, the worth of a one-day sdDPT is highlighted. Literature indicates that a negative sdDPT is strongly predictive of both immediate and non-immediate reactions, providing conclusive evidence that most individuals who initially develop hypersensitivity can be safely re-exposed under the advice of medical professionals (Genis et al., 2024). These evaluations are mandatory, especially in children in which misdiagnosis is not unexpected due to the fact that viral infections may mimic allergic reactions. Through proper evaluations, clinicians can minimize the inappropriate avoidance of effective medications, ensuring patients receive optimal therapeutic results. Apart from diagnosis, treatment of the acute HSRs also necessitates recognition of the different degrees of severity and potential for recurrence with exposure to drugs. Breakthrough reaction analysis indicates that the reactions can even occur following a prior allergic reaction to the same medication, and thus, precautions must be taken during drug administration. A multicenter study reported that, although most reactions were mild, a significant percentage of cases presented with moderate to severe symptoms (Beiner et al., 2024). Such findings highlight the need for a standardized procedure for managing acute allergic reactions, ranging from epinephrine for anaphylaxis to antihistamines for its milder forms. Continuous education for both patients and health workers is hence imperative in making people aware of immediate HSRs, and its recognition and response accordingly (Figure 5.5).

5.1.2. Delayed Hypersensitivity Reactions

Delayed hypersensitivity reactions (DHRs) pose a significant challenge within the broader category of hypersensitivity reactions, particularly due to their complex immunological underpinnings. While immediate reactions to drugs show up right away, DHRs usually happen at least six hours after the drug is taken. Such a delayed reaction often makes it difficult to diagnose and treat the patient, as symptoms may not appear for several days or even weeks after exposure. According to Villarreal-González et al. (2024), these reactions can arise as a result of Type B ADRs, which are primarily immune-mediated. Knowing about these mechanisms matters to healthcare providers, since the late start of symptoms can result in dangerous clinical issues, including life-threatening situations. Therefore, determining which drug caused the reaction is necessary for handling and preventing further problems. Delayed HSRs happen when T-cells interact with drug antigens in a complicated way. Mostly, these reactions happen when $CD4^+$ and $CD8^+$ T-lymphocytes are triggered by drug-modified self-proteins that form hapten-protein complexes. The fact that T-cells come in different subtypes can result in different symptoms in patients. Various models explain the antigen presentation processes responsible for DHRs, including the hapten hypothesis and the pharmacological interaction of drugs with immune receptors (Chen et al., 2023). Additionally, genetic factors may play a pivotal role in predisposing individuals to these reactions, as certain human leukocyte antigen (HLA) alleles have been identified as risk factors for specific drug-related hypersensitivity reactions.

It is essential to understand these mechanisms, as they inform the approaches to diagnosing and treating DHRs. If HSRs are delayed, they may lead to serious problems for patients and compromise the quality of healthcare. At times, DHRs can cause severe skin reactions that should be treated right away by a doctor. It is essential to be aware of the various clinical signs of DHRs to develop more effective treatment methods. As highlighted in current research, next-generation sequencing technologies have facilitated the discovery of genetic susceptibility to these reactions, providing an avenue for personalized medicine approaches (Chen et al., 2023). Because of this genetic information, doctors can both diagnose delayed hypersensitivity and help high-risk patients avoid it, which significantly benefits patients. Since many factors are involved in DHRs, it is essential to employ a multidisciplinary approach to enhance both the treatment outcomes and patient outcomes (Figure 5.6).

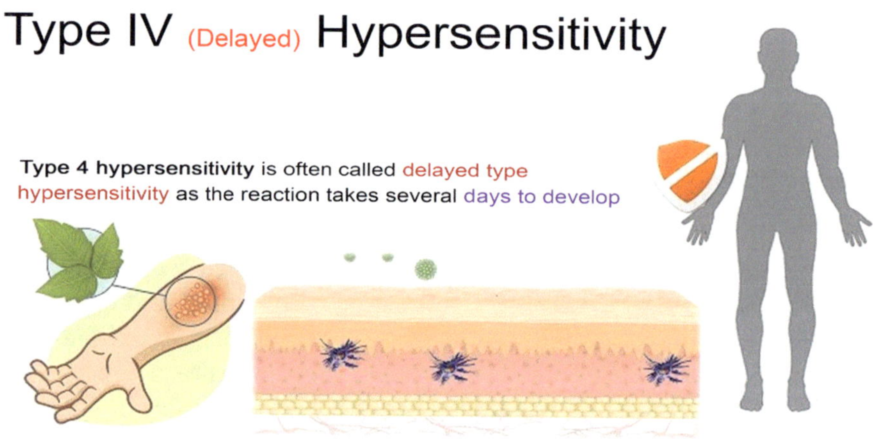

Figure 5.6. Delayed hypersensitivity.

Source: https://i.ytimg.com/vi/H_YQ8sB9nb4/sddefault.jpg.

5.1.3. Mixed Hypersensitivity Reactions

In the setting of DHRs, mixed HSRs represent a complex and dynamic response to pharmacologic drugs. These reactions suggest the occurrence of greater than one immunologic mechanism, which may be both IgE-mediated and non-IgE-mediated. This blend may present with varied clinical findings, ranging from cutaneous rashes to respiratory compromise, which can severely complicate diagnosis and treatment. As such, clinicians must also gain an insight into the mechanisms of these mixed reactions. This becomes vital in accurately identifying the culprit drugs, so that effective management strategies can be implemented to minimize patient risk and maximize therapeutic gains. The classification of mixed HSRs has been extended to other drug categories, including the non-steroidal anti-inflammatory drugs (NSAIDs). In clinical practice, it is not uncommon for patients to exhibit a combination of respiratory and dermatological symptoms following NSAID administration. For instance, the European Network on Drug Allergy (ENDA) acknowledges that reactions may not always fit neatly into established categories, giving rise to blended reactions that encompass symptoms from multiple organ systems. Infected patients may also express urticaria or angioedema with secondary respiratory distress, which is a reflection of the interconnectedness of HSRs. This highlights the importance of careful clinical evaluation and investigation to enable proper diagnosis and the direction of appropriate, individualized treatment modalities for infected patients (Doña et al., 2018). Moreover, the best management of simultaneous HSRs requires careful control in the event of future drug administration. For instance, in anti-TB DILI, adherence to set guidelines is paramount. Such guidelines demand minimal re-exposure to the causative agents, especially when a severe reaction has already been encountered (N/A, 2024). Physicians also have to consider genetic predisposition, past history, as well as alternative therapy that may minimize the risk of re-exposure. It recognizes varying presentations, such as with mixed NSAID reactions or anti-TB drug complexities, by requesting ongoing study to maximize classification models and intervention programs to enhance patient safety and therapeutic results among patients with mixed HSRs (Figure 5.7).

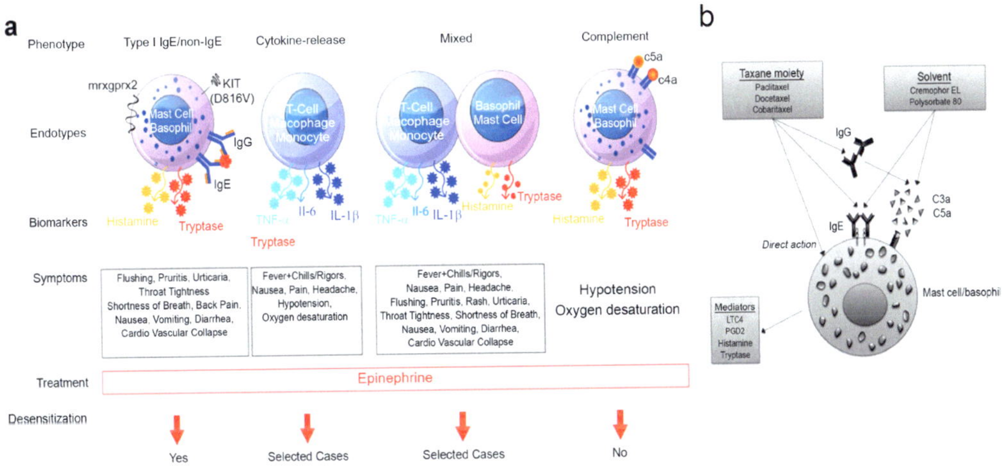

Figure 5.7. Hypersensitivity reactions.

Source: https://media.springernature.com/lw1200/springer-static/image/art%3A10.1007%2Fs12016-021-08877-y/MediaObjects/12016_2021_8877_Fig1_HTML.png.

5.2. Mechanisms of Drug Hypersensitivity

DHRs occur due to complex and multifaceted factors that involve both the immune system and metabolic processes. While type A reactions are caused by the amount of drug taken, type B reactions, like drug hypersensitivity, happen unpredictably and are not related to how much of the drug is given. This type of reaction occurs when the immune system responds abnormally to certain drugs, and the metabolites of these drugs bind to proteins, triggering the immune system to react with hypersensitivity. During this immune response, T cells and dendritic cells are important for spotting and presenting the drug-modified antigens to the immune system. That's why understanding these mechanisms is crucial for identifying patients at risk and developing strategies to manage ADRs caused by hypersensitivity. Pharmacogenomics has become an important area for understanding why some individuals are more susceptible to certain drugs. Genetic changes in the genes encoding drug-metabolizing enzymes, particularly those in the cytochrome P450 pathway, can significantly impact how drugs are processed and the risk of adverse reactions in patients. Apart from age, gender, and pre-existing conditions, differences in how these enzymes function can also lead to variations in drug bioactivation and detoxification, which are important for deciding an individual's risk of HSRs. Some biomarkers can help predict if a person might have an ADR and guide treatment; however, most studies have concentrated on type A reactions, leaving little known about type B reactions such as drug-induced hypersensitivity. This knowledge could drive future advancements in clinical practice. Also, the signs and symptoms of drug hypersensitivity are varied, which is a sign of the complexity of the process involved. Some allergic reactions are just rashes, but others can be very serious and may lead to anaphylaxis. The Gell and Coombs system categorizes HSRs into four main types, highlighting the distinct immune reactions associated with each. These reactions are affected by a person's genes, the environment they are in, and how the drug is processed in their body, showing that they can be unpredictable. A deeper understanding of the processes that lead to drug hypersensitivity is necessary for accurate diagnosis, confirmation, and the development of effective prevention and treatment strategies. The new approach in this area shows that teamwork in research and practice is important and leads to better ways of managing DHRs.

5.2.1. Immune System Involvement

The role of the immune system in DHRs is complex and multifaceted as it represents the complexity of such unexpected reactions. Most DHRs form type B ADRs, i.e., they are not dose-dependent and typically happen independent of the pharmacologic properties of the drugs. Such unexpectedness necessitates a thorough clarification of the underlying immune mechanisms. Evidence has shown that DHRs have the potential to involve several immune mechanisms, whereby the body's immune mechanisms, such as the T cells and the B cells, react abnormally to drug components with the resulting of undesirable clinical phenomena. Evidence demonstrating these mechanisms has shifted the paradigm for understanding drug allergy and revealed the immune system's pivotal role in mediating these phenomena (Trayer et al., 2024).

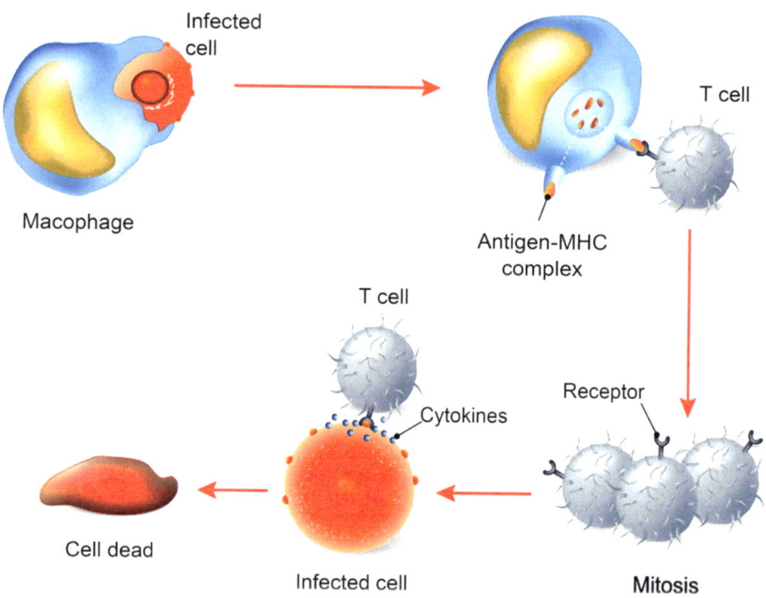

Figure 5.8. Immune response.

Source: https://healthjade.com/wp-content/uploads/2019/03/immune-response.jpg.

Neutrophils, being part of innate immunity, have emerged as key players in DHRs-related allergic reactions. Previously regarded as transient cells primarily responsible for antimicrobial protection, recent evidence depicts their diversity and role as key players beyond their usual functions. In drug allergy, neutrophils may function as amplifiers of immune response, particularly in type 1 HSRs that have the potential to result in anaphylaxis. These cells undergo rapid migration to areas of inflammation, where they perform actions such as phagocytosis and degranulation, further adding to the allergic milieu. The role of neutrophils in other mechanisms of DHRs, such as food allergy and respiratory conditions, is a firsthand example of their role as orchestrators in the immune response, indicating an extended role of immune cells in allergic diseases (Trayer et al., 2024). This exploration of immune system involvement is also complicated by several hypotheses that explain how low-molecular-weight drugs can trigger immune responses. The initial "hapten" hypothesis remains fundamental; however, more recent paradigms such as the reactive metabolite hypothesis and the pharmacological interaction (p-i) concept have emerged, shedding light on the multiple mechanisms of DHR pathophysiology. Later theories, including the inflammasome activation hypothesis, broaden the understanding of these complex interactions by proposing that immune activation in DHRs is not only reliant on the drug but also on the degree of the proinflammatory setting. This perspective promotes an integrative consideration of the understanding of DHRs as theories suggest that parts of the immune system operate within a dynamic interaction that dictates an individual's reaction to drugs (Abdelbaset et al., 2022) (Figure 5.8).

5.2.2. Role of Pharmacogenomics

The relationship between pharmacogenomics and DHRs provides a valuable approach to enhancing the safety and effectiveness of treatments for patients. Pharmacogenomics studies how an individual's genes can influence their reaction to drugs, which affects the likelihood of experiencing adverse reactions, such as hypersensitivity. Differences in genes that help metabolize drugs, such as cytochrome P450, can result in significant changes in drug levels in the body.

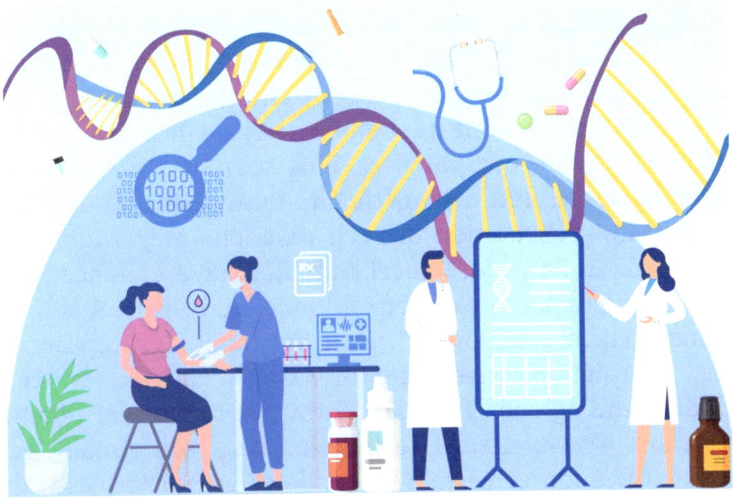

Figure 5.9. Pharmacogenomics.

Source: https://coreprescribingsolutions.co.uk/wp-content/uploads/2024/03/PHARMACOGENOMICS-scaled.jpg.

Such genetic differences may make some individuals more susceptible to adverse reactions to certain medications. With knowledge of these genetic factors, healthcare providers can select the most effective drug therapy for each patient, thereby improving outcomes and reducing side effects. Moreover, advancements in pharmacogenomic research have led to the development of comprehensive resources, such as the Pharmacogenomics Knowledgebase (PharmGKB), which plays a crucial role in informing clinical practices. PharmGKB provides clinicians and researchers with valuable information on how drugs interact with genes and how to implement personalized medicine. The resource helps HCPs decide on drug treatment and management, especially for people who have had HSRs before. When pharmacogenomic data are included in healthcare systems, the selection of medications becomes more precise, there is less trial-and-error prescribing, and patient outcomes improve significantly. Offering pharmacogenomic advice can change the way we prevent HSRs from medications. With the increasing use of pharmacogenomic testing, people are now discussing the ethical and accessibility issues associated with it. Personalized medicine relies on ensuring that pharmacogenomic services and insights are shared equally among individuals from all backgrounds. A lack of genetic testing for some groups can stop them from getting therapies that help avoid DHRs. For this reason, we must address these inequalities to ensure that every patient receives the best care. It is also important to keep providing healthcare providers with up-to-date information about pharmacogenomics. With new developments in pharmacogenomics, providers will need to continually learn to effectively utilize it in their work, thereby helping to ensure safer and more successful treatment for individuals at risk of HSRs (Figure 5.9).

5.2.3. Pathophysiological Processes

An understanding of the pathophysiologic mechanisms of DHRs is critical to successful diagnosis and management. DHRs are of two broad categories, depending on whether or not they are IgE-mediated, each of which has its own immunologic mechanism. In IgE-mediated reactions, initial exposure to a drug sensitizes the immune system to develop specific IgE antibodies. On re-exposure, these antibodies induce the degranulation of basophils and mast cells, spilling histamines and other mediators into the fluid, which results in allergic manifestations. Non-IgE-mediated reactions, however, are intricate immune responses that do not rely on IgE antibodies, often involving T cells or other immune components. This variation in pathophysiologic processes underscores the imperative for tailored diagnostic and treatment approaches, particularly among pediatric age groups, wherein presentation of such reactions may widely vary from their adult counterparts (Timothy et al., 2024). More recent studies have enhanced our understanding of the specific pathophysiologic foundations of non-IgE-mediated DHRs. A subset of these responses has been shown to include critical functions of particular immune receptors and cell components, such as the Mas-related G protein-coupled receptor X2 on mast cells, which may influence their severity and onset. Understanding such intricate pathways can reveal potential biomarkers that predict reaction severity and inform clinical decision-making. Additionally, genetic predisposition research, such as the identification of certain HLA alleles associated with drug hypersensitivity causing SCAR, has uncovered new pathways for the prevention and therapeutic management of DHRs. The application of these findings into practice is ready to improve patient outcomes through early identification and intervention strategies based on individualized risk profiles (Timothy et al., 2024). In exploring the importance of pathophysiological knowledge on drug hypersensitivity, it is clear that it must be approached from a complex viewpoint for effective management. For instance, with a sufficient appreciation for the mechanisms, clinicians can better forecast the likelihood of a reaction when exposed to the same drugs in the future. Additionally, recent research into breakthrough reactions (BTRs) suggests that risk for hypersensitivity is perhaps relative and not absolute. For instance, a study indicates that most patients can tolerate repeated exposures to allergenic drugs, especially when other drugs are administered concurrently or when skin tests for allergy reappear as negative. Thus, the variability of drug hypersensitivity underscores the need for ongoing research and refinement of clinical practice, ensuring that advances in knowledge are effectively implemented (Figure 5.10).

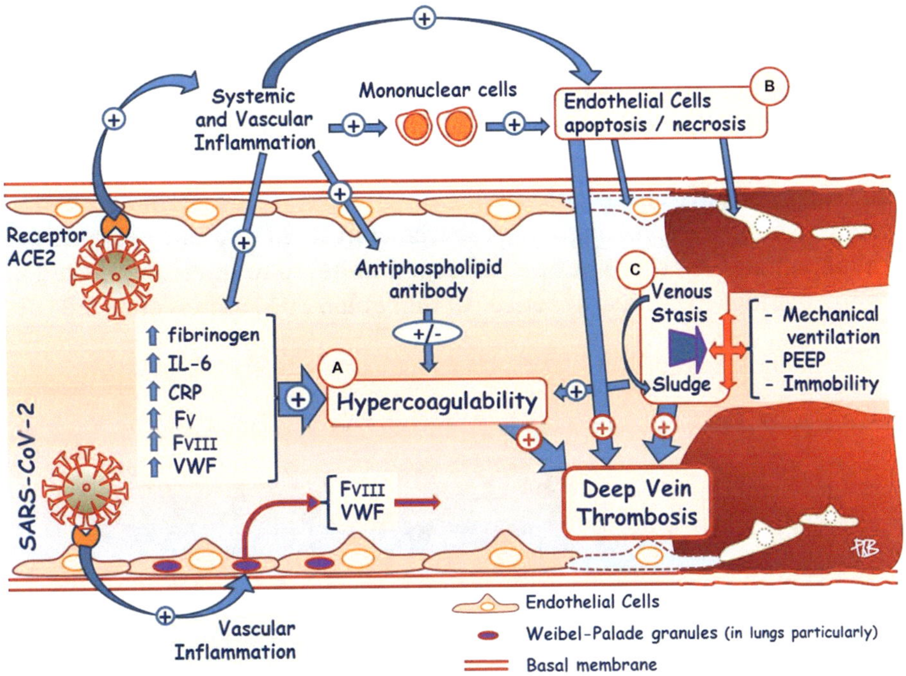

Figure 5.10. Pathophysiological processes.

Source: https://www.frontiersin.org/files/Articles/608788/fphys-11-608788-HTML-r1/image_m/fphys-11-608788-g001.jpg.

5.3. Common Drugs Associated with Hypersensitivity

Drug hypersensitivity shows that a range of medications can lead to negative reactions, and some categories are more common than others. Among these, beta-lactam antibiotics, such as penicillin and cephalosporins, along with NSAIDs, are frequently implicated. Different people may have mild skin reactions or severe allergic reactions when taking these drugs. In particular, healthcare providers in pediatrics should possess a thorough understanding of these medications. Most of the time, HSRs are identified by reviewing the patient's history and symptoms, but it is still important to perform confirmatory tests to avoid mistakes. The Italian Pediatric Society has emphasized that sdDPTs are vital for evaluating tolerance to suspected allergens, especially for antibiotics and NSAIDs, in order to minimize exposure to potentially harmful drugs (Arasi et al., 2018). AEDs also warrant attention as significant agents associated with HSRs. These medications, including carbamazepine, phenytoin, and lamotrigine, are known to precipitate SCAR, such as SJS and toxic epidermal necrolysis (TEN). These hypersensitivity syndromes are typically characterized by symptoms such as fever and skin rashes, which typically appear within weeks after exposure. Research indicates that specific genetic factors, including the presence of the HLA-B*1502 allele, contribute to an increased risk for reactions in certain populations, particularly among Han Chinese patients. Furthermore, assays such as the lymphocyte toxicity assay (LTA) have shown promise in identifying potential hypersensitivity, helping to predict outcomes better and guide treatment protocols (Cohen et al., 2011). Apart from beta-lactam antibiotics and AEDs, there are other drugs that may cause HSRs. Just like antibiotics, sulfonamides, and some chemotherapeutic agents have also been reported to cause side effects in certain people. The results of these reactions indicate that HCPs should exercise greater caution and adopt preventive measures. Proper training of medical staff on dealing with drug hypersensitivity can greatly decrease the risk of related health problems. Additionally, educating patients about potential drug allergies and alternative therapies is crucial for preventing adverse outcomes. As ongoing research continues to identify prone populations and mechanisms of hypersensitivity, there lies an increased impetus to develop tailored approaches for prevention and management in clinical practice (Cohen et al., 2011; Arasi et al., 2018) (Figure 5.11).

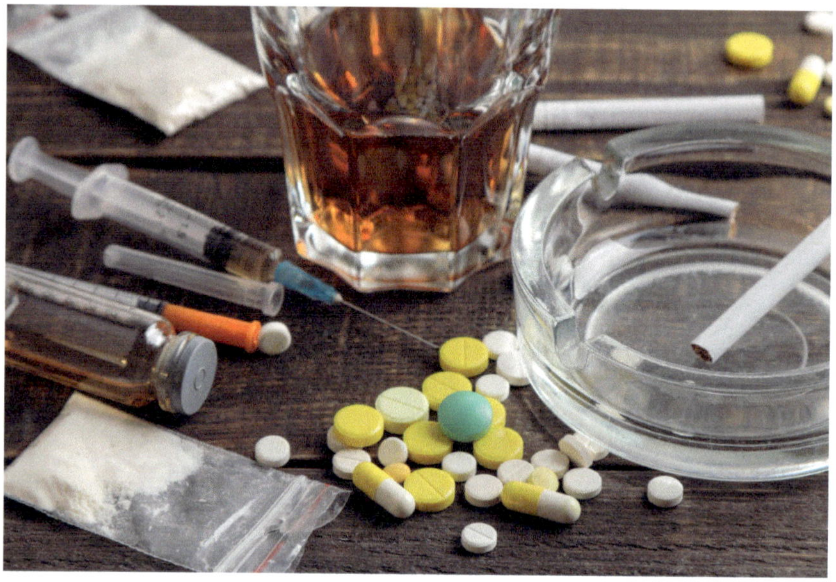

Figure 5.11. Common drugs associated with hypersensitivity.

Source: https://www.turnbridge.com/wp-content/uploads/2022/07/AdobeStock_244539544-scaled.jpeg.

5.3.1. Antibiotics

The extensive use of antibiotics has transformed the landscape of medical treatment by improving the success rate of most bacterial infections. However, this widespread practice has triggered a corresponding upsurge in DHRs, which might complicate therapy strategies. These unwanted reactions can manifest as superficial rashes or severe syndromes of drug reaction with eosinophilia and systemic symptoms (DRESS) and DILI. While they are of clinical significance, diagnosis and treatment present challenges since the relationship between the offending antibiotic and hypersensitivity is generally not well understood. It is even more complex when patients concurrently receive multiple drugs, hence it is particularly challenging to isolate the offending drug (Rizzi et al., 2023). Clinicians thus face daunting dilemmas that entail serious considerations of both short- and long-term implications for patient health. Antibiotic prophylaxis—like the judicious use of beta-lactams—is an essential part of surgery regimens, employed to prevent infection after surgery. However, their reliance is tainted with drug allergic complications. Guidelines emphasize the use of first- and second-generation cephalosporins and aminopenicillins, with a preference for surgical environments. However, clinical experience suggests that discrepancies exist between documented allergies and actual hypersensitivity cases. Several patients self-label as allergic based on a misunderstanding of previous reactions, overestimating the risks of these antibiotics. The danger of underestimating real allergy rates can undermine patient management by inducing unnecessary avoidance of successful treatments and augmenting the risk of adverse effects due to untreated infections (Zyryanov et al., 2022). Knowledge of the patterns of such reactions is essential for maximizing the benefits of antibiotic use and reducing hypersensitivity responses. The management of DHRs requires an integrated framework that incorporates both diagnostic and therapeutic approaches. Since tests for allergies also carry certain limitations, other methods, such as desensitization procedures, have emerged but vary greatly in practice and recognition. The first action in the management of serious reactions such as DRESS and DILI would often involve the immediate cessation of all suspected antibiotics, followed by the administration of corticosteroids to alleviate symptoms. Unfortunately, identification of the culpable drug remains a complex issue, often confounded by patients' previous history of antibiotics and background drugs (Rizzi et al., 2023). Thus, clinical practice guidelines and research must strive to enhance knowledge of hypersensitivity mechanisms, diagnostic accuracy, and therapeutic algorithms in order to provide better care for antibiotic-induced hypersensitivity reactions (Figure 5.12).

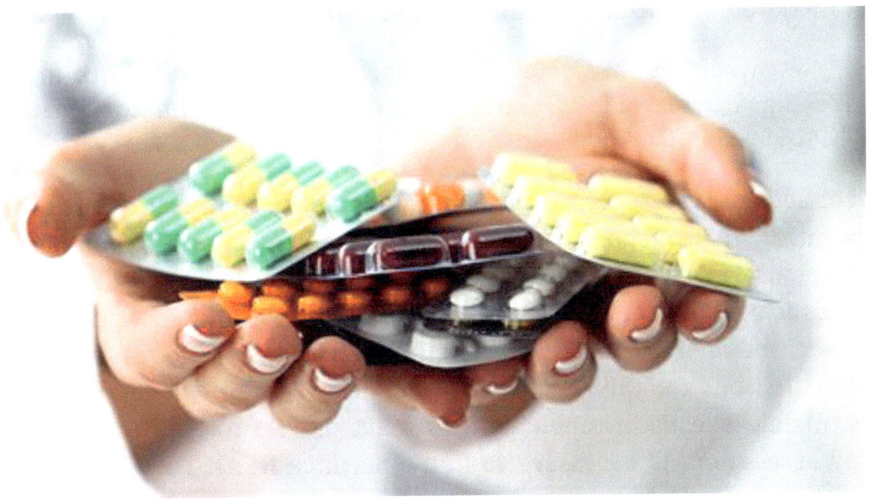

Figure 5.12. Antibiotics.

Source: https://external-content.duckduckgo.com/iu/?u=https%3A%2F%2Ftse2.mm.bing.net% 2Fth%3Fid%3DOIP.ps6kARqD66VuEVZlwcYBGAHaD5%26pid%3DApi&f=1&ipt=25dd60daca1d2abf9bece39131296c6c8d69d2a4494c1e323288d1ae48fcfb04.

5.3.2. Non-Steroidal Anti-Inflammatory Drugs (NSAIDs)

The widespread use of NSAIDs for pain management and inflammation control has raised significant concerns regarding DHRs. Medications for arthritis and headaches can cause HSRs, so they are the second most common reason for these drug-related events. Notably, the mechanism underlying these reactions often involves the inhibition of cyclooxygenase type 1 (COX-1), which may contribute to cross-HSRs among different NSAID subgroups. It is very important to understand the symptoms of these reactions, since they can range from minor hives to a life-threatening anaphylactic shock. So that therapists can choose safer options, more research is required to find out how NSAID hypersensitivity works and to identify new treatments.

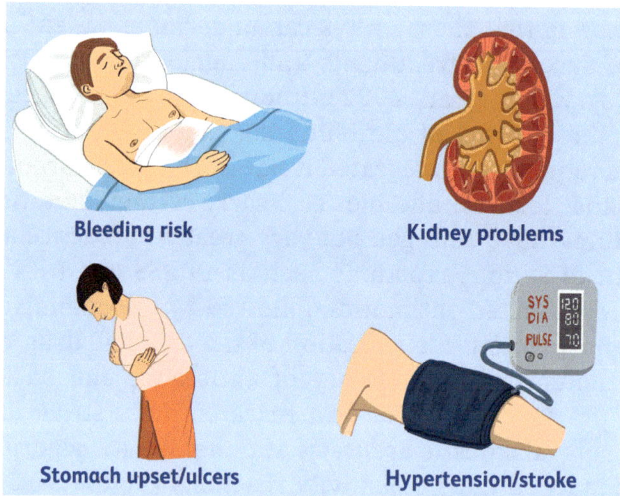

Figure 5.13. Non-steroidal anti-inflammatory drugs (NSAIDs).

Source: https://www.verywellhealth.com/thmb/FwSyuuRY_ficRu0rTdts_mDqQo8=/1500x0/filters:no_upscale():max_bytes(150000):strip_icc()/best-anti-inflammatory-medication-2548734-c7ad2c0e99d8424b95ce54ef0cb1a041.png.

A study conducted over several years revealed that a significant portion of patients with immediate-type drug hypersensitivity reactions (IDHRs) to NSAIDs experienced reactions characterized by urticaria or angioedema (CRs-UA). A single institution's study found that 307 patients with suspected NSAID hypersensitivity were seen, and 237 of them were confirmed to have IDHRs. It was found that women experienced CRs-UA more often than men, which could point to biological reasons for this. For this reason, therapies should be personalized to include sex differences, mainly because women tend to react more slowly. The study points out that a thorough allergy assessment is necessary to find out which NSAIDs trigger allergic reactions and help manage people who have been diagnosed with hypersensitivity. The tolerability of NSAIDs for people with hypersensitivity depends on the drug taken and the patient's background. A retrospective analysis demonstrated that skin testing followed by oral provocation tests (OPTs) can effectively identify safe alternatives for patients with known NSAID reactions. In the study, 398 patients were included, and although a few reacted well to the first NSAID, most patients experienced no problems with acetaminophen and celecoxib. Clinicians can use controlled challenges to determine the safety of alternative NSAIDs and learn about each patient's reaction, which helps improve their pharmacological care. For this reason, it is important to test patients thoroughly and prescribe analgesics carefully to those who have been diagnosed with NSAID hypersensitivity, so they are safe and their pain is effectively managed (Figure 5.13).

5.3.3. Anticonvulsants

Anticonvulsants represent a diverse group of drugs primarily employed in the management of seizure disorders but also for off-label use, like mood stabilization and neuropathic pain. Despite the proven efficacy of these medications, their use is shrouded by the risk of DHRs ranging from mild cutaneous eruptions to fulminant and life-threatening disease. Notably, aromatic anticonvulsants such as carbamazepine and phenytoin are the most frequent to be involved in HSRs. Increasing evidence reveals that newer non-aromatic anticonvulsants like levetiracetam are also not exempt from this risk, thereby necessitating a sense of caution among health practitioners to monitor patients for side effects while on treatment carefully (Roseni et al., 2024). Severe HSRs to anticonvulsants are severe clinical problems, particularly in diagnosis and treatment. Among the reactions are DRESS syndrome, which is a severe but rare condition associated with anticonvulsant therapy. Patients may present with a cluster of symptoms including fever, lymphadenopathy, rash, and systemic involvement of organs, particularly the liver (Lee et al., 2023). DRESS syndrome's complexity demands a high level of suspicion to allow timely detection, as this is central in preventing complications and improving patient outcomes. Management typically consists of withdrawal of the offending drug and initiation of corticosteroid therapy, which is effective in eliminating the symptoms and halting further decline of the patient's condition (Roseni et al., 2024). Furthermore, the prevention of DHRs in patients undergoing anticonvulsant therapy requires a multidisciplinary approach. This entails careful selection of patients on the basis of genetic predisposition and prior allergic history, since certain groups could be particularly vulnerable to the development of adverse effects. Educating the patients and doctors about the clinical presentation of hypersensitivity could facilitate early intervention and reduce the risk of adverse outcomes. Continuous updating of guidelines, according to new research, is at the heart of directing prescribing practice and optimizing safety profiles of these medications in clinical practice. Overall, information regarding DHRs is essential for both neurologists and primary physicians (Lee et al., 2023) (Figure 5.14).

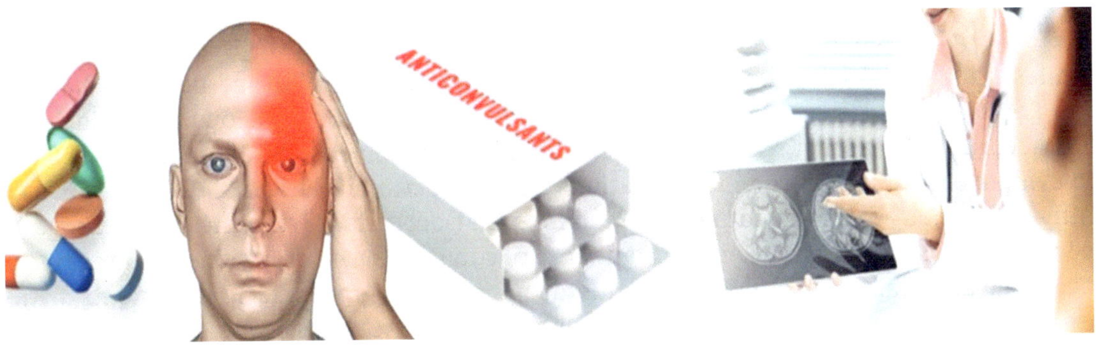

Figure 5.14. Anticonvulsants.

Source: https://www.internationaldrugmart.com/wp-content/uploads/2024/03/28022024-blog-image-What-anticonvulsants-are-used-for-migraine-1024x236.webp.

5.4. Clinical Manifestations

There are many symptoms of drug hypersensitivity, and they are usually sorted by the time they appear and how severe they are. Type B HSRs happen within a short period of time after exposure and usually lead to urticaria, angioedema, or anaphylactic shock. These rapid responses involve the release of immunoglobulin E (IgE) and the activation of mast cells, leading to the release of histamine and other mediators. At the same time, delayed hypersensitivity can cause symptoms to appear after several days and may result in problems such as maculopapular rashes or blisters. The variability in clinical presentation underscores the necessity for HCPs to establish robust diagnostic criteria and maintain a high index of suspicion when faced with potential drug allergies, as understanding these manifestations is crucial for effective management of ADRs (Villarreal-González et al., 2024). Among the severe forms of DHRs are SJS and DRESS. Both conditions represent extreme responses that can be life-threatening. The main symptoms of SJS include painful sores on the mucous membranes and widespread rashes, which typically begin as flu-like symptoms and then progress rapidly. Alternatively, DRESS syndrome is characterized by fever, a rash, swollen lymph nodes, and organ dysfunction, particularly in the liver, resulting from an immune response. Since these conditions have complex symptoms, they are challenging to diagnose and often require hospitalization and assistance from various specialists. Given the potential severity, recognizing early signs of SJS and DRESS syndrome is paramount to minimizing morbidity and mortality associated with these DHRs (Sura, 2024). The wide range of symptoms observed in DHRs suggests a delicate connection between drugs and the immune system. Things like a person's genes, other drugs they are taking, and any health problems they have can increase the chances and seriousness of these reactions. When healthcare providers notice different signs of the disease, they can respond with the right treatment promptly. Additionally, understanding the immune system's role in these diseases is crucial for developing more effective treatments and prevention strategies. The field of research is still growing, showing why it is necessary to educate people about drug hypersensitivity. In doing so, the healthcare community can work towards reducing the incidence of such ADRs and improving patient outcomes (Villarreal-González et al., 2024).

5.4.1. Skin Reactions

The manifestation of skin reactions in DHRs is of the highest significance both clinically and in research. The reactions vary from minor rashes and eruptions to more serious forms, including SJS and TEN. According to current studies, cutaneous presentation is observed in nearly 97.5% of DHR cases, playing a crucial role in the manifestation of such reactions (Şule et al., 2024). It is essential to identify the various forms of cutaneous reactions that occur following the use of drugs for the effective management of patients. The predominance of cutaneous manifestations requires meticulous monitoring for all cutaneous changes following drug exposure, particularly in patients with prior histories of atopic disorders, because such individuals can acquire accentuated drug sensitivity. Furthermore, the pathogenesis of cutaneous reactions can often be multifactorial, involving multiple underlying mechanisms, including both immunologic and non-immunologic factors. Urticaria and angioedema are common immediate HSRs that occur minutes to hours following exposure to the offending drug. Delayed HSRs, however, can occur days to weeks following administration and frequently manifest as exanthematous drug eruptions. The literature has established that certain drugs, such as antibiotics, are most commonly associated with skin reactions, which occur in a high number of cases (Şule et al., 2024). Identification of these reactions is necessary; appropriate diagnostic testing, including skin testing and provocation protocols, is justified to accurately identify the causative agent and prevent potentially hazardous future medication regimens. More recent research has expanded our understanding of the genetic basis for drug-induced skin reactions, particularly with nonionic iodinated contrast media (ICMs). A genome-wide association study identified several candidate risk loci for both immediate and delayed HSRs. This genetic data provides a potential avenue for designing targeted treatments and preventing life-threatening skin reactions in individuals at risk. Notably, immediate and delayed hypersensitivity responses may be mediated by distinct genetic and biological pathways, as suggested by pathway enrichment analyses. This growing body of evidence supports the need for careful assessments within clinical practice, which enable accurate diagnoses and informed treatment plans, ultimately addressing the complexity associated with drug-induced cutaneous reactions in vulnerable patient populations (Figure 5.15).

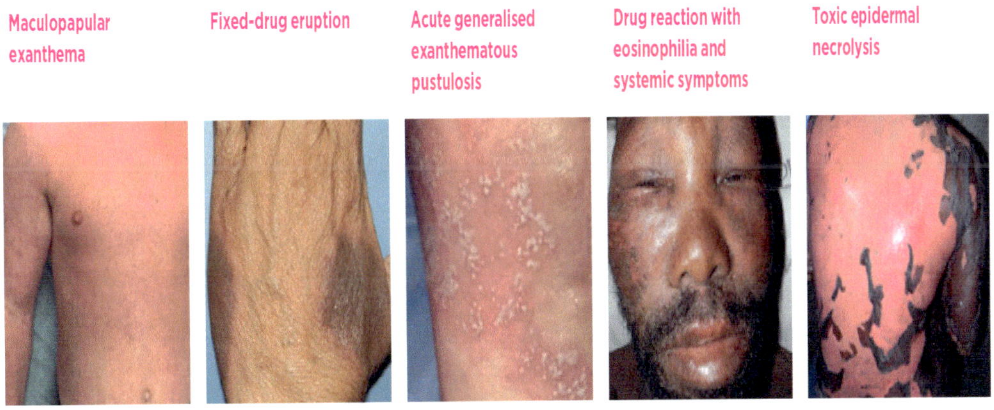

Figure 5.15. Reactions in drug.

Source: https://www.nps.org.au/assets/AP/images/Fig_p43-Copaescu-Trubiano-2.png.

5.4.2. Respiratory Symptoms

Respiratory symptoms are significant in DHRs and often result in serious health problems and, in the worst cases, death. These symptoms can range from mild respiratory discomfort to severe conditions such as acute respiratory distress syndrome (ARDS). Antibiotics and chemotherapy agents are well-known for causing breathing problems, so doctors closely watch patients' breathing when they take these drugs. It is often difficult to tell if someone's breathing problems are due to drugs or to infections or other health conditions, since this knowledge is essential for proper treatment. For instance, daptomycin, an antibiotic used for resistant infections, has been associated with HSRs that include eosinophilic pneumonia, complicating the diagnostic process due to symptom overlap with other respiratory illnesses, as highlighted in recent literature (Shakour et al., 2025). When evaluating respiratory symptoms in drug-induced hypersensitivity, doctors review the patient's medical history, the drugs to which they have been exposed, and the type of symptoms they are experiencing. Acute hypoxemic respiratory failure (AHRF), a serious presentation linked to drug hypersensitivity, necessitates immediate attention and intervention. A person with respiratory distress may experience wheezing, have trouble breathing, and show a significant drop in oxygen saturation levels. So, health care providers must decide which possible illnesses to focus on, mainly when patients are taking several drugs at the same time for chemotherapy. The complexity of these situations is underscored by the fact that various chemotherapeutic agents, including platinum compounds and taxanes, are known to provoke respiratory HSRs, further complicating therapeutic decisions (Atias et al., 2024). Additionally, managing DHRs that involve breathing difficulties often requires the collaboration of multiple medical professionals. This may require the assistance of allergists, pulmonologists, and the primary healthcare team to manage care effectively. When airway disease or other respiratory problems occur, the offending agent must be removed, and drugs such as bronchodilators or corticosteroids may be needed to help ease inflammation and open the airways. In cases where desensitization is possible, particularly in chemotherapy-induced hypersensitivity, careful protocols are established to reintroduce the drug while minimizing the risk of adverse reactions (Atias et al., 2024). This highlights the importance of managing these cases effectively, as unaddressed respiratory complications can significantly impact both the patient's health and the treatment's effectiveness. Therefore, it is crucial to remain vigilant and respond promptly to any suspected DHR (Figure 5.16).

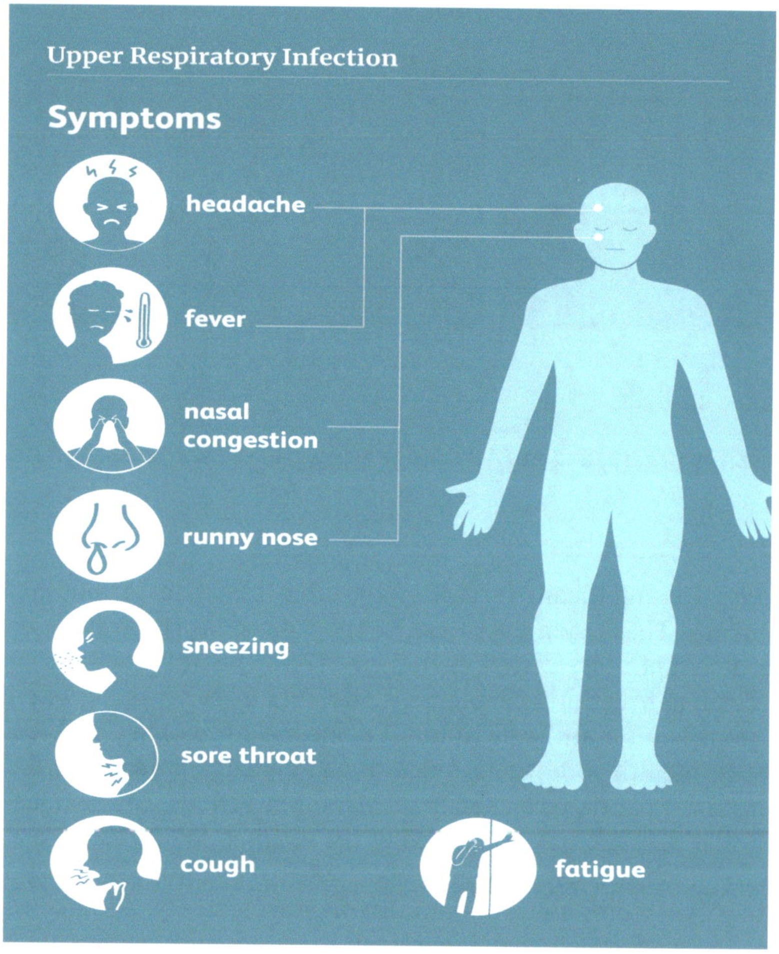

Figure 5.16. Respiratory symptoms.

Source: https://www.verywellhealth.com/thmb/t4KoSyyIskGFGgTh8zR6VL6vpNE=/1500x0/filters:no_upscale():max_bytes(150000):strip_icc()/upper-respiratory-infection-overview-4582263-5c7016c2c9e77c000149e4ae.png.

5.4.3. Systemic Reactions

Systemic DHRs mean a variety of reactions that are found throughout the body, typically with a significant impact on patient health. Systemic reactions typically occur when the immune system responds abnormally to a drug, causing extensive symptoms with variable intensity. For instance, beta-lactam antibiotics are designed to produce systemic reactions such as anaphylaxis and serious cutaneous adverse reactions. The presentation can range from mildly symptomatic, e.g., maculopapular exanthema or urticaria, to possibly lethal in a few instances. Understanding the mechanisms behind these systemic responses is vital for effective diagnosis and control because they are more likely to incorporate complex immune mechanisms in which the T cells play a central role in mediating the responses, which suggests cautious evaluation when patients present with hypersensitivity to drugs, particularly antibiotics and NSAIDs as has been observed in literature (Arasi et al., 2018; Ballmer-Weber et al., 2022). The immune mechanisms responsible for inducing systemic reactions can be categorized into two broad patterns: the hapten concept and the pharmacological interaction with immune receptors (p-i concept). Clinical observations reveal that patients with immediate reactions frequently exhibit T-cell activation through the predominantly hapten mechanism, where drug molecules covalently bind to proteins to form new antigenic structures. In contrast, those individuals with more intense reactions characterized by systemic symptoms and eosinophilic infiltration have largely positive responses due to the p-i mechanism. This is significant for making treatment and risk decisions for future drug exposures. A shift in reactivity patterns away from hapten-mediated and toward p-i-mediated reactions suggests that the severity of clinical effects is inextricably linked to the underlying immunological mechanisms involved, thus informing the development of targeted interventions and prevention measures to mitigate drug hypersensitivity risks (Ballmer-Weber et al., 2022). The clinical relevance of these systemic reactions highlights the necessity for stringent diagnostic protocols, particularly in pediatric patients who may be more susceptible to toxic drug reactions. Current laboratory tests are often not discriminative enough to unequivocally diagnose drug allergies; hence, the drug provocation test (DPT) is the method of choice for diagnosis. The DPT employs a stratified approach in establishing allergen tolerance through the application of controlled doses of the supposed medication, enabling medical professionals to correctly identify the causative agent of the hypersensitivity reaction. DPT protocols can vary based on the type of drug and the onset of the reaction, taking into account the patient's history and clinical presentation. As outlined in regulations by health authorities, the systematic approach to DPT emphasizes the importance of clear guidelines in identifying hypersensitivity, aiming to ensure safety and efficacy in treating drug allergies in children and adolescents (Arasi et al., 2018).

5.5. Diagnosis of Drug Hypersensitivity

The diagnosis of DHRs is a complex process that necessitates a thorough understanding of both clinical history and various diagnostic techniques. Initially, physicians need to collect a comprehensive anamnesis by asking about any previous medications taken and the symptoms that followed. It is essential to understand the many different mechanisms that cause these reactions for proper diagnosis. For instance, certain drugs, like NSAIDs, can provoke a variety of HSRs, leading to diverse clinical manifestations. As noted by Cucu et al. (2019), physicians must assess patients to evaluate the likelihood of DHR based on clinical analysis and may need to pursue further diagnostic steps for confirmation, such as in vitro tests or oral provocation challenges, as recommended by allergy specialists. Skin testing is now often used to find out if a person has allergies to drugs. However, its accuracy may be affected by the possibility of false positives and the fact that every person's immune response is unique. Although fluoroquinolones are less likely to cause HSRs, they may still cause reactions immediately upon exposure. Given the complexity of diagnosing fluoroquinolone hypersensitivity, Malagón et al. (2018) emphasize that accurate interpretation of clinical history is often inadequate on its own. However, allergists should keep in mind that provocation tests may sometimes exacerbate the patient's condition. Therefore, new in vitro tests are being developed to assess specific IgE antibodies more accurately and safely for individuals who may have drug allergies. Ultimately, drug hypersensitivity is diagnosed by reviewing the patient's medical history and utilizing advanced diagnostic testing methods. It is essential for clinicians to monitor for allergic reactions, particularly in patients taking NSAIDs and fluoroquinolones. Better immunoassay techniques are enhancing the process, and they may lead to more reliable diagnostic methods in the future. As highlighted by Malagón et al. (2018), the development of solid-phase assays for detecting specific IgE linked to fluoroquinolone exposure reflects the ongoing evolution of diagnostic practices in this field. As researchers continually refine these methods, it becomes increasingly easier to diagnose DHRs promptly and manage patients effectively.

5.5.1. Patient History and Clinical Evaluation

Patient history taking forms one of the cornerstones of DHR clinical diagnosis. The history not only encompasses the history of exposure to drugs by the patient but also details about the time, nature, and severity of previous exposure. The history of the patient should receive prime consideration from the clinician, such as the history of asthma or cystic fibrosis, which puts the patient at risk for certain HSRs. For example, allergic bronchopulmonary aspergillosis (ABPA) patients would otherwise be more sensitive to Aspergillus fumigatus and may experience ADRs of an extreme nature when they receive inappropriate antibiotics. Thus, awareness of a patient's history of drug reaction can assist clinicians in formulating a differential diagnosis and planning subsequent therapy, thereby making patients safer and improving treatment outcomes (Reza et al., 2025). Clinical evaluation also attests to the value of pharmacologic history, as evidenced by references to a broad range of diagnostic tests and rating scales. Pharmacovigilance—the surveillance of drug action following drug licensure—is a central function in identifying potentially toxic drug interactions in at-risk groups. For instance, some allergy tests to measure serum levels of IgE, while accurate clinical scoring systems are able to estimate the chances of a hypersensitivity reaction. Where patients have complicated histories of drug reactions, such tools are extremely important. They assist clinicians in being able to determine whether symptoms are causally related to drug hypersensitivity or not, but rather are being caused by other concomitant pathologies, like somatoform disorders. This distinction is critical, as noted in evaluating a patient with ABPA whose complications were the result of mismanaged antibiotic interventions, which underscores the importance of advanced clinical maneuvers (Reza et al., 2025). Beyond identifying a patient's drug history and using clinical scoring approaches, it is essential to understand the broader consequences of microbial interaction when evaluating HSRs. For instance, patients with a previous history of multiple drug hypersensitivity, such as those influenced by *Cutibacterium avidum* infection due to pacemaker implantation, illustrate the complexities faced in effective treatment protocols. The biofilm formation is chronic and hence poses a hindrance for antibiotics to become effective, leading to a cycle of infection and hypersensitivity. This highlights the necessity of an integrated process in the clinical assessment procedure where patient history must be harmoniously interfaced with an awareness of microbial pathogenicity and host susceptibility. Through such a synthesis of these aspects, treating doctors can formulate holistic treatment protocols to address not only the presenting drug reactions but also the underlying infectious processes, thereby refining patient outcomes (Figure 5.17).

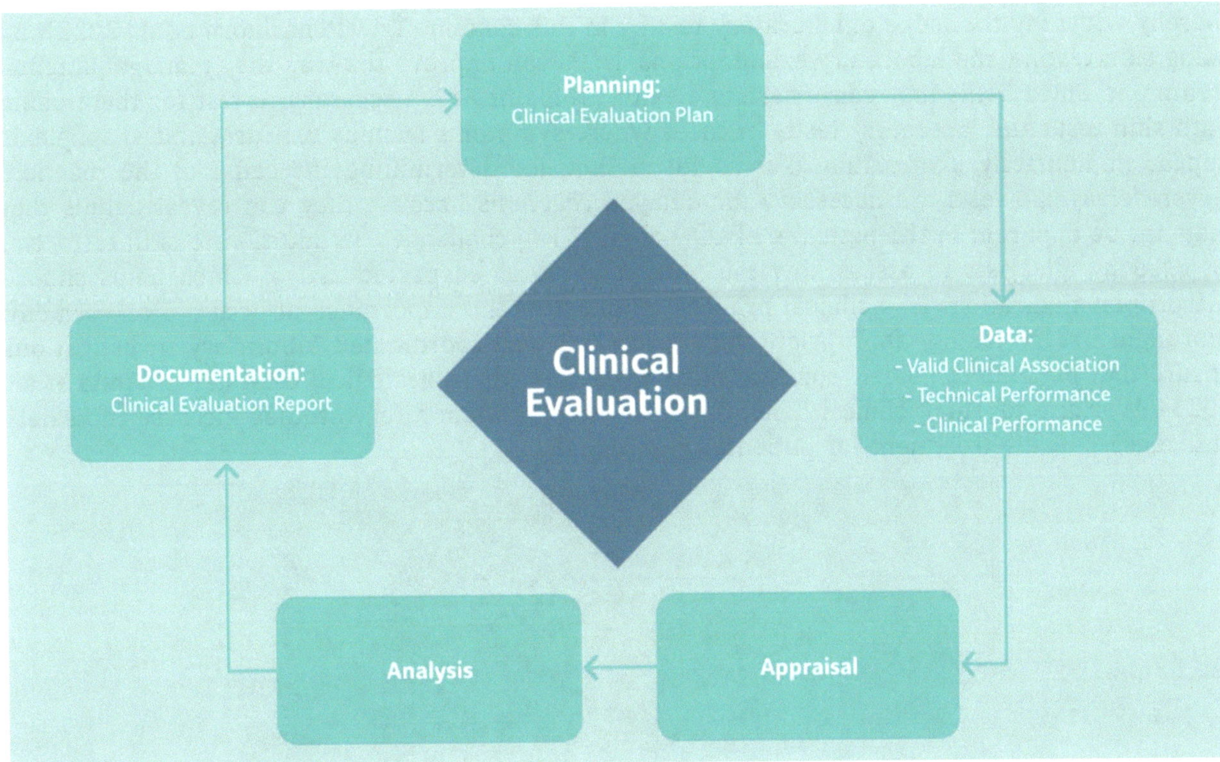

Figure 5.17. Clinical evaluation.

Source: https://congenius.ch/wp-content/uploads/2022/03/Overview-of-Clinical-Evaluation-stages.jpg.

5.5.2. Skin Testing and Laboratory Tests

In the diagnosis of IgE-mediated reactions, skin testing plays a crucial role. When allergens are applied to the skin by clinicians, immediate reactions can show if someone is sensitive to them. For drugs such as penicillin, this approach is widely used since standard skin tests are available. Still, when examining other medications, the situation becomes more complicated, as there are not many established testing protocols. Alternatively, immunological tests and a complete review of the patient's history are still the main methods for diagnosing drug-induced HSRs. By employing these various approaches, it becomes easier to identify the cause of the disease and select safer treatments. Therefore, using skin tests and reviewing the patient's history is a key method in diagnosing drug allergies and determining the best treatment for affected individuals. Besides skin tests, laboratory tests can give important information about how DHRs occur. For example, finding drug-specific T cells with different immunological methods makes it easier to diagnose delayed-type HSRs. With these techniques, it is possible to uncover the mechanisms at work, especially in cases of drug-related immune complex reactions that are not always readily apparent. Measuring specific immunoglobulins, for example IgE and IgG, gives valuable information that helps identify the type of hypersensitivity a patient has. As indicated by recent findings, the use of skin tests with delayed readings may further confirm certain types of immune complex-mediated hypersensitivity, thereby widening the scope of laboratory testing in this context (Triwatcharikorn et al., 2022). By using skin testing and laboratory examinations, HCPs can improve the way they manage patients' treatment. Since DHRs may cause serious health problems, it is necessary to test for them using both skin tests and laboratory tests. In cases where symptoms such as urticaria and anaphylaxis appear immediately, skin testing is a useful method for determining the cause of the reaction. Nevertheless, lab tests are necessary for delayed reactions because they can reveal details that may not be apparent in the patient's history alone. Drug challenges, in addition to skin tests, can be used by allergists to assess how the patient tolerates suspected drugs, which helps choose the proper medication. This clinical practice emphasizes the importance of accurate assessment; thorough history taking, appropriate skin tests, and well-coordinated laboratory investigations ensure that patients can safely continue their necessary pharmacological treatments (Anna et al., 2021). Working together, clinical history, skin testing, and laboratory studies increase the safety and success of the treatment for patients (Figure 5.18).

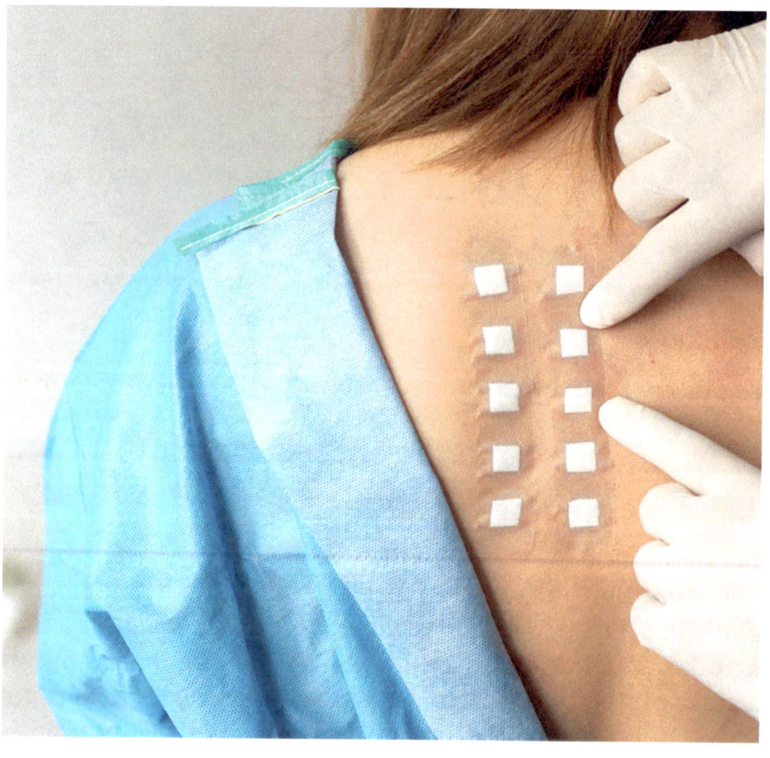

Figure 5.18. Skin testing.

Source: https://mascotspincontrol.in/cdn/shop/files/PATCHTESTFORSENSITIVESKIN.jpg?v=1683347078.

5.5.3. Drug Provocation Tests

Drug provocation tests (DPTs) are an important diagnostic tool in the evaluation of suspected allergic reactions to drugs in DHR evaluation. During the process of such tests, the drug is given in a controlled setting to monitor patients for any adverse reactions. The significance of DPTs is that they can differentiate between true hypersensitivity and other non-allergic adverse effects that can typically present similarly. For example, research has established that various drugs, most commonly antibiotics and analgesics, are frequently implicated in hypersensitivity cases, and rigorous testing procedures must be followed to ensure patient safety and guide treatment decisions appropriately (Audicana et al., 2022). DPTs, when done in clinical healthcare environments, add a critical facet to understanding individual patient responses to drugs that were previously avoided. DPTs, in addition, can shed light on the character of DHRs and enhance therapeutic counsel in patients with a history of ADR. They are of most tremendous significance in individuals who have shown responses to particular drugs, as the results can inform clinicians whether there are safe alternatives or if the administered drug can be tolerated when the conditions are being managed. Other research has shown that most individuals develop urticaria or angioedema when exposed to known allergens, highlighting the importance of DPTs in elucidating the exact mechanism of hypersensitivity and identifying cross-reactivity of therapeutic drugs (Audicana et al., 2022). The approach enables clinicians to make an objective clinical choice and administer maximum drug therapy to patients while preventing recurrent HSRs. The implementation of drug provocation testing into practice necessitates that multiple factors be considered in depth, including patient selection, test protocol, and monitoring methods. As highlighted in the literature, thorough patient evaluation is necessary to prevent undue reaction in testing, particularly in subjects at high risk of anaphylactic reaction. It is supremely crucial for health professionals to be thoroughly trained in administering DPT, as proficiency in this skill has a direct implication for patient outcomes. Positive test results not only confirm drug tolerance but also make setting procedures for future medication handling possible. With ongoing studies on the safety and efficacy of DPTs, it is evident that these tests are an essential part in the overall framework of managing DHRs, enhancing patient safety, and contributing to better therapeutic practices (Ebru, 2022).

5.6. Management and Treatment

Effective management and treatment strategies for DHRs are crucial in mitigating patient distress and ensuring continuity of care. In cases of immediate drug hypersensitivity reactions (IDHRs), rapid drug desensitization (RDD) has emerged as a viable option, particularly for patients undergoing antineoplastic therapy. RDD could be more useful in certain areas, but it is not used as extensively in Northern Europe as in Southern Europe and the United States, where allergists play a larger role in managing allergic reactions. In Denmark, a study found that 2.5% of patients had IDHRs while receiving antineoplastic therapy; therefore, it is necessary to include allergy testing and RDD in the management of these patients. The findings suggest that a substantial number of patients, particularly those with gynecologic cancers, may benefit from more effective treatment strategies to minimize disruptions caused by DHRs (Rasmussen et al., 2025). The treatment of severe drug reactions, such as DRESS syndrome, necessitates a nuanced pharmacological approach tailored to individual patient needs. The primary feature of DRESS syndrome is that the delayed hypersensitivity reaction results in severe skin and systemic symptoms. During the use of unfractionated heparin in a clinical case, a patient suffered a DRESS episode and had severe problems following surgery. Using bivalirudin, a direct thrombin inhibitor, during cardiopulmonary bypass surgery was very important in an urgent situation. Because there is no reversal agent for bivalirudin, it is essential to closely monitor patients and use the appropriate anticoagulation approach to prevent worsening the hypersensitivity reaction. This case highlights the importance of considering the clinical context and the need for a flexible management plan that minimizes adverse effects through suitable treatment options (Pe Lña-Blanco et al., 2024). The primary objective of managing DHRs is to ensure patient safety while still allowing for effective treatment. Some strategies include giving stronger premedication, paying close attention to the patient, and ensuring that all healthcare providers are working together. If a patient stops taking a drug because of an IDHR, as happened with 45% of patients, giving them a different drug or using a desensitization protocol may help prevent more treatment breaks. It is essential to consider a patient's medical history and the type of reaction they experience when selecting the appropriate medication. As HCPs continue to grapple with the implications of DHRs on patient outcomes, increasing awareness of alternative therapeutic options and employing proactive management tactics will be vital in reducing the incidence of HSRs and promoting overall patient well-being (Pe Lña-Blanco et al., 2024; Rasmussen et al., 2025) (Figure 5.19).

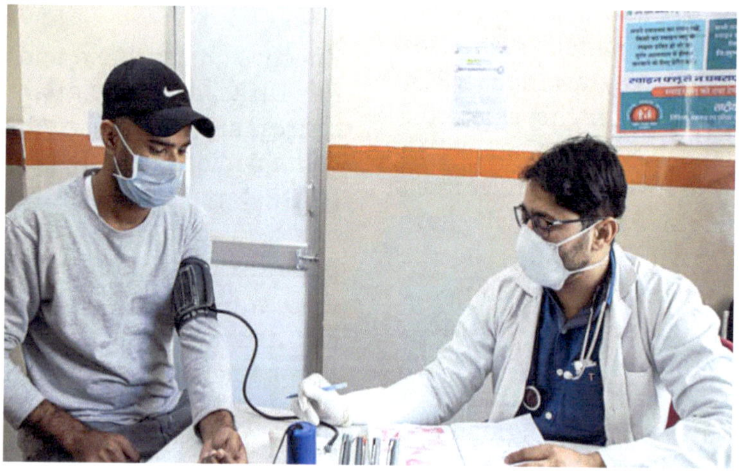

Figure 5.19. Medical treatments.

Source: https://www.indiaspend.com/h-upload/old_images/1500x900_342694-overpricing1440.jpg.

5.6.1. Avoidance of Offending Drugs

Avoiding offending drugs is important in the treatment of drug HSRs. After an established diagnosis of drug allergy, patients should avoid the offending agent entirely to prevent recurrence of the adverse effects. Not only does this type of avoidance enhance patient safety, but it also improves the quality of life in general by preventing life-threatening or even lethal HSRs. Successful avoidance also involves not just the removal of the offending allergen, but also demands careful consideration of substitute drugs. Patients must be educated by health care practitioners about their specific drug allergies and instructed on cross-reactive drugs to enable them to make informed decisions in obtaining care. As underscored by Jeimy et al. (2025), proper clinician-directed avoidance is key to the successful treatment of this patient population. Moreover, the choice of alternative drugs must involve a rigorous examination of chemical structure and mechanisms of action. Healthcare providers are responsible for identifying alternatives that lower the risk of such HSRs, while still continuing to treat the patients' underlying medical conditions. This could be a complex undertaking when dealing with systemic medications known for cross-reactivity within the same drug classes. Clinicians must understand these connections when prescribing. When an essential medication is required but previously determined substitutes are found to have the same risks, clinicians may resort to more advanced methods, such as desensitization protocols. Although avoidance is the primary method for the majority of patients, as shown by Stan (2023), judicious application of desensitization can make it feasible to safely administer the offending drug when no other solution is available. The use of avoidance techniques also entails practicing necessary precautions within the healthcare environment. For instance, healthcare facilities must put strong measures in place for recording and reporting drug allergies by patients in their medical records. Additionally, training staff courses have to emphasize the importance of such records in prescribing regimens in avoiding inadvertent exposure to offending drugs. Educational initiatives are not only reserved for healthcare staff; patients must also be empowered so that they can accurately convey their allergies to all the members of their care team, i.e., pharmacists and emergency medical staff. By inducing a culture of cooperation and vigilance, the likelihood of DHRs can be effectively minimized. Such a group effort to prevent offending drugs serves as the foundation for much of the guidelines and advice reported in literature, e.g., (Jeimy et al., 2025), thereby promoting patient safety and therapeutic success.

5.6.2. Pharmacological Interventions

In the context of DHRs, pharmacological interventions play a pivotal role in managing symptoms and preventing future occurrences. Antihistamines are commonly given to patients to reduce the impact of histamine release when they have an allergic reaction. They are helpful in most cases, but when a severe reaction, such as anaphylaxis, occurs, epinephrine must be administered immediately. Since fast action is important in these cases, doctors have investigated using steroids and additional drugs to help patients. In addition, following complete premedication plans has been proven to decrease the number of DHRs, mainly among people using high-risk medicines. Still, it is essential to explore how these interventions can be applied to various patient groups. In children, health professionals must use specialized medications because their bodies are not the same as those of adults, and they may develop unusual immune responses. Antihistamines and corticosteroids given beforehand are being highlighted as ways to help children avoid or reduce HSRs when they take antibiotics or chemotherapy. Still, since studies on using epinephrine for pediatric patients, mainly those with non-IgE-mediated allergies, are not very common, it is recommended to approach each case with care and an individual plan. Klain et al. (2025) emphasize the importance of developing guidelines that are informed by rigorous studies within this demographic, as many existing interventions are derived from adult populations. Therefore, additional studies are required to develop guidelines that guarantee the safety and effectiveness of these drugs for children. RDD represents a pharmacological intervention gaining traction as a solution for patients experiencing immediate drug hypersensitivity reactions (IDHRs) during necessary treatments, mainly with antineoplastic agents. Researchers have found that RDD protocols can yield different results, as they gradually increase the dose to induce tolerance. In Denmark, for instance, the integration of RDD within cancer treatment protocols is limited, highlighting a disconnect between practices in different regions. Rasmussen et al. (2025) demonstrate the significant impact of IDHRs on treatment adherence among cancer patients. Although adjusting premedication and infusion rates can be beneficial, the occurrence of major reactions suggests that we should further enhance our efforts to identify allergies and standardize the RDD process. Since DHRs are a major issue in oncology, further studies are needed to help improve how patients take their medicines without putting them at risk (Figure 5.20).

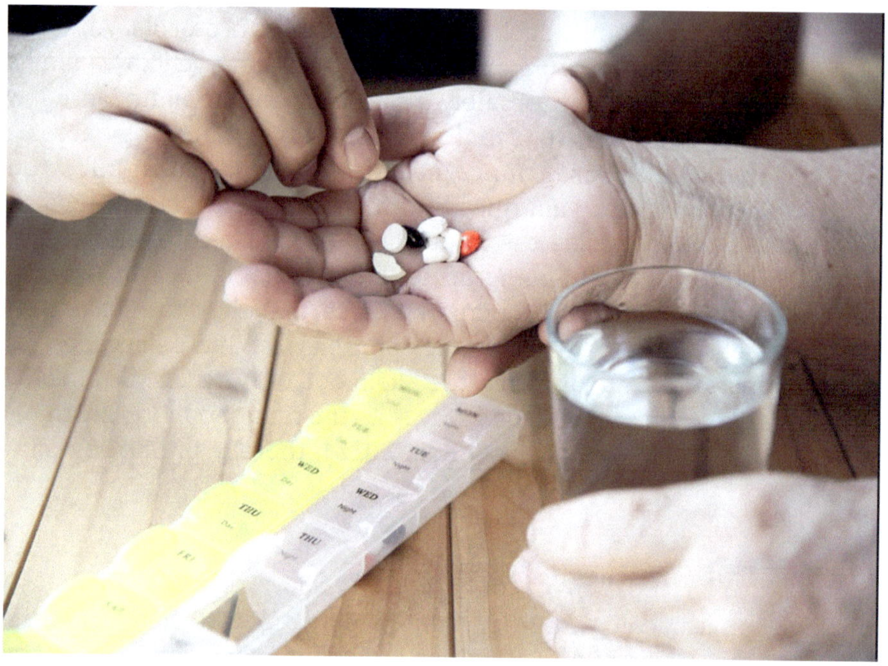

Figure 5.20. Pharmacological treatments.

Source: https://nirvanhospital.com/wp-content/uploads/2023/12/Integrating-Medication-Management.png.

5.6.3. Patient Education and Counseling

In the context of DHRs, patient counseling and education become key factors in preventing negative health outcomes. When patients are well-informed about drugs and potential allergic reactions, they will be better equipped to recognize and report symptoms in a timely manner. With an understanding of the importance of adherence to medications and the risks associated with drug hypersensitivity, patients can get engaged in their treatment. Effective communication between patients and physicians can facilitate candid discussion about the side effects of medication, an anticipatory management strategy. The role of pharmacists becomes particularly central, as they can provide patient-specific counseling tailored to individual needs, ultimately enhancing overall therapeutic outcomes by reducing the frequency and severity of HSRs (Newar et al., 2025). Further, application of specific strategies such as motivational interviewing (MI) in patient counseling can facilitate learning and memory for significant drug hypersensitivity information. This can be achieved by pharmacists providing tangible tools such as customized medication calendars or information on identifying signs and symptoms of hypersensitivity. This tangible assistance not only empowers patients but also reinforces patients' roles in drug safety. By integrating education interventions that focus on patient-centered care, healthcare practitioners can minimize the potential risks of HSRs, leading to improved patient compliance and satisfaction. Regular assessment of patient comprehension through following up during consultation is essential so that patients are in a position to apply what they have gained effectively, thereby improving the quality of care being administered to them and reducing adverse drug effects (Lu et al., 2025). Additionally, patient education involves the use of comprehensive care plans that incorporate pharmacist-led practice within outpatient settings. Through the integration of systematic counseling into routine care, patients gain a solid understanding of their medications, including potential interactions and hypersensitivity risks. This proactive training can be utilized to bridge the gap in treatment, often found in patients, and particularly in elderly patients, who are prone to DHRs. By establishing a collaborative partnership among patients and pharmacists, healthcare providers can identify individual coping styles and preferences and further individualize the process of education. As evidence shows, intervention by pharmacists enhances patient outcomes. It reduces the frequency of ADRs, which is a significant step forward in patient safety and medication management practices within the healthcare system (Newar et al., 2025).

Summary

In conclusion, the prevalence of DHRs represents a significant public health concern, particularly among younger adults. Research shows that approximately 12% of individuals aged 18 to 25 experience such adverse reactions, predominantly linked to antibiotics and NSAIDs (Barajas et al., 2017). It shows that both healthcare workers and patients should be better informed about DHRs. If medical practitioners are aware of the usual signs and causes, they can identify at-risk individuals earlier and take action, which may help reduce the number and severity of these reactions. Additionally, when examining the history of allergies in a patient and their family, it becomes clear that personalized medicines are necessary to mitigate the risk of drug-related problems. Since drug hypersensitivity has many aspects, strong systems for diagnosis and treatment are needed. Differentiating between immunological and non-immunological mechanisms is crucial for effectively addressing NSAIDs-induced hypersensitivity, a prevalent concern among various patient populations (Cucu et al., 2019). Therefore, clinicians should start their diagnosis by carefully reviewing a patient's history and conducting thorough clinical examinations. Although a thorough anamnesis is very helpful for identifying DHRs, it must be supported by proper diagnostic tests and, if necessary, oral provocation challenges performed by experts. Such strategies help doctors understand the leading causes, which results in better management plans for each patient. Effects of drug hypersensitivity are seen in public health, the cost of healthcare, and the entire healthcare system. As highlighted in recent studies, the relationship between specific drug classes and allergic reactions, particularly concerning antibiotics and NSAIDs, necessitates ongoing research into the epidemiology of DHRs (Barajas et al., 2017; Cucu et al., 2019). Being aware of the things that increase the risk of HSRs, for example, genetic background and atopic history, can help with preventing and treating them. All in all, dealing with DHRs calls for teamwork among HCPs, the pharmaceutical sector, and efforts to educate both patients and providers about this important issue in today's medicine.

Since DHRs can be complicated, it is essential to understand their various symptoms and the conditions under which they occur. Even though many substances can cause hypersensitivity, the frequency and severity of the reactions depend on the patient, their genetic background, and the drug being used. It has become clear that using the same definitions and classifications for these reactions would facilitate the management and reporting of them across different clinical areas. The assessment and agreement on the acute toxic effects of treatments for acute lymphoblastic leukaemia show that clinicians need to handle each patient's particular hypersensitivity differently. This underscores the importance of integrating standardized definitions that can guide future research and enhance therapeutic strategies in DHRs (Attarbaschi et al., 2016). When looking at anaphylaxis, which is a dangerous hypersensitivity reaction, guidelines agree that immediate action is necessary to avoid serious consequences. Experts from various countries are now emphasizing that epinephrine should be used first in treating anaphylaxis. It is also crucial to properly identify and treat affected individuals, demonstrating once again the importance of swift action in emergencies. The guidelines indicate that using antihistamines or glucocorticoids should not be done instead of giving epinephrine, since it can significantly affect the outcome. An extensive review of epidemiological data and patient risk factors has fueled discussions on potential improvements in both clinical practice and patient education regarding the prevention and management of anaphylaxis (Alvarez-Twose et al., 2014). The creation of detailed guidelines helps individual patients and also supports bigger studies on drug hypersensitivity. It is crucial to understand the causes, risk factors, and triggers of these reactions to develop effective methods for prevention. The recent push for joint research efforts indicates a global effort to address missing information and develop effective methods for handling DHRs. The effort aims to provide similar care across different healthcare systems and prevent the same issue from recurring in patients. Ultimately, the insights gleaned from these research endeavors have the potential to transform clinical practice, making it essential for HCPs to remain vigilant and informed about the evolving landscape of DHRs (Alvarez-Twose et al., 2014; Attarbaschi et al., 2016).

CLOSER LOOK

NEXT-GENERATION SEQUENCING TECHNOLOGIES

Next-generation sequencing (NGS) technologies have revolutionized genomics by enabling the rapid and cost-effective sequencing of DNA and RNA. Unlike traditional Sanger sequencing, which is labor-intensive and time-consuming, NGS allows for massively parallel sequencing, processing millions of fragments simultaneously. This high-throughput capability has expanded the scope of genomic research, enabling whole-genome sequencing, transcriptome profiling, and metagenomic analysis with unprecedented speed and accuracy. The primary platforms—such as Illumina, Ion Torrent, Pacific Biosciences (PacBio), and Oxford Nanopore—differ in chemistry, read length, and accuracy, catering to diverse research needs. Illumina dominates the market with short-read sequencing known for its high accuracy and low cost, while long-read technologies like PacBio and Oxford Nanopore are instrumental in resolving complex genomic regions and structural variants.

NGS technologies have had profound implications in biomedical research, clinical diagnostics, and personalized medicine. In oncology, they help identify mutations driving cancer, enabling targeted therapies. In infectious disease, NGS enables rapid pathogen identification and tracking of antimicrobial resistance. Additionally, it plays a key role in prenatal screening, rare disease diagnosis, and pharmacogenomics. Despite its transformative power, challenges such as data storage, bioinformatics analysis, and interpretation remain significant, requiring robust computational infrastructure and expertise.

Continued innovation is driving the next phase of NGS development, with third-generation sequencing promising real-time analysis, greater portability, and single-molecule resolution. As costs decline and accuracy improves, NGS is poised to become a routine part of clinical practice and public health surveillance. The integration of artificial intelligence and machine learning into NGS data interpretation is also enhancing the ability to derive meaningful insights from vast datasets. Overall, next-generation sequencing technologies are not only reshaping the landscape of genetic research but also paving the way for more precise, predictive, and personalized healthcare.

References

1. Ajon, A. R. S., & Camara, P. T. A. (2024). Drug rash with eosinophilia and systemic symptoms (DRESS) due to multiple Anti-Epileptic Drug hypersensitivity. *Cureus*. https://doi.org/10.7759/cureus.65417Al-Bayati, S. F. (2024). Severe hypersensitivity reactions with oral manifestations: Case reports on Stevens-Johnson syndrome and DRESS syndrome. *Journal of Pharmacy & Bioallied Sciences, 16*, S4935–S4939. https://www.semanticscholar.org/paper/6075af61be0b2846f1699f1cbf4e6ab0b018ab05 (accessed on 9 June 2025).
2. Alvarez-Twose, I., Muraro, A., Arga, M., Armstrong, K., Arroabarren, E., Sheikh, A., Barnett, D., et al. (2014). International consensus on (ICON) anaphylaxis. https://core.ac.uk/download/28978204.pdf (accessed on 9 June 2025).
3. Andrade, R. J., Carvajal, A., Cueto, R., Lucena, M. I., et al. (2007). Genetic and molecular factors in drug-induced liver injury: A review. https://core.ac.uk/download/13100800.pdf (accessed on 9 June 2025).
4. Arasi, S., Barni, S., Bottau, P., Caffarelli, C., et al. (2018). SIAIP position paper: Provocation challenge to antibiotics and non-steroidal anti-inflammatory drugs in children. https://core.ac.uk/download/188829702.pdf (accessed on 9 June 2025).
5. Atias, E. S., & Šematonytė, J. (2024). The role of the allergist in the management of chemotherapy-induced hypersensitivity reactions. *Pulmonology and Allergology*. https://www.semanticscholar.org/paper/79a2f211d732bbdc59c589090b8e781f421f3e9d (accessed on 9 June 2025).
6. Attarbaschi, A., Barzilai, S., Escherich, G., Frandsen, B., et al. (2016). Consensus definitions of 14 severe acute toxic effects for childhood lymphoblastic leukemia treatment: A Delphi consensus. https://core.ac.uk/download/42370388.pdf.
7. Audicana, M. T., & Ortega, N. R. (2022). Spanish Society of Allergology and Clinical Immunology (SEAIC) vision of drug provocation tests: Reply. *Journal of Investigational Allergology & Clinical Immunology, 32*(3), 242–243. https://www.semanticscholar.org/paper/36e5c1db5ee393267c728f4f63d6cf79b565efee (accessed on 9 June 2025).
8. Ballmer-Weber, B., Jörg, L., Schlapbach, C., Wuillemin, N., et al. (2022). The activation pattern of drug-reacting T cells has an impact on the clinical picture of hypersensitivity reactions. https://core.ac.uk/download/527937402.pdf (accessed on 9 June 2025).
9. Bangerl, T., Zahel, B., Lueger, A., Guenova, E., Angelova-Fischer, I., & Hoetzenecker, W. (2020). Hypersensitivity reactions to non-steroidal anti-inflammatory drugs: Results of an Austrian cohort study. *Allegro Journal International, 29*, 227–232. https://www.semanticscholar.org/paper/b5c6fcbdb3c7ad6fab7700836ce6f98701060299 (accessed on 9 June 2025).
10. Barbarino, J. M., Whirl-Carrillo, M., Altman, R. B., & Klein, T. E. (2018). PharmGKB: A worldwide resource for pharmacogenomic information. *WIREs Systems Biology and Medicine, 10*. https://doi.org/10.1002/wsbm.1417.
11. Bedolla Barajas, M., Dominguez Garcia, M. V., et al. (2017). Self-report prevalence and associated factors to drug hypersensitivity in Mexican young adults. https://core.ac.uk/download/154795675.pdf (accessed on 9 June 2025).
12. Begum, S. H., Venugopal Reddy, M., Sharon Sonia, S., Sahayaraj, K., et al. (2022). Texans induced hypersensitivity reactions in cancer chemotherapy patients reported at adverse drug reaction

monitoring center at a tertiary care hospital. https://core.ac.uk/download/552654483.pdf (accessed on 9 June 2025).

13. Beiner, L., Jeong, J., Kang, D., Lombardo, P., Kang, H., & Boehm, I. B. (2024). Immediate hypersensitivity reactions to iodinated contrast media despite drug prophylaxis—a comparative retrospective cohort study of breakthrough reactions in Bern (Switzerland) and Seoul (South Korea). *Quantitative Imaging in Medicine and Surgery, 14*, 3326–3338. https://www.semanticscholar.org/paper/f1f0c12ab29c85cc307dd8299152bd0509150958 (accessed on 9 June 2025).

14. Büyük Yaytokgil, Ş., & Vezir, E. (2024). Characteristics of drug hypersensitivity reactions in children: A retrospective analysis in an allergy outpatient clinic. *Turkish Journal of Pediatric Disease.* https://www.semanticscholar.org/paper/c6402fe1f08171baceba9e63a2d9739eb8c4a237 (accessed on 9 June 2025).

15. Cankat Genis, F., Kuzucu, Z., Şengül Emeksiz, Z., & Dibek Mısırlıoğlu, E. (2024). Negative predictive value of single-day drug provocation test for immediate and non-immediate beta-lactam hypersensitivity reactions in children. *International Archives of Allergy and Immunology, 186*, 150–158. https://www.semanticscholar.org/paper/9fa506965057840d95b4193eb18bb4b2fadbc14a (accessed on 9 June 2025).

16. Carter, A. (2021). *Importance of Understanding Genetic Predisposition.* https://core.ac.uk/download/426969023.pdf (accessed on 9 June 2025).

17. Chen, C. B., Lee, C. C., Wang, C. W., & Hung, W. (2023). Genetic associations of human leukocyte antigen alleles in cutaneous delayed drug hypersensitivity reactions: An updated review. *Dermatological Sinica, 41*, 183–198. https://www.semanticscholar.org/paper/f2627a859fde0dc773c563fb9b058d6597c79b35 (accessed on 9 June 2025).

18. Chinese Journal of Tuberculosis and Respiratory Diseases. (2024). Guidelines for diagnosis and management of drug-induced liver injury caused by anti-tuberculosis drugs (2024 version). *Zhonghua Jie He He Hu Xi Za Zhi = Zhonghua Jiehe He Huxi Zazhi = Chinese Journal of Tuberculosis and Respiratory Diseases, 47*(11), 1069–1090. https://www.semanticscholar.org/paper/e9b6e7c0517d144c8ec8fe079d1a377589fa3bf6 (accessed on 9 June 2025).

19. Chow, T. G., Muzaffar, A. F., & Alvarez-Arango, S. (2024). Non-IgE-mediated drug-induced hypersensitivity reactions in pediatrics. *Current Opinion in Pediatrics, 36*, 674–683. https://www.semanticscholar.org/paper/008145915c1cbaec61e025cac10889a7fc205703 (accessed on 9 June 2025).

20. Cohen, L., Neuman, M. G., Hwang, P. A., & Nanau, R. M. (2011). *Genetic and Immune Predictors for Hypersensitivity Syndrome to Antiepileptic Drugs.* https://core.ac.uk/download/pdf/290366.pdf (accessed on 9 June 2025).

21. Corsini, E., García, E., Agú, J. A. G., Golka, K., & Selinski, S. (2017). Biomarkers in drug hypersensitivity. https://core.ac.uk/download/187979798.pdf (accessed on 9 June 2025).

22. Cucu, A., Ghiciuc, C. M., Turliuc, D., Veres, D., et al. (2019). Nonsteroidal anti-inflammatory drugs-induced hypersensitivity reactions: Algorithm for the diagnostic and management. https://core.ac.uk/download/276556441.pdf (accessed on 9 June 2025).

23. Daubner, B., Groux-Keller, M., Kawabata, T., Naisbitt, D., Park, K. B., Thomas, W., Lerch, M., et al. (2011). Multiple drug hypersensitivity: Role of T regulatory cells (55.15). *The Journal of*

Immunology. https://www.semanticscholar.org/paper/407c63c5967d75963847ff0628af643d8a1b8a4d (accessed on 9 June 2025).

24. Doña, I., Barrionuevo, E., Salas, M., Laguna, J., Agúndez, J., García-Martín, E., & Bogas, G., et al. (2018). NSAIDs-hypersensitivity often induces a blended reaction pattern involving multiple organs. *Scientific Reports, 8*. https://www.semanticscholar.org/paper/a69e9d09ac99995eed6ae759199ed10374451196 (accessed on 9 June 2025).
25. Elzagallaai, A. A., & Rieder, M. (2022). Pathophysiology of drug hypersensitivity. *British Journal of Clinical Pharmacology, 90*, 1856–1868. https://www.semanticscholar.org/paper/bac335ee5e98ca1113dae135631fe6df3b0e51c6 (accessed on 9 June 2025).
26. Jeimy, S., Wong, T., Ben-Shoshan, M., Copaescu, A., Isabwe, G., & Ellis, A. (2025). Drug allergy. *Allergy, Asthma, and Clinical Immunology, 20*. https://www.semanticscholar.org/paper/9b2158e420fd0738c56301d5a077aa334afc0774 (accessed on 9 June 2025).
27. Klain, A., Galletta, F., Mori, F., Bettini, I., Tomei, L., Senatore, A. A., Manti, S., et al. (2025). Challenges and preventive strategies in pediatric drug hypersensitivity reactions: Where do we stand? *Italian Journal of Pediatrics, 51*. https://www.semanticscholar.org/paper/ce3f1270962db334bfb0c9adebfe8267c778320a (accessed on 9 June 2025).
28. Lee, E. H., & Jang, Y. (2023). Cutaneous adverse drug reactions. *Journal of the Korean Medical Association*. https://www.semanticscholar.org/paper/e5d381daebd2f60179e37f69206f79aa8e616c8d (accessed on 9 June 2025).
29. Lin, M. R., Liu, T. Y., Hsu, H. Y., Hsieh, Y. W., Palupi, P. D., Lau, P. P., Chang, W. C., et al. (2024). Genome-wide association study of hypersensitivity skin reactions induced by nonionic iodinated contrast media. *Asian Pacific Journal of Allergy and Immunology*. https://www.semanticscholar.org/paper/14dcc3a6789451a8c023c8db79b6da5ceee943c6 (accessed on 9 June 2025).
30. Lu, J., Luo, Y., Cai, D., & Wang, Y. (2025). A study protocol for exploring and implementing a surgical pharmaceutical service model in drug treatment management for patients with osteoporosis fracture in China. *Frontiers in Medicine, 12*. https://www.semanticscholar.org/paper/470f0e6dfce43e90d790037c5f82c416c60863f4 (accessed on 9 June 2025).
31. Malagón, P., Montañez, M. I., & Vazquez, S. (2018). *Synthesis and Characterization of New Carrier Molecule-Antibiotic Conjugates for Its Study in The Diagnosis of Drug Allergy*. https://core.ac.uk/download/287245350.pdf (accessed on 9 June 2025).
32. Myasnikova, T. N., Nekrasova, T., Romanova, T. S., Smirnov, V., & Latysheva, T. (2024). Cross-hypersensitivity reactions to non-steroidal anti-inflammatory drugs, manifested as urticaria and/or angioedema, anaphylaxis. *Russian Journal of Allergy*. https://www.semanticscholar.org/paper/2e29369622fa031494fa6c8553d31264966b9271 (accessed on 9 June 2025).
33. Newar, N., Kumari, P., & Das, C. (2025). Reconciliation of medication counseling by pharmacists for improving outpatient adherence: A review. *International Journal of Medical Sciences and Nursing Research*. https://www.semanticscholar.org/paper/be40f215c2ede6c5ff02ce0033bc160dbc3c9328 (accessed on 9 June 2025).
34. Özdemir, E. (2022). Review of patients with immediate-type drug reactions and test results: Retrospective study from the Malatya Province. *Annals of Medical Research*. https://www.semanticscholar.org/paper/7ce960475b2a0cec080274ce5511b1d22a64b026 (accessed on 9 June 2025).

35. Özden, Ş., Tepetam, F. M., & Atik, Ö. (2024). One-bag 8-step ferric carboxymaltose desensitization protocol for patients with a history of hypersensitivity reactions to iron preparations. *International Archives of Allergy and Immunology, 185*, 449–455. https://www.semanticscholar.org/paper/8eed7dc0f62547955b69c2a11a271fbaa7922d1b (accessed on 9 June 2025).

36. Pagani, S., Lombardi, N., Crescioli, G., Vighi, V. G., Spada, G., Andreetta, P., Capuano, A., et al. (2022). Drug-related hypersensitivity reactions leading to emergency department: Original data and systematic review. *Journal of Clinical Medicine, 11*. https://www.semanticscholar.org/paper/23310dea6f9b6923539f7a2dd36bed59776716ad (accessed on 9 June 2025).

37. Peña-Blanco, L., Gutiérrez-Soriano, L., Montes, F. R., Barragán-Méndez, A., Beltrán-Villegas, S., López-Reyes, J. J., & Villa-Hincapié, C. A., et al. (2024). Heparin-induced DRESS syndrome in a pediatric patient and successful anesthetic management in cardiovascular bypass surgery: Case report. *Journal of Cardiothoracic Surgery, 19*. https://www.semanticscholar.org/paper/15783e2bd406dabb5622a22c87bd03d04d47d9fe (accessed on 9 June 2025).

38. Popov, D. A., Osokina, R. A., Vostrikova, T., Serguladze, S., Kvasha, B. I., Shishkina, N. M., & Filippova, S. G. (2024). Infectious endocarditis caused by *Cutibacterium avidum* in a patient with endocardial pacemaker and multiple drug hypersensitivity reactions: A clinical case. *Clinical Microbiology and Antimicrobial Chemotherapy*. https://www.semanticscholar.org/paper/c5b5caa27c76e08e9be19f331b58f05a292c1d60 (accessed on 9 June 2025).

39. Rasmussen, T. H., Mortz, C., Pfeiffer, P., Andersen, N., & Bindslev-Jensen, C. (2025). Prevalence and management of immediate drug hypersensitivity observed during antineoplastic drug therapy. *Acta Oncological, 64*. https://www.semanticscholar.org/paper/5590efdc21781082efca675456c5bf885bfad94d (accessed on 9 June 2025).

40. Reza, M., Thakare, V., Langade, D., & Jain, M. (2025). Somatoform disorder presenting as serious adverse drug reaction with Inj. Ceftazidime and Tazobactam combination in a patient of allergic bronchopulmonary aspergillosis–seropositive (ABPA-S): A case report. *Global Journal for Research Analysis*. https://www.semanticscholar.org/paper/421acfb875c99213d95d9babbf58e06223a99e6d (accessed on 9 June 2025).

41. Rizzi, A., Nucera, E., Urbani, S., Longhino, D., Lohmeyer, F., Gambassi, G., Krishnamra, N., et al. (2023). Antituberculosis drug-induced non-blistering systemic severe reactions: A 10-year (2012–2022) literature review. *Asian Pacific Journal of Allergy and Immunology*. https://www.semanticscholar.org/paper/cce72dc138a343fc7237d1b0467a06df3f7c7284 (accessed on 9 June 2025).

42. Shakour, H., Mumtaz, R., & Abu-Samra, A. G. (2025). A diagnostic dilemma: Daptomycin-induced drug reaction with eosinophilia and systemic symptoms (DRESS) syndrome and eosinophilic pneumonia with concurrent COVID-19. *Cureus, 17*. https://www.semanticscholar.org/paper/e0a7b1e3e4dc38f52ee126a6e447595fb925daad (accessed on 9 June 2025).

43. Stan, R. (2023). Erroneous detection of desensitization doses in the prevention of hypersensitivity reactions. *BMC Research Notes, 16*. https://www.semanticscholar.org/paper/586c91806a8779d92a82b5e7e9b4bd0a7c92043f (accessed on 9 June 2025).

44. Trayer, J., Isaza-Correa, J. M., Kelly, L., Kelleher, M., Hourihane, J., Byrne, A., & Molloy, E. (2024). The role of neutrophils in allergic disease. *Clinical and Experimental Immunology, 219*. https://www.semanticscholar.org/paper/92e88629356bae29e5bc669ebf3c68fe83902148 (accessed on 9 June 2025).

45. Triwatcharikorn, J., Pholmoo, N., Ratanasutiranont, N., Rerknimitr, P., & Klaewsongkram, J. (2022). Skin testing might have a diagnostic role in immune complex-mediated hypersensitivity reactions. *Clinical and Experimental Dermatology, 48*(1), 27–30. https://www.semanticscholar.org/paper/eb23e06ef0297ac783614ae647f76642ff99cdba (accessed on 9 June 2025).

46. van den Anker, J., Reed, M. D., Allegaert, K., & Kearns, G. L. (2018). Developmental changes in pharmacokinetics and pharmacodynamics. *The Journal of Clinical Pharmacology, 58*. https://doi.org/10.1002/jcph.1284.

47. Villarreal-González, R., Ortega-Cisneros, M., Cadenas-García, D., Canel-Paredes, A., Fraga-Olvera, A., Delgado-Bañuelos, A., Rico-Solís, G. A., et al. (2024). [Delayed hypersensitivity reactions to drugs: Group Report of the Drug Allergy Committee of the Mexican College of Clinical Immunology and Allergy (CMICA).] *Revita Alegria México, 71*(3), 169–188. https://www.semanticscholar.org/paper/553bcbf378631e2960f2cd1b1e048e03ff19543d (accessed on 9 June 2025).

48. Wolfson, A. R., & Banerji, A. (2021). Skin testing and drug challenge in the evaluation of drug hypersensitivity reactions. *Allergy and Asthma Proceedings, 42*(1), 16–21. https://www.semanticscholar.org/paper/520b2b2fa986582eb1653bb457b0b82408e9c27a (accessed on 9 June 2025).

49. Zyryanov, S., & Butranova, O. (2022). Surgical antibiotic prophylaxis: Current issues of beta-lactams use. *Hirurg (Surgeon)*. https://www.semanticscholar.org/paper/5595201feb67bc1c256124b99af89b62e22cf6e3 (accessed on 9 June 2025).

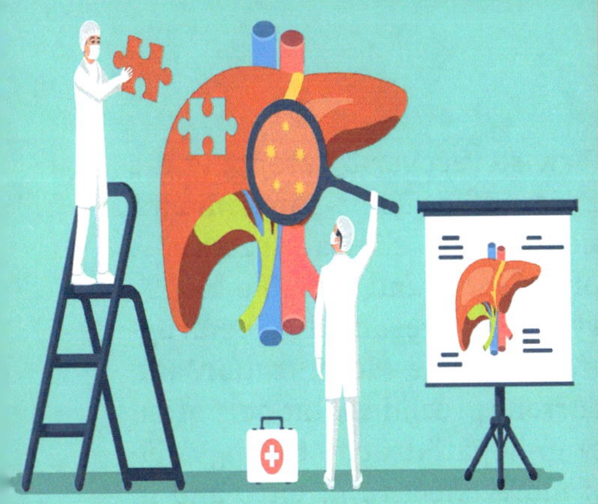

Chapter 6

DRUG-INDUCED LIVER INJURY (DILI)

Contents

Introduction

The drug-induced liver injury (DILI) phenomenon is a serious condition in the clinical and public health field of hepatology. DILI is presented as a range of liver damage due to varied drugs, food supplements, and herbal medicines, making it idiosyncratic when drug-induced and lacking in predictable responses (iDILI). The complexity of DILI is highlighted by the fact that it presents with multiple clinical features, which can be atypical of other liver diseases, making early diagnosis and treatment challenging. Timely identification of DILI is important because the disease tends to worsen rapidly and can cause serious complications like acute liver failure. The high incidence of DILI emphasizes the need for increased awareness among clinicians for early presentation and distinguishing it from other liver diseases. One of the most difficult subtypes of DILI is Drug-Induced Autoimmune-Like Hepatitis (DI-ALH), which shares features with autoimmune hepatitis (AIH). Due to this overlap, it is a challenging condition to diagnose, and thorough clinical evaluation is necessary to differentiate between them effectively. The value of familiarization with DI-ALH is appreciated in a paradigm of patient management in which misdiagnosis leads to unnecessary and perhaps toxic long-term immunosuppressive treatment of patients who may otherwise recover by stopping the drug. It has been established by research that over 40 medications, as well as some supplements, have been implicated in DI-ALH, indicating its wide-ranging applications in clinical practice. A combined approach involving clinical experience, directed laboratory testing, and possible biopsy may thus be needed to separate the pathologic cause of liver injury that is presumed to be drug-induced (Raúl et al., 2023). The lack of well-defined biomarkers to guide the identification and treatment of DILI is the biggest challenge to clinical practice. The current preclinical models often fail to replicate human responses, leading to a lack of predictability in hepatotoxicity during drug development. This gap has created a demand for an exploration of more effective in vitro and in vivo models and patient-derived cellular models to understand susceptibility and mechanisms of iDILI better. Moreover, advances in computational methods are poised to enhance drug safety predictions. Lastly, ongoing research and collaboration are necessary to refine efforts to reduce the incidence of DILI, expedite the identification of at-risk patients, and foster a culture of safety in pharmacotherapy (Segovia et al., 2021) (Figure 6.1).

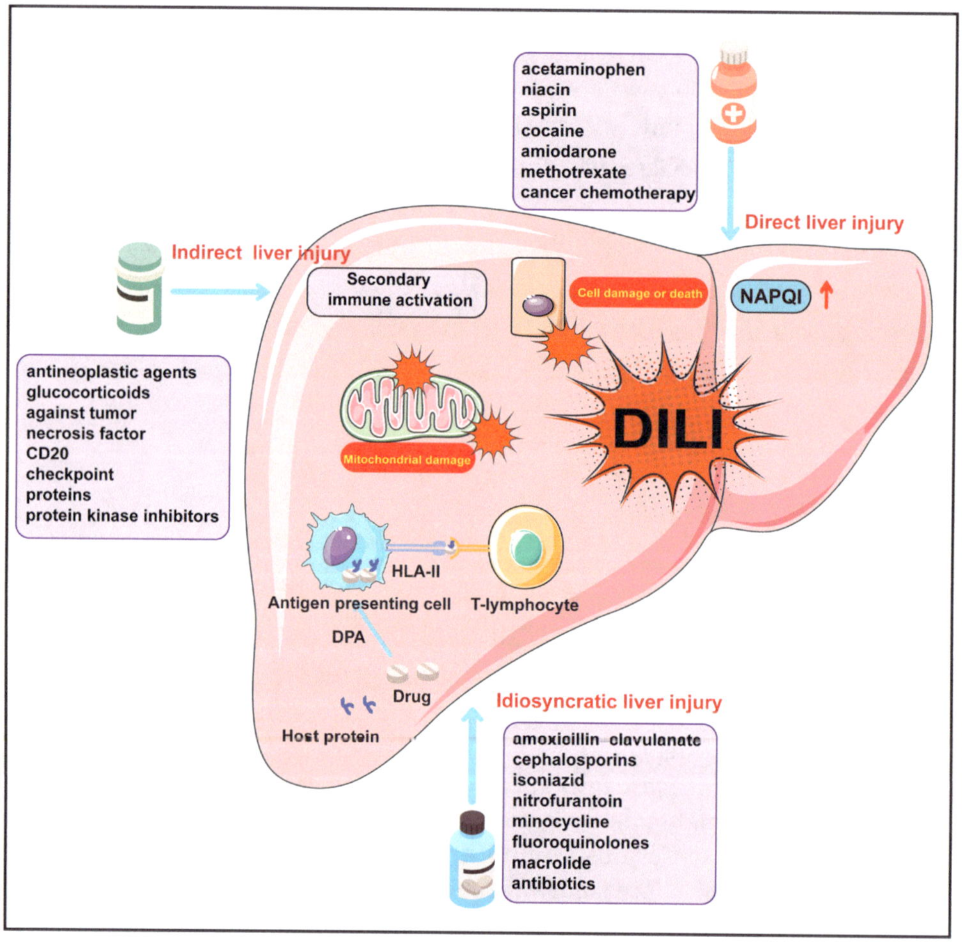

Figure 6.1. Drug-induced liver injury (DILI).

Source: https://thumbs.dreamstime.com/z/conceptual-image-drug-induced-hepatotoxicity-d-illustration-conceptual-image-drug-induced-liver-damage-106151349.jpg.

Definition of Drug-Induced Liver Injury

The concept of DILI encompasses a range of hepatic complications that arise as an adverse reaction to pharmacological agents. It is not just a unique reaction, but it takes into account how the body handles drugs and the person's chances of being affected. One of the liver's main jobs is to help change xenobiotics into metabolites. Still, some of these metabolites can be toxic to the liver, potentially leading to inflammation and cell damage. DILI can only be understood by considering all the factors that play a role, such as the patient's genes, previous liver problems, and other drugs taken at the same time. This points out that spotting DILI early is necessary, because if it is not treated, the disease can advance to serious liver damage and may call for a liver transplant. Recently, discussions about liver disease terminology have revealed a significant shift in the way DILI is categorized and understood. The emergence of terms like metabolic dysfunction-associated steatotic liver disease (MASLD) underscores a growing recognition of metabolic contributors to hepatic injury, which could encompass cases of DILI where metabolic dysfunction intersects with pharmacological hepatotoxicity.

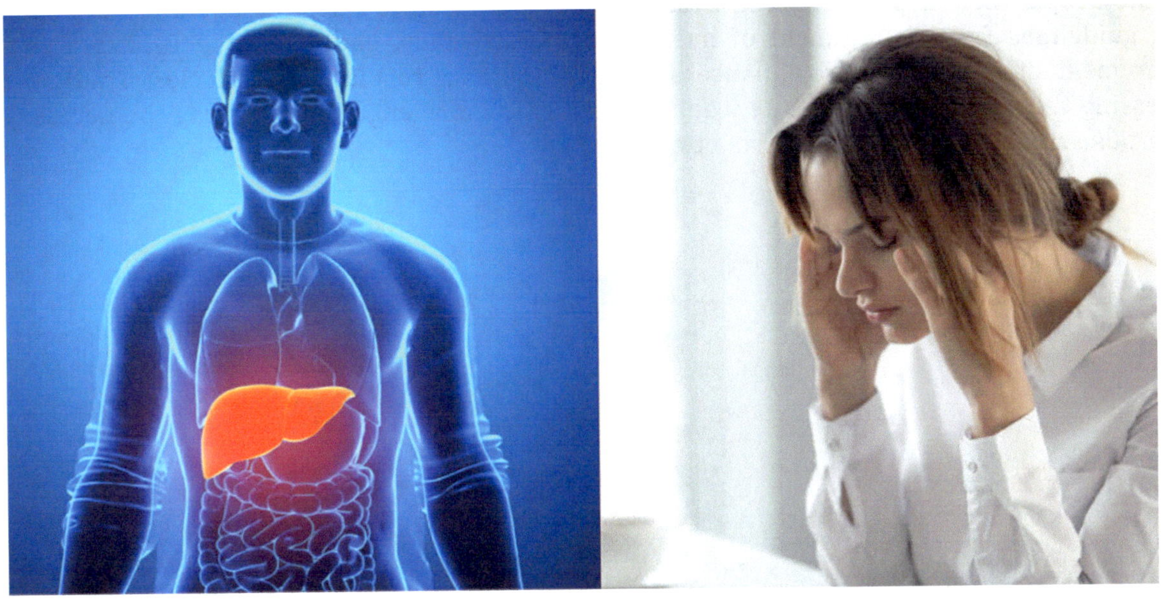

Figure 6.2. Definition of drug-induced liver injury.

Source: https://healthjade.net/wp-content/uploads/2022/10/drug-induced-liver-injury.jpg.

The systematic effort by international liver associations to establish newer, more inclusive classifications derives from the understanding that existing terminologies, including non-alcoholic fatty liver disease (NAFLD), carry stigmatizing connotations, thereby potentially limiting patient awareness and engagement. Using a term that encompasses various causes but also emphasizes metabolic aspects is a sign of how hepatic medicine is evolving and why it's essential to employ a detailed strategy for DILI management. As a result of these changes, it is necessary to use strict guidelines for diagnosing DILI. Experts have recommended that a patient's evaluation should include both the symptoms they show and their biochemical test results. Since healthcare professionals (HCPs) do not relate to traditional nomenclature, it is important to introduce new educational programs to increase their awareness of DILI. Since steatotic liver disease covers different causes of liver damage, doctors can now identify and handle the risks linked to drug therapy more effectively. By redefining these classifications, DILI can be contextualized within a broader spectrum of liver diseases, ultimately aiming to refine patient management strategies and improve outcomes in those affected by drug-induced hepatic injury (Gi-Kim et al., 2023; Mary et al., 2023) (Figure 6.2).

Importance of Studying DILI

Understanding the importance of DILI stems from its vital role in both drug development and patient safety. DILI poses a significant challenge, not only due to its clinical significance but also due to its relevance to pharmaceutical companies. The adverse effects of DILI can lead to drug withdrawals, loss of money, and health damage to the public, necessitating better preventive and monitoring strategies. According to the literature, anti-tubercular treatment (ATT) DILI is particularly difficult, especially in developing countries where resources for monitoring and managing such patients are generally limited (Chakrawarty et al., 2017). Thus, emphasizing research in DILI is to enable deeper mechanistic insight in DILI and ultimately lead to safer therapeutics development and guidelines for the treatment of liver injury. Additionally, understanding DILI is a critical component of both pharmacovigilance and drug approval regulatory strategies. Traditionally, assessing the hepatotoxicity of a new drug poses critical challenges, highlighting the necessity of rigorous screening procedures (Aerts et al., 2017).

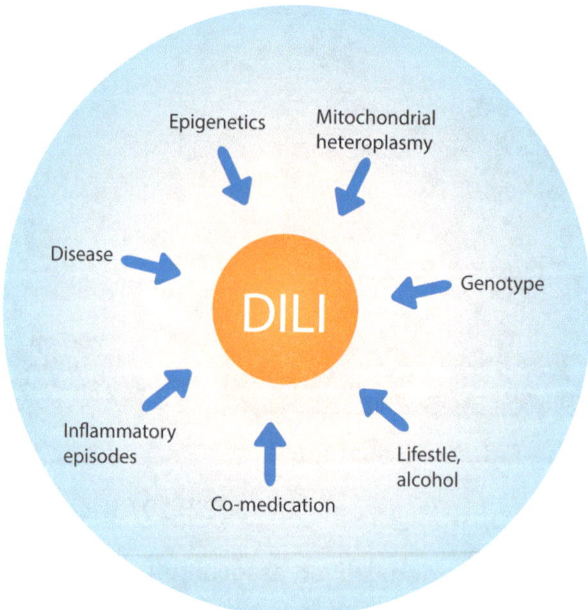

Figure 6.3. Importance of studying DILI.

Source: https://www.researchgate.net/publication/281682691/figure/fig2/AS:11431281276361881@1725629097784/Determinants-of-susceptibility-to-drug-induced-liver-injury-DILI-A-number-of.tif.

Current protocols using other cell models exhibit considerable inter-laboratory variability, making it challenging to establish standardized safety testing protocols. The variability highlights the need to enhance in vitro models so that they become more consistent in distinguishing between DILI-implicated and non-DILI compounds. Along with advancements in technology and an enhanced understanding of molecular events in DILI, scientists can improve early-stage drug safety assessment and ultimately decrease the risk of medication-related liver injury. Moreover, studies of DILI are essential for developing knowledge on genetic and environmental determinants of individual susceptibility to liver damage. This study has implications for public health, as specific populations are likely to be at greater risk of liver injury due to co-morbid or genetic risk factors. Such comprehensive studies, which mention these variables, would allow for risk stratification and a personalized medicine approach, offering clinicians the opportunity to individualize their therapy based on liver function and genetic status. Risk factor assessment and recommended monitoring strategies for DILI, particularly in high-burden scenarios such as ATT drugs, reveal the importance of the coordination of researchers, health care providers, and public health authorities in reducing the risks of DILI and ultimately drug safety and patient care improvement (Chakrawarty et al., 2017) (Figure 6.3).

6.1. Mechanisms of Drug-Induced Liver Injury

The mechanisms underlying DILI are multifaceted and complex, involving various biochemical pathways that can lead to hepatotoxicity. Oxidative stress is a main cause, and it happens when the number of free radicals exceeds the body's ability to fight them with antioxidants. As a result of drug exposure, reactive oxygen species (ROS) are generated, which can damage lipids, proteins, and DNA within hepatocytes. As a result of this chain of events, the cell's structure is damaged, and inflammation is initiated, which exacerbates the injury to the liver. Additionally, factors such as drug dose, duration of exposure, and genetic predispositions further complicate the susceptibility to oxidative stress-induced liver damage, highlighting the need for a deeper understanding of individual variances in response to hepatotoxic agents (Anuj et al., 2025).

Mitochondrial problems are also significant in DILI, since they affect energy production and the process of cell death. The health of hepatocytes depends on mitochondria, and if they are impaired, it can trigger several harmful effects, such as a drop in ATP production and the release of more pro-apoptotic factors. Several drugs can disrupt mitochondrial function by either inhibiting oxidative phosphorylation or allowing toxic metabolites to accumulate within the mitochondria. As a result of bioenergetic failure, cells die, and hepatic stellate cells may be activated, which encourages fibrosis and harms the liver. Understanding these mitochondrial alterations offers significant insights into the pathophysiology of DILI and emphasizes the importance of considering these effects during drug development (Anuj et al., 2025). Lastly, the immune system can play a significant role in DILI, since damage to the liver from drugs may lead to an unusual immune reaction. At times, drugs can alter the proteins in liver cells, causing the immune system to perceive these cells as foreign and attack them with T cells. The strength of the immune response may vary significantly from one person to another, depending on their genetic makeup and medical history. Researchers have identified specific immune markers and cytokines that support the immune system, leading to new approaches for treating diseases. Researchers are working to elucidate these immune-related pathways in order to develop methods for predicting who is likely to suffer from DILI and enhance the monitoring of patients during drug treatment (Figure 6.4).

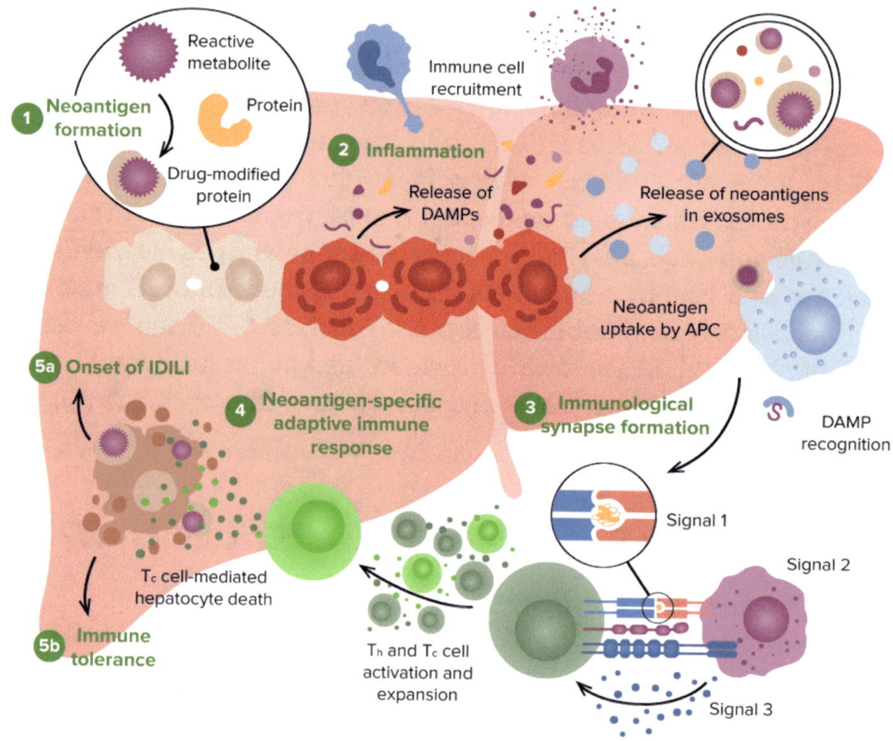

Figure 6.4. Mechanisms of drug-induced liver injury.

Source: https://cdn.lecturio.com/assets/Drug-induced-liver-injury-1-01.png.

6.1.1. Metabolic Activation of Drugs

The metabolism of drugs is a central role in the development of DILI, as it not only determines the effectiveness of pharmacotherapeutic drugs but also their toxicity potential. The majority of drugs are primarily biotransformed within the liver, where they can be converted into reactive metabolites that have the ability to interact with cellular macromolecules in a detrimental manner. This metabolic transformation, typically catalyzed by cytochrome P450 enzymes, metabolizes inert molecules into reactive species that can induce oxidative stress, inflammation, and tissue damage. A good case in point of such a phenomenon is that of acetaminophen (APAP), which, at therapeutic levels, is generally nontoxic. However, toxicity upon overdose can lead to the generation of highly reactive metabolites that result in acute liver failure, underscoring the fine line between drug efficacy and toxicity (Li et al., 2022). In addition, drug metabolism-mediated hepatotoxicity is often compounded by underlying individual genetic variability, pre-existing liver disease, and co-medications. Polymorphisms involving drug-metabolizing enzymes may lead to differences in metabolic activation rates among individuals and thus increased vulnerability to DILI in specific populations. Moreover, concomitant medications may enhance or suppress the metabolic reactions, further raising the risk profile for liver injury. For instance, the simultaneous use of cytochrome P450 enzyme inducers can enhance the generation of harmful metabolites, thereby increasing the risk of DILI. Identification of such differences is significant for physicians when formulating individualized treatment plans, avoiding the risk of liver injury while maintaining therapeutic efficacy. Current data have pointed to potential protective measures against DILI, with antioxidants and other mitigating measures prominently placed in the context of metabolic activation. The antioxidant potential of chemicals such as α-asarone is demonstrated to counteract the oxidative stress and inflammation typically triggered by reactive metabolites. Experiments indicate that α-asarone can trigger signaling pathways, such as the Keap1/Nrf2 pathway, which is crucial in defensive mechanisms against oxidative damage in liver cells. By managing metabolic pathways and inducing antioxidant defenses, the agent has demonstrated potential as a promising therapeutic candidate in DILI prevention (Chen et al., 2025). These innovations, along with others, point not only to increased understanding of DILI but also towards the creation of drugs that are protective against metabolic activation-induced toxicity.

6.1.2. Immune-Mediated Liver Injury

The intricate relationship between the immune system and liver function plays a critical role in understanding immune-mediated liver injury, particularly in the context of DILI. Since the liver is involved in removing toxins, it can easily be harmed by the adverse effects of various drugs. A mistake by the immune system can cause liver cells to be damaged, which may result in symptoms ranging from mild enzyme changes to severe liver failure. This dysregulation can arise from a range of triggers, including pharmaceuticals, herbal supplements, and dietary components that provoke an immune response, highlighting the necessity for a comprehensive understanding of the underlying mechanisms involved in such injuries (Anuj et al., 2025). It is essential for clinicians to realize that immune-mediated damage plays a significant role in DILI for proper treatment. Immune-mediated liver injury is further demonstrated to be complex because numerous pathways are involved, particularly those related to oxidative stress and mitochondrial dysfunction. If drugs cause the immune system to react, the liver can be seriously damaged by pro-inflammatory cytokines. For instance, tumor necrosis factor-alpha (TNF-α) has been shown to exacerbate liver injury in the presence of certain compounds, such as bavachin and epimedin B, which are derived from traditional herbal medicines (Lin et al., 2024). They are known to cause idiosyncratic DILI by setting off an inflammation process that leads to more liver enzymes being released and a sign of damage. It is essential to study these interactions so that we can predict and minimize the dangerous effects of immune-related liver injury in patients undergoing treatment. Because of immune-mediated liver injury, people may require serious treatments such as liver transplantation. Since DILI is often the reason for acute liver failure and transplants, exploring how the immune system works in these cases may open new ways to treat these conditions. Current research focuses on identifying biomarkers that may predict susceptibility to DILI, with insights on metabolic pathways disrupted during immune responses offering promising avenues for patient-specific management (Lin et al., 2024). When healthcare providers understand immune-related problems, they can design more effective treatment and monitoring plans to help patients and prevent major liver injury from certain drugs. It is essential to employ this approach to address issues related to DILI in today's clinical settings.

6.1.3. Direct Hepatotoxicity

The mechanism of direct hepatotoxicity is of critical relevance in the context of DILI. Direct hepatotoxicity refers to the liver's adverse reaction to a drug or its metabolites that leads to cellular damage and inflammation. The toxicity may be initiated by multiple mechanisms, like metabolic activation of the drug, leading to the formation of reactive metabolites, which bind covalently with cellular components of hepatocytes. For example, rifampicin, a widely used antibiotic, has a very high hepatotoxicity profile; thus, its clinical usage is limited, despite its efficacy against tuberculosis (TB). DILI mechanistic paradigms are commonly the interaction of drug metabolites with the liver's endogenous detoxifying processes, and thus it is necessary to understand the molecular mechanisms of action in order to develop safer pharmacological treatments (Hou et al., 2024). The liver is particularly vulnerable to drug-induced damage owing to the central role it plays in drug metabolism and detoxification.

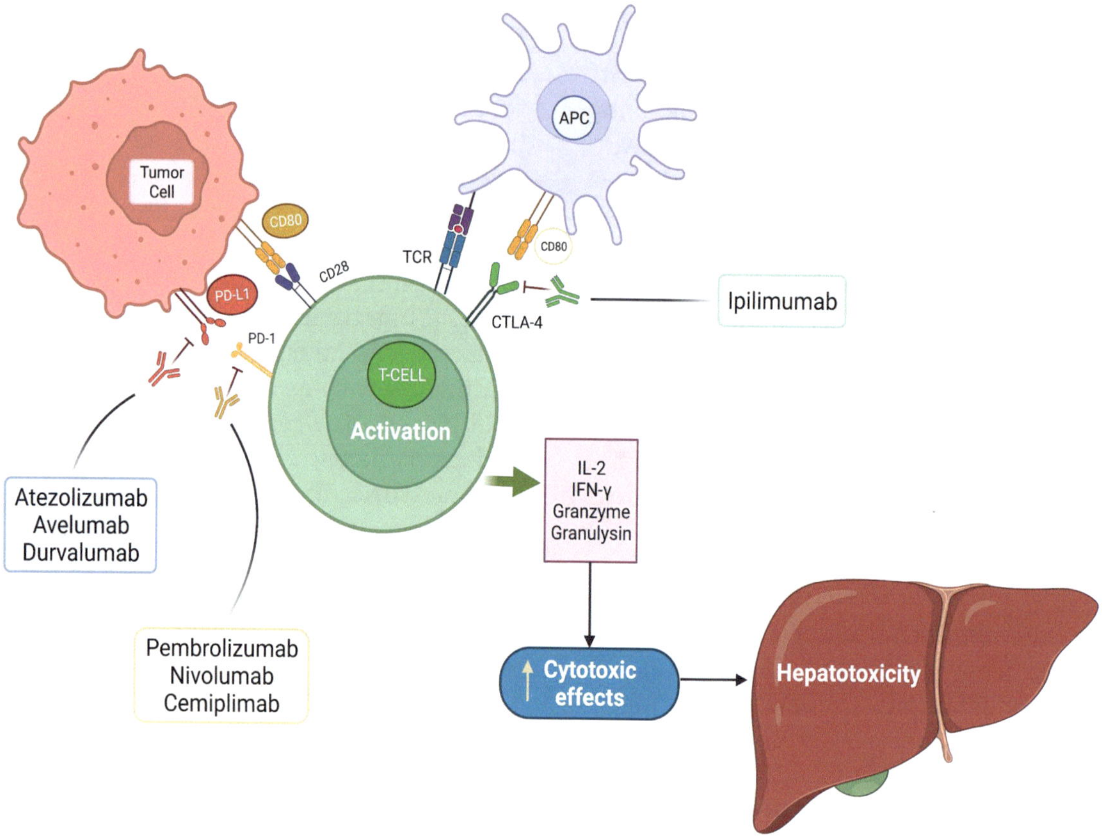

Figure 6.5. Direct hepatotoxicity.

Source: https://publinestorage.blob.core.windows.net/4d091aa5-d823-417d-a627-84794f5911da/jcth-d-22-00105-g002.jpg.

Hepatocytes are equipped with various enzymes responsible for the biodegradation of drugs; however, this activity can also lead to toxicity when the metabolites are harmful. For instance, in critical infections such as COVID-19, patients will often present with increased liver enzyme levels, which are markers of hepatocellular injury that can be caused by direct hepatotoxicity of antiviral medication like lopinavir and ritonavir. The etiology of liver damage in these conditions is multifactorial, making diagnosis and treatment of DILI challenging and often necessitating a comprehensive evaluation of the drug-pre-existing liver state of disease interaction. Thus, identifying risk factors for direct hepatotoxicity is crucial for protecting vulnerable populations and informing therapeutic decisions (Naeem et al., 2023). In the study of direct hepatotoxicity, priority must be given to designing novel therapeutic interventions to neutralize liver damage. For instance, identifying the role of specific transcription factors, such as Krüppel-like factor 15 (KLF15), can inform strategies to encourage drug detoxification processes. Evidence shows that the modulation of expression levels of detoxifying enzymes like Cyp3a11 can significantly constrain hepatotoxicity, providing a potential intervention for the prevention of drug-induced liver damage from drugs like rifampicin. Additionally, within the broader context of global health issues, such as the COVID-19 outbreak, the importance of rigorous research and clinical procedures to effectively maintain liver health in the face of drug-induced toxicity is now imperative. By prioritizing these factors, the clinical practice of the future can be directed towards limiting the public health impact of DILI (Hou et al., 2024) (Figure 6.5).

6.2. Common Drugs Associated with DILI

The landscape of DILI is often complicated by the variety of pharmaceuticals that can trigger hepatic damage. Acetaminophen is often recognized as a typical offender, because it can lead to liver damage, mainly when taken in high doses. Chronic drinking of alcohol can make the liver damage from the drug even more serious. The combination of acetaminophen and alcohol shows why people who are at risk should be cautious, which is an important point in DILI epidemiology. For this reason, it is necessary to study the factors that lead to DILI and develop methods to protect patients who are taking acetaminophen. Moreover, it is critical to acknowledge the role of antiepileptic drugs (AEDs) as significant contributors to DILI cases.

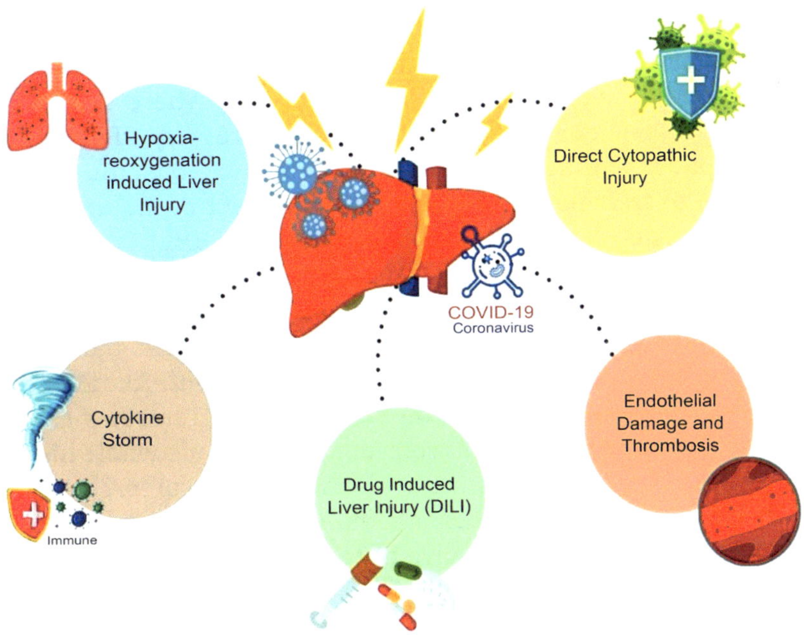

Figure 6.6. Common drugs associated with DILI.

Source: https://media.springernature.com/lw1200/springer-static/image/art%3A10.1186%2Fs43066-024-00381-0/MediaObjects/43066_2024_381_Fig1_HTML.png.

Carbamazepine and phenytoin are linked to hypersensitivity syndrome, which commonly leads to serious skin issues and problems with the liver. Clinical evidence suggests the presence of specific genetic markers, such as HLA-B*1502, that increase susceptibility to these adverse effects in certain populations, particularly among individuals of Han Chinese descent. Therefore, when prescribing these drugs, it is necessary to be extra cautious since the risk of DILI is connected to a patient's genetic background. By understanding the link, clinicians can select the most effective therapy for patients, thereby reducing the risk of DILI. Lastly, NSAIDs, particularly those used over extended periods, also warrant attention in the discussion of common drugs associated with DILI. Although these drugs are valued for reducing inflammation, using them for a long time may cause unusual liver problems. The immune system causes most of the time, NSAID-related liver injury, and patients may experience different reactions. It is essential to note that a proinflammatory state can increase the risk of injury, highlighting the importance of the patient's overall health in developing DILI. Further research is essential to elucidate the environmental and genetic factors that contribute to NSAID-associated liver injury, as a comprehensive understanding of these elements is vital in crafting safer therapeutic protocols and fostering preventive measures in populations at risk of drug-induced liver damage, supporting the imperative need for ongoing vigilance in pharmacotherapy (Cohen et al., 2011; Chalasani et al., 2017;) (Figure 6.6).

6.2.1. Over-the-Counter Medications

The field of over-the-counter (OTC) medications has subtleties that have not been adequately appreciated, above all concerning their ability to cause liver injury. While OTC drugs offer instant relief from a variety of ailments without a doctor's prescription, they are not without risk, DILI among them. Acetaminophen, a well-used analgesic, is prominently known for its hepatotoxicity, especially when taken in overdose or when combined with alcohol. The risk is also compounded for patients with pre-existing liver disease or polypharmacy, where multiple drugs are taken simultaneously to enhance their effect. Because OTC drugs are very often used indiscriminately, HCPS must educate the patient on dosages and the necessity of consulting medical professionals prior to an amalgamation of treatments so the collective impact of the drugs has extreme effects on the liver and as well." The diagnosis of OTC drug-induced DILI is clinically challenging for the doctor due to its overlap with other liver diseases. The presentation of hepatic damage, i.e., jaundice, abdominal pain, and lethargy, can easily misdirect the diagnosis because these signs are not observed in drug toxicity alone. Moreover, the capability of the OTC drugs to present with autoimmune-like hepatitis, whose characteristics overlap with idiopathic AIH, compels this further. Pharmacologic agents like ibuprofen and certain herbal remedies have been reported to induce this phenotype. Thus, clinicians should consider the patient's whole history of medications, including OTC and herbal preparations, during evaluations. This comprehensive research is vital for differentiating DILI from other liver conditions, enabling effective management measures. Such measures are crucial, given that DILI can resolve after withdrawal of the causative factor, as seen in the case of DI-ALH (Raúl et al., 2023).

The explanation of the mechanisms of DILI from OTC drugs forms the core of designing prevention measures. Hepatotoxicity results from several mechanisms, including metabolic activation and immune-mediated injury, which are generally dose-dependent. Studies have shown that some OTC medications, particularly drugs subjected to hepatic metabolism, lead to hepatocyte damage by the production of reactive metabolites or cholestasis. Moreover, the additive hepatotoxic impact of the combined use of several OTC medications heightens the risk of DILI. Thus, routine follow-up of liver function tests (LFTs) in those with chronic use of these medications is essential. Resources like LiverTox provide important data on the risk of hepatotoxicity from over 1,400 medications, including OTC drugs, and thereby enable clinicians to identify patients at risk and create treatment plans on an individual basis (Paul et al., 2024). Implementing this proactive approach can potentially substantially decrease the threat posed by DILI from OTC drug use (Figure 6.7).

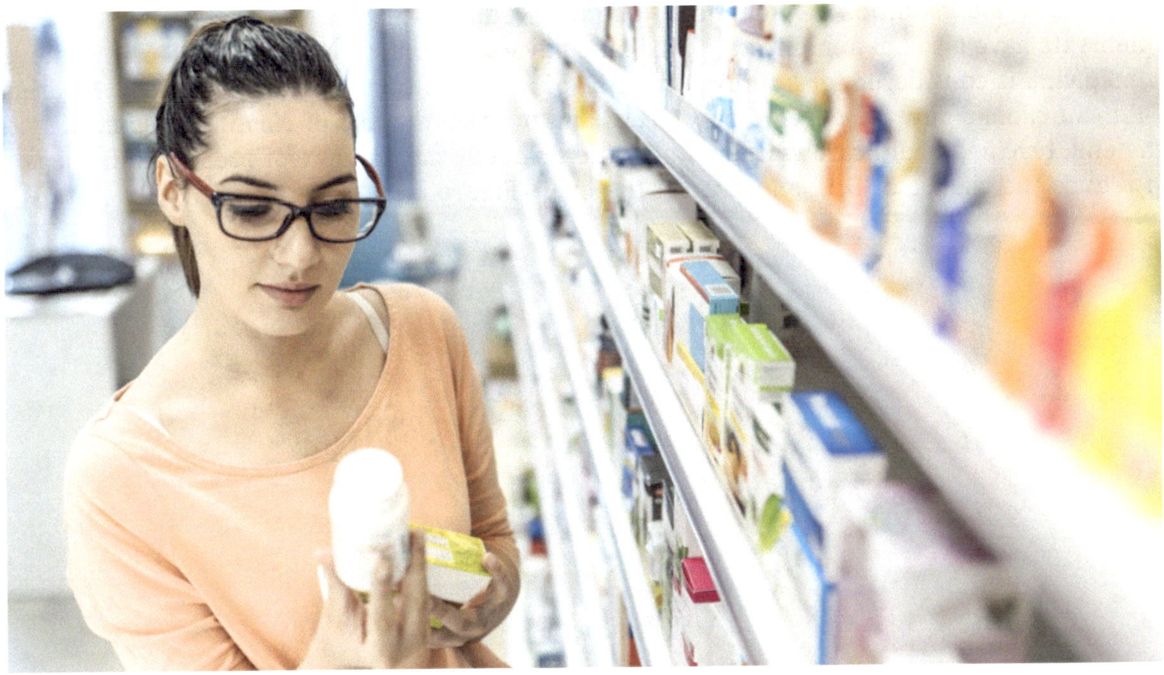

Figure 6.7. Over-the-counter medications.

Source: https://images.ctfassets.net/4f3rgqwzdznj/3Qzxk78gKhSbGKE3Cz4Vl0/2469f0a23329dcf6368def4d1dbd670a/reading_otc_labels_pharmacy_aisle-983235484.jpg.

6.2.2. Prescription Drugs

Modern medicine relies heavily on prescription drugs because they are important for treating various health issues. However, the rise in pharmaceutical consumption has brought about significant concerns regarding the prevalence of DILI. Since more patients take a combination of drugs and herbal supplements, the frequency of DILI has gone up in medical settings. Since DILI is a significant reason for acute liver failure around the world, healthcare workers should stay alert. Recognizing and taking away drugs suspected of causing liver damage early is very important for effective DILI management. By adopting a comprehensive understanding of the drugs used and their potential liver-related side effects, clinicians can play a crucial role in minimizing risks and optimizing patient safety during drug administration (Haque et al., 2016). DILI is mainly divided into two groups: intrinsic and idiosyncratic. When DILI happens due to the drug itself, it is usually dose-related and easy for clinicians to expect risks linked to drugs such as acetaminophen. Conversely, idiosyncratic DILI appears unpredictably, often affecting a small subset of patients who possess genetic or environmental predispositions (Licata et al., 2016). Because of this, it becomes difficult for doctors to diagnose and manage cases, as the clinical guidelines do not always provide advance warning. Amoxicillin-clavulanate is one of the drugs that frequently causes idiosyncratic DILI. HCPS need to know how these types of DILI occur, since it highlights the need to assess patients individually and learn about possible drug interactions and liver toxicity. Since prescription medications are essential for public health, the appearance of DILI creates significant issues. More and more, registries and studies on drug use are needed to spot drugs that often cause DILI and to understand the condition's epidemiology better. Notably, various NSAIDs, statins, and herbal supplements have also been implicated in hepatic adverse events (Licata et al., 2016). Whenever a new medicine is considered for approval, the risk of DILI is always carefully examined. Awareness of DILI can change how we develop new drugs and oversee the use of existing ones in hospitals. In the end, teaching healthcare workers and patients about the dangers of prescription drugs will help reduce the chance of DILI and protect the liver (Figure 6.8).

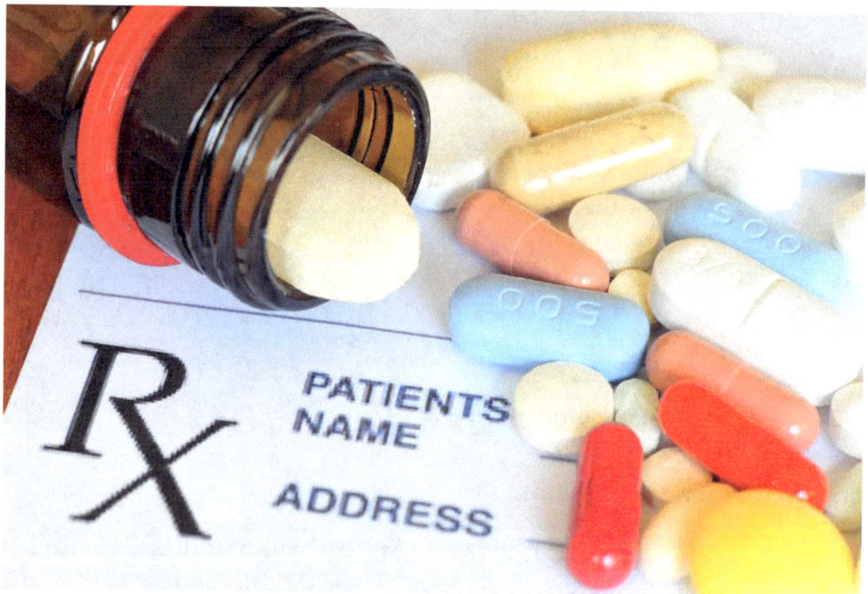

Figure 6.8. Prescription drugs.

Source: https://www.ariafl.com/wp-content/uploads/2022/08/prescriptions-drug-abuse.jpg.

6.2.3. Herbal Supplements

An even greater increase has matched the growing popularity of herbal supplements in concerns regarding their capacity to cause DILI. Herbal remedies, widely conceived as natural and hence safe alternatives to conventional medication, actually contain active constituents with hepatotoxic properties. The catch is that the pharmacological activity of such supplements can be unpredictable. For instance, constituents may vary significantly depending on cultivation practices, harvesting seasons, and manufacturing processes, which may expose them to risks of contamination with toxic substances or adulterants. The products are unknowingly ingested by patients when they attempt to treat liver diseases, which instead exacerbate the conditions and risk additional liver damage. Understanding these complexities is crucial for physicians in counseling patients who are inclined towards herbal supplements in maintaining liver health. In addition, the idiosyncratic character of DILI caused by herbal remedies makes it challenging to diagnose and treat. While most individuals using herbal supplements remain free from adverse effects, a proportion can end up with severe liver injury, challenging clinicians to pinpoint the offending agent in the absence of a high level of suspicion. According to recent studies, herbal and dietary supplements are increasingly being recognized as causative agents of DILI, most often competing with traditional drugs when it comes to impact on liver function (Amacher et al., 2016). Diagnosis typically involves excluding other potential causes of hepatic impairment, considering the patient's history of taking herbal supplements. Without diagnostic tests or biomarkers to confirm herbal-induced liver injury, healthcare providers are forced to rely significantly on good patient history taking and clinical acumen when managing this complication, ultimately targeting patient-centered practice and educated decision-making. Healthcare providers need to employ teamwork and communication-based practice when discussing herbal supplement use with patients, especially those with compromised liver function. The majority of the patients take such supplements under the illusion that they are safe, and they are not even aware of their hepatotoxicity. The clinicians' issue is not merely to provide the correct information but also to establish a culture where patients freely discuss all the supplements. Having an evaluation framework for the risks and benefits of herbal supplements will assist physicians in advising the use of herbal supplements in patients with chronic liver diseases (Dhruva et al., 2024). By applying the principles of integrative medicine, clinicians can teach patients to make informed choices about the use of herbal supplements, ensuring that their consultations about health are holistic and evidence-based. This collaboration can help reduce the risks associated with the unmonitored intake of herbal products and promote overall patient safety and well-being (Figure 6.9).

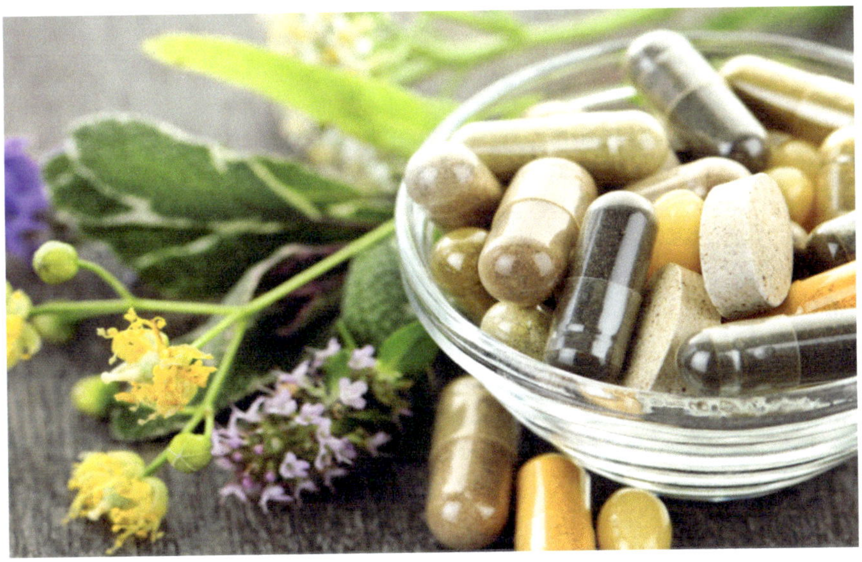

Figure 6.9. Herbal supplements.

Source: https://www.murrayaco.com/wp-content/uploads/2015/09/services-herbal-supplements.jpg.

6.3. Risk Factors for DILI

Understanding the risk factors associated with DILI is pivotal for enhancing patient safety and improving therapeutic outcomes. Several features in people's lives and health play a key role in causing DILI. Having a liver condition, for example, gallbladder disease, can make DILI much more severe. Also, initial total bilirubin levels and prothrombin time in the laboratory have become independent risk factors. They help doctors assess the liver's health and estimate the chances of DILI in people who are at risk. The interplay of these variables underscores the necessity for vigilant monitoring in populations considered high-risk, particularly those with existing liver pathology, ensuring timely intervention when liver injury is detected (Wei et al., 2024). Investigations carried out recently have pointed out that certain drugs can increase the risk of DILI, showing how drugs can interact with the liver. It has been observed through studies that traditional Chinese medicines, responsible for a large number of DILI cases, can damage the liver because of their complex ingredients and the risk of hepatotoxicity. According to the analysis, more than half of the cases of DILI were linked to the use of these herbal remedies, showing that people should be more aware of their safety. If there are extended periods between the highest enzyme levels, it may be an indication of chronic DILI. This knowledge is essential for clinicians prescribing these medicines, as it offers insights into safe usage and monitoring protocols (Wei et al., 2024). In the context of anti-TB therapies, additional risk factors have been identified that contribute specifically to anti-TB drug-induced liver injury (ATB-DILI). Studies done recently suggest that malnutrition and low hemoglobin levels are significant factors that predict moderate to severe ATB-DILI in those with TB. The connection between malnutrition and liver injury points out that a weak nutritional state may intensify the liver damage caused by some drugs. This discovery is significant for populations dealing with TB, since helping them with malnutrition could be a useful way to prevent liver problems during the treatment. All in all, these results highlight that DILI is caused by multiple factors, so it should be managed and assessed comprehensively.

6.3.1. Genetic Predisposition

In the discussion of DILI, mention must be given of genetic predisposition as an etiologic risk factor. Genetics can dictate how one metabolizes drugs, making them sensitive or resistant to hepatotoxic effects. For instance, polymorphisms of genes responsible for drug metabolism, such as cytochrome P450 enzymes, can lead to aberrations in enzymatic activity. This alteration can improve the toxicity of certain drugs and make liver damage more likely. Furthermore, individuals with prior liver disease or on chronic medication, combined with their genetic predisposition, are also at higher risk for DILI. The determination of genetic risk factors can enable clinicians to better predict and diagnose DILI, thereby facilitating early interventions to prevent potential damage (Gantsgorn et al., 2025). Investigations have elucidated how genetic susceptibility is associated with idiosyncratic reactions to certain NSAIDs, revealing a subgroup of patients who are particularly vulnerable to NSAID-induced DILI. Some of these genetic markers have been associated with adverse effects, with implications for a hereditary component that could guide clinical decision-making. As an example, gene polymorphisms in glutathione S-transferase have been associated with an increased risk for acute liver injury related to NSAID exposure. This genetic background not only highlights population variation in drug response but also underscores the need for personalized approaches in pharmacotherapy. Clinicians should consider these genetic risk factors when they prescribe NSAIDs since they can inform safer drug choice in patients with a susceptibility to liver injury (Herbert et al., 2024). It is crucial to learn more about the genetic predisposition to DILI in order to improve patient care and outcome. Integrating genomics into practice enables HCPs to risk-stratify liver injury more effectively, changing drug selection and dosage following specific genetic profiles. Furthermore, with augmented access to pharmacogenomic testing, the potential for DILI prevention through preemptive screening and goal-oriented interventions can become a reality. Incorporating such policies has the potential to enable the design of safer treatment regimens, minimizing side effects and augmenting patient protection. Lastly, the identification of the influence of genetic predisposition on drug metabolism provides an opportunity for innovation in clinical practice to reduce DILI risk and enable more personalized medicine (Gantsgorn et al., 2025).

6.3.2. Pre-Existing Liver Conditions

Pre-existing liver conditions significantly influence the risk and outcomes associated with DILI. Patients diagnosed with chronic liver diseases, including cirrhosis, hepatitis B or C, and nonalcoholic fatty liver disease, have damaged and less effective livers. Hence, they are more likely to respond negatively to hepatotoxic drugs. Because of how their bodies handle drugs, these patients may receive more of the medication and have a greater chance of liver problems. It is necessary to assess the patient's liver health before diagnosing DILI, as any underlying liver problems can make the results of liver enzyme tests unclear. Because of the link between liver disease and DILI, healthcare providers should use different assessment methods to catch and address ADRs as soon as possible. Various studies have pointed out that liver conditions can cause unique issues during the testing of new drugs in clinical trials.

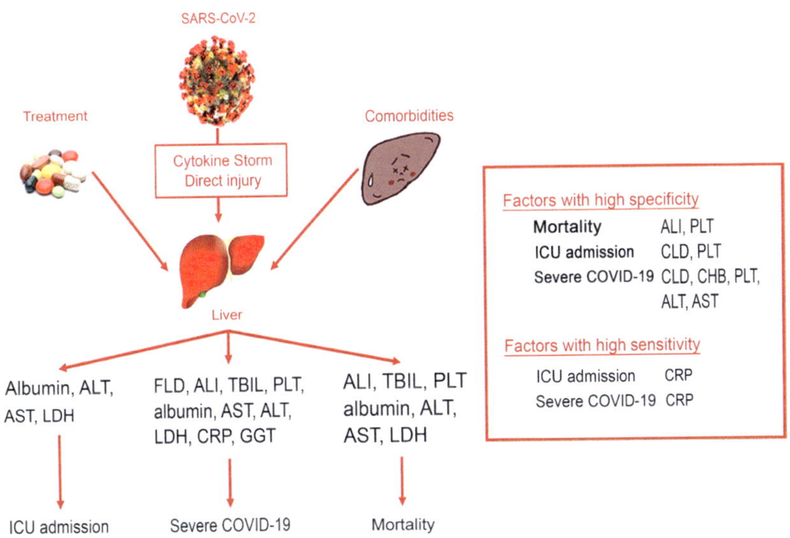

Figure 6.10. Pre-existing liver conditions.

Source: https://www.frontiersin.org/files/Articles/572115/fmed-07-572115-HTML/image_m/fmed-07-572115-g002.jpg.

For instance, patients suffering from nonalcoholic steatohepatitis (NASH) demonstrate unique responses to drugs that may not be observed in individuals with healthy livers. Even though more clinical trials have focused on this group in the last decade, the rules for assessing DILI in such studies are still insufficient. The current guidelines do not clearly explain the best ways to manage and monitor DILI in NASH patients, which could result in more issues. It is essential that pharmaceutical companies and researchers collaborate with hepatology experts to develop comprehensive strategies that incorporate hepatic inclusion and exclusion criteria, causality assessments, and protocols for detecting acute DILI during clinical assessments, particularly for individuals with compromised liver function (Adams et al., 2019)—taking pre-existing liver conditions into account in DILI matters for both doctors and those who make drugs and rules for their use. Considering that chronic liver diseases increase the risk of liver damage, clinical trials can be planned with special attention to liver health monitoring. It is also essential for pharmaceutical firms, regulators, and medical professionals to communicate more effectively to design and implement strategies that safeguard vulnerable individuals. Efforts involving different groups should concentrate on making DILI guidelines suitable for patients with pre-existing liver conditions, so that these patients can receive the most secure treatment. By integrating insights regarding pre-existing liver health into DILI strategies, stakeholders can work toward mitigating risks and enhancing the overall safety profile of new and existing medications (Licata et al., 2016) (Figure 6.10).

6.3.3. Drug Interactions

The intricacy of drug interactions plays a significant role in the risk of DILI, as many drug agents are metabolized through the liver. If more than one drug is taken simultaneously, the risk of negative interactions increases, potentially causing altered pharmacokinetics (PK) and pharmacodynamics. An example of this is that drugs might induce or inhibit a range of cytochrome P450 enzymes, resulting in enhanced hepatotoxicity. The intraindividual variation in the expression of enzymes, as influenced by the genetic variations, can also make these interactions more complicated, and thus, the monitoring of polypharmacy patients becomes crucial. Physicians need to sense well the synergistic effect of combination drugs, particularly in comorbid patients with illnesses such as HIV or TB where DILI risk is already high, such that familiarity with predictors of associated liver injury is necessary, as studies of antiretroviral drug-treated patients and their genetic backgrounds highlighted (Habtewold et al., 2012). Research has identified specific drug interactions that enhance the incidence and severity of DILI, specifying the biochemical pathways underlying. Some drug classes, such as HIV treatment, have adverse interactions with other drugs, particularly anti-TB medication, causing elevated levels of liver enzymes. Drug metabolism pathways typically denote that commonly used drugs will compete with the same metabolic enzymes, leading to increased levels of drugs in the plasma that have the potential for causing liver injury. Lifestyle variables such as alcohol further alter the disease process, particularly when patients are being administered drugs such as acetaminophen, which is renowned for its intrinsic hepatotoxicity. Understanding how such interactions play a role in the domain of DILI is essential for clinicians managing patient care to effectively avoid the risk of liver injury and provide safer therapeutic options (Chalasani et al., 2017). Clinical presentations of drug interactions regarding DILI necessitate an integrative approach towards the management of the patient. Enhanced attention during the monitoring of LFTs will allow for the detection of early signs of potential liver injury, so that early intervention can be initiated to prevent further damage. Education of patients on the importance of adherence to prescribed medication schedules, along with illumination of the extreme dangers of self-medication and consumption of alcohol, will prevent the development of DILI. Along with this, physicians must stay current regarding new studies on drug-drug interactions and the ability to cause liver injury. Through this lifelong learning, clinicians will be able to make rational choices in prescribing drugs and adjusting them based on patients genetic backgrounds, concomitant drugs, and overall health condition and thereby optimize patient safety and drug efficacy in patients at risk for DILI (Habtewold et al., 2012) (Figure 6.11).

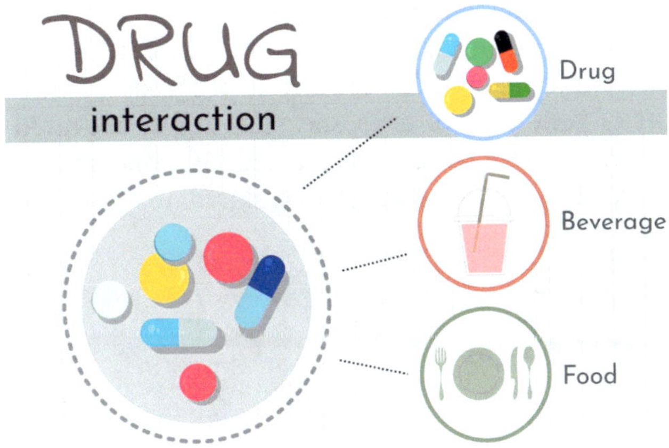

Figure 6.11. Drug interactions.

Source: https://yourislandnews.com/wp-content/uploads/2023/06/medication-interactions.webp.

6.4. Clinical Presentation of DILI

The clinical presentation of DILI can vary significantly between patients, complicating timely diagnosis and management. Usually, patients may experience only mild and vague symptoms like tiredness and low energy, or they may develop more serious ones such as jaundice, pain in the abdomen, and blood clotting problems. If laboratory results show high liver enzymes, increased bilirubin, and changes in coagulation, these symptoms may point to acute liver failure in serious cases. Besides, there are cases where patients complain of nausea or rashes, which may hide the actual liver problem. So, because liver dysfunction may have unusual signs, doctors should be more cautious when noticing new cases, mainly in those who have recently started using medicines that can harm the liver. It becomes harder to diagnose DILI when patients have other diseases or complications that are linked to it. In some cases, having TB along with another infection can be difficult because the main symptoms are similar. A case that demonstrates this complexity was about a young patient who got liver damage from the drugs used to treat central nervous system (CNS) TB. Even with proper TB treatment, the patient's liver and brain functions worsened, which shows that doctors should use different approaches and tailor treatment for every patient. Doctors are expected to deal with these complex issues to avoid missing the effects of DILI on patients' health. It is still essential to identify unusual forms of DILI in both emergency and outpatient care, since polypharmacy is becoming more common among patients. A condition called iliopsoas abscess, which can cause back pain and fever, can occur with DILI, making it hard to diagnose. The authors of the case report pointed out that reviewing the patient's history and symptoms helped them find out about hepatotoxicity caused by using the wrong medication. It points out that HCPs in emergency departments must evaluate patients carefully, as time is usually significant. A better understanding of the various symptoms of DILI can help doctors make an accurate diagnosis, which can benefit patients and reduce the risks associated with delayed recognition of this condition.

6.4.1. Symptoms and Signs

Symptoms and signs of DILI presence are crucial components of the clinical diagnosis and management of the disease. Nonspecific symptoms, whether severe or mild, will be present in the majority of DILI patients. Fatigue, nausea, and stomach discomfort are the first signs, which may be mistakenly attributed to other benign conditions. As the condition progresses, jaundice is a prominent sign that is manifested in terms of yellowing of eyes and skin due to elevated bilirubin. Tests for liver function should be closely monitored in such scenarios, as abnormal findings in transaminases and alkaline phosphatase typically indicate hepatocellular damage.

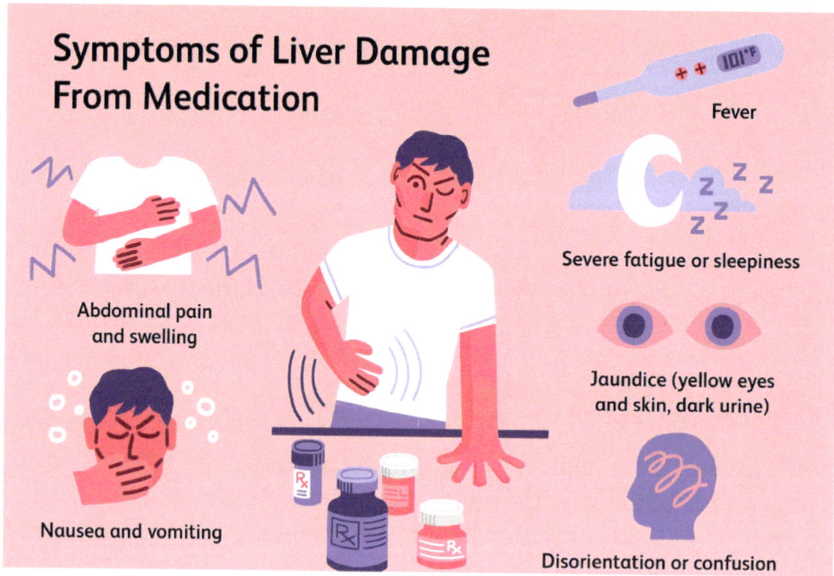

Figure 6.12. Symptoms and signs.

Source: https://www.verywellhealth.com/thmb/z1C12qI4G0d80CxafKt5pnQK6sQ=/3000x2000/filters:no_upscale():max_bytes(150000):strip_icc()/SymptomsLiverDamage_1943023_Final_1-ea70d54025564870bd9ac7aabbfca921.jpg.

Recognition of these early warning signs is key to early management, serving to underscore the need for prescribers to be highly attuned to the potential for liver damage due to prescription and OTC medications. In some instances, the presentation may involve more than the typical markers of liver dysfunction. For instance, the use of certain drug classes has been linked to more severe presentations, such as ascites and hepatic encephalopathy, which are indicators of advanced liver disease. A study highlighted the importance of some targeted therapy medications, noting that CDK4/6 inhibitor patients, such as those receiving ribociclib, frequently had clinical presentations of DILI, and a reporting odds ratio (ROR) of 2.60, indicating considerable risk for liver side effects. Apart from liver-oriented studies, other patients may exhibit a variety of different clinical signs, ranging from pruritus to periumbilical swelling. As the results indicate, understanding the variability of symptoms associated with different drugs may facilitate early intervention and customized treatment regimens, thereby preventing harm and enhancing patient outcomes (She et al., 2024). Moreover, the increasing problem of herbal supplements adds complexity to the matrix of DILI symptoms and diagnosis. New cases of turmeric-induced liver damage demonstrate this phenomenon, as patients may present with symptoms identical to drug-induced hepatotoxicity. For instance, a single case report of a female patient who consumed turmeric-flavored tea manifested acute hepatitis and shows the danger that seemingly harmless supplements can present for the development of massive liver damage. The symptoms of presentation in this patient—such as pain in the abdomen, lethargy, and jaundice—are similar to the classical DILI presentations, emphasizing the role of the health care professional to take into account all the factors of a patient's drug history, including dietary supplements. The shift in understanding symptomatic presentations is essential to render judicious care and also promotes a sensitivity that complements the clinic practice for DILI management (David et al., 2023) (Figure 6.12).

6.4.2. Laboratory Findings

The analysis of laboratory findings is crucial in understanding DILI, as these findings often serve as the first indication of hepatotoxicity. Laboratory tests focused on liver function typically measure serum enzyme levels, including alanine aminotransferase (ALT) and aspartate aminotransferase (AST). When these enzymes are significantly elevated, it usually means the liver is damaged, which might be caused by specific drugs. According to data extracted from the United States Food and Drug Administration Adverse Events Reporting System (FAERS), nefazodone emerges as a primary contributor to DILI, with a notable ROR of 7.79 for cholestatic injury and 18.67 for severe drug-related hepatic disorders. Such laboratory findings not only assist in identifying affected patients but also inform clinicians of potential therapy modifications based on the metabolic impact of specific medications (Jiang et al., 2024). Besides, studying the genes that play a role in DILI helps explain the results seen in laboratory tests. Changes in genes that help break down drugs and those involved in the immune system can have a significant impact on how the liver responds to medication. For example, changes in the HLA-DQB1 gene have been linked to a higher chance of liver injury caused by anti-TB drugs. Notably, a study identified a significant association between the HLA-DQB1*05:02 allele and increased susceptibility to DILI.

When genotyping is added to regular laboratory tests, it helps doctors understand a patient's risks related to medications and plan the most effective treatment. Such integrative analyses reflect the growing recognition of personalized medicine in managing DILI (Prayuni et al., 2023). In addition, laboratory results in DILI call for careful monitoring and reporting systems. The use of routine LFTs should be included in the treatment plans for people who are given potentially harmful drugs for the liver. Reviewing data from FAERS proves that it is necessary to monitor for any adverse drug events. The discovery of issues related to antidepressants points out that it is important to keep studying and regulating these drugs. Early detection of DILI can be achieved by being proactive in monitoring laboratories, which may help protect the patient's health. Therefore, laboratory findings not only reflect the immediate impact of pharmaceuticals on liver function but also warrant further investigation to elucidate causal relationships and improve clinical outcomes (Jiang et al., 2024) (Figure 6.13).

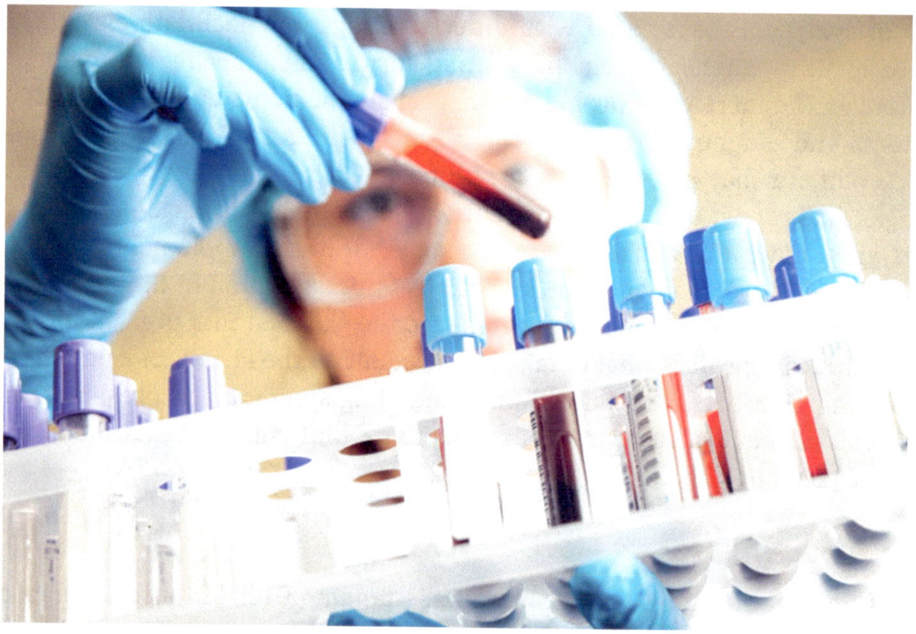

Figure 6.13. Laboratory findings.

Source: https://medlineplus.gov/images/LaboratoryTests_share.jpg.

6.4.3. Severity Classification

Severity grading of DILI is crucial in determining the potential risks associated with various pharmacological interventions. Severity grading enables the stratification of liver injury based on clinical presentation, laboratory findings, and LFTs. DILI will be graded as mild, moderate, or severe in the majority of cases, which will enable clinicians to make informed decisions regarding patient care. An essential part of this grouping relies on the understanding of the mechanisms by which some drugs induce hepatotoxicity. Immune checkpoint inhibitors (ICIs), e.g., which have been at the forefront of cancer treatment, are now recognized to have the capacity to induce significant hepatotoxicity, hence making strict monitoring and grading of liver damage severity among such treated individuals a necessity (Hountondji et al., 2024). New research further highlights the need for more precise severity grading in the development of therapeutic agents. Comparative analysis of drugs like CDK4/6 inhibitors has established dramatic contrasts in hepatobiliary toxicity, leading to a more nuanced interpretation of drug-associated risk. With the incorporation of data from the FDA Adverse Event Reporting System (FAERS), scientists can establish the causal relationship between drugs and liver injury more effectively, thereby facilitating better risk stratification. In these studies, the character of liver injury—from liver tissue damage to loss of function—is often classified under a broader regulatory mechanism to ensure patient protection. Evidence reveals that there are high risks of liver injury for ribociclib and abemaciclib, supporting the requirement of using severity classification in clinical assessment (She et al., 2024). The application of severity classification in the DILI framework also enhances the decision to provide therapy. In clinicians who are managing patients on possibly hepatotoxic drugs, the degree of liver injury must be known so that decision-making in terms of continuance of the drug, modification of dosage, or instituting alternative therapy can be made. Furthermore, severity grading may guide risk-profile-specific monitoring strategies for each drug's hepatotoxicity. Since DILI is a primary focus for the pharmacovigilance of new medicines, ongoing revisions to severity classification will further result in better patient outcomes. This dynamic system not only facilitates enhanced monitoring but also fosters a safety culture within clinical practice, where the early identification of severe cases could greatly improve the management of patients and outcome.

6.5. Diagnosis of DILI

The diagnosis of DILI is a complex process that necessitates meticulous attention to clinical history, LFTs, and diagnostic criteria specific to liver injury. The first step is to conduct a thorough review of a patient's medical history, including the medications they have taken, any existing liver issues, and their current symptoms. The guidelines suggest that R-value is used to identify the type of liver injury by calculating the ratio of ALT to ALP. The result of this calculation helps decide the outlook and further care for possible DILI cases. It is essential to utilize liver biochemical tests, which should include checking ALT, AST, ALP, GGT, total bilirubin, and albumin, to obtain a comprehensive assessment of the patient's liver function. Without careful adherence to these diagnostic strategies, misdiagnosis could lead to inappropriate therapeutic interventions, underscoring the importance of precision in diagnosis (N/A, 2024). A DILI diagnosis depends on identifying the different types of liver injury, which is achieved by examining both the lab results and the patient's overall medical history. Doctors use certain guidelines to confirm that liver injury is caused by drugs. Among these are a past history of drug use, fast return of liver enzymes to normal after stopping the drug, no other possible causes for liver injury, and a reaction when the drug is used again. When three of these criteria are met, the diagnosis is stronger; however, if only the first two are met, it is merely a suspicion of DILI. This rigorous approach is crucial for effective diagnosis and ensures that clinicians make informed decisions, particularly given the varied manifestations of liver injury that different drugs can cause (Wang et al., 2023). In addition, the management of possible DILI depends on quick actions taken after the diagnostic results. Taking the offending drug away is the main priority and has been found to affect how well someone recovers strongly. Studies have shown that the rapid removal of potential toxins helps the liver recover; however, the regular use of hepatoprotective drugs is still being debated. Research suggests that using multiple hepatoprotective agents simultaneously does not yield better results than using only one, suggesting that relying on these drugs may not be necessary. For this reason, it is crucial to closely monitor and evaluate patients during treatment, as their reactions can vary significantly. Establishing clear diagnostic protocols and management strategies is essential to navigate the complexities of DILI effectively (N/A, 2024).

6.5.1. Clinical Assessment

The clinical assessment of DILI is a comprehensive process that requires a thorough approach to diagnose and treat the condition accurately. The focal point of this assessment is taking a thorough medical history which would identify any potential risk factors and previous drug exposures. The idiosyncratic nature of DILI makes it a complex condition to diagnose, and hence, other etiologies of liver injury need to be excluded. Based on current evidence, factors such as the onset time, clinical presentation, and laboratory findings are crucial in determining causality in cases of suspected DILI. Additionally, standardized nomenclature and terminology are crucial for facilitating communication between health professionals involved in the diagnostic process. Ultimately, an effective clinical assessment can pave the way for appropriate management programs, thereby mitigating the adverse effects of DILI (Aithal et al., 2010). In all situations where DILI is suspected, laboratory procedures cannot be overemphasized. LFTs are included in the fundamental diagnostic methods used to assess the extent of damage caused to the liver. Enzyme activity abnormalities, such as ALT and AST, can be indicative of the onset of hepatic distress. Additionally, the inclusion of advanced testing methods and biomarkers can aid in distinguishing DILI from other liver disorders and enhance the accuracy of diagnosis. Determination of causality is particularly challenging in multimedicated individuals or patients with chronic liver disease because these parameters skew laboratory value interpretation. Hence, medical professionals must employ a holistic approach when evaluating both laboratory and clinical data (Alvarez-Alvarez et al., 2021). Moreover, identification of offending drugs associated with DILI remains at the focus of investigation at the clinical level. Recent studies have suggested a chain of drugs, including antibiotics and anti-epileptics, as common causatives of liver injury. The challenge lies not only in recognizing these drugs but also in recognizing the genetic and immunologic determinants that make an individual susceptible to subsequent adverse reactions. There are some specific HLA alleles, for example, which have been identified as critical risk factors for DILI, and thus, pharmacogenomic screening needs to be implemented in such populations. In addition, the evolving climate of drug development and increased use of herbal supplements create challenges in making the diagnosis with the unstandardized criteria used for assessment. Hence, a collaborative endeavor on the part of clinicians to implement updated guidelines and share resources will be essential to enhancing the treatment and understanding of DILI (Aithal et al., 2010) (Figure 6.14).

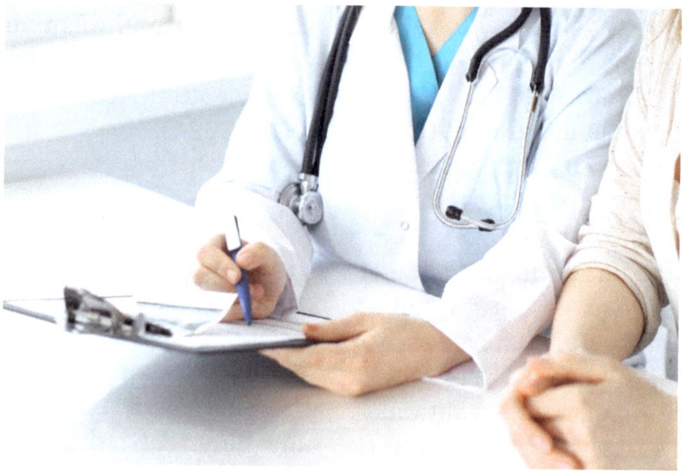

Figure 6.14. Clinical assessment.

Source: https://pamentalhealth.com/wp-content/uploads/2022/08/Clinical-Assessments-Individual-Therapy.jpg.

6.5.2. Liver Function Tests

Liver function tests (LFTs) are critical tools in the detection and evaluation of liver health, particularly in cases of DILI. They check the levels of several enzymes and proteins in the blood to see how well the liver can function. The most commonly assessed parameters include ALT and AST, which are indicative of hepatocellular damage. When these enzymes are found in high levels, it could indicate that the liver is still being harmed so that doctors may investigate the reason. Quick and correct interpretation of LFT results in DILI is necessary to tell if liver damage is reversible or severe, which helps decide on the best medical care.

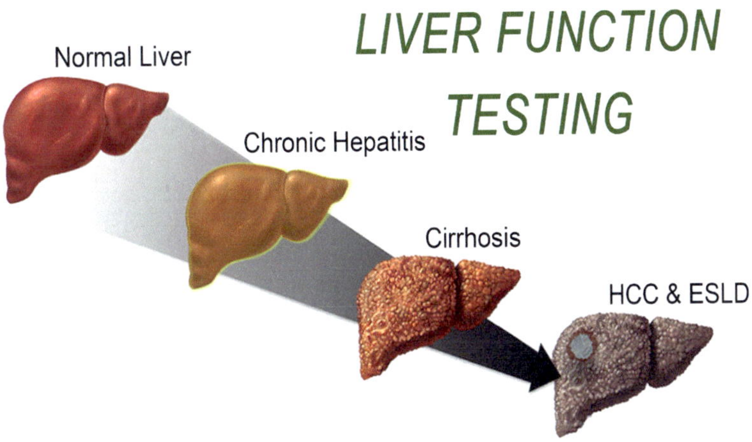

Figure 6.15. Liver function tests.

Source: https://mughallabs.com/wp-content/uploads/2023/07/Liver-Function-Test.jpg.

The meaning of LFT results changes significantly depending on the cause of abnormal liver function. Enzyme levels can exhibit specific patterns when an injury is caused by drugs. As an illustration, when a patient has cholestatic liver injury, their ALT and AST levels may be higher along with alkaline phosphatase, making it important to think about the impact of bile flow. The process of the liver absorbing and metabolizing drugs can result in various reactions and may lead to the formation of toxic substances that can harm cells and cause inflammation. Understanding these enzymatic changes allows for better stratification of risk in patients undergoing pharmacotherapy, ultimately contributing to more informed clinical decision-making regarding the continuation or cessation of suspect medications (Chen et al., 2025). In addition, LFTs are important for monitoring the recovery of the liver after the harmful agent is removed. For instance, in a documented case involving hydroxychloroquine (HCQ), elevated LFTs prompted the modification of treatment plans, leading to a gradual decline in enzyme levels after discontinuation.

This suggests that the liver is capable of responding and healing when faced with challenges. Additionally, emerging research highlights the potential of dietary components, such as polyphenols found in green tea, as protective agents against hepatotoxicity (Winiarska-Mieczan et al., 2024). This means that non-drug approaches can be used in conjunction with traditional medicines to protect the liver (Figure 6.15) better.

6.5.3. Histological Evaluation

The assessment of DILI needs a detailed histological investigation, which is a crucial assistance in the identification of structural changes in liver tissue brought about by hepatotoxic agents. Histological investigations provide data on cellular and tissue architecture within the liver, with data on abnormalities such as necrosis, inflammation, and steatosis. These histological alterations commonly are the earliest manifestations of DILI and can be employed to distinguish between drug-induced damage and other conditions of liver disease. Such evaluations are justified because they can confirm the presence of an injury not revealed by laboratory tests in isolation, which provides supporting evidence for the value of histological techniques in the early detection and diagnosis of DILI. By integrating histological findings and clinical data, clinicians can tailor individual treatment strategies to prevent injury and enhance patient care. Moreover, technological advances in histology have improved DILI assessment, particularly with the aid of new human liver models. These models exhibit liver phenotypes and functions for extended periods, thereby facilitating the in vitro recapitulation of hepatotoxicity events. This capacity is particularly important in preclinical drug discovery, where DILI risk can halt the development of a lead therapy. Histological evaluation of these models reveals a wealth of information, which, when combined with biochemical and toxicogenomic readouts, enhances the predictive capability for liver safety liabilities. The proper integration of these disparate data types is crucial, as it enables scientists to better predict idiosyncratic drug responses, potentially saving costly clinical trial setbacks and advancing progress in public health protection (Zhou et al., 2025). The diagnostic utility of histological evaluation is further enhanced by the discovery of novel biomarkers of DILI. Earlier LFTs are grossly lacking in sensitivity and specificity, and they lead to delayed diagnosis and poorer patient outcomes. New biomarkers, such as osteopontin and cytokeratin-18, provide a second level of measurement, supporting the histological information and enhancing diagnostic accuracy. They enable the detection of hepatocellular damage at an early stage and present the severity of liver pathology more accurately than conventional tests. Consequently, combining these new biomarkers within a histological context raises diagnostic precision and overall understanding of DILI mechanisms, thereby paving the way for enhanced monitoring and patient management of affected patients (Cueto-Sánchez et al., 2023).

6.6. Management and Treatment of DILI

The management of DILI is a complex process that necessitates a careful and systematic approach. It is essential for clinicians to determine which drug caused the problem by reviewing the patient's history and employing standard methods. It is vital at this point since DILI may develop suddenly or slowly, and its symptoms can be quite different for each person and drug. It is essential to follow guidelines that recommend clinicians with experience in liver diseases lead the care of patients with liver injuries. In this regard, the consensus among experts emphasizes the importance of adherence to US Food and Drug Administration (FDA) guidelines, which outline the essential clinical and laboratory measures for assessing DILI risk in new therapeutics (Chien et al., 2019).

Doing LFTs is important in this care, as it helps doctors determine the extent of liver damage and whether further treatment is needed. Stopping the drug or medicine that caused DILI is the primary treatment, and this action usually leads to improvement in most cases. Still, this procedure should be done with extra care in patients who are being treated for serious diseases with life support. There are cases where doctors use additional therapies based on the patient's condition and the type of liver injury. In severe cases, such as those involving vanishing bile duct syndrome (VBDS) related to specific drugs like pexidartinib, advanced management strategies may be required, including liver transplantation (Chien et al., 2019). Since transplantation is a complex matter, it requires a team of specialists to weigh the pros and cons of the procedure. It is essential to continually monitor the patient's condition while managing their care to achieve the best possible results. New studies and training sessions have highlighted that collecting data in a standardized manner is crucial for managing DILI. Consistency in clinical measures, lab specimens, and evolving clinical terminology is critical in assessing DILI risk within clinical trials (Andrade et al., 2014). Using this approach makes it easier for healthcare workers to communicate and respond quickly in cases of liver injury. Moreover, the latest discussions have highlighted the importance of examining pharmacogenomic and proteomic markers that may reveal an individual's risk of developing DILI.

As these biomarkers are used in clinical practice, they may improve how patients are managed, which could result in finding people at high risk and reducing drug-related liver problems. All in all, using methods such as monitoring, early diagnosis, and clear communication is key to handling DILI well.

6.6.1. Discontinuation of the Offending Drug

Withdrawal of the causative drug is of prime concern in the treatment of DILI. Because the liver is responsible for metabolizing a vast array of drugs, hepatotoxicity is an exaggerated danger. As soon as DILI is suspected or diagnosed, withdrawal of the causative drug is unavoidable to prevent further hepatic damage. This step not only stops further progression of liver injury but also initiates the body's own healing process. Evidence indicates that patients demonstrate significant improvement in LFTs within days following drug cessation, thereby again emphasizing the importance of early treatment. Proper management of DILI relies on the vigilance of clinicians regarding the safety profiles of medicines, so that patients can be advised on potential risks associated with specific medications. Hence, drug cessation of the offending agent is an immediate, crucial step and a core component of the overall strategy in managing DILI. Drug withdrawal of one suspected to cause DILI necessitates meticulous planning of the patient's history and any other form of treatment that may minimize further risk to the liver.

The physician must weigh the risk-benefit of continuing the drug, particularly if the causative drug is required for treating a chronic medical condition. In this situation, the doctor may be forced to explore other treatments with a lower risk of hepatotoxicity. It can be highly challenging to balance between treating the underlying disease and preventing drug-induced liver disease. Extremely careful monitoring of the LFTs is required during this transition period. By being alert and offering appropriate follow-up care, clinicians can bring in a safer recovery for the patient without exposing them to the risk of ADRs. These assumptions also substantiate the use of personalized medicine in the treatment of DILI. After the immediate withdrawal of the offending drug, supportive care plays an important role in the overall management of DILI. Depending on the severity of liver injury, the patients may require interventions such as nutritional supplementation, rehydration, and management of any emerging complications with symptomatic treatment.

The physicians may also consider the use of adjunctive therapies, such as antioxidants, to support hepatic recovery. For example, N-acetylcysteine (NAC) has been studied for its potential in the management of DILI, particularly that induced by acetaminophen overdose. The NAC treatment intervention emphasizes the broader context of treating DILI, wherein stopping the offending drug, coupled with supportive therapy, will significantly reduce patient outcomes. Notably, identification and awareness of the risk of hepatotoxic drugs remain core elements of prevention strategies that will help clinicians prevent recurrence of DILI in their patients (Figure 6.16).

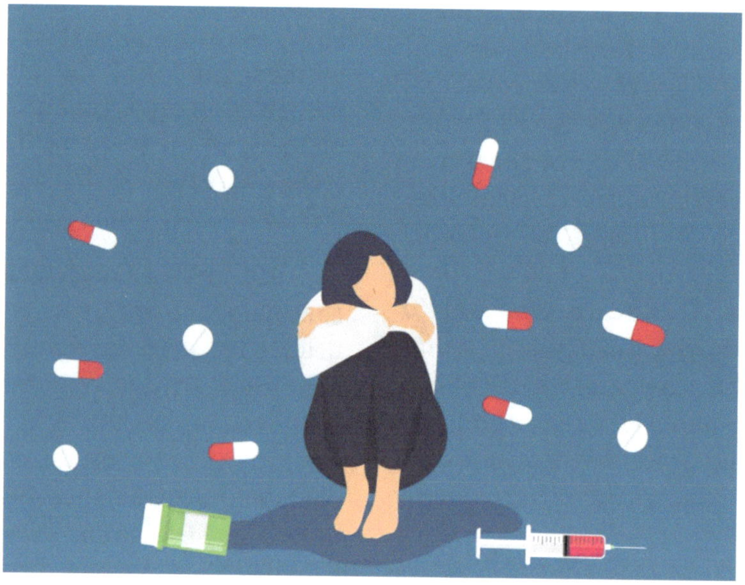

Figure 6.16. Discontinuation of the offending drug.

Source: https://musetreatment.com/wp-content/uploads/2024/05/Treatment-for-Drug-Withdrawal-1536x1152.jpg.

6.6.2. Supportive Care

Supportive care plays a pivotal role in the management of DILI, addressing the immediate and underlying needs of affected patients. When the diagnosis is made, the first step is to discontinue the medication that caused the problem to prevent further liver damage. Although this action can be beneficial in many simple cases, supportive care primarily focuses on alleviating symptoms and facilitating the liver's proper functioning. Similar symptoms to those of other liver diseases may be present in patients, which means they need to be carefully monitored and treated. The primary goal of supportive care is to provide comfort and alleviate discomfort caused by symptoms such as jaundice, fatigue, and abdominal pain, thereby enhancing the patient's overall quality of life during recovery from DILI (Roy et al., 2024). Ensuring the patient is adequately hydrated and receives proper nutrition is crucial in DILI. Because many patients may not feel hungry, lose weight, and feel tired, it is important to help them eat enough calories. Drinking water is particularly important when the liver is not functioning well, as it helps alleviate general symptoms and supports the body's detoxification process. Moreover, it is important to use monitoring methods, including regular LFTs, to check the patient's progress and spot any signs of acute or chronic liver failure. Effective supportive care also aligns with individualized treatment plans that consider the patient's medical history, previous liver conditions, and potential for genetic susceptibilities to DILI, thus paving the way for tailored interventions that optimize outcomes (Xiao et al., 2024). Taking care of psychological needs is a crucial aspect of managing DILI. The effects of liver injury on people's emotions and mental state can be very serious, often causing anxiety and depression. Therefore, mental health check-ups and easy access to counseling should be incorporated into the care team's overall approach. Attending peer support groups can make patients feel supported and provide them with an opportunity to discuss their problems and how they manage them. When both the body and mind are supported, the patient's recovery chances increase and they become stronger. Ultimately, the incorporation of multifaceted supportive care strategies is essential to improving the overall health outcomes and well-being of patients suffering from DILI (Roy et al., 2024) (Figure 6.17).

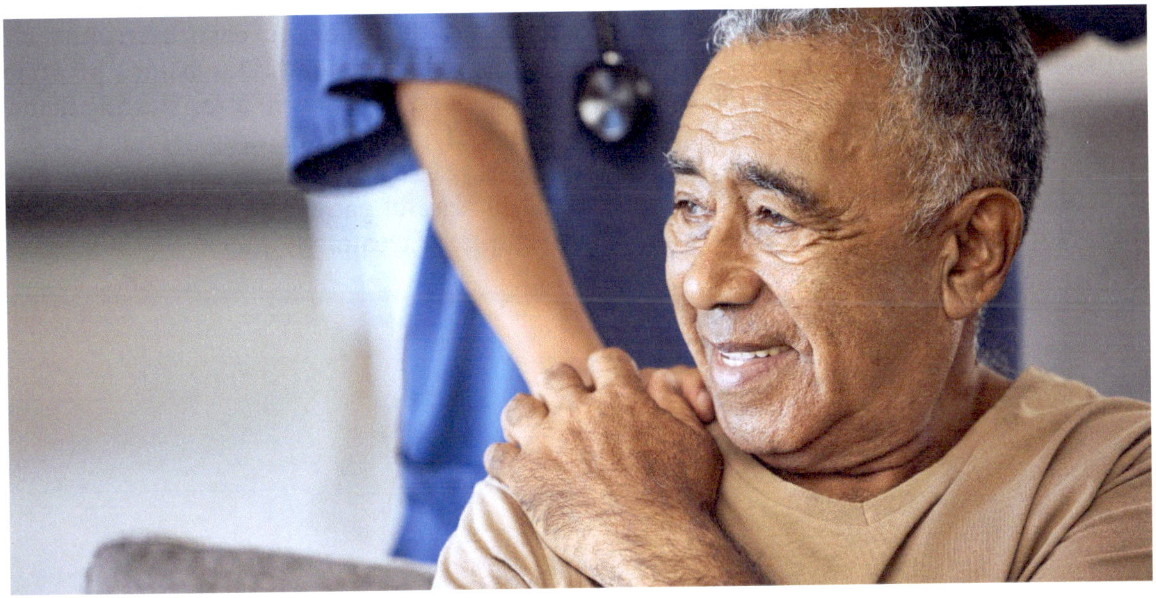

Figure 6.17. Supportive care.

Source: https://osf-p-001.sitecorecontenthub.cloud/api/public/content/Supportive-Care-hero?v=3e5458ee?t=w800.

6.6.3. Potential Use of Corticosteroids

Corticosteroids have proved to be a potential therapeutic agent in the treatment of DILI, particularly when the disorder takes a chronic course. These agents are known for their potent anti-inflammatory and immunosuppressive properties, which can be utilized for the treatment of liver damage resulting from drug-induced injury. In particular, corticosteroid administration can reverse immune-mediated mechanisms that cause liver damage, thereby reducing inflammation and promoting recovery. Clinicians have documented an increase in liver function when corticosteroids are administered, particularly in cases diagnosed early and treated promptly. They are therefore an essential component of DILI treatment regimens, with evidence based on systematic investigation of their effectiveness in various scenarios. Research has shown that corticosteroid therapy is likely to be effective in treating chronic DILI, as indicated by previous randomized controlled trials. One significant study showed that those on an SSR therapy for 48 weeks had notable improvements, confirming the drug's promise to address extensive liver inflammation. However, there are questions about what the appropriate duration of steroid therapy should be to ensure patient protection and the effectiveness of treatment. For instance, recent research has been exploring whether a shorter, 36-week SSR can be as effective as the standard 48-week treatment without compromising patient outcomes. The complete ramifications of such research are considerable, as determining the optimal ratio between effective therapy and preventing the potential hazards of prolonged corticosteroid treatment can significantly enhance clinical outcomes for DILI patients (Huang et al., 2024). Even as corticosteroids present a thrilling therapeutic choice for DILI, it is also crucial to be mindful of their innate side effects, considering the role of the liver in metabolizing drugs. Immunosuppression, increased susceptibility to infection, and metabolic disturbances are common risks associated with corticosteroid treatment. Moreover, reactivation of latent infection, such as TB, continues to be a fatal risk among patients treated with prolonged corticosteroid therapy. Thus, healthcare providers must carefully evaluate the risk-to-benefit ratio before prescribing these medications for DILI. The case of a patient with cholestatic jaundice after starting lisinopril illustrates the complexity involved in the management of DILI, where drug withdrawal led to significant amelioration in liver function (Georgeina et al., 2024). Therefore, while corticosteroids might be a potentially helpful adjunct in managing DILI, careful patient assessment and ongoing monitoring are still necessary to achieve the most significant treatment effect.

Summary

The investigation of DILI has underscored the critical interplay between pharmaceutical therapies and hepatic health. The available literature reveals a concerning incidence of DILI among diverse patient populations, particularly highlighting its prevalence in pediatric oncology settings, as evidenced by a study that reported a 21.34% occurrence of DILI in children undergoing chemotherapy for acute lymphoblastic leukemia (ALL) (Bai et al., 2024). It is crucial to understand the risk factors that can cause DILI to improve patient care. It was found that body mass index, vitamin D levels, and blood transfusion frequency were significant risk factors for DILI in this group, making it essential to monitor for liver problems and provide targeted care. People receiving treatment for TB in adulthood also face serious outcomes from DILI. A prospective study identified malnutrition and low hemoglobin levels as independent risk factors for the occurrence of moderate to severe anti-TB drug-induced liver injury (ATB-DILI), with an incidence of 2.0% reported (Liu et al., 2024). Because of this, healthcare providers should start using nutrition assessment and management as a preventative strategy. Since DILI is complicated, it is important to understand both the patient's and the treatment's influence on liver health during drug therapy. For DILI to be managed and prevented, HCPs need to be proactive. Strategies that work well are those that help find and address potential liver problems early, when using medications that may be harmful. Healthcare workers should develop plans for patients by considering their dietary needs and the medications they are taking. Additionally, both doctors and patients should be informed about the symptoms and signs of liver injury, allowing for timely adjustments to treatment plans. In short, dealing with DILI requires us to work together to identify what causes it and carry out strategies that protect the liver and make sure that important medicines are effective.

The discussion surrounding DILI highlights several critical aspects imperative for understanding this public health issue. Among the most important factors is the ability to identify biomarkers and liver-specific variables that can suggest DILI, primarily with the aid of Hys Law. This guideline uses extreme levels of LFTs to estimate the chances of severe liver damage from drugs. The usefulness of this model proves that careful testing in labs is essential before drugs are used, because finding DILI early can change the approval and use of medications. The insights provided by models such as Heffernan and Tawn's conditional dependence model further elucidate how certain doses may correlate with the occurrence of adverse effects, enhancing the pharmaceutical industry's capacity to manage risk effectively and safeguard patient safety (Box et al., 2014). When it comes to clinical care, keeping track of DILI incidents and their timing matters a lot, especially for those who are using antiretroviral drugs. A recent study on HIV patients found out how different drug regimens are linked to DILI. It was found that the rate of DILI was 7.8%, and the increase was mostly seen in patients who were treated for HIV and TB at the same time. The evidence suggests that it is crucial to closely monitor liver function in co-infected patients, as DILI may develop within the first few weeks of treatment initiation. Understanding the nuances of how demographic and genetic factors, such as the CYP2B6 genotype, can predispose individuals to liver injury during treatment is imperative in tailoring therapeutic approaches and advancing personalized medicine (Habtewold et al., 2012). Additionally, the findings from these studies have implications for public health and pharmaceutical approaches. If genetic screening and monitoring are added to the usual treatment plans, it could help patients and lower the risk of DILI. Earlier use of these measures may help avoid serious outcomes that could result in the need to end treatment. In addition, it is essential to regularly assess the safety of drugs in development to ensure that the benefits of new therapies outweigh the risks of DILI. All in all, these main points show how DILI is complex, so it requires wide-ranging efforts in drug assessment, caring for patients, and research to address this issue.

CLOSER LOOK

RISK-PROFILE-SPECIFIC MONITORING STRATEGIES

Risk-profile-specific monitoring strategies are tailored surveillance and management approaches designed to align with the individual risk levels of patients or populations. These strategies are increasingly utilized in healthcare, public health, and clinical research to enhance precision, improve outcomes, and allocate resources more efficiently. By assessing various risk factors—such as age, genetic predisposition, comorbidities, lifestyle behaviors, or environmental exposures—patients can be stratified into risk categories (low, moderate, or high), each with corresponding monitoring protocols. For instance, individuals at high risk for cardiovascular disease may undergo more frequent blood pressure and cholesterol checks, while those at lower risk might only need annual assessments.

In oncology, risk-profile-specific monitoring is crucial in surveillance of cancer recurrence or progression. Patients with higher genetic risk (e.g., BRCA mutations) may require more intensive imaging and biomarker testing than average-risk individuals. Similarly, in infectious disease management, such as HIV or tuberculosis, monitoring frequency and intervention strategies vary based on viral load, immune status, or exposure history. These customized protocols reduce unnecessary testing for low-risk individuals and ensure timely interventions for high-risk groups, optimizing both clinical efficiency and patient care.

The implementation of such strategies depends heavily on data analytics, electronic health records, and risk prediction models. Advances in machine learning and AI have further enhanced risk stratification accuracy, enabling dynamic and real-time monitoring plans. However, challenges remain, including ensuring data privacy, avoiding disparities in access to tailored care, and maintaining the accuracy of risk assessment tools across diverse populations. Despite these hurdles, risk-profile-specific monitoring represents a major shift toward proactive, personalized medicine. By aligning surveillance intensity with individual risk, these strategies not only improve clinical outcomes but also contribute to more sustainable and equitable healthcare systems.

References

1. Regev, A., Palmer, M., Avigan, M. I., Dimick-Santos, L., Treem, W. R., Marcinak, J. F., Seekins, D., Krishna, G., Anania, F. A., Freston, J. W., Lewis, J. H., Sanyal, A. J., & Chalasani, N. (2019). Consensus: guidelines: best practices for detection, assessment and management of suspected acute drug-induced liver injury during clinical trials in patients with nonalcoholic steatohepatitis. *Alimentary Pharmacology & Therapeutics*, *49*(6), 702–713. https://doi.org/10.1111/apt.15153
2. Aerts, H., Alexandre, E., Antherieu, S., Dorau, M., et al. (2017). A multicenter assessment of single-cell models aligned to standard measures of cell health for prediction of acute hepatotoxicity. https://core.ac.uk/download/80779109.pdf (accessed on 9 June 2025).
3. Aithal, G. P., Andrade, R. J., Arimone, Y., Begaud, B., Benichou, C., Bjornsson, E. S., et al. (2010). Standardization of nomenclature and causality assessment in drug-induced liver injury: Summary of a clinical research workshop. http://deepblue.lib.umich.edu/bitstream/2027.42/77985/1/23696_ftp.pdf (accessed on 9 June 2025).
4. Alvarez-Alvarez, I., Andrade-Bellido, R. J., Lucena, M. I., Medina-Caliz, I., et al. (2021). Critical review of gaps in the diagnosis and management of drug-induced liver injury associated with severe cutaneous adverse reactions. https://core.ac.uk/download/489431958.pdf (accessed on 9 June 2025).
5. Amacher, A., Chalasani, N., Chen, M., Chien, J., El Sherrif, Y., Hillman, L., et al. (2016). Drug-induced liver injury. https://core.ac.uk/download/74226387.pdf.
6. Andrade, R. J., Aithal, G. P., de Boer, Y. S., Liberal, R., Gerbes, A. L., Regev, A., Beretta-Piccoli, B. T., et al. (2023). Nomenclature, diagnosis and management of drug-induced autoimmune-like hepatitis (DI-ALH): An expert opinion meeting report. *Journal of Hepatology, 79*, 853–866. https://doi.org/10.1016/j.jhep.2023.04.033.
7. Andrade, R. J., Avigan, M. I., Bjornsson, E. S., Cooper, G. S., et al. (2014). Liver safety assessment: Required data elements and best practices for data collection and standardization in clinical trials. https://core.ac.uk/download/38282943.pdf (accessed on 9 June 2025).
8. Bai, T., Hong, L., Na, L., Qian, N., & Jiao, F. (2024). A single-center clinical analysis of drug-induced liver injury in children with acute leukemia. *Asian Journal of Pediatric Research*. https://www.semanticscholar.org/paper/14a8f7a2d03a670cee7d8f5db747fab1b276ba0c (accessed on 9 June 2025).
9. Bonkovsky, H. L., Ghabril, M., Nicoletti, P., Dellinger, A., Fontana, R. J., Barnhart, H., Gu, J., et al. (2024). Drug-induced liver injury (DILI) ascribed to non-steroidal anti-inflammatory drugs (NSAIDs) in the USA—Update with genetic correlations. *Liver International, 44*, 1409–1421. https://www.semanticscholar.org/paper/358641dd884c214887a1e30ca4289d930492e052 (accessed on 9 June 2025).
10. Box, G., Coles, S., Cox, D. R., Davison, A. C., Eastoe, E. F., et al. (2014). Stochastic ordering under conditional modelling of extreme values: Drug-induced liver injury. http://arxiv.org/abs/1210.6003 (accessed on 9 June 2025).
11. Chakrawarty, A., Kumar, J., Mohan, R., Nandhini, R., & Ranjan, A. (2017). Comprehensive review of anti-tubercular treatment induced liver injury. https://core.ac.uk/download/544390300.pdf (accessed on 9 June 2025).

12. Chalasani, N. P., & Stine, J. G. (2017). Drug hepatotoxicity: Environmental factors. https://core.ac.uk/download/228066166.pdf (accessed on 9 June 2025).

13. Chen, D., Pham, C., Kaur, M., & Yip, K. (2025). Hydroxychloroquine-induced hepatotoxicity in systemic lupus erythematosus: A case report and literature review. *Cureus, 17*. https://www.semanticscholar.org/paper/cb1fb86b36417887549f4b58e6dda79696e55759 (accessed on 9 June 2025).

14. Chen, L., Li, J., Li, Q., & Sun, Q. (2025). α-Asarone enhances antioxidant capacity and modulates metabolic pathways of sodium valproate-induced liver injury in mice. *Traditional Medicine Research*. https://www.semanticscholar.org/paper/7e688ca050c3479833fc0745316e75d2ead1e409 (accessed on 9 June 2025).

15. Chien, A. J., Esserman, L. J., Hyland, C., Piawah, S., et al. (2019). A case report of vanishing bile duct syndrome after exposure to pericarditis (PLX3397) and paclitaxel. https://core.ac.uk/download/323072463.pdf.

16. Chinese Medical Association Tuberculosis Branch. (2024). Guidelines for diagnosis and management of drug-induced liver injury caused by anti-tuberculosis drugs (2024 version). *Zhonghua Jie He He Hu Xi Za Zhi = Chinese Journal of Tuberculosis and Respiratory Diseases, 47*(11), 1069–1090. https://www.semanticscholar.org/paper/e9b6e7c0517d144c8ec8fe079d1a377589fa3bf6 (accessed on 9 June 2025).

17. Cohen, L., Neuman, M. G., Hwang, P. A., & Nanau, R. M. (2011). Genetic and immune predictors for hypersensitivity syndrome to antiepileptic drugs. https://core.ac.uk/download/pdf/290366.pdf (accessed on 9 June 2025).

18. Cueto-Sanchez, A., Niu, H., Álvarez-Álvarez, I., López-Longarela, B., Del Campo-Herrera, E., Ortega-Alonso, A., García-Cortés, M., et al. (2023). Evaluation of diagnostic and prognostic candidate biomarkers in drug-induced liver injury vs. other forms of acute liver damage. *British Journal of Clinical Pharmacology, 89*, 2497–2507. https://www.semanticscholar.org/paper/99b866fff373d0c9deebde0ebdd2ddf45bbd7382 (accessed on 9 June 2025).

19. Dhruva, A., Lai, J. C., Ring, M., Yeh, G. Y., et al. (2024). A patient-centered approach to dietary supplements for patients with chronic liver disease. https://core.ac.uk/download/622528881.pdf (accessed on 9 June 2025).

20. Gantsgorn, E. V., Bozhko, A. V., & Yarchenko, S. V. (2025). Diagnosis and prognostic assessment of drug-induced liver injury: What are the outpatient options? (Review). *Safety and Risk of Pharmacotherapy*. https://www.semanticscholar.org/paper/9d954df082efa57b3b9944e5bd4c215d4d10e9fc (accessed on 9 June 2025).

21. Habtewold, A., Kwara, A., Patel, A., Tostmann, A., Turkova, A., et al. (2012). Liver enzyme abnormalities and associated risk factors in HIV patients on efavirenz-based HAART with or without tuberculosis co-infection in Tanzania. https://core.ac.uk/download/pdf/16666841.pdf (accessed on 9 June 2025).

22. Haque, T., Hayashi, P. H., & Sasatomi, E. (2016). Drug-induced liver injury: Pattern recognition and future directions. https://core.ac.uk/download/304663756.pdf (accessed on 9 June 2025).

23. Hayashi, P. H., & Hoofnagle, J. H. (2024). Diagnostic challenges in drug-induced liver injury. *Clinical Liver Disease, 23*. https://doi.org/10.1097/cld.0000000000000206.

24. Hou, W., Huo, K. G., Guo, X., Xu, M., Yang, Y., Shi, Z., Xu, W., et al. (2024). KLF15-Cyp3a11

axis regulates rifampicin-induced liver injury. *Drug Metabolism and Disposition, 52*, 606–613. https://www.semanticscholar.org/paper/9afd5f9453b375ea9935895d7833a85d476cd810 (accessed on 9 June 2025).

25. Hountondji, L., Faure, S., Palassin, P., Witkowski, P., Durand Viel, M., Dupuy, M., Larrey, D., Lamoureux, A., et al. (2024). Time to use the right classification to predict the severity of checkpoint inhibitor-induced liver injury, as assessed for causality using the updated RUCAM. *Alimentary Pharmacology & Therapeutics, 60*, 1561–1572. https://www.semanticscholar.org/paper/bfeeeb3638a048a344df236531453a53f85a4a08 (accessed on 9 June 2025).
26. Huang, A., Zhu, Y., Liu, S., Sun, Y., Liu, Z., Liang, Q., Zhao, J., et al. (2024). An optimized short-term steroid therapy for chronic drug-induced liver injury: A prospective randomized clinical trial. *Liver International, 44*, 1435–1447. https://www.semanticscholar.org/paper/01a0fd6426c3473483454a1fa7e4320d2b70e5e7 (accessed on 9 June 2025).
27. Jarman, G. L., & Webb, G. (2024). Delayed drug-induced liver injury (DILI) and flare of chronic plaque psoriasis secondary to lisinopril use. *Drug and Therapeutics Bulletin, 62*, 189–191. https://www.semanticscholar.org/paper/a25bfc472aa528ab288fcfc269088494fff24b39 (accessed on 9 June 2025).
28. Jiang, A. M., Wei, C., Zhu, W., Wu, F., & Wu, B. (2024). Adverse event profiles of drug-induced liver injury caused by antidepressant drugs: A disproportionality analysis. *Therapeutic Advances in Drug Safety, 15*. https://www.semanticscholar.org/paper/ae66668d130cdc91ddadedc6da61ea5fbce0ff26 (accessed on 9 June 2025).
29. Keshari, A. C., Thitame, S., Aher, A., & Keshari, U. (2025). Drug-induced liver injury: Mechanisms, diagnosis, and management: A review. *Journal of Pharmacy and Bioallied Sciences*. https://www.semanticscholar.org/paper/f9e608e3b5a19cd2d71f1b045c145171a999de00 (accessed on 9 June 2025).
30. Kim, G. A., Moon, J. H., & Kim, W. (2023). Critical appraisal of metabolic dysfunction-associated steatosis liver disease: Implication of Janus-faced modernity. *Clinical and Molecular Hepatology, 29*, 831–843. https://doi.org/10.3350/cmh.2023.0277.
31. Li, Q., Chen, F., & Wang, F. (2022). The immunological mechanisms and therapeutic potential in drug-induced liver injury: Lessons learned from acetaminophen hepatotoxicity. *Cell & Bioscience, 12*. https://www.semanticscholar.org/paper/8804b0da7293f019690e31f69495c1799284755d (accessed on 9 June 2025).
32. Licata, A. (2016). Adverse drug reaction and organ damage: The liver. https://core.ac.uk/download/53305996.pdf (accessed on 9 June 2025).
33. Lin, M., Li, Y., Cao, B., Xu, J., Xiao, X. H., Li, G., & Li, C. Y. (2024). [Pseudo-targeted metabolomics study of immune stress-mediated idiosyncratic liver injury induced by synergistic effects of bavachin and epimedin B]. *Zhongguo Zhong yao za zhi = China Journal of Chinese Materia Medica, 49*(2), 443–452. https://www.semanticscholar.org/paper/bd73b8b981b6fa5f5f1b535b7336bc59fdc3b59e (accessed on 9 June 2025).
34. Liu, Q., Huang, L., Yan, H., Zong, Z., Chen, Z., Wu, X., Chen, L., et al. (2024). Clinical risk factors for moderate and severe antituberculosis drug-induced liver injury. *Frontiers in Pharmacology, 15*. https://www.semanticscholar.org/paper/7a80023a6bb7af917c597b3d598a6e43414d422c (accessed on 9 June 2025).

35. Mederle, O. A., Sima, L., Popa, D., Williams, C., Mîțu, D. A., Șutoi, D., Trebuian, C., et al. (2024). Primary iliopsoas abscess and drug-induced liver injury in the emergency department: A case report. *Diseases, 12*. https://www.semanticscholar.org/paper/35ecc14822d660369d1fe41594fc9e615fed310f (accessed on 9 June 2025).

36. Naeem, M., Bano, N., Manzoor, S., Ahmad, A., Munawar, N., Abd Razak, S. I., Lee, T. Y., et al. (2023). Pathogenetic mechanisms of liver-associated injuries, management, and current challenges in COVID-19 patients. *Biomolecules, 13*. https://www.semanticscholar.org/paper/9c0f01be51a6ea8cbf6b57df9930592a323e33a9 (accessed on 9 June 2025).

37. Niu, C., Xie, X., Liu, R., Liang, X., Hu, Y., & Lai, Y. (2024). CYP7A1 gene induction via SHP-dependent or independent mechanisms can increase the risk of drug-induced liver injury independently or in synergy with BSEP inhibition. *Drug Metabolism and Disposition, 52*, 432–441. https://www.semanticscholar.org/paper/90f5b049f84feb85587cac6467fbfc99956c4d1a (accessed on 9 June 2025).

38. Ntchana, A., & Muhumza, R. (2024). Use of N-acetylcysteine in the management of isoniazid-induced liver injury in a tuberculosis patient: A case report. *Cureus, 16*. https://www.semanticscholar.org/paper/3053d4ec74f1119de7e18374871434a3895d1735 (accessed on 9 June 2025).

39. Prayuni, K., Zahroh, H., Syafrizal, S., & Yuliwulandari, R. (2023). HLA-DQB1*05:02 allele association with anti-tuberculosis drug-induced liver injury: A single-hospital based study in Jakarta, Indonesian population. *Medical Laboratory Technology Journal*. https://www.semanticscholar.org/paper/e4a404458be7686812f7cd28549d532b8333cf27 (accessed on 9 June 2025).

40. Rinella, M. E., Lazarus, J. V., Ratziu, V., Francque, S., Sanyal, A. J., Kanwal, F., Romero, D., et al. (2023). A multisociety Delphi consensus statement on new fatty liver disease nomenclature. *Annals of Hepatology, 29*, 101133. https://doi.org/10.1016/j.aohep.2023.101133.

41. Roy, S., Shah, Z., & Chakraborthy, G. S. (2024). A brief overview of drug-induced liver damage. *The Egyptian Journal of Internal Medicine*. https://www.semanticscholar.org/paper/71519e4ec922a4de01dbd3ff774769e3f5455d2c (accessed on 9 June 2025).

42. Segovia-Zafra, A., Di Zeo-Sánchez, D. E., Lopez-Gómez, C., Pérez-Valdés, Z., García-Fuentes, E., Andrade, R. J., Lucena, M. I., et al. (2021). Preclinical models of idiosyncratic drug-induced liver injury (iDILI): Moving towards prediction. *Acta Pharmaceutica Sinica B, 11*, 3685–3726. https://doi.org/10.1016/j.apsb.2021.11.013.

43. She, Y., Guo, Z., Zhai, Q., Liu, J., Du, Q., & Zhang, Z. (2024). CDK4/6 inhibitors in drug-induced liver injury: A pharmacovigilance study of the FAERS database and analysis of the drug–gene interaction network. *Frontiers in Pharmacology, 15*. https://www.semanticscholar.org/paper/db9d8962cd5e91dc89a42ce1e4d6117faab08503 (accessed on 9 June 2025).

44. Smith, D. N., Pungwe, P., Comer, L. L., Ajayi, T. A., & Suarez, M. G. (2023). Turmeric-associated liver injury: A rare case of drug-induced liver injury. *Cureus, 15*. https://www.semanticscholar.org/paper/29d61444f6a811f62b61da2d4f6028cbc83c4dec (accessed on 9 June 2025).

45. Veeramachaneni, A., Rangaswamy, D. R., Kamble, N., & Kumar, V. S. (2024). Thalidomide as an adjunctive therapy in complex childhood neuro-tuberculosis: A case report. *Bulletin of the National Research Centre, 48*, 1–4. https://www.semanticscholar.org/paper/f3cec66478f9b878fe9475cac5ddba5cfd8488a7 (accessed on 9 June 2025).

46. Wang, X., Huang, A., Gao, S., Hu, W., Wu, J., & Cheng, H. (2023). Association between the treatment pattern of drug-induced liver injury and clinical outcomes: A retrospective study. *Journal of Clinical Pharmacy and Therapeutics.* https://www.semanticscholar.org/paper/577969a97d8110426bc2c6433ed8ad8b75bb52f8 (accessed on 9 June 2025).

47. Wei, Q., Li, L., Zeng, X. Q., Abidan, B., Yin, J., Gao, H., & Guo, J. S. (2024). [An analysis on clinical characteristics and prognosis-related risk factors in patients with drug-induced liver injury]. *Zhonghua Gan Zang Bing Za Zhi = Chinese Journal of Hepatology, 32*(3), 214–221. https://www.semanticscholar.org/paper/36311313bdec47506c7e037b1ff0ca78e6022208 (accessed on 9 June 2025).

48. Wijaya, L., Adevita, S., Alvianto, S., Christiani, Y., & Yolanda, R. (2024). Drug-induced hypersensitivity syndrome with liver injury due to phenytoin: A case report. *Journal of General–Procedural Dermatology & Venereology Indonesia*. https://www.semanticscholar.org/paper/2f04975d0ca91b85d6dfc8a3d2c91ff192ef4277 (accessed on 9 June 2025).

49. Winiarska-Mieczan, A., Jachimowicz-Rogowska, K., Kwiecień, M., Borsuk-Stanulewicz, M., Tomczyk-Warunek, A., Stamirowska-Krzaczek, E., Purwin, C., et al. (2024). Regular consumption of green tea as an element of diet therapy in drug-induced liver injury (DILI). *Nutrients, 16.* https://www.semanticscholar.org/paper/21d5b2310e1ff4babc49d51669e870105bc32f40 (accessed on 9 June 2025).

50. Xiao, Y., Chen, Y., Huang, R., Jiang, F., Zhou, J., & Yang, T. (2024). Interpretable machine learning in predicting drug-induced liver injury among tuberculosis patients: Model development and validation study. *BMC Medical Research Methodology, 24.* https://www.semanticscholar.org/paper/6645fa2f8a25ff31f560f1764319ef62a7e06141 (accessed on 9 June 2025).

51. Zhou, Y., Zhong, Y., & Lauschke, V. (2025). Evaluating the synergistic use of advanced liver models and AI for the prediction of drug-induced liver injury. *Expert Opinion on Drug Metabolism & Toxicology, 21*, 563–577. https://www.semanticscholar.org/paper/93c718c986426c1071362aaa205c847b430c5a72 (accessed on 9 June 2025).

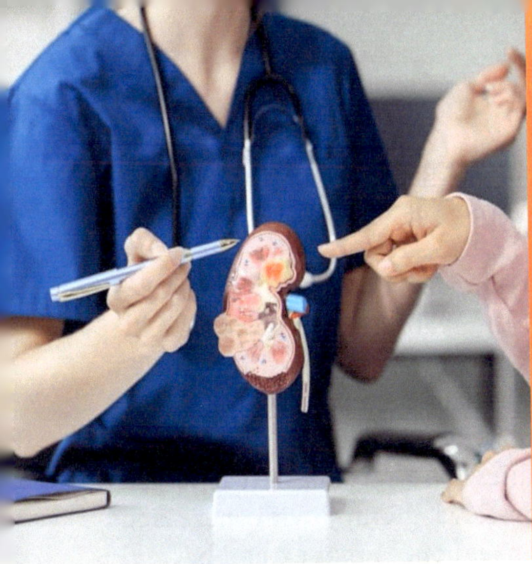

Chapter 7

DRUG-INDUCED NEPHROTOXICITY

Contents

Introduction

The topic of drug-induced nephrotoxicity has gained widespread attention in clinical practice and research settings because various drug agents possess the potential to cause adverse effects on kidney function. Healthcare providers should understand the mechanisms of this condition, particularly as nephrotoxicity has the potential to cause severe morbidity and may necessitate modifications to treatment. By understanding the pharmacological properties of different drugs, one comes to realize that certain drugs, specifically those with a narrow therapeutic index, require strict monitoring to minimize risks. The occurrence of nephrotoxic side effects is exacerbated in children because their renal systems are not fully developed yet and are therefore especially vulnerable to side effects of such widespread medications such as acyclovir, which has caused acute renal failure even though otherwise it has a very favorable safety profile (Vella et al., 2013). Such cases underscore the importance of ongoing research into the safety profile of drugs.

In the area of organ transplantation, the requirement for addressing nephrotoxicity is more urgent because immunosuppressants are employed in order to avoid rejection of transplanted organs. The drugs, although essential to successful transplants, present a unique challenge because they possess narrow therapeutic margins and differential responses in individuals. Under-immunosuppression can initiate rejection episodes, compromising the viability of the graft, while over-immunosuppression makes one susceptible to infections and malignancies (Abboudi et al., 2012). This is the kind of balance that needs tight therapeutic drug monitoring (TDM) and individualized therapy to balance their potency as well as their nephrotoxic potential. Thus, recent developments in pharmacogenetics and biomarker-assisted risk-stratification strategies have emerged as prospective avenues to maximizing the safety of immunosuppressive therapy with increased patient advantages. Nephrotoxicity induced by drugs has clinical consequences that extend beyond the transient effect on renal function and encompass additional systemic impacts and final health outcomes. These patients may have a chain of complications, including electrolyte derangements and cardiovascular disturbance, further rendering their management medical. Besides, early identification of the manifestations and signs of nephrotoxicity will, enable quick interventions that can correct renal injury if the issue is addressed on schedule. With more information becoming available through continued research, the healthcare community is awaiting the adoption of new approaches to the prevention and treatment of nephrotoxicity, with an increasing interest in individualized measures during medication administration. Such a shift in practice is essential to advancing patient safety and outcomes in an era of compounded pharmaceutical therapies aimed at treating complex disease states (Figure 7.1).

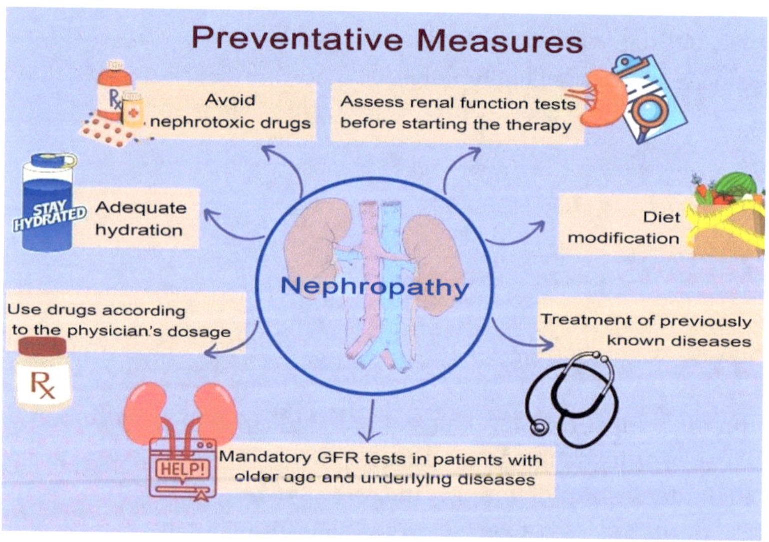

Figure 7.1. Drug-induced nephrotoxicity.

Source: https://s3.amazonaws.com/images.icliniq.com/infographics/What+Are+the+Preventative+Measures+for+Nephropathy+Using+effective+but+not+nephrotoxic+drugs.+Estimation+of+underlying+risk+factors+like+diabetes+mellitus%2C+high+blood+pressure%2C+and+immunocompromised+conditions+due+.jpg.

Definition of Nephrotoxicity

Pharmacology is concerned with nephrotoxicity, which refers to the adverse effects certain substances have on the kidneys. The kidneys are essential for maintaining the body's stability by regulating electrolytes and removing waste. When exposed to nephrotoxic agents, the kidneys can suffer acute or chronic damage, leading to conditions such as acute kidney injury (AKI) and chronic kidney disease (CKD). Nephrotoxicity should not only be seen in the immediate effects on patients; it involves a range of kidney injuries caused by drugs and toxins, which can be sorted into different types. These include glomerular, tubular, and interstitial nephritis types, each characterized by specific histopathological changes and functional impairments, thereby necessitating a comprehensive understanding of the underlying mechanisms involved in drug-induced nephrotoxicity (Awdishu et al., 2015). The mechanisms by which drugs induce nephrotoxicity vary significantly, depending on the agent and the kidney's physiology. Chemotherapeutic drugs, especially cisplatin, are famous for causing cytotoxicity and having a strong potential to harm the kidneys. Cisplatins mechanism involves the formation of ROS and subsequent oxidative stress, leading to cellular apoptosis and damage to renal tubular cells. Due to the interplay between genes and environment, it is crucial to treat individuals with personalized medicine for this type of nephrotoxicity. For instance, certain genetic polymorphisms have been linked to an increased risk of cisplatin-induced nephrotoxicity, underscoring the importance of understanding patient-specific risk factors (Dinh et al., 2019). Such knowledge is necessary for both medical experts who treat patients with potentially harmful drugs and for researchers who aim to develop new, safer drugs. Having set definitions and types of drug-induced kidney disease makes it easier for HCPs and regulators to discuss the issue. They enable the more effective detection and measurement of nephrotoxicity, leading to improved patient outcomes. Additionally, studying the ways nephrotoxicity affects the kidneys and its various forms can help identify effective biomarkers, making it possible to detect and address the condition earlier. By refining our understanding of nephrotoxicity, the medical community can better address the challenges posed by drug-induced kidney injuries and enhance therapeutic practices in the treatment of various diseases (Awdishu et al., 2015) (Figure 7.2).

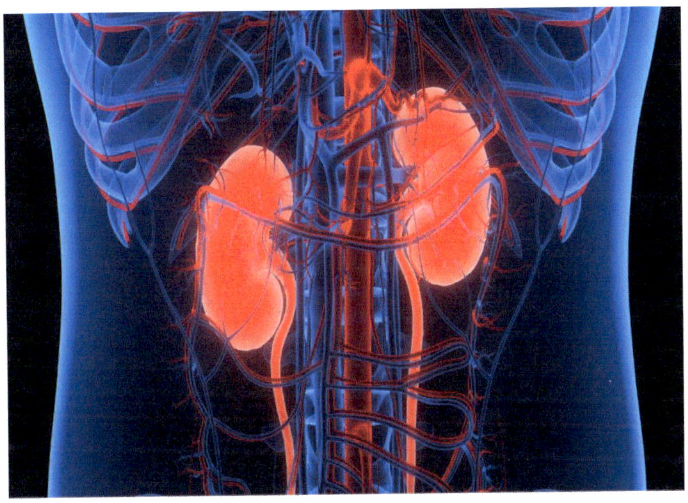

Figure 7.2. Nephrotoxicity.

Source: https://www.evotec.com/toxicology/nephrotoxicity.

Importance of Studying Drug-Induced Nephrotoxicity

It is essential to recognize the significance of studying drug-induced nephrotoxicity, as the kidneys play a vital role in the metabolism and excretion of drugs. With the increased prescribing of numerous pharmacological treatments by healthcare practitioners, nephrotoxic events are a severe problem. For example, chemotherapeutic agents like cisplatin used in the treatment of various cancers are increasingly recognized to have nephrotoxic side effects. Such side effects may necessitate dose reduction or the exploration of therapeutic alternatives, ultimately impacting patient outcomes. This research into the mechanisms of nephrotoxicity may also provide insight into genetic vulnerabilities to such complications in certain patients, enabling more personalized treatment protocols. Therefore, a more profound understanding of drug-induced nephrotoxicity not only enhances therapeutic strategies but also ensures improved patient safety and overall quality of healthcare, underlining the importance of continued research in this crucial area of pharmacology. In addition, control of drug-induced nephrotoxicity is particularly relevant to public health, particularly in the case of vulnerable groups. More specifically, patients with CKD form a group that is most at risk for adverse effects due to exposure to nephrotoxic drugs. The PK of such drugs as vancomycin needs to be strictly followed and the dosing regimen modified in order to avoid further kidney damage. One such recent study stressed that dosing models need to be developed for CKD patients with the aim of evading risks of nephrotoxicity and achieving effective outcomes (Chae et al., 2019). This emphasizes the importance of understanding how various drugs affect compromised renal function so that the safety and effectiveness of drug therapy can be enhanced. Ultimately, enhancing knowledge in this field serves to protect the health of vulnerable patients and achieve the maximum therapeutic effect through evidence-based clinical practice. Secondly, the investigation into drug-induced nephrotoxicity can lead to improvement in drug development and regulatory practice. With increasingly sophisticated complexities of drug interactions with renal physiology, the pharmaceutical industry can transform its approach to designing new drugs. Inclusion of nephrotoxicity testing in drug development can facilitate the identification of potentially toxic compounds at the early phases of drug development. Development in the form of predictive models and biological screening helps in establishing nephrotoxic risk, which ultimately results in safer therapeutic options. These advancements serve not only the health of the patient but also a maximized healthcare system through the potential relief of the burden of drug complications. The relationship between research, clinical practice, and regulatory guidelines plays a crucial role in advancing the understanding of nephrotoxicity, providing opportunities to enhance patient care in the evolving context of pharmaceutical therapies.

7.1. Mechanisms of Drug-Induced Nephrotoxicity

Nephrotoxicity caused by drugs is typically the result of several biological processes acting in concert. One primary pathway is the activation of oxidative stress, where ROS overwhelm the kidney's antioxidant defenses, leading to cellular damage. This kind of injury can cause inflammation and apoptosis, which worsen the renal problems. It has been demonstrated that anticancer drugs can cause nephrotoxicity, leading to cell death and inflammation. By promoting the release of damage-associated molecular patterns (DAMPs), these drugs can elicit an immune response that worsens kidney injury. As evidenced by recent systematic reviews, therapeutic strategies aimed at reducing oxidative stress can potentially mitigate these adverse effects, highlighting the importance of understanding these mechanisms in developing protective interventions against nephrotoxic agents (Asadi-Samani et al., 2017). Aging is another critical factor contributing to the susceptibility of the kidneys to drug-induced damage. It has been observed that aging increases the risk of nephrotoxic injury to the kidneys due to certain age-related changes. Specifically, hemodynamic changes in the aging population lead to reduced renal blood flow, predisposing older adults to AKI when exposed to various drugs. What is more, the weakening of cellular repair and the rise in inflammation in old age make pharmaceuticals more harmful to the kidneys. Such changes increase the amount of oxidative stress and apoptosis in kidney tissues, thereby exacerbating the damage caused by nephrotoxic agents. Given that the elderly population is increasingly prescribed medications, understanding how aging impacts these nephrotoxic mechanisms is crucial in clinical settings (Bonventre et al., 2014). Furthermore, the role of inflammation in drug-induced nephrotoxicity cannot be overstated. Many nephrotoxic drugs induce inflammation by activating pro-inflammatory cytokines and recruiting immune cells into the kidneys. Oxidative stress is a common cause of this inflammatory process, which can lead to further cell damage and death. For example, anticancer drugs that harm the kidneys can damage cells and also stimulate the immune system, leading to ongoing kidney inflammation. A constant link between inflammation and oxidative stress may eventually result in CKD if the inflammatory response is not controlled. Investigative studies focusing on modulating inflammatory pathways may pave the way for new therapeutic strategies aimed at minimizing drug-induced nephrotoxicity (Asadi-Samani et al., 2017).

7.1.1. Direct Cellular Damage

The mechanism of direct cell injury is particularly important in the pathogenesis of drug-induced nephrotoxicity, especially with drugs such as cisplatin. The chemotherapeutic drug, while useful in the treatment of numerous cancers, has been found to induce profound renal injury by interacting with renal tubular cells. Once internalized into these cells, cisplatin is transformed into reactive species, which in turn are implicated in the formation of oxidative free radicals. This oxidative stress is the primary cause of producing cellular damage, apoptosis, and extensive functional impairment of the renal tubules. With progressive nephrotoxicity, disturbances in electrolyte homeostasis, including sodium, potassium, and magnesium wasting, become evident, indicating the extensive impact of cisplatin on renal cell integrity and function. With an understanding of the mechanisms of cell damage caused by cisplatin, methods can be designed to neutralize its toxic action and preserve renal function. Cell mechanisms of nephrotoxicity also involve alterations in the pathways governing cell survival and death. Cisplatin exposure triggers a cascade of events, one of which is the activation of pro-apoptotic proteins and the disruption of survival signaling. Specifically, the p53 tumor suppressor protein has been demonstrated to be implicated in cell responses to cisplatin, such that increases in its activity lead to increased cell death in renal tissues. New renoprotective interventions include p53 inhibition and modulation of mitogen-activated protein kinases. These strategies, in addition to mitigating the direct cellular damage caused by cisplatin, also aim to enhance the therapeutic ratio of this chemotherapeutic agent. Investigating these pathways holds promise for preserving renal function during cancer therapy. Antioxidants have been investigated as potential therapeutic agents against direct cellular damage caused by drug-induced nephrotoxicity. High antioxidant content, nature-derived products have been revealed to detoxify the ROS formed in the course of cisplatin treatment and thereby decrease oxidative damage in renal cells. The evidence indicates that antioxidants not only suppress oxidative stress but also augment the protective mechanisms in the kidneys, which is significant in preventing tubular damage. For instance, studies with ferulic acid show that the compound can potentially reduce lipid peroxidation and improve antioxidant status in renal tissue, thereby preserving cell function and integrity. These findings pinpoint the twofold role of antioxidants; they are shielding from drug-induced cellular injury but possess the ability to preserve the drug's efficacy towards cancer. Hence, the addition of antioxidant regimens to cisplatin chemotherapy treatment may effectively mitigate nephrotoxicity and improve the outcomes of cancer patients (Figure 7.3).

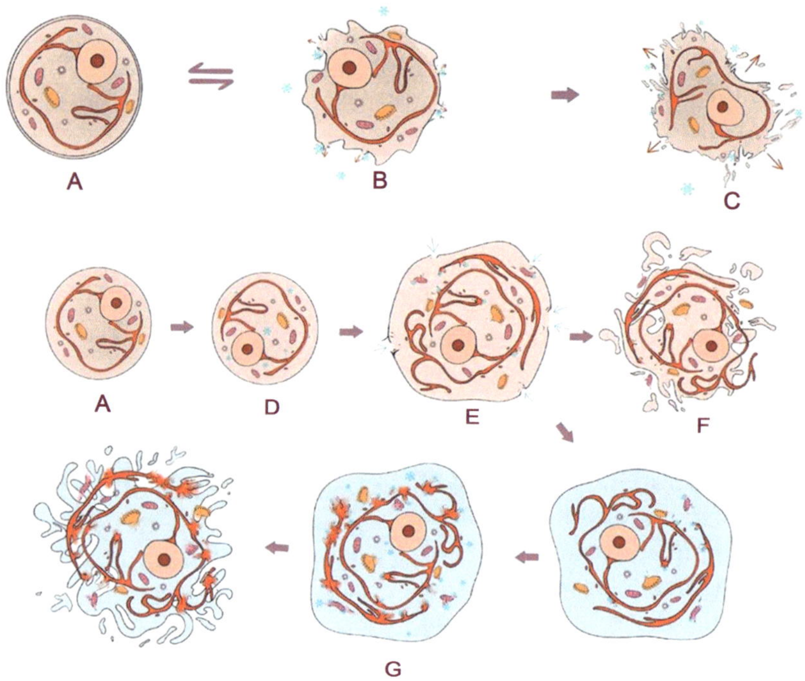

Figure 7.3. Direct cellular damage.

Source: https://www.researchgate.net/figure/Direct-damage-Normal-structure-of-the-cell-When-the-temperature-drops-slowly-and-does_fig4_353550468.

7.1.2. Alteration of Renal Hemodynamics

Changes in blood flow through the kidneys are a primary factor in drug-induced nephrotoxicity, since they can seriously affect kidney function and the body's balance. Medications can initiate hemodynamic changes that lead to renal dysfunction through various mechanisms, including the modulation of glomerular filtration rate (GFR) and renal blood flow. As an example, drugs may tighten the afferent or efferent arterioles, which changes the pressure inside the kidney and can result in AKI. When blood flow to the kidneys is reduced, waste is not filtered out as effectively, which can lead to numerous negative effects and ultimately, serious health problems. Thus, understanding the interplay between drug exposure and renal hemodynamics is crucial for preventing nephrotoxicity and preserving renal function in susceptible populations (Sari et al., 2019). Furthermore, certain classes of drugs, particularly those that affect nitric oxide pathways, have been shown to induce notable changes in renal hemodynamics. For instance, the administration of cyclosporine A (CsA) is associated with an initial phase of renal vasoconstriction due to an imbalance between vasodilators, such as nitric oxide, and vasoconstrictors, including endothelins. CsA appears to inhibit the function of nitric oxide synthase, resulting in reduced nitric oxide production and potentially leading to issues with kidney function and blood circulation. Research suggests that L-arginine, essential for nitric oxide synthesis, may help protect the kidneys from CsA by replenishing nitric oxide and enhancing blood flow to the kidneys. The alteration of renal hemodynamics induced by such drugs underscores the need to monitor renal function meticulously in patients receiving nephrotoxic therapy (Amore et al., 1995). In conclusion, the investigation into the alteration of renal hemodynamics as a result of drug exposure highlights the intricate mechanisms of nephrotoxicity and the potential for preventive strategies. Clinicians should pay attention to symptoms of altered renal blood flow, since they may signal the start of drug-induced kidney damage. It could require changing the amount of medication or using vasodilatory agents together with other drugs. It is vital to do more research to find out how drugs impact the kidneys, so we can better understand the reasons for kidney damage. Such insights not only improve patient care but also contribute to the development of safer pharmacological agents that mitigate the risk of renal injury while providing therapeutic benefits (Sari et al., 2019) (Figure 7.4).

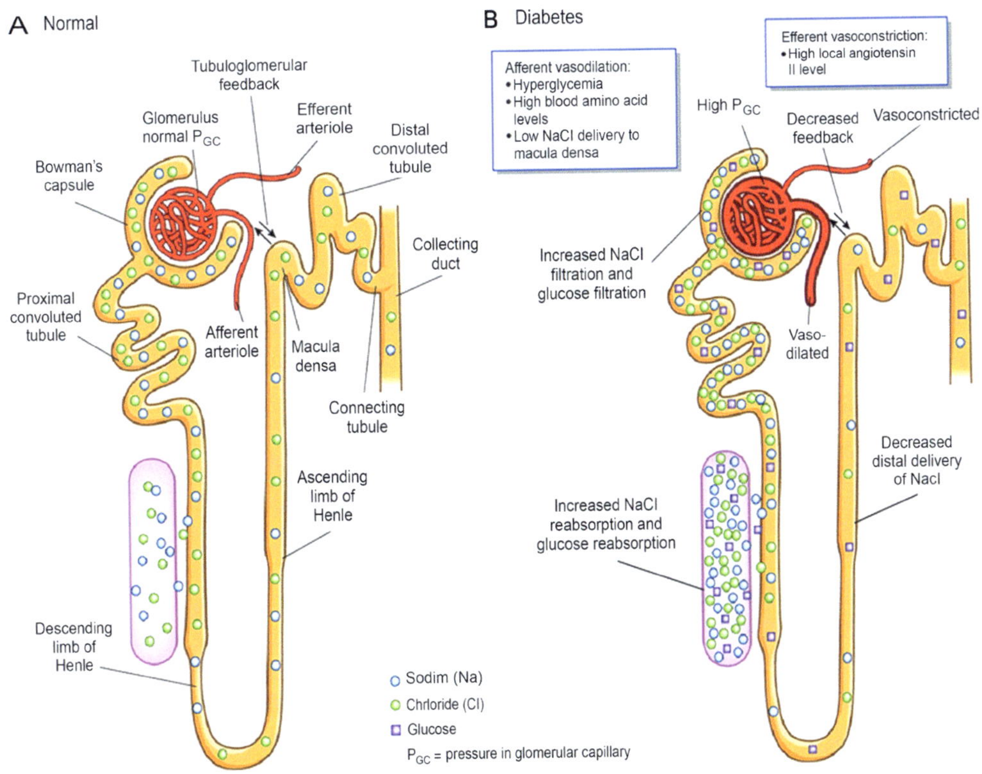

Figure 7.4. Alteration of renal hemodynamics.

Source: https://www.researchgate.net/profile/Radica-Alicic/publication/317033947/figure/fig4/AS:550543623561217@1508271236441/Normal-and-diabetic-nephron-with-altered-renal-hemodynamics.png.

7.1.3. Immune-Mediated Injury

Immunemediated injury is a critical component of drug-induced nephrotoxicity, as it results from the body's overactive immune response to pharmacologic agents. Nephrotoxicity may be differentiated into types such as AKI or CKD based on patient susceptibility as well as the type of drugs involved. When drugs are considered as extraneous antigens, the immune response may cause a reaction that leads to antibody or T-cell activation, which can mistakenly attack renal tissue. The resulting immunological responses can lead to inflammation and cellular damage, characteristic manifestations of immune-mediated injury that complicate the diagnosis and treatment of nephrotoxicity. Understanding the processes of these immune reactions is crucial for both researchers and clinicians in formulating specific therapeutic strategies and counteracting the harmful effects of most nephrotoxic substances on kidney function. Recent research has underscored the role of some cytotoxic mechanisms in immune-mediated kidney injury, particularly with chemotherapy drugs like cisplatin. Cisplatin, as potent an anticancer agent as it is, is notorious for its nephrotoxicity. Activation of inflammatory processes following exposure to cisplatin increases the injury to renal epithelial cells, leading to further cell death and manifesting as renal impairment in patients. This is not an isolated event; this inflammation occurs within the overall context of immune-mediated damage resulting from drug therapy. These interactions are designed to show the necessity for a better understanding of the immunologic fundamentals of nephrotoxicity, as they not only determine the extent of the renal damage but also delineate the potential for prevention in clinical oncology. To effectively treat immune-mediated injury in drug-induced nephrotoxicity, a systematic method is needed for identifying and classifying the manifestations of nephrotoxic reactions. By defining specific phenotypes based on clinical presentation, medical practitioners will be better equipped to recognize, anticipate, and treat such complications. Awdishu et al. (2015) emphasize the importance of distinguishing between various phenotypes, such as glomerular and tubular injury, in order to tailor treatments for the afflicted individuals. By precisely designing diagnostic parameters and treatment outcomes within this structured system, practitioners will be better equipped to mitigate the risk of nephrotoxicity. Additionally, continued research into drug-induced renal injury and immune interactions, as noted by Akbari et al. (2010), is crucial for ongoing learning and ultimately implementing successful prevention strategies in clinics.

7.2. Common Drugs Associated with Nephrotoxicity

Since many drugs used in hospitals can harm the kidneys, it is important to notice and control their risks. Common medications known to cause renal damage include NSAIDs, certain antibiotics, and chemotherapeutic agents. NSAIDs, such as ibuprofen and naproxen, can lead to AKI primarily through reductions in renal blood flow due to their inhibition of prostaglandin synthesis. It is especially noticeable in people who already have kidney problems or are dehydrated. Antibiotics called aminoglycosides can be harmful to the kidneys by damaging tubular cells; therefore, it is essential to monitor the serum creatinine level to detect any early issues with kidney function. Awareness of these risks is crucial for clinicians prescribing these common medications, as patient safety depends on implementing preventive measures and seeking alternatives when appropriate (Bhagat et al., 2017). Antineoplastic agents also present a significant risk for inducing nephrotoxicity, complicating cancer treatment regimens. Cisplatin and methotrexate have been proven to frequently damage the kidneys' tubules. Cisplatin, which is frequently used in chemotherapy, is known to produce ROS that cause oxidative stress and lead to the death of renal tubular cells by apoptosis. For this reason, the advantages of therapy must be carefully weighed against the risk of kidney damage. To mitigate these risks, clinicians employ hydration plans and administer nephroprotective drugs, such as amifostine. Understanding the mechanisms through which these drugs exert their nephrotoxic effects is paramount for devising effective treatment plans that minimize renal complications in cancer patients (Awdishu et al., 2015). Additionally, the clinical landscape recognizes the varying susceptibilities among patients to drug-induced nephrotoxicity, influenced by both intrinsic and extrinsic factors. Having a genetic risk, existing kidney conditions, and using several nephrotoxic drugs increases the chance of harming the kidneys. When assessing risk, it is essential to evaluate the patient's baseline kidney function and determine if they have any other underlying health conditions that may increase the risk of toxicity. It is important to give counseling on hydration and adjust the drug dosage for those with kidney problems. Following the established guidelines, healthcare workers can be more alert and act sooner, helping patients who use nephrotoxic drugs. Hence, a deeper understanding of PK and nephrotoxicity is essential for effective clinical practice (Bhagat et al., 2017) (Figure 7.5).

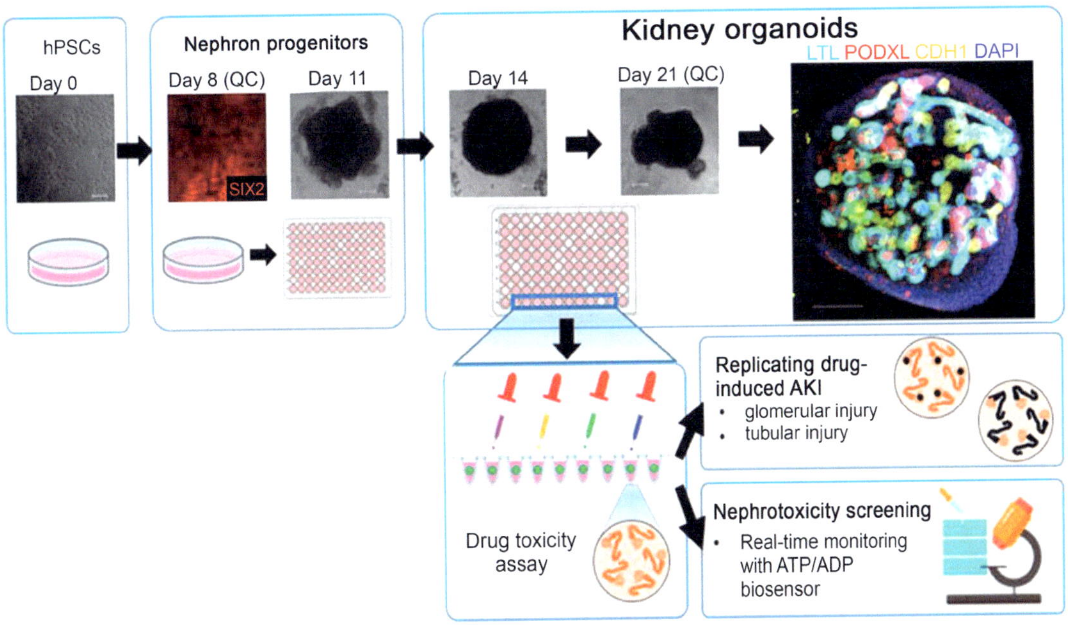

Figure 7.5. Common drugs associated with nephrotoxicity.

Source: https://www.frontiersin.org/files/Articles/1138504/fcell-11-1138504-HTML-r1/image_m/fcell-11-1138504-g001.jpg.

7.2.1. Nonsteroidal Anti-Inflammatory Drugs (NSAIDs)

Nonsteroidal anti-inflammatory drugs (NSAIDs) are widely employed for their analgesic and anti-inflammatory properties in a variety of clinical states, most frequently for the alleviation of acute and chronic pain of disorders such as arthritis and musculoskeletal trauma. As effective as they are, however, the use of NSAIDs is currently firmly recognized as a significant risk factor for drug-induced nephrotoxicity. This is a harmful effect produced by such drugs when they impair renal function, cause conditions such as AKI and CKD. The mechanisms by which NSAIDs produce their nephrotoxicity are many, one of them being inhibition of the cyclooxygenase enzymes, leading to reduced renal blood flow. These pharmacodynamic actions are in a position to induce renal ischemia, and therefore, the necessity of monitoring renal function during NSAID use, especially in individuals with susceptibility to renal impairment, such as the elderly or patients with pre-existing renal disease. Laboratory experiments have established that certain NSAIDs, such as mefenamic acid, are able to induce various histopathological changes to the kidney, ranging from mild glomerular necrosis to inflammation and atrophy of the tubules. Preclinical studies have shown that the intraperitoneal administration of mefenamic acid in animal models results in significant alterations in renal histology and biomarkers of nephrotoxicity, including elevated plasma blood urea nitrogen (BUN) and creatinine levels. These findings emphasize the need for characterizing the distinctive nephrotoxic profiles of distinctive NSAIDs because varied compounds can be risky to varying degrees. As emphasized by recent consensus guidelines, phenotypic separation of drug-induced kidney injury into renal or tubular damage and AKI assists in characterizing and managing NSAID-related nephrotoxicity, which aids in clinical decision-making and limits patient risks (Awdishu et al., 2015). In light of such considerations, it is apparent that the proper use of NSAIDs must assume an all-encompassing approach that includes assessment of underlying risk factors, dose, and patient education regarding renal impairment signs. It is the clinicians' responsibility to carry out routine monitoring of renal function in patients on NSAIDs, particularly when administered at high doses or for prolonged durations. Having good guidelines for proper NSAID usage can help significantly in minimizing cases of nephrotoxicity from NSAIDs. Sustained research activities to elucidate the specific mechanisms of NSAID-induced nephrotoxicity will be essential for future therapeutic strategies, as well as for the creation of safer analgesic agents (Sanat et al., 2014). As increasing trends in NSAID usage continue, resolution of the intrinsic nephrotoxic potential inherent to these drugs continues to be a public health issue (Figure 7.6).

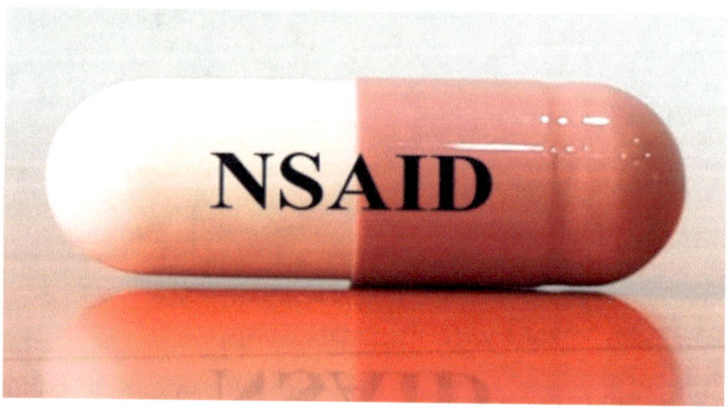

Figure 7.6. Nonsteroidal anti-inflammatory drugs (NSAIDs).

Source: https://complete-physio.co.uk/prophylactic-nsaids-usage-in-sports/.

7.2.2. Antibiotics and Antimicrobial Agents

Antibiotic resistance is causing many infections, mainly when caused by Klebsiella pneumoniae and Acinetobacter baumannii, and this has led to the need for new treatments. Since they are resistant to common antibiotics, these pathogens cause a unique problem in hospitals and clinics. One of the most concerning aspects of managing infections due to carbapenemase-resistant Klebsiella pneumoniae (CR-Kp) is the high mortality rate coupled with limited treatment options. Since traditional treatments have failed, scientists are trying combinations with colistin, a powerful antibiotic that, however, may seriously harm the kidneys. As healthcare practitioners navigate these complexities, balancing the efficacy of antibiotic treatments against potential renal harm becomes imperative to preserve kidney function while combating severe infections (Angelis et al., 2017). The interplay between antibiotic efficacy and nephrotoxicity is particularly evident in the clinical use of colistin. Even though it is a primary treatment for CR-Kp infections, its harmful effects on the kidneys require close monitoring of patients. When colistin is used in combination with other antibiotics, it can more effectively combat resistant bacteria, but it may also increase the risk of kidney problems. Studies indicate that combining colistin with other agents, such as meropenem or tigecycline, may enhance therapeutic success without significantly increasing nephrotoxic risk—although close patient monitoring remains critical (Angelis et al., 2017). It is crucial to develop new antibiotics and treatment methods as healthcare systems strive to preserve kidney function in patients susceptible to drug-resistant infections. Increasingly, doctors are utilizing ceftazidime-avibactam and ceftolozane-tazobactam as alternatives to traditional antibiotic regimens. They are being used worldwide to tackle bacteria that are resistant to antibiotics and to keep harmful effects to a minimum. Additionally, further research on bacteriophage therapy and the use of biocidal agents may help enhance current antibiotic treatments and potentially reduce the risk of nephrotoxicity. The pressing need for advancements in antibiotic therapy highlights the importance of ongoing research efforts aimed at managing complex infections without compromising kidney health (Angelis et al., 2017).

7.2.3. Chemotherapeutic Agents

The development of chemotherapeutic drugs has arrived as a source of hope for millions of cancer patients. However, their nephrotoxicity causes enormous issues in clinical practice. Cisplatin, one of the most widely used chemotherapeutic drugs, is notorious for its dose-related nephrotoxicity, lowering its therapeutic index many-fold. It has been reported that cisplatin-induced nephrotoxicity occurs via oxidative stress, inflammation, and apoptosis of renal cells. These mechanisms disrupt renal function and may lead to AKI, necessitating tight monitoring of renal parameters during therapy. In addition, the absence of reversal-specific interventions for these toxicities means that clinicians are frequently obliged to resort to dose reduction or discontinuation, which jeopardizes the general efficacy of a cancer treatment regimen (Manavi et al., 2024). Therefore, it is crucial to comprehend the nephrotoxic potential of chemotherapeutic agents in order to deliver optimal patient care and treatment. Another significant chemotherapeutic agent, doxorubicin (DOX), also poses a high risk of developing nephrotoxicity. DOX-caused nephrotoxicity is attributed to its capacity to induce oxidative injury and inflammation in renal tissues, leading to both structural and functional injury. In experimental studies, DOX treatment was found to cause generalized inflammation and tubular damage, significantly impacting renal homeostasis (Antar et al., 2023). Interestingly, protective agents such as metformin have been used to counteract this effect. Evidence indicated that metformin may decrease markers of inflammation and restore antioxidant balance in DOX-damaged kidney tissues. As an antidiabetic agent and a potential renal protector, metformin represents a promising area of investigation focused on preserving renal function in the context of chemotherapy. This also highlights the significance of elucidating both the potency and the systemic toxicity of chemotherapeutic agents. Evaluations focused on drug-induced nephrotoxicity need to involve a comprehensive comprehension of the cellular pathways involved in these toxicities. Activation of apoptosis and inflammatory pathways is at the core of dose-limiting toxicities associated with many chemotherapeutic agents. Activation of the nuclear factor-kappa B pathway, for instance, has been suggested to be involved in DOX-induced kidney injury, leading to detrimental histological changes and renal dysfunction (Antar et al., 2023). Utilization of these pathways with protective agents and targeted therapy could be an important part in preventing nephrotoxic risk. There is still an immense gap in the approaches for maintaining renal function during potentially life-saving chemotherapy drug administration, highlighting the imperative to conduct further studies. Investigating the unique molecular mechanisms at play can lead the way for new approaches for ensuring renal integrity, thereby enhancing the safety and efficacy of cancer treatment protocols (Manavi et al., 2024) (Figure 7.7).

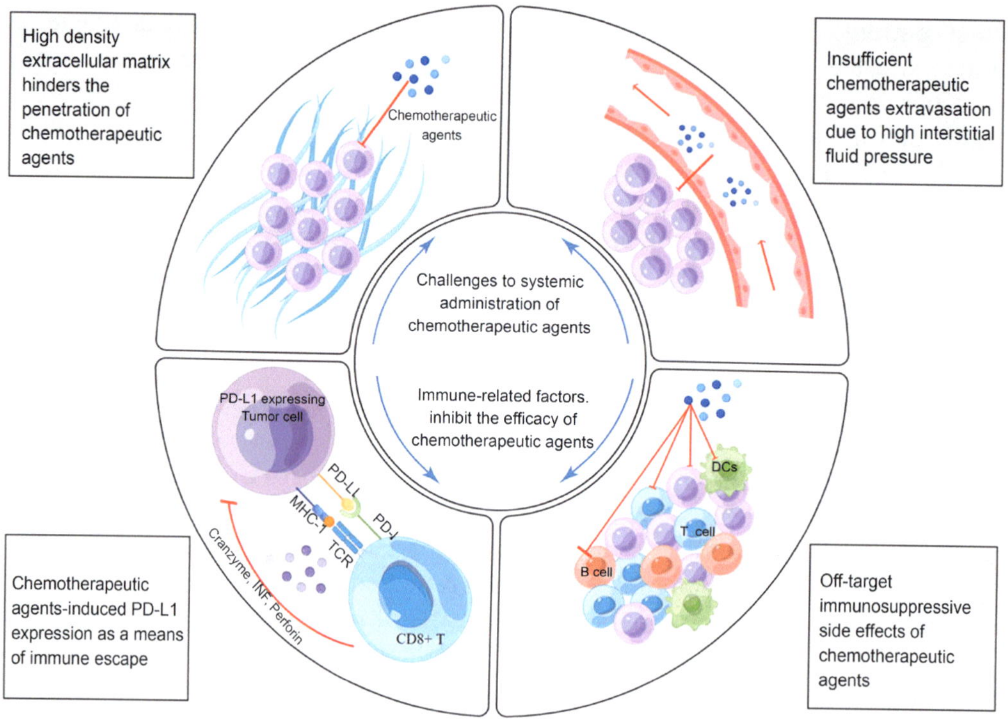

Figure 7.7. Chemotherapeutic agents.

Source: https://www.frontiersin.org/files/Articles/1035954/fphar-13-1035954-HTML/image_m/fphar-13-1035954-g002.jpg.

7.3. Risk Factors for Developing Nephrotoxicity

Several risk factors can make treating drug-induced nephrotoxicity much more challenging. Among these, the patient's age, any pre-existing kidney problems, and other health issues are particularly important. Many elderly patients are more likely to suffer from nephrotoxic effects because their kidneys do not function as well as they age. Moreover, people with chronic renal disease are more likely to be harmed since their kidneys may already be impaired and cannot handle these dangerous substances well. Concurrent medical conditions, such as diabetes mellitus and hypertension, may also predispose patients to renal impairment when exposed to certain medications, underscoring the importance of careful patient assessment before initiating drug therapy in these high-risk populations (Bhagat et al., 2017). Furthermore, the choice of medication itself can significantly affect the likelihood of developing nephrotoxicity. Specific drug classes, particularly antibiotics, have been closely linked to AKI. Aminoglycosides and vancomycin are known to cause kidney damage, and the way this happens depends on the drugs' actions. The way these drugs are given, for how long, and the dosage can all play a significant role in the risk they carry. In addition, using several nephrotoxic drugs at the same time can cause greater toxicity because the effects add up. Understanding the PK and pharmacodynamics of these drugs is essential for clinicians to mitigate risks and tailor therapeutic strategies accordingly (Abishek et al., 2023). In addition to individual patient characteristics and the properties of the administered drugs, environmental and contextual factors can influence the occurrence of drug-induced nephrotoxicity. Patients in the hospital are at greater risk since they are usually given many medications, some of which may be harmful to the kidneys. Since many healthcare-related infections occur, using broad-spectrum antibiotics is important, but it may cause damage to the kidneys. Also, if renal function is not carefully monitored in the hospital, it can go unnoticed when nephrotoxicity occurs, causing the problem to be addressed too late. For this reason, prevention plans should involve selecting the appropriate medications and adjusting their dosages according to the patient's kidney function. A proactive approach to understanding the multifaceted risk factors for nephrotoxicity is vital in improving patient outcomes (Bhagat et al., 2017; Abishek et al., 2023) (Figure 7.8).

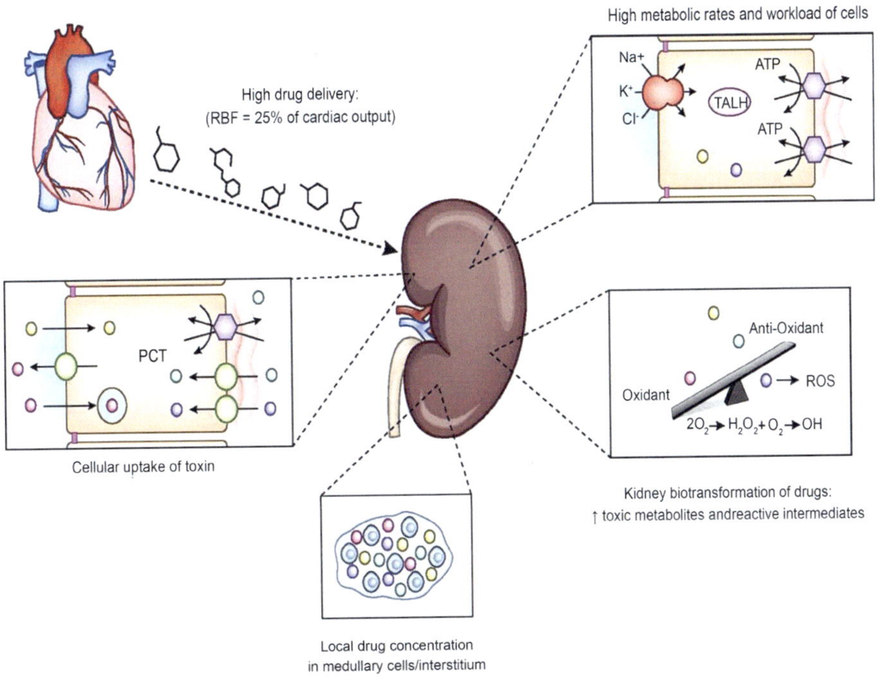

Figure 7.8. Risk factors for developing nephrotoxicity.

Source: https://healthjade.net/wp-content/uploads/2019/11/Kidney-factors-for-drug-induced-nephrotoxicity.jpg.

7.3.1. Pre-Existing Kidney Conditions

Pre-existing kidney disease greatly influences drug-induced nephrotoxicity, and such diseases may enhance the severity of adverse effects of some drugs. CKD and AKI patients possess compromised renal function, and therefore, they are most susceptible to nephrotoxic agents. The decrease in kidney function among such patients enhances drug and metabolite storage in the body, thereby enhancing the risk for further renal damage. Factors involved are the patient's age, simultaneous drug use, and comorbidities, which also cause variable responses to nephrotoxic drugs and complicate treatment regimens. Understanding how existing kidney disease increases the risks of drug therapy is essential in minimizing adverse effects and ensuring that pharmacologic intervention is safely administered in this vulnerable population. The phenotypic categorization of drug-induced kidney disease can help identify the relevance of underlying conditions to patient management. Four large phenotypes have been proposed by more recent evidence on clinical presentation: AKI, glomerular, tubular, and nephrolithiasis (Awdishu et al., 2015). Each of these phenotypes is characterized by specific properties that clinicians must consider when assessing the likelihood of nephrotoxicity associated with the drug. For example, patients with AKI might already have decreased renal function, and therefore, the choice of drug and dose becomes particularly critical. Just as knowledge of the particular type of pre-existing kidney disease will inform which drugs carry the highest risks, it will allow clinicians to individualize treatment regimens that balance efficacy with safety. Furthermore, the scope of pre-existing kidney disease implications reaches into clinical practice and drug-induced nephrotoxicity management guidelines. Kidney Disease: Improving Global Outcomes (KDIGO) has formulated evidence-based practice guidelines for the recognition, prevention, and treatment of AKI with a significant focus on the thorough evaluation of underlying renal conditions (Kellum et al., 2013). The guidelines emphasize the importance of active search for patients with underlying renal diseases prior to initiating potentially nephrotoxic therapies. Appropriate management of the existing conditions not only prevents acute exacerbations but also facilitates better overall results in the medication-managed patient. Thus, integrating an understanding of the patients' renal status into pharmacologic decision making is important to maximize both safety and efficacy in clinical practice (Figure 7.9).

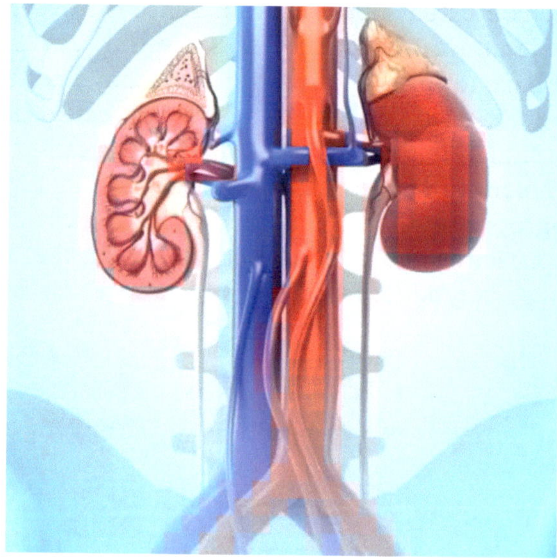

Figure 7.9. Pre-existing kidney conditions.

Source: https://healthify.nz/assets/Health-A-Z/Kidney-topics/kidney-location-and-cross-section-canva-500x500.jpg

7.3.2. Age and Gender Considerations

When assessing drug-induced nephrotoxicity, it is essential to consider age and gender, since they both play a significant role in renal function and how drugs are processed. Age-related physiological changes can affect drug metabolism and excretion. For instance, elderly patients typically experience a decline in GFR, which may render them more susceptible to nephrotoxic agents. Because this group is often affected by other diseases and takes many medicines, it is more likely to suffer from kidney damage. Due to their growing kidneys, young adults and children might react differently to nephrotoxic drugs. For this reason, unique treatment plans are required to address the possible kidney damage that can happen in different age groups. Gender should also be considered because it can influence the occurrence and severity of drug-induced kidney damage. Due to hormonal and anatomical differences, females and males can respond differently to the same medications. For example, males are more likely to suffer from drug-related kidney problems because they have more cases of hypertension and diabetes, which worsen the effects of nephrotoxic agents. When examining groups exposed to nephrotoxic agents, such as pemetrexed (Bhavya et al., 2021), studies reveal a predominance of male patients with abnormal renal function. Therefore, it is important to include gender-specific guidelines to help predict and handle drug-induced kidney damage. When people with diabetes and hypertension take nephrotoxic drugs, the risk of AKI increases. Besides, what we eat and drink can affect the health of our kidneys. For example, not drinking enough water can exacerbate the effects of nephrotoxic drugs, making them more harmful. Therefore, it is essential to educate patients about the importance of hydration. The integration of metabolic profiling methods, such as those discussed in metabolomics research (Heillier et al., 2011), may offer insights into individual susceptibility, facilitating personalized approaches to avoid nephrotoxic outcomes. Recognizing the various aspects of drug-induced nephrotoxicity enables doctors to provide more effective and personalized care for different patients.

7.3.3. Concurrent Use of Multiple Medications

The concomitant use of many drugs, called polypharmacy, is hazardous regarding drug-induced nephrotoxicity, particularly in patients with underlying renal impairment. With increasing age or the development of chronic illness, the likelihood of being on multiple drugs is increased, and so is the risk of adverse interactions between drugs. Pathophysiologically, the basis for nephrotoxicity can often be enhanced by the combination of pharmacologic agents, leading to increased toxicity to renal cells. This is a relevant consideration outlined in recent literature, which points out that causality in drug-induced kidney disease must be demonstrated through a multifactorial approach, including the analysis of alternative risk factors and the biological possibility of nephrotoxic agents, as discussed by Awdishu et al. (2015). Wherever possible, polypharmacy should be avoided. If it cannot be avoided, careful administration and monitoring of the drug are essential to prevent these risks and preserve renal function. Numerically on the verge of immediate risk of nephrotoxicity, the long-term consequence of concomitant drug use mandates careful evaluation of patient management strategies. Chronic exposure to nephrotoxic drugs, particularly when used simultaneously, can lead to the development of AKI and irreversible CKD. The clinicians must balance the interactions of drugs on the renal system and apply standardized protocols in the diagnosis and classification of drug-induced kidney disease as an effective strategy. The novel recommendations for phenotyping drug-induced kidney disease based on clinical presentation provide a framework to address such risks, enabling healthcare providers to more systematically screen and evaluate patient responses to concomitant drugs, as demonstrated by Awdishu et al. (2015). Therefore, effective communication among health professionals and vigilant monitoring of patients play a critical role in minimizing the potential for nephrotoxicity from polypharmacy. Additionally, patient education and involvement in their drug regimens are also crucial for the prevention of the development of nephrotoxicity due to polypharmacy. Noting all medications, such as prescription drugs, OTC preparations, and supplements, and requesting that patients report them, health professionals are better able to identify interactions likely to lead to renal impairment. Furthermore, explaining to the patients the purpose of every drug, the possibility of side effects, as well as proof of renal impairment can facilitate their active participation in treatment. A multidisciplinary team comprising the nephrologist and pharmacist is vital to the development of a personalized care plan that decreases risk factors while addressing the patient's health needs. These collective efforts demonstrate how the development and adherence to guidelines, as presented by Awdishu et al. (2015), can ensure safer medication practices and improved outcomes for patients at risk of nephrotoxicity due to the use of concomitant medications (Figure 7.10).

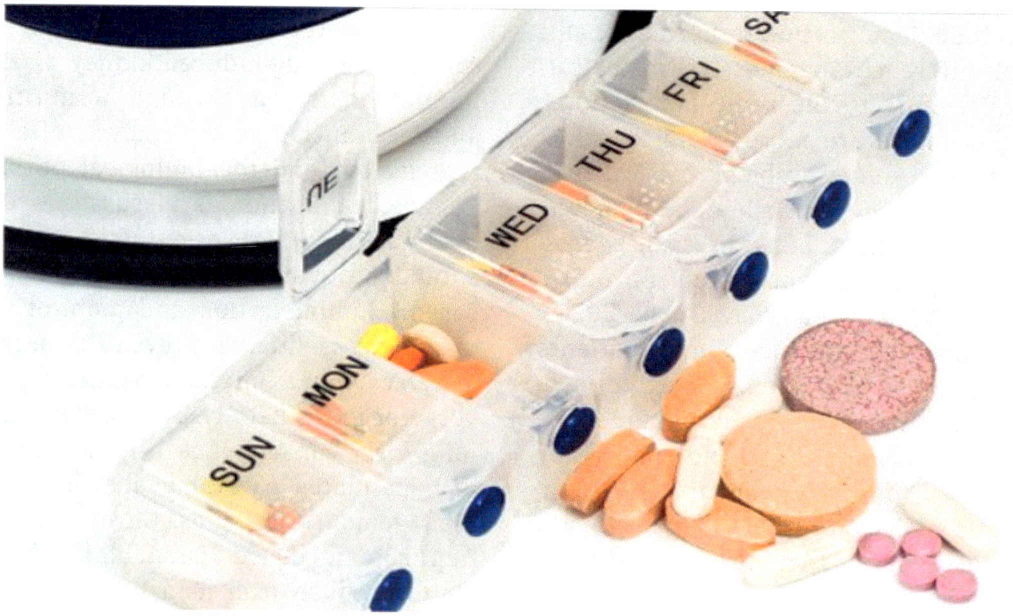

Figure 7.10. Concurrent use of multiple medications.

Source: https://www.physio-pedia.com/Polypharmacy.

7.4. Clinical Manifestations of Nephrotoxicity

Healthcare providers have to deal with the varied symptoms of nephrotoxicity when it results from drug use. Toxicity of this kind may appear quickly, slowly, or over time, damaging the glomeruli, tubules, and blood vessels in the kidneys. The presentation of AKI, a notable complication, is characterized by a rapid decline in renal function, evidenced by an increase in serum creatinine and alterations in urine output. AKI is a serious condition for patients since it may result in lasting kidney damage and higher death rates, mainly in people who receive nephrotoxic drugs for cancer or already have kidney problems. It is essential to understand these changes to implement effective monitoring and risk reduction strategies, which ultimately improve patient outcomes in such critical situations. Recent studies have shown that urinary transferrin levels may suggest possible kidney damage before it is noticeable, especially when patients are treated with cisplatin or gentamicin.

When transferrin levels are elevated, it indicates that the tubules have a reduced ability to reabsorb, revealing early changes in their function before serious problems develop. The use of these biomarkers is highly beneficial, as it enables the grouping of patients according to their risk of complications from nephrotoxicity. Furthermore, identifying high-risk populations—such as those undergoing oncological treatments—can facilitate personalized medicine approaches, improving safety and therapeutic effectiveness for patients at risk of drug-induced renal damage (Casanova et al., 2020). In clinical practice, managing drug-induced nephrotoxicity requires a multifaceted approach, emphasizing early detection, risk assessment, and evidence-based preventive measures. The international clinical practice guidelines established by Kidney Disease: Improving Global Outcomes provide a structured framework for clinicians to assess and manage AKI, including the evaluation of nephrotoxicity risks associated with specific pharmacotherapies (Kellum et al., 2013). When these guidelines are followed in routine examinations, healthcare providers can detect AKI earlier and initiate actions to protect the kidneys from permanent damage. Thus, doctors should constantly monitor kidney function and carefully review whether patients have been exposed to nephrotoxic drugs. If the signs of kidney damage are recognized and proper care is provided, it can greatly improve patients' health and reduce the number of renal disease cases in healthcare.

7.4.1. Acute Kidney Injury (AKI)

The syndrome of AKI constitutes an important problem in the area of drug-induced nephrotoxicity due to the fact that its development implies significant morbidity and health costs. AKI is characterized by a sudden decline in renal function, typically measured in terms of a lowering of GFR and an increase in serum creatinine concentrations. This condition may be due to a variety of causes, among which exposure to drugs accounts for a high proportion of AKI in the hospital environment. Identification of nephrotoxic agents and the mechanisms by which such drugs lead to renal injury will inform clinical management and patient outcomes. For instance, certain antibiotics, especially the polymyxins, have been shown to induce AKI at rates of renal impairment ranging between 5% and 13%, a fact that justifies caution when issuing such medications (Liu et al., 2024). In examining the specific mechanisms involved in drug-induced AKI, researchers have made a differentiation between two broad categories of adverse drug reactions (ADRs): type A and type B. Type A reactions correlate predictably with dose about a drug's pharmacology and have a tendency to cause acute tubular necrosis (ATN). Type B reactions are idiosyncratic, unpredictable, and dose-independent, manifesting as syndromes such as acute interstitial nephritis (AIN). The intricacy of these reactions demands a sophisticated understanding of the biological response to various drugs along with patient-dependent factors that predispose a patient to increased susceptibility to nephrotoxicity. More specifically, retrospective study of patient records has established that drug-induced AKI is an immense and distinctive category of kidney injury, emphasizing the clinical importance of early detection and treatment of such cases (Garcia et al., 2024). Early treatment of acute nephrotoxic drug-induced kidney injury is dependent on a multi-targeted approach consisting of early detection and alteration of the offending drug. HCPS must identify AKI in its initial phases and take appropriate measures to slow its course, including dosing adjustments or discontinuation of the causative agent. Monitoring and patient education cannot be overstated; however, as educated patients who are aware of probable nephrotoxicity are more likely to adhere to recommendations for protecting kidney function. Additionally, recent research into the pathophysiologic mechanisms of drug-induced AKI, such as polymyxin B nephrotoxicity, highlights the necessity of uniform methodologies in studying such responses in order to yield reproducible and usable findings (Liu et al., 2024). Addressing these elements is essential in maximizing patient outcomes and reducing drug-induced nephrotoxicity-related complications (Figure 7.11).

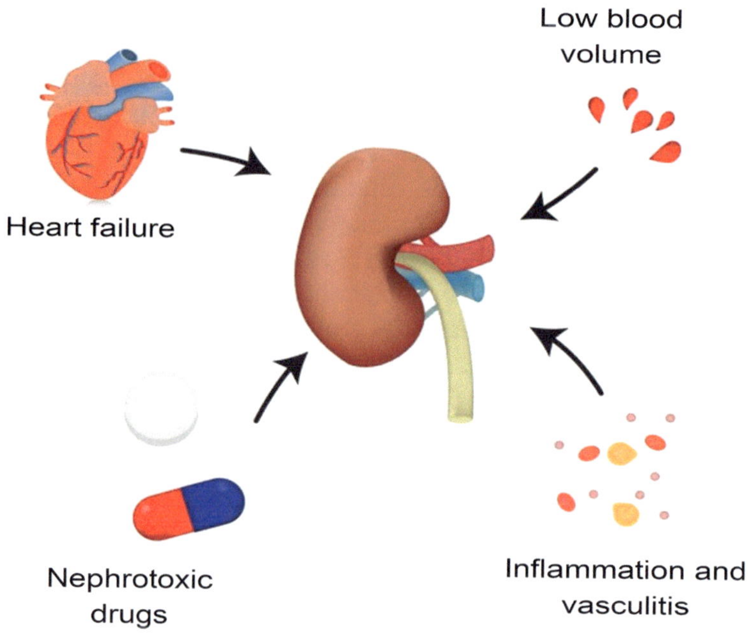

Figure 7.11. Acute kidney injury (AKI).

Source: https://kidneycareep.com/images/page/aki-acute-kidney-injury-elpaso.jpg.

7.4.2. Chronic Kidney Disease (CKD)

Chronic kidney disease (CKD) represents a significant health challenge, particularly as it relates to drug-induced nephrotoxicity. Since the kidneys play a crucial role in drug processing, any damage to them can exacerbate the effects of drugs. Taking certain nephrotoxic drugs may accelerate the progression of CKD, as the kidneys are unable to remove harmful substances as effectively. When kidney function decreases, patients become more likely to have adverse reactions to drugs, which makes CKD even worse and adds more damage from drugs. It has been recognized that the link between aging and CKD is important, especially when it comes to nephrotoxicity, so healthcare providers should check kidney function regularly in elderly patients taking such medications. As individuals age, they frequently exhibit enhanced vulnerability to AKI, which can subsequently result in CKD. Experts have found that changes in kidney pathways with age increase the kidneys' susceptibility to injury by toxins. Because of this, older people are more likely to experience serious CKD, especially since they are often given multiple medications. Understanding the mechanisms underlying this increased susceptibility is essential for developing targeted strategies in preventing and managing CKD among older adults, especially in the context of polypharmacy where the cumulative effects of multiple medications may lead to significant renal impairment (Bonventre et al., 2014). Developing standardized phenotypes of drug-induced kidney diseases is critically important for both clinical practice and research. The four main types of drug-related kidney problems are called AKI, glomerular, tubular, and nephrolithiasis. Every phenotype is linked to certain clinical signs and criteria that help with diagnosing and treating the patient. Noticing these phenotypes enables healthcare providers to understand the relationship between drugs and CKD progression. Establishing a causative relationship requires comprehensive assessments that consider biological plausibility, mechanisms of action, and individual patient risk factors (Awdishu et al., 2015). This way of studying drug-induced nephrotoxicity can improve our knowledge and help develop strategies to reduce the number of CKD cases in vulnerable groups (Figure 7.12).

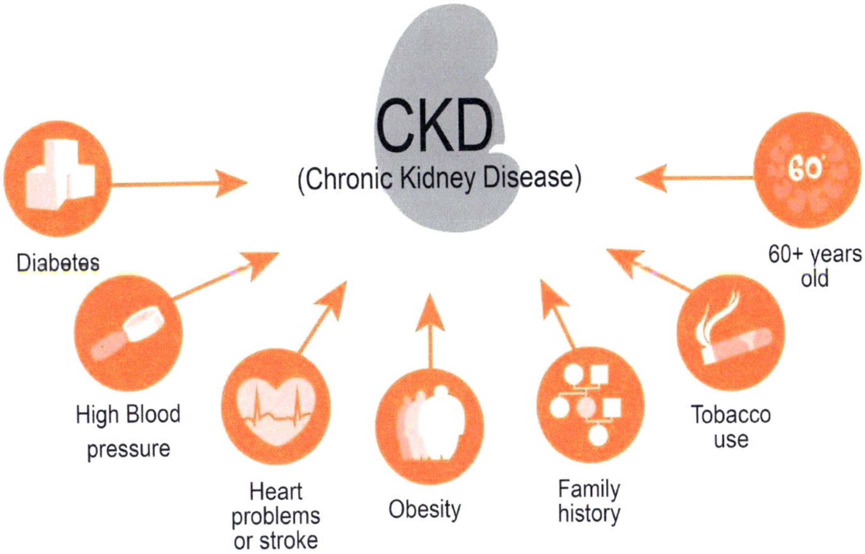

Figure 7.12. Chronic kidney disease (CKD).

Source: https://en.wikipedia.org/wiki/Chronic_kidney_disease.

7.4.3. Symptoms and Signs of Renal Impairment

Renal impairment can be caused by a myriad of signs and symptoms, which tend to be subtle or overt, depending on the degree of impairment. Presentation in the early stages may be non-specific in nature, such as fatigue, weakness, and loss of appetite, and thus readily overlooked or blamed on other illnesses. As renal function decreases, symptoms are more specific, including edema due to fluid retention, changes in urine output, and urine color. Most importantly, patients develop hypertension due to impaired renal function, which also contributes to worsening cardiovascular status. The clinical detection of such symptoms is critical in drug-induced nephrotoxicity, as timely intervention can prevent potential chronic renal damage (Attarbaschi et al., 2016). Progressive renal impairment is typically preceded by a more specific constellation of clinical signs, which can be identified through laboratory tests. For instance, elevated serum creatinine levels are a significant indicator of renal function, signaling nephron damage when they increase above the normal range. Furthermore, the presence of albumin, or proteinuria, in the urine signifies additional renal impairment (cited in management guidelines). Monitoring changes in electrolyte balance, i.e., hyperkalemia, may also indicate renal impairment as the kidneys are now unable products (Burger et al., 2002). Hence, distinguishing the levels of renal impairment through such laboratory tests is essential to identifying vulnerable people to drug-induced nephrotoxicity as well as to appropriate therapeutic management. In the clinic, symptomatology combined with laboratory findings allows for complete assessment of the effects of renal dysfunction on patients on potentially nephrotoxic drugs. Enhanced sensitivity to these phenomena among clinicians leads to more rigorous patient monitoring recommendations, which enable the early detection and treatment of patients with drug-induced renal insults. For example, patients on therapy for acute lymphoblastic leukemia (ALL) can develop specific toxicities that need careful monitoring of renal function along with standard treatment. Hence, defining uniform definitions of such toxicities through consensus guidelines is important, as it offers the same assessment and reporting across different therapeutic regimens. This multifold strategy ultimately yields improved outcomes in renal function, particularly in the at-risk population of drug-induced nephrotoxicity (Attarbaschi et al., 2016) (Figure 7.13).

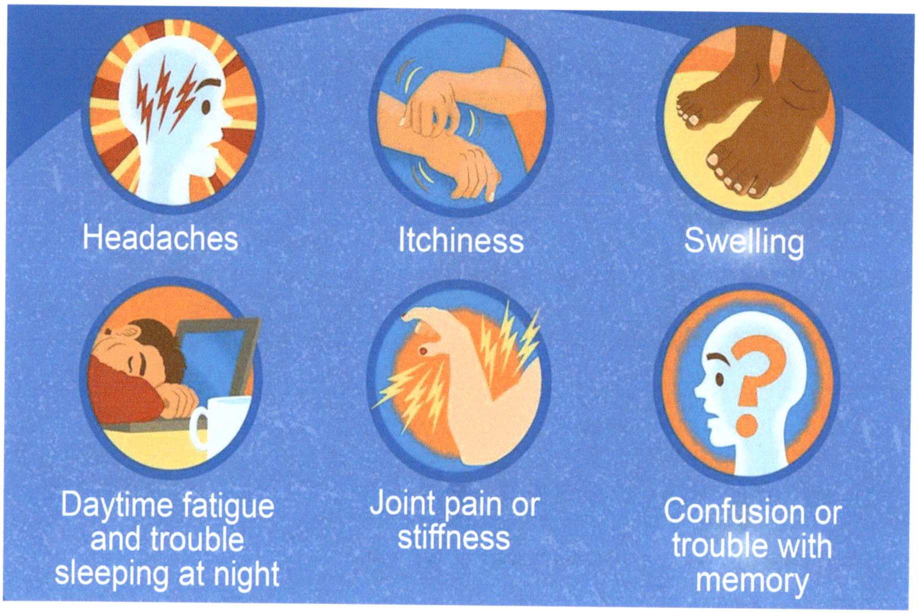

Figure 7.13. Symptoms and signs of renal impairment.

Source: https://www.verywellhealth.com/signs-and-symptoms-of-kidney-failure-5212918.

7.5. Diagnosis of Drug-Induced Nephrotoxicity

A proper diagnosis of drug-induced nephrotoxicity requires checking the patient's symptoms, laboratory tests, and the list of medications they are taking. The initial assessment typically begins with monitoring renal function through serum creatinine levels and estimating the glomerular filtration rate (eGFR). A significant rise in serum creatinine during or shortly after the administration of a suspected nephrotoxic agent serves as a crucial indicator of AKI. Furthermore, urinalysis may reveal the presence of proteinuria or hematuria, which can indicate kidney damage. Grouping AKI into prerenal, intrinsic, and postrenal categories helps to understand the particular cause of the nephrotoxic event. Systematic interpretation of these findings, in conjunction with the KDIGO guidelines, facilitates the establishment of a clear diagnosis and guides management strategies to mitigate renal impairment (Andreoli et al., 2018). In cases involving chemotherapy agents like ifosfamide, careful longitudinal follow-up is essential for early detection of potential renal impairment.

A recent study illustrated that survivors of childhood sarcoma treated with ifosfamide showed no significant long-term glomerular or tubular dysfunction, suggesting that some nephrotoxic agents may not lead to enduring renal damage when monitored appropriately (Andreoli et al., 2018). This points out that clinicians need to assess a person's risk of nephrotoxicity when choosing cancer therapies. Early identification of patients at higher risk of kidney damage enables doctors to employ targeted strategies, including dose adjustments, additional kidney-protective measures, and regular monitoring of kidney function. Novel renal biomarkers, such as neutrophil gelatinase-associated lipocalin (NGAL) and kidney injury molecule-1 (KIM-1), have shown promise in detecting early renal injury before traditional markers like creatinine become elevated. These biomarkers may help identify nephrotoxicity in individuals at risk, allowing for timely treatment to prevent kidney disease. In addition, scientists are exploring how a person's genes and medication responses can be used to identify their risk of nephrotoxicity better. Collectively, these advancements present an opportunity for improved clinical outcomes by fostering early detection and tailored management in patients susceptible to drug-induced renal damage (Kellum et al., 2013).

7.5.1. Laboratory Tests and Biomarkers

Drug-induced nephrotoxicity is significantly enhanced by laboratory tests and biomarkers that provide significant hints regarding kidney injury and function. Biomarkers are biological markers or measurable molecules present in the body that provide insight into renal damage-related pathological events. Traditional renal biomarkers such as serum creatinine and BUN are used routinely to assess AKI. However, their limitations, such as baseline level variability and delayed post-injury rise, suggest the necessity of more precise and sensitive biomarkers. New biomarkers such as urinary NGAL and interleukin-18 (IL-18) are increasingly emerging as hopeful markers of early kidney injury, with their timely treatment and potential prevention of nephrotoxic effects of certain drugs. These advancements underscore the ongoing effort to enhance diagnostic tools in nephrology, particularly in the context of drug safety. During research that quantified the impact of specific nephrotoxic drugs, such as cisplatin, laboratory tests and biomarkers have been important factors in determining the extent of kidney injury. Cisplatin is an anticancer drug that exhibits nephrotoxic properties, necessitating close monitoring of kidney function (Tidholm et al., 2014). Experiments have established that subclinical doses of cisplatin can elicit measurable physiological effects through biomarkers. Plasma creatinine, for instance, may not markedly change but may yield a gauge of bone marrow suppression after renal stress, as demonstrated by alterations in the granulocyte number. The identification of these effects not only enhances the beauty of the pharmacodynamic profile of cisplatin but also demonstrates how research tests can serve as reference markers in the clinic, guiding dose adjustments and tailoring patient treatment strategies in cancer. The landscape of biomarker research, therefore, is much larger than nephrotoxicity and also encompasses transplant, where they are pivotal elements in monitoring allograft function and patient status. The ability to analyze genomic, transcriptomic, and proteomic profiles, in addition to clinical presentation, represents a multidimensional approach to renal health after transplant (Khatri et al., 2011). Current studies have found potential pre- and post-transplantation biomarkers, including specific cytokine gene expression and the development of new non-HLA antibodies, that may be linked with allograft damage. Such research is pointing towards the potential capability of these biomarkers to facilitate personalized medicine strategies, tailoring immunosuppression therapy to individual risks and therefore optimizing longevity and function of transplanted organs. This use of biomarkers in practice has the potential to optimize outcomes for patients at risk for nephrotoxicity from both pharmacologic treatment and transplantation pathology (Figure 7.14).

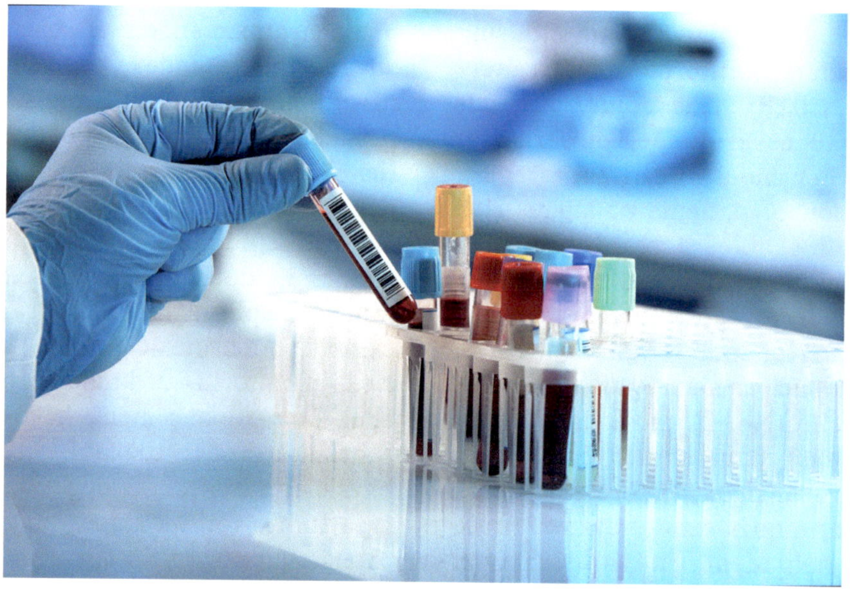

Figure 7.14. Laboratory tests and biomarkers.

Source: https://www.apdaparkinson.org/article/new-laboratory-tests-for-parkinsons-disease/.

7.5.2. Imaging Studies

Imaging tests are essential for spotting and assessing damage to the kidneys caused by drugs, which allows for early action and might reduce future harm to the kidneys. With these techniques, doctors can visualize kidney structures and assess their health without invasive methods, which helps them understand how medications affect the kidneys. Non-invasive methods, such as ultrasound and magnetic resonance imaging (MRI), have been employed to identify morphological changes associated with nephrotoxicity. Additionally, attaching targeted probes to renal injury markers can significantly enhance the effectiveness of these imaging techniques in assessing damage caused by drugs. By detecting changes in the structure and blood flow of the kidneys, imaging studies help determine the degree of nephrotoxicity and support the need for immediate adjustments in drug dosage or discontinuation of the offending medication. According to recent research, bioluminescence imaging makes it possible to monitor kidney conditions in real-time and observe how the kidneys react to different drugs. Notably, the use of a reporter gene system, such as the Saa3 promoter-driven luciferase reporter, has enabled the detection of early signals of kidney injury induced by substances. More bioluminescent signals from renal tissues treated with cisplatin indicate that localized injury and inflammation have occurred, confirming the technique's ability to detect these conditions early on. This non-invasive indicator offers a promising tool for researchers and clinicians alike, facilitating a deeper understanding of nephrotoxic mechanisms and ultimately improving patient outcomes through the timely diagnosis and management of renal impairment (Kudo et al., 2024). However, challenges remain in standardizing imaging techniques for diagnosing drug-induced nephrotoxicity across various clinical settings. At present, there are no standard definitions and criteria for drug-induced nephrotoxicity, which makes it challenging to understand imaging findings. It is mentioned in the literature that drug-induced nephrotoxicity involves several mechanisms, including immune system changes and reduced renal blood flow, and each may manifest differently on imaging tests. Because individuals react differently to drugs and imaging is not uniform everywhere, thorough testing of imaging markers in multiple groups is crucial. By establishing more precise diagnostic criteria and enhancing imaging methodologies, healthcare providers can improve the recognition and management of nephrotoxic risks associated with pharmacotherapy (Dobrek, 2023) (Figure 7.15).

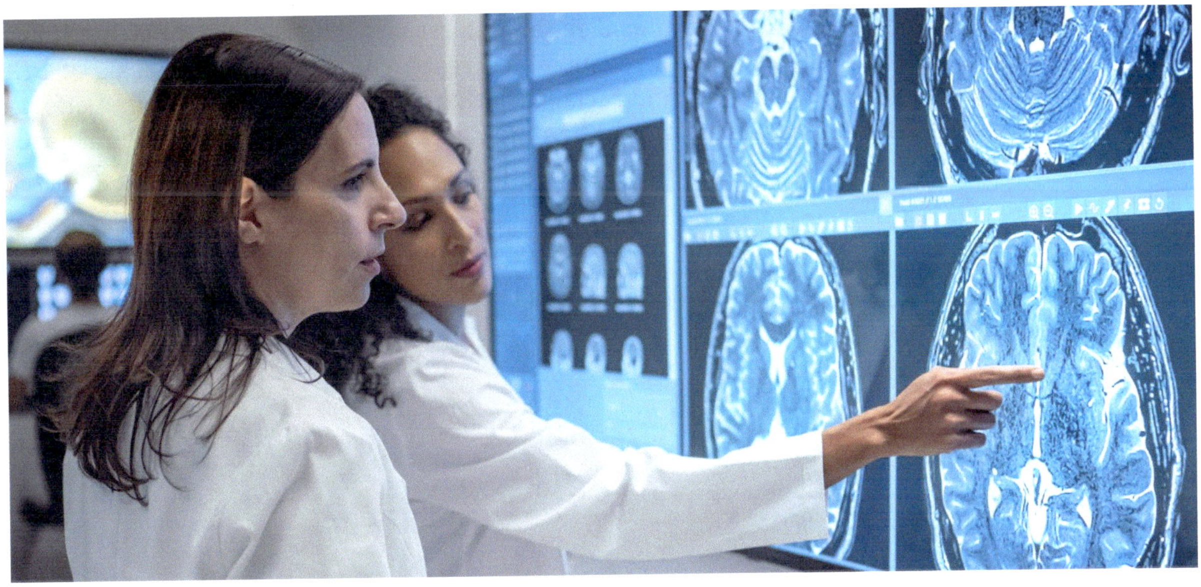

Figure 7.15. Imaging studies.

Source: https://ezra.com/blog/understanding-diagnostic-imaging-tests-a-comprehensive-guide.

7.5.3. Patient History and Medication Review

Good patient history-taking and attention to detail in medication review are vital in the prevention and treatment of drug-induced nephrotoxicity. Adequate knowledge of a patient's medical history might provide information on underlying conditions that might predispose such a patient to renal injury upon exposure to some drugs. Other information about previous reactions to drugs, allergies, and the temporal relationship of symptoms is also essential for clinicians to make viable diagnoses. By establishing an extensive medication history, prescribed, OTC, and herbal medications, providers can identify potential nephrotoxic agents. This initiative is particularly crucial since early detection of harmful drug-drug interactions will significantly reduce exposure-related AKI, ultimately contributing to patient safety and outcome. The importance of accurately documenting a patient's medication regimen is even more significant with the increased complexity of modern-day pharmacotherapeutics. Because the patients have commonly been treated with more than one medication for several diseases, the potential for interaction and consequent nephrotoxicity is enhanced. An evidence-based review of medicines should consider therapy length, dose alteration, and baseline and follow-up renal function. New technology, such as electronic drug calendars, can facilitate this by providing clinicians with immediate access to a patient's complete medication history, potentially identifying any causative agents of nephrotoxicity. The calendars can also provide information regarding the timing of side effects or drug reactions, offering valuable insights that enhance clinical decision-making (Cohen et al., 2020). Lastly, a thorough medication review is an indispensable part of protecting renal function through pharmacotherapy. Knowledge on the role of genetics to drug-induced nephrotoxicity also becomes an important area of research that will inform patient management. Studies have established that genetic predisposition may be a factor in putting someone at risk of developing drug-induced kidney disease (DIKD) (Awdishu et al., 2016). By integrating genetic testing into routine patient assessments, clinicians may be able to identify individuals at risk and tailor medication regimens to minimize nephrotoxic risk. For example, pharmacogenomic data can guide the selection of alternative drugs that offer therapeutic efficacy with less kidney damage. Furthermore, sustained research on the genetic basis of DIKD will further elucidate drug response ethnic and racial variations toward more specific and effective treatment regimens. Therefore, incorporation of patient history, medication assessment, and genetic knowledge is an integrated approach for avoiding drug-induced nephrotoxicity (Figure 7.16).

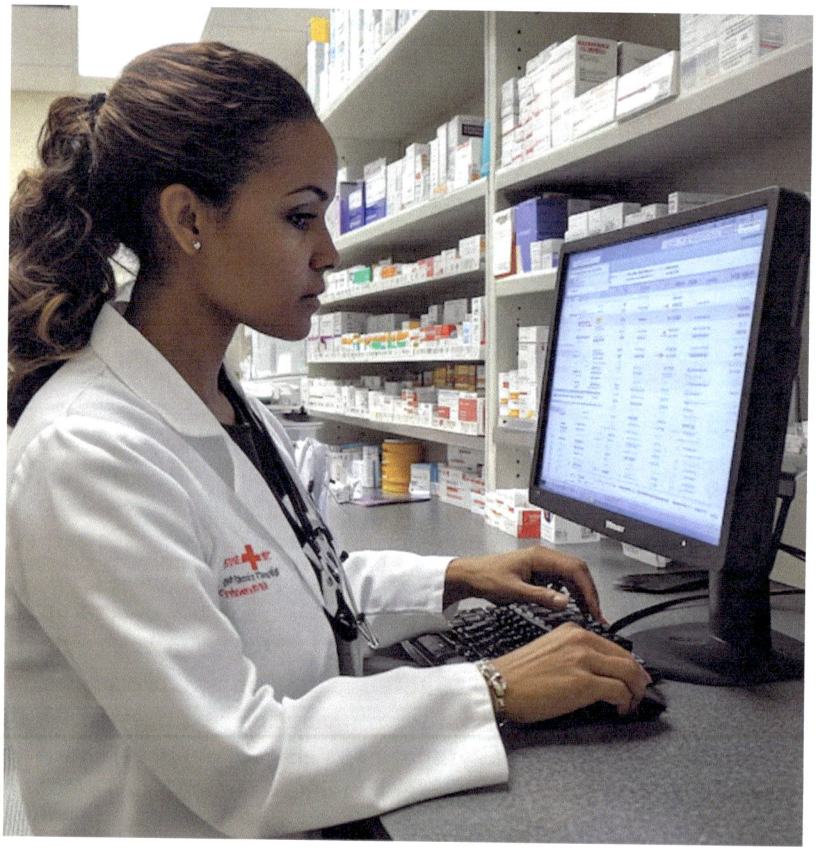

Figure 7.16. Patient history and medication review.

Source: https://img.freepik.com/premium-photo/pharmacist-using-digital-chart-review-patients-medication-history_1327465-57186.jpg.

7.6. Management and Prevention Strategies

Effective management and prevention strategies for drug-induced nephrotoxicity are pivotal in clinical practice, particularly given the prevalence of AKI associated with various pharmacological agents. In 2012, the Kidney Disease: Improving Global Outcomes guidelines were created to guide the identification and management of this serious problem. These recommendations highlight that it is important to check for patients who are likely to suffer nephrotoxicity due to their age, how well their kidneys are functioning, and any other health problems they have. After the assessment, HCPs should take steps such as changing the drug dose, carefully observing kidney function, and avoiding drugs that can harm the kidneys whenever they can. By applying these evidence-based strategies, healthcare providers can significantly mitigate the risk of AKI and enhance patient outcomes (Kellum et al., 2013). In the context of specific nephrotoxic agents, strategies must be tailored to the pharmacodynamics and PK of the drugs involved.

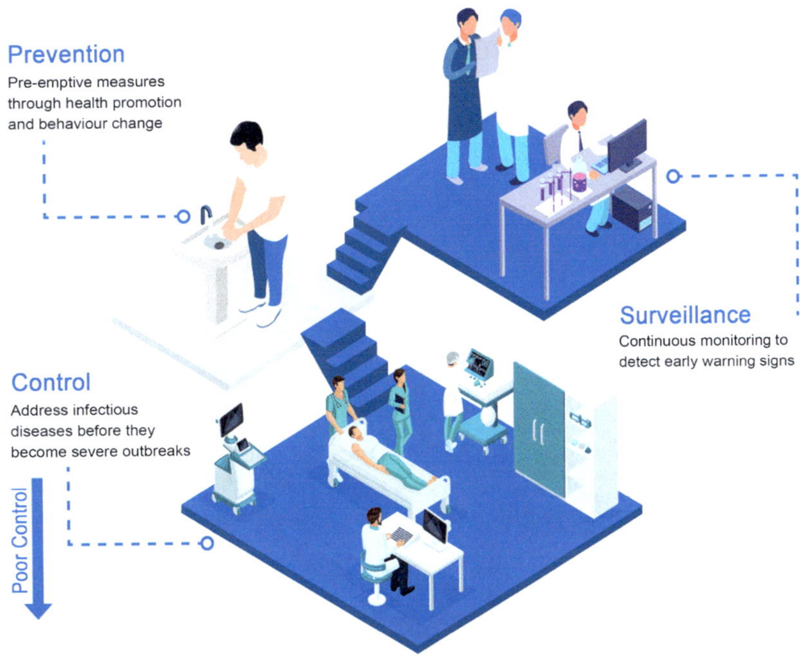

Figure 7.17. Management and prevention strategies.

Source: https://www.hindustantimes.com/lifestyle/health/tackling-non-communicable-diseases-prevention-tips-and-management-strategies-101684566617215.html.

Cisplatin is a chemotherapy drug that is effective against various cancers, but it is also known for causing kidney damage. To mitigate the toxic side effects, it is essential to use hydration protocols before and after cisplatin administration, as they help maintain kidney function and reduce the concentration of harmful substances. Additionally, research on biomarkers has enabled doctors to identify patients at high risk and take preventive measures. Studies done recently have pointed out that some genetic variations can make people more likely to suffer kidney damage from cisplatin. This approach underscores the necessity of personalized medicine in managing drug-induced nephrotoxicity (Dinh et al., 2019). The implementation of supportive therapies also plays a crucial role in managing drug-induced nephrotoxicity. Using antioxidants as agents that protect the kidneys is being studied as a way to reduce oxidative stress caused by nephrotoxic drugs. In addition, new ways to identify and treat nephrotoxic events early make it possible to reduce the seriousness of AKI. Checking the serum creatinine and monitoring urine output are helpful methods for detecting early renal problems. Such approaches help care for patients and protect their kidneys while they take medicines, allowing the drugs to be used effectively without harming the kidneys. So, being attentive, encouraging patients to drink enough, and managing them according to their needs is a complete approach to prevent drug-induced nephrotoxicity (Figure 7.17).

7.6.1. Dose Adjustment and Medication Review

One of the key interventions in the management of drug-induced nephrotoxicity is dose adjustment and full review of the drugs. Nephrotoxic drugs, such as certain antibiotics, typically need to have their dosages adjusted to avoid the onset of AKI. For instance, one has to consider the drug's PK and pharmacodynamics about the renal function of the patients. Proper monitoring with renal function tests enables healthcare providers to adjust dosing appropriately, ensuring therapeutic drug levels without increasing the risk of toxicity.

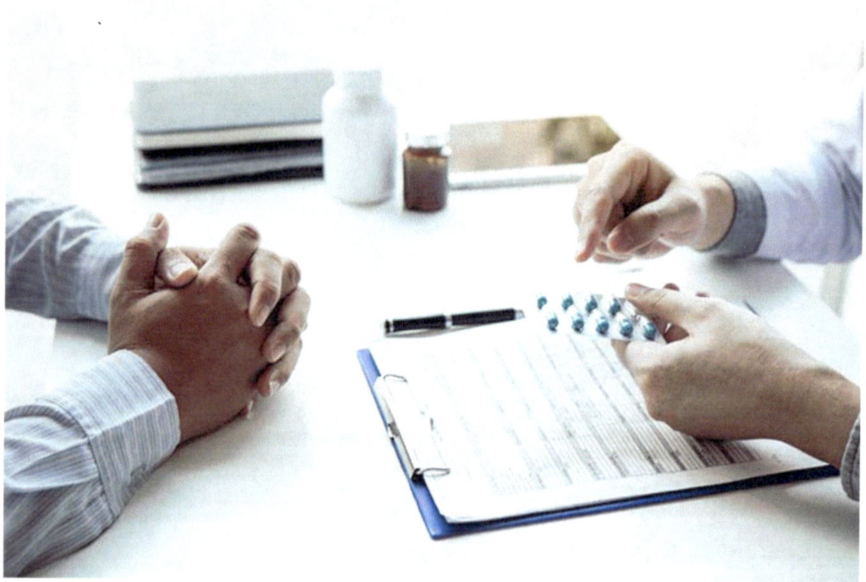

Figure 7.18. Dose adjustment and medication review.

Source: https://ausmed-images.s3-ap-southeast-2.amazonaws.com/ausmed.com/ausmed-articles/20200915_body_3.jpg.

This preventative step is important, given that 20–60% of AKI in hospitalized patients is drug-induced nephrotoxicity, and therefore, there is a high importance placed on careful monitoring of medication in clinical practice (Abishek et al., 2023). The medication review role is not merely pharmacological optimization; it entails careful exploration of the patient's entire medication regimen. This approach not only detects drugs with nephrotoxicity but also detects potential drug-

drug interaction that further compromises renal function. Healthcare providers are encouraged to implement systematic reconciliation of medications at the point of hospital admission or on follow-up outpatient visit. Through careful review of the patient's current medication and their pre-existing renal impairment, healthcare providers are able to develop an individualized plan of care. Such an assessment is critical because concomitant disorders such as pre-existing chronic renal impairment can intensify drug-induced nephrotoxicity, and avoiding such risks may lead to better patient outcomes (Awdishu et al., 2016). Lastly, ongoing monitoring and patient education are key components of effective medication use in patients at risk for nephrotoxicity. Following the adjustment of the dose, a follow-up schedule should be established to monitor renal function and ensure that the adjustments made have had the desired effect without compromising the patient's overall treatment plan. Educating the patient on the signs of renal impairment and the importance of adhering to prescribed dosages can go a long way in enhancing safety. In short, the integration of dose adjustment, medication review, and patient education provides a framework that prioritizes renal protection, with the ultimate goal of reducing the incidence and severity of drug-induced nephrotoxicity in at-risk groups (Abishek et al., 2023) (Figure 7.18).

7.6.2. Hydration and Supportive Care

When it comes to drug-induced kidney damage, making sure the patient is well hydrated and receiving proper care is very important. Keeping the kidneys well-hydrated is vital for preventing AKI, particularly in patients exposed to nephrotoxic agents. Taking in enough fluids helps the kidneys by diluting the dangerous substances in the urine.

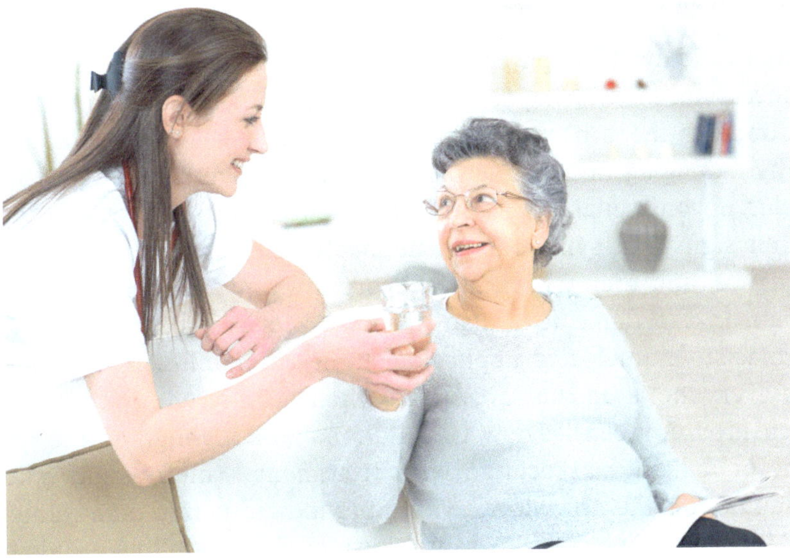

Figure 7.19. Dose adjustment and medication review.

Source: https://assistinghands.com/54/wp-content/uploads/sites/82/2021/03/How-to-Prevent-Dehydration-in-the-Elderly.jpg.

When a patient cannot drink enough or drinking is not permitted, intravenous (IV) fluids can be administered in hospitals. This active fluid management helps the kidneys work better, so that kidney function is less likely to deteriorate during any drugs given as part of the patient's treatment plan. Supportive care should include checking electrolytes, kidney function, and urine output to help detect problems early. Thanks to these measures, healthcare providers can act promptly, which may prevent kidney disease from worsening. Additionally, educating the patient helps them recognize renal impairment by noticing fatigue or changes in urination patterns, allowing them to seek medical help promptly. As a result, providing adequate hydration and supportive measures forms a comprehensive plan for patient care that addresses both physical and mental needs. Investigations into the renal protective effects of substances like Aloe vera have revealed promising results, particularly in the context of nephrotoxicity induced by drugs such as Amphotericin B. Studies have shown that Aloe vera demonstrates significant renal protective benefits, leading to reduced BUN and creatinine levels in affected individuals (Allan et al., 2024). This suggests that combining additional treatments with hydration may lead to better outcomes for patients. When healthcare providers ensure adequate hydration and help patients employ protective strategies, it becomes easier for renal recovery and overall health, highlighting the importance of using multiple approaches to manage drug-induced nephrotoxicity (Figure 7.19).

7.6.3. Monitoring and Follow-Up Protocols

For nephrotoxicity caused by drugs, detailed follow-up and monitoring are essential to neutralize possible adverse kidney impacts. These practices are recommendations for identifying renal damage at an early stage, particularly in patients undergoing nephrotoxic therapy. Utilization of systematic monitoring strategies enables medical professionals to establish baseline kidney function prior to beginning treatment, which can subsequently be used in identifying deviations that may signify AKI.

Monitoring renal function through continuous measurement of serum creatinine and urine output is vital in successful monitoring as defined by guidelines designed to manage AKI (Kellum et al., 2013). By adopting these best practices, clinicians will be in a position to enhance the patient outcomes by managing in a timely fashion, thereby averting long-term renal damage by nephrotoxic therapies. Beyond renal biomarker assessment, follow-up processes need to incorporate patient education on signs and symptoms of nephrotoxicity. Patient participation in their own care promotes vigilance, and they will notify if there are any abnormal changes such as altered urine output or pain in the flank. It is also necessary to establish a multidisciplinary system that includes pharmacists, nurses, and nephrologists in the monitoring system. Multidisciplinary care would ensure everyone is on the same page when dealing with potential nephrotoxic risks and prevention measures. A recent review in childhood ALL highlighted the immediate need for uniform definitions of toxicities associated with treatment, which would guide follow-up care guidelines in this population, thereby allowing for more individualized management and prevention of nephrotoxicity (Attarbaschi et al., 2016). In addition, regular follow-up visits are essential in ongoing monitoring of patients exposed to nephrotoxic substances. These consultations provide comprehensive evaluations that extend beyond immediate renal function to encompass the patient's overall health status and quality of life. Clinicians should be cautious when establishing final follow-up timelines based on the specific nephrotoxic agent used, since different drugs exhibit different levels of risk and recovery timelines. Implementation of evidence-based follow-up periods also aligns with care recommendations, ensuring patients receive proper surveillance for potential late-onset nephrotoxicity. The development of these routine follow-up and monitoring practices ultimately forms a proactive healthcare environment, in which drug-induced nephrotoxicity risks are minimized and patient care is optimized (Figure 7.20).

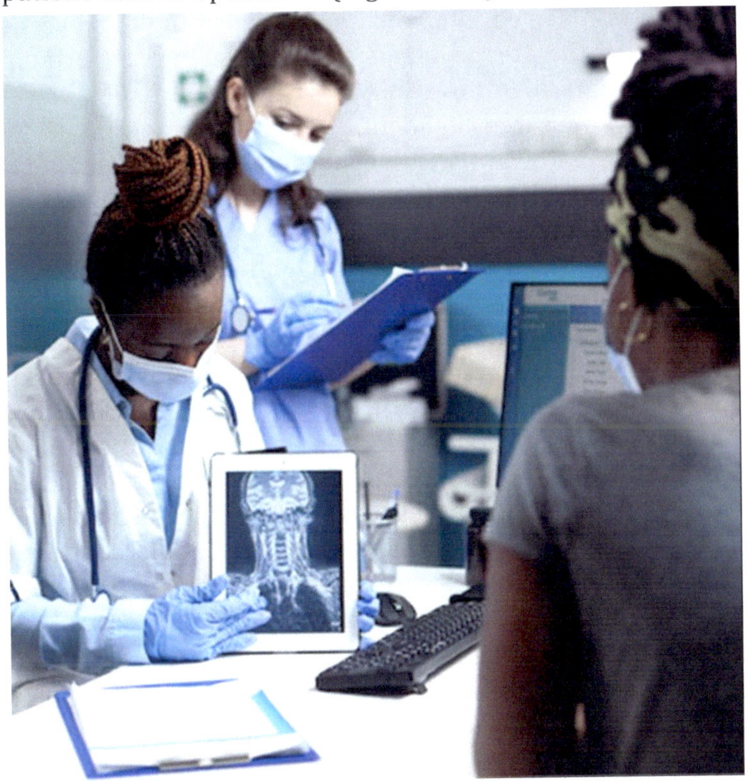

Figure 7.20. Monitoring and follow-up protocols.

Source: https://www.askdogood.com/wp-content/uploads/2024/04/Follow-up-Thyroid-Monitoring.png.

Summary

Looking into drug-induced kidney damage highlights why it is important to pay close attention in clinical settings. Since many drugs used in medicine may harm the kidneys, nephrotoxicity brings both short-term and long-term health problems. Understanding the primary causes, including fibrosis and alterations in glomerular filtration, is crucial for developing effective prevention strategies. For instance, recent research highlights the role of integrins in the fibrotic response, suggesting that targeting these pathways with small-molecule antagonists may have therapeutic potential in mitigating drug-induced kidney damage (Basta et al., 2020). Clinicians can mitigate the effects of CKD and improve outcomes for patients by preventing renal fibrosis. It has been discovered that ifosfamide and other chemotherapy agents may result in renal impairment even after many years. In a cohort of childhood sarcoma survivors, renal dysfunction was evident in a notable number, revealing the lasting effects of nephrotoxic therapies (Andreoli et al., 2018). This discovery highlights the importance of regular health checks and monitoring for early signs of kidney disease that may develop after treatment. In short, managing nephrotoxicity requires various strategies, including prevention, careful observation, and patient education. Continued study of how nephrotoxicity happens and the creation of treatments for specific cases is very important. When clinicians, researchers, and patients join forces, they can learn more about safe medication and reduce the dangers linked to nephrotoxic drugs. Researchers should continue to study the effects of certain drugs on kidney function to help create more effective guidelines and improve care for patients at risk of kidney damage. Taking care of the kidneys is crucial for providing the best possible care to patients who use potentially harmful medications. Drug-induced kidney damage is an important topic in pharmacotherapy today, since it can seriously affect patients taking different medications. A thorough examination of PK reveals that factors such as absorption, distribution, metabolism, and excretion play pivotal roles in determining drug safety. New research highlights that drug-metabolizing enzymes and transporters play a crucial role in causing kidney damage, underscoring the importance of recognizing individual variations in how drugs affect people. Moreover, advancements in understanding xenobiotic receptors and noncoding RNAs provide new insights into how these factors modulate nephrotoxicity, underscoring the need for individualized treatment approaches in mitigating risks associated with renal impairment (Abduljalil et al., 2019). In pediatric populations, the management of drug-induced nephrotoxicity becomes even more challenging, particularly in the context of ALL treatment. Even though survival rates in children with ALL have gone up, the use of chemotherapy causes many side effects, among them nephrotoxicity. A recent study pointed out that several acute toxic effects are linked to ALL protocols, and high-dose methotrexate-related kidney damage is one of the main ones. Because there are many ways to define and assess nephrotoxicity in treatment, it becomes difficult to manage these effects well. Establishing standardized criteria is crucial in facilitating reliable comparisons across studies and optimizing the safety of therapeutic regimens for this vulnerable population (Attarbaschi et al., 2016). Ultimately, the integration of emerging research findings into clinical practice highlights the importance of ongoing vigilance regarding drug-induced nephrotoxicity. As new methods to predict kidney damage and assess drug interactions are being developed, healthcare providers must stay current with the latest information. It is essential to closely watch and prevent kidney damage by using drugs, as the patient's condition plays a significant role. All in all, it will be crucial for medical experts, scientists, and regulators to collaborate in designing safe treatments for ALL and similar diseases that do not harm the kidneys.

CLOSER LOOK

DOSE-LIMITING TOXICITIES ASSOCIATED

Dose-limiting toxicities (DLTs) are adverse effects of a drug or therapy that are severe enough to prevent an increase in dose or continuation of treatment. They play a critical role in determining the maximum tolerated dose (MTD) during clinical trials, especially in oncology and other high-risk therapeutic areas. DLTs are typically identified in early-phase clinical trials, where the primary aim is to assess safety and establish a safe dosage range. These toxicities can include severe hematological effects (like neutropenia or thrombocytopenia), gastrointestinal disturbances (such as persistent vomiting or diarrhea), hepatotoxicity, neurotoxicity, and organ-specific damage. The occurrence of DLTs helps researchers balance the therapeutic efficacy of a drug with its safety profile.

In cancer treatment, DLTs are particularly significant due to the aggressive nature of chemotherapy and targeted therapies. For instance, cisplatin may cause nephrotoxicity and ototoxicity, while paclitaxel can lead to peripheral neuropathy. In immunotherapy, such as checkpoint inhibitors, immune-related adverse effects like colitis, pneumonitis, or hepatitis may emerge as DLTs. These toxicities not only affect the patient's quality of life but also influence the design and progression of clinical trials, making their identification and management essential for drug development.

Effective management of DLTs involves dose modifications, supportive care, or the use of prophylactic measures to prevent severe reactions. Increasingly, predictive biomarkers and pharmacogenomic profiling are being explored to anticipate patient susceptibility to DLTs, allowing for more personalized treatment regimens. While DLTs pose a limitation, they also offer valuable insights into a drug's safety window, guiding regulatory decisions and clinical practice. Ultimately, a deeper understanding of dose-limiting toxicities enhances patient safety and contributes to the development of more effective and tolerable therapeutic options.

References

1. MacPhee, I., & Abboudi, N. (2012). Individualized immunosuppression in transplant patients: potential role of pharmacogenetics. *Pharmacogenomics and Personalized Medicine*, 63. https://doi.org/10.2147/pgpm.s21743Abduljalil, M., Aghazadeh-Habashi, A., Aigrain, P., Aitman, T., Al Za'abi, M., Alegre, M. L., Alnaqeeb, M. A., et al. (2019). *Current trends in drug metabolism and pharmacokinetics*. https://core.ac.uk/download/286361678.pdf.
2. Abishek, A., & Venkateswaramurthy, N. (2023). A review on antibiotics-induced nephrotoxicity. https://core.ac.uk/download/570905256.pdf (accessed on 9 June 2025).
3. Akbari, O., Akbari, A., Al-Sarraf, N., Apetoh, L., Appendroth, D., Arany, Z., Arany, I., et al. (2010). Mechanisms of cisplatin nephrotoxicity. https://core.ac.uk/download/pdf/8605063.pdf.
4. Allan, K. W., & Wycliffe, R. O. (2024). Renal biochemical marker changes in renal protective effects of different doses of Aloe vera on Amphotericin B-induced nephrotoxicity in albino rats: An animal study. *Mediterranean Journal of Basic and Applied Sciences*. https://www.semanticscholar.org/paper/4eddd08eaabdc31f65c3349b183e3eea9534a070 (accessed on 9 June 2025).
5. Amore, A., Bussolino, F., Cacace, G., & Coppo, R. (1995). *A Possible Role for Nitric Oxide in Modulating the Functional Cyclosporine Toxicity by Arginine*. https://core.ac.uk/download/pdf/82439284.pdf.
6. Andreoli, G., Bonci, E., Celani, C., Marrucci, L., et al. (2018). Long-term renal function and hypertension in adult survivors of childhood sarcoma. https://core.ac.uk/download/159268194.pdf (accessed on 9 June 2025).
7. Anitha, C. T., & Divakaran, S. A. (2021). *Treatment With Ferulic Acid Ameliorated CisplatinInduced Nephrotoxicity and Oxidative Stress in Tumor-Bearing Mice*. https://core.ac.uk/download/539886834.pdf (accessed on 9 June 2025).
8. Antar, S., Abd-Elsalam, M. M., Abdo, W., Abdeen, A., Abdo, M., Fericean, L., Raslan, N., et al. (2023). Modulatory role of autophagy in metformin therapeutic activity toward doxorubicin-induced nephrotoxicity. *Toxics, 11*. https://www.semanticscholar.org/paper/aec8cdcd0aedcdcb13dae047864da72eaff2f273 (accessed on 9 June 2025).
9. Asadi-Samani, M., Heidari-Soureshjani, S., Saeedi-Boroujeni, A., & Yang, Q., et al. (2017). Phytotherapy of nephrotoxicity induced by cancer drugs: An updated review. https://core.ac.uk/download/143840266.pdf (accessed on 9 June 2025).
10. Asenjo, A., Iglesias-Freire, O., Kazakova, O., Lartsev, A., et al. (2008). Antibiotic adverse reactions and drug interactions. https://core.ac.uk/download/pdf/35276650.pdf (accessed on 9 June 2025).
11. Attarbaschi, A., Barzilai, S., Escherich, G., Frandsen, T. L., et al. (2016). *Consensus Definitions Of 14 Severe Acute Toxic Effects for Childhood Lymphoblastic Leukaemia Treatment: A Delphi Consensus*. https://core.ac.uk/download/42370388.pdf.
12. Awdishu, L., Cerda, J., Chakaravarthi, R., Davenport, K., et al. (2015). *Phenotype Standardization for Drug-Induced Kidney Disease*. https://core.ac.uk/download/323065889.pdf.
13. Awdishu, L., Cerda, J., Chakaravarthi, R., Davenport, K., et al. (2016). *Rationale and design of the Genetic Contribution to Drug Induced Renal Injury (DIRECT) Study*. https://core.ac.uk/download/pdf/82035256.pdf.

14. Basta, J., Griggs, D. W., Prinsen, M. J., Rauchman, M., et al. (2020). *Pharmacologic Inhibition of RGD-Binding Integrins Ameliorates Fibrosis and Improves Function Following Kidney Injury.* https://core.ac.uk/download/322802289.pdf (accessed on 9 June 2025).
15. Bhagat, S. B., Dhodi, D. K., Patel, S. B., Pathak, A., et al. (2017). Drug-Induced Nephrotoxicity. https://core.ac.uk/download/552654433.pdf (accessed on 9 June 2025).
16. Bhavya, C., Harichandana, P., Kallem, S. V. R., Thota, S., et al. (2021). A retrospective study on pemetrexed-induced nephrotoxicity in non-small cell lung carcinoma patients. https://core.ac.uk/download/539896090.pdf (accessed on 9 June 2025).
17. Bonventre, J. V., Parrish, A. R., & Wang, X. (2014). The aging kidney: Increased susceptibility to nephrotoxicity. https://core.ac.uk/download/28951924.pdf (accessed on 9 June 2025).
18. Burger, D. M., Cransberg, K., Dieleman, J. P., Fraaij, P. L. A., et al. (2002). Persistent sterile leukocyturia is associated with impaired renal function in HIV-1-infected children treated with indinavir. https://core.ac.uk/download/19185172.pdf (accessed on 9 June 2025).
19. Casanova, A. G., Cruz González, I., Cruz, J. J., del Barco, E., et al. (2020). *Urinary Transferrin Pre-Emptively Identifies the Risk of Renal Damage Posed by Subclinical Tubular Alterations.* https://core.ac.uk/download/610668534.pdf.
20. Chae, J. W., Chan, A., Dorajoo, S. R., Goh, B. C., et al. (2019). *Optimizing Vancomycin Dosing in Chronic Kidney Disease by Deriving and Implementing a Web-Based Tool Using a Population Pharmacokinetics Analysis.* https://core.ac.uk/download/323066264.pdf.
21. Cohen, P. R., & Grossman, M. E. (2020). *The Use of Drug Calendars for The Diagnosis of Cutaneous Drug Eruptions in The Age of Electronic Medical Records.* https://core.ac.uk/download/288432494.pdf.
22. De Angelis, M., Mascellino, M. T., & Oliva, A. (2017). Multi-drug-resistant Gram-negative bacteria: Antibiotic resistance and new treatment strategies. https://core.ac.uk/download/227029142.pdf (accessed on 9 June 2025).
23. Dinh, P. C. Jr., Dolan, M., El Charif, O., Travis, L. B., et al. (2019). Genetic and modifiable risk factors contributing to cisplatin-induced toxicities. https://core.ac.uk/download/299809037.pdf (accessed on 9 June 2025).
24. Dobrek, L. (2023). A synopsis of current theories on drug-induced nephrotoxicity. *Life, 13.* https://www.semanticscholar.org/paper/690830d56675816fc1b698835e630df96a0dfd06 (accessed on 9 June 2025).
25. Garcia, G., Pacchini, V., Zamoner, W., Balbi, A., & Ponce, D. (2024). Drug-induced acute kidney injury: A cohort study on incidence, identification of pathophysiological mechanisms, and prognostic factors. *Frontiers in Medicine, 11.* https://www.semanticscholar.org/paper/d03104f2b21d27a38bc74c12fe941e7675db17fb (accessed on 9 June 2025).
26. Hajian, S., Nasri, H., & Rafieian-Kopaei, M. (2014). Renoprotective effects of antioxidants against cisplatin nephrotoxicity. https://core.ac.uk/download/143841487.pdf (accessed on 9 June 2025).
27. Heillier, J. F., Junot, C., Lison, D., Roux, A., et al. (2011). Applications of liquid chromatography coupled to mass spectrometry-based metabolomics in clinical chemistry and toxicology: A review. https://core.ac.uk/download/52690308.pdf (accessed on 9 June 2025).
28. Kellum, J. A., & Lameire, N. (2013). *Diagnosis, Evaluation, And Management of Acute Kidney*

Injury: A KDIGO Summary (Part 1). https://core.ac.uk/download/55846642.pdf (accessed on 9 June 2025).

29. Khatri, P., Roedder, S., Sarwal, M. M., Vitalone, M. J., et al. (2011). *Biomarkers in Solid Organ Transplantation: Establishing Personalized Transplantation Medicine.* https://core.ac.uk/download/323074810.pdf.
30. Kudo, A., Osedo, H., Aisyah, R., Yazawa, N., Saliu, T., Miyata, K., Kumrungsee, T., et al. (2024). Serum amyloid A3 promoter-luciferase reporter mice are useful for early drug-induced nephrotoxicity detection. *International Journal of Molecular Sciences, 25.* https://www.semanticscholar.org/paper/4e33501219cafbff5f26cca5fae81465fed10c3d (accessed on 9 June 2025).
31. Liu, L., Liu, Y., Xin, Y., Liu, Y., Gao, Y., Yu, K., & Wang, C. (2024). An early and stable mouse model of polymyxin-induced acute kidney injury. *Intensive Care Medicine Experimental, 12.* https://www.semanticscholar.org/paper/1bc78e1f25c83bf62c6e7037334f1b1c08dbe231 (accessed on 9 June 2025).
32. Manavi, M. A., Fathian Nasab, M. H., Mohammad Jafari, R., & Dehpour, A. (2024). Mechanisms underlying dose-limiting toxicities of conventional chemotherapeutic agents. *Journal of Chemotherapy, 36*, 623–653. https://www.semanticscholar.org/paper/0fecc23acce1193e50372f7a86c4d5a61269a414 (accessed on 9 June 2025).
33. Roy, S., Shah, Z., & Chakraborthy, G. S. (2024). A brief overview of drug-induced liver damage. *The Egyptian Journal of Internal Medicine.* https://www.semanticscholar.org/paper/71519e4ec922a4de01dbd3ff774769e3f5455d2c (accessed on 9 June 2025).
34. Sanat, F., Hui, G. E., Somchit, M. N., Wahab, S. I., & Ahmad, Z. (2014). Mefenamic acid-induced nephrotoxicity: An animal model. https://core.ac.uk/download/pdf/26977623.pdf (accessed on 9 June 2025).
35. Sari, A. (2019). *Nephrotoxic Effects of Drugs.* https://core.ac.uk/download/322440908.pdf (accessed on 9 June 2025).
36. Tidholm, A., Rose, B. D., Horn, C. C., Limebeer, C. L., Dale, D. C., Vail, D. M., Portillo, E., et al. (2014). Assessment of low-dose cisplatin as a model of nausea and emesis in beagle dogs: Potential for repeated administration. https://core.ac.uk/download/36777715.pdf (accessed on 9 June 2025).
37. Vella, C. (2013). Acyclovir-induced nephropathy: A case report. https://core.ac.uk/download/46602400.pdf (accessed on 9 June 2025).

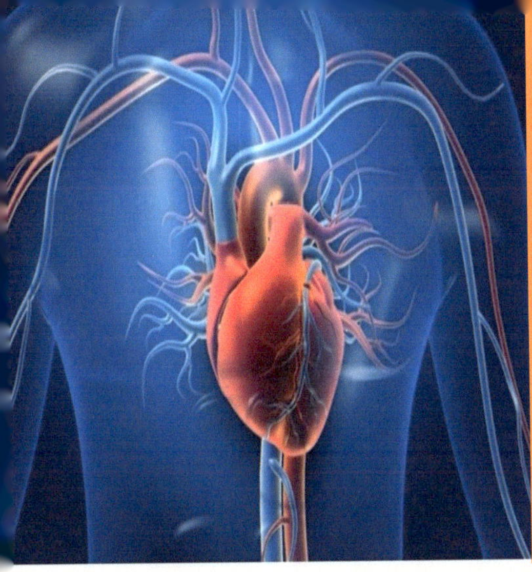

Chapter 8

CARDIOVASCULAR AND HEMATOLOGIC ADVERSE DRUG REACTIONS

Contents

Introduction

The science of pharmacological therapeutics has advanced significantly over the last few decades, particularly in the context of treating complex illnesses such as cancer and chronic conditions. The advancement in drug discovery has, therefore, revealed a pivotal underlying factor overshadowed by cure: the risk of adverse drug reactions (ADRs). Cardiovascular and hematologic ADRs are a particular concern since these could potentially lead to severe complications and reduce the level of patient health outcomes. These adverse effects should be familiar to healthcare practitioners, as managing these complications has an immediate impact on patient safety, adherence to treatment, and overall quality of life. With the increasing prevalence of aging populations and comorbidities, the early detection and prevention of adverse drug reactions become increasingly important. Therefore, an in-depth exploration of their mechanisms, frequency, and management is all the more imperative. Most recent studies project the omnipresence of cardiovascular and hematologic adverse reactions with commonly used therapies. For instance, in therapeutic regimes like bortezomib-based therapy, the patients typically develop complications of peripheral neuropathy and thrombocytopenia during therapy, which are of utmost priority for pre-existing patients. The increased vulnerability for cardiovascular complications in advanced-age patients receiving aggressive multiplex therapy raises alerts about the safe incorporation of such therapy in clinics. In addition, patients with comorbidities and polypharmacy are most susceptible to suffering from side effects, further necessitating careful observation and personalized treatment protocols. As quoted by recent studies, patients with multiple myeloma typically present with multifaceted comorbidities, including cardiovascular disease, thereby making it necessary to have better information regarding drug interactions and individualized risk assessment to improve patient outcomes (Lee et al., 2016). Furthermore, the landscape of drug-related side effects has broadened with the introduction of new cancer therapies like immune-based therapy. These newer modalities also present some special challenges, offering a distinct profile of side effects that require specialized skills to handle effectively. Immune-related toxicities, involving a cascade of symptoms impacting greater than one organ system, are another challenge in monitoring patient safety with treatment. In this context, it is crucial that clinicians consider both the benefits and potential side effects of such treatments, as well as the necessity to intervene immediately in the event of adverse effects. The balance between therapeutic efficacy and patient safety is one of the key battlegrounds in modern medicine, which requires extensive clinician education in the diagnosis and management of cardiovascular and hematologic ADRs for enhancing patient care and therapeutic efficacy (Brém et al., 2020) (Figure 8.1).

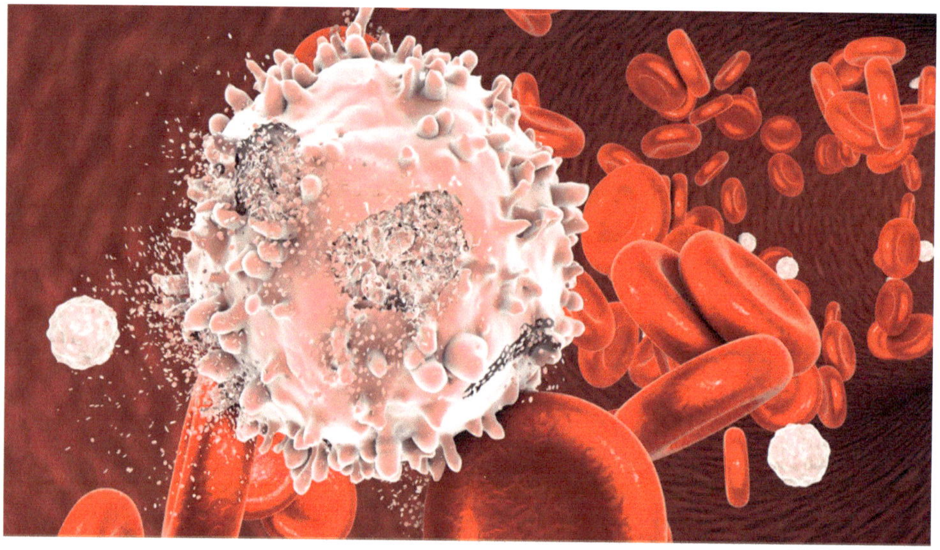

Figure 8.1. Cardiovascular and hematologic adverse drug reactions.

Source: https://www.sriramakrishnahospital.com/wp-content/uploads/2022/05/Hematological-Risks.png.

Definition of Adverse Drug Reactions (ADRs)

The concept of ADRs encompasses a range of unintended and harmful responses to medications administered for therapeutic purposes. ADRs may appear as mild effects or as serious ones that force people to be treated in the hospital or can be fatal. Healthcare providers must understand what ADRs are, as they can significantly impact both patient safety and the effectiveness of treatment. According to research, a substantial percentage of ADR-related hospital admissions stem from complications associated with pharmacological treatments, thereby imposing a considerable burden on healthcare systems. This is evidenced by findings related to antiretroviral therapies in Africa, which have documented high rates of hospitalization due to ADRs (Moirana et al., 2023). To summarize, this highlights the importance of paying closer attention and improving monitoring in clinics to prevent these adverse reactions. ADRs can be categorized into Type A (predictable) and Type B (idiosyncratic) reactions, based on their relationship to the pharmacological activity of the drug. Type A reactions depend on the dose and can occur in any patient, but Type B reactions are not guaranteed and may only affect some patients. There is a need to pay extra attention to cardiovascular and hematologic ADRs because they can be quite severe and affect a patient's health. It is especially important to recognize these specific ADRs, since the way medicines are used today is more complicated and involves more types of drugs for long-term conditions. Therefore, all individuals involved in healthcare should be aware of the unique characteristics of these drug reactions. Managing ADRs can lead to more hospital stays and longer treatments, placing significant pressure on the healthcare system. For instance, the occurrence of ADRs related to antiretroviral therapy (ART) demonstrates the economic burden associated with drug side effects, which complicate treatment regimens and result in additional medical costs (Moirana et al., 2023) as new drugs are being introduced, for example, using antibody-drug conjugates, the importance of monitoring their effects increases. A good understanding of ADR definitions and their types enables healthcare workers to develop more effective treatment plans and educate both patients and other medical staff, ultimately leading to improved healthcare outcomes (Figure 8.2).

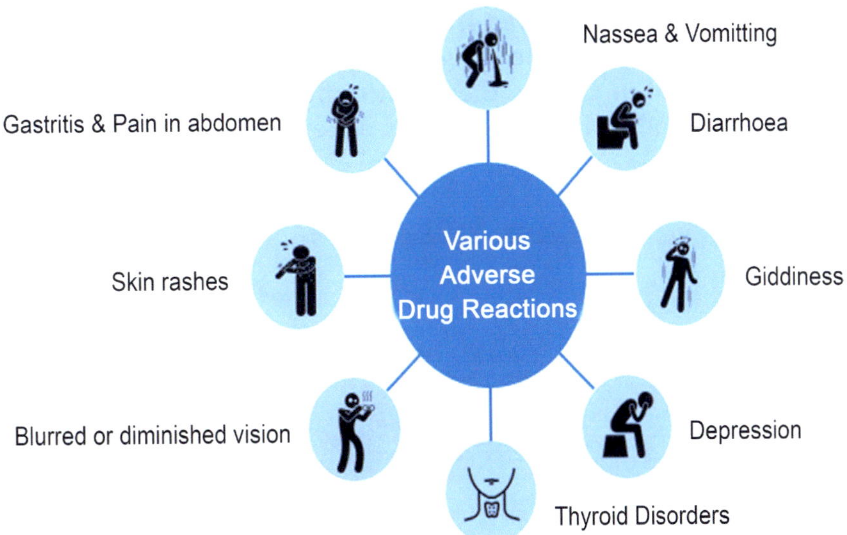

Figure 8.2. Adverse drug reactions (ADRs).

Source: https://ntep.in/node/5654/mopp-adrs-att.

Importance of Studying Cardiovascular and Hematologic ADRs

The significance of learning cardiovascular and hematologic ADRs is highlighted because they do happen and have a profound effect on patient outcomes. Cardiovascular ADRs, from arrhythmias to myocardial infarction, represent an integral challenge in clinical practice because these can lead to extreme morbidity and mortality. Perhaps more importantly, the introduction of complex pharmacotherapies added to this risk, particularly in those with comorbid disease. As reflected by Jacobs et al. (2016), the management of elderly patients with cancer, possibly on more than one agent, emphasizes prudence for potential cardiovascular responses to therapy. Given the complexity of patient profiles these days, health professionals need to stay informed on which specific drugs pose heightened risk, so they can design treatment regimens that minimize adverse effects while maximizing therapeutic benefit. Beyond cardiovascular conditions, hematologic ADRs also require a concerted effort due to what they imply on patients' general well-being. The hematologic system, which is responsible for maintaining immune processes and transporting oxygen, can be significantly affected by certain drugs. Familiar responses like thrombocytopenia, leukopenia, or anemia not only may worsen existing disease but also can influence adherence to treatment and patient quality of life. The consequences of such responses are considerable, considering that studies have shown adverse reactions related to ART, for instance, to lead to hospitalization and high death rates, especially among vulnerable populations (Moirana et al., 2023). As treatments evolve, it is paramount that clinicians understand the hematologic profile of their pharmacologic agents and play an active role in monitoring for these potentially fatal reactions. In the end, the studies of cardiovascular and hematologic ADRs are paramount to optimizing patient safety and optimizing therapeutic effectiveness. Through establishing an intimate acquaintance with these side effects, clinicians will be in a position to adopt important prevention strategies, thereby curtailing the development of severe complications. Education aimed at enhancing clinician sensitivity regarding the interaction between different drug therapies and their cardiovascular or hematologic implications is critical. Apart from this, as healthcare frameworks drive the agenda for precision medicine and personalized treatment, the insights derived from such ADRs will inform interventions to achieve healthier outcomes. Therefore, acknowledging the relevance of such adverse effects not only contributes to the management of current therapeutics but also spurs future research to explore safer drug development methods for heterogeneous patient groups (Figure 8.3).

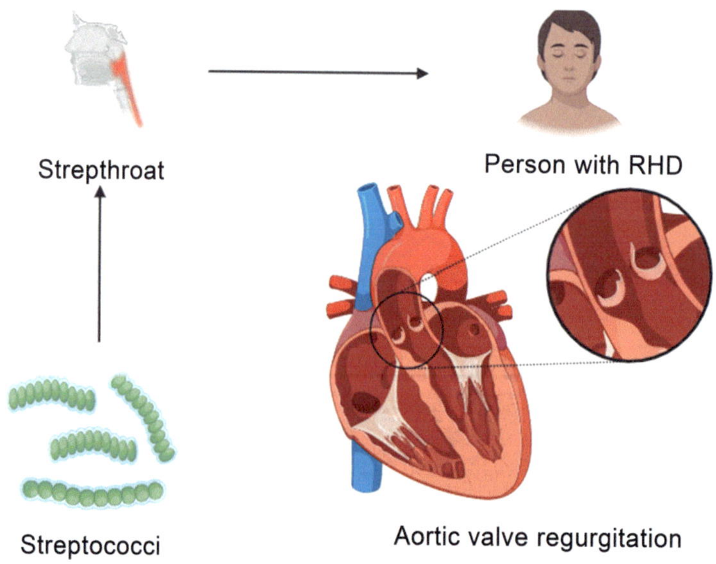

Figure 8.3. Studying cardiovascular and hematologic ADRs.

Source: https://www.mdpi.com/2073-4409/13/17/1471.

8.1. Mechanisms of Cardiovascular Adverse Drug Reactions

The mechanisms underlying cardiovascular ADRs are complex and multifaceted, often involving a combination of pharmacological effects, individual patient characteristics, and interactions with other medications. Some drugs can harm the heart directly or disturb the heart's circulation, which may result in arrhythmias, high blood pressure, or heart failure. For instance, specific antivirals prescribed during the COVID-19 pandemic, such as remdesivir and molnupiravir, have been associated with significant cardiovascular effects despite their therapeutic benefits in combating viral infections like SARS-CoV-2 (Chen et al., 2024). Recognizing these processes is essential for healthcare providers to assess the risks and benefits of using medications in patients with heart problems or those who may be at risk of developing further issues. How drugs are broken down in the body by the body's systems depends a lot on pharmacogenomics. For example, a patient's genetic makeup may affect how they respond to cardiovascular medications, leading to either therapeutic success or adverse events, including skin reactions and altered cardiovascular function (Anika et al., 2024). It is becoming clear that using personalized medicine based on a patient's genetic data may help reduce the chances of ADRs. Since there are now more medications available, clinicians need to stay aware of the risk of side effects, mainly for more vulnerable people. More cases of dermatologic and systemic reactions caused by cardiovascular medications have been noticed as new ones are approved. For instance, while these drugs are designed to improve cardiovascular outcomes, they are not without risk, as evidenced by emerging literature detailing both common and rare adverse effects (Anika et al., 2024). Doctors and nurses should be aware of these possible complications to spot and treat drug-induced reactions. The relationship between the beneficial and adverse effects of cardiovascular drugs highlights the importance of understanding how these medications work, which enables doctors to use them more safely in treating heart diseases.

8.1.1. Pharmacological Mechanisms

The pharmacologic mechanisms of cardiovascular and hematologic ADRs are multifactorial and complex, typically consisting of complex drug-biologic interactions. Direct effects on cardiac myocytes, alteration in vascular tone, or disruption of hemostasis may cause cardiovascular ADRs. For instance, certain antihypertensive agents, such as angiotensin-converting enzyme inhibitors, may induce hyperkalemia, which in turn can affect cardiac electrical activity and lead to arrhythmias. Anticoagulants, in a similar context, predispose patients to bleeding complications by inhibiting coagulation mechanisms, underscoring the need for a thorough understanding of their pharmacodynamics. Understanding such mechanisms is significant, as it informs clinicians of the delicate balance of achieving therapeutic effectiveness without inducing side effects. Beyond direct actions on cardiovascular physiology, certain drugs induce hematologic effects through immune-mediated mechanisms or effects on hematopoiesis. Drugs such as NSAIDs may lead to gastrointestinal bleeding, subsequent effects on blood volume, and associated cardiovascular stability. Some antibiotics also lead to thrombocytopenia by eliciting immune reactions against platelet antibodies. These hematologic reactions could not only compromise the efficacy of treatment protocols but also the health status of patients, subsequently requiring robust pharmacovigilance. As highlighted by the evolving field of drug development, it is critical that a complete comprehension of these pharmacologic mechanisms is appreciated for prevention and anticipation of future ADRs and to enhance patient safety finally. Moreover, pharmacogenetics' role provides critical insight into the variability of drug response with cardiovascular and hematologic ADRs. Gene polymorphisms can influence metabolism and make individuals susceptible to adverse effects, thus affecting treatment outcomes. For instance, certain patients may have alleles that affect the potency of anticoagulants, leading to ineffective anticoagulation or an increased bleeding risk. This observation highlights the importance of personalized medicine, where genetic information is used to tailor drug therapy to an individual's unique biochemistry. As emerging developments in pharmacogenomics progress, they hold the potential to decrease the risk of cardiovascular and hematologic ADRs by making the selection and dosing of drugs more informed. These mechanisms of pharmacology must be understood, as they correspond to practice for further improving patient outcomes in the field of pharmacotherapy.

8.1.2. Genetic Predispositions

Understanding genetic predispositions is essential in the context of cardiovascular and hematologic ADRs. The way a person responds to certain medications may depend on their genetic makeup, especially those that affect the heart and blood. The genes, for example, CYP450, are important in the metabolism of drugs and can change how effective and safe they are. A patient whose genes differ can respond differently to anticoagulants or antihypertensive drugs, which may result in either poor effects or side effects.

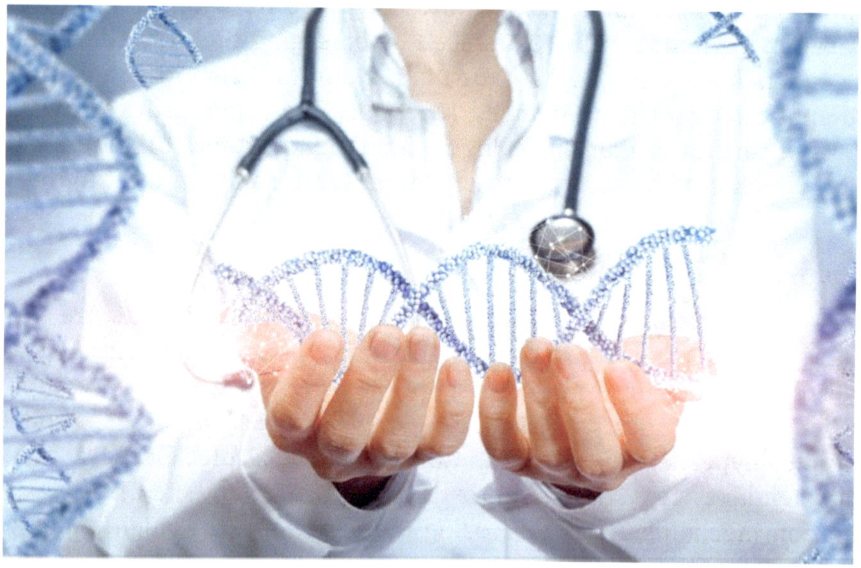

Figure 8.4. Genetic predispositions.

Source: https://centerforfamilymedicine.com/general-health/what-does-it-mean-to-have-a-genetic-predisposition-family-history-and-your-health/.

As a result, doctors can use this information to provide patients with the best treatment and reduce the likelihood of adverse drug reactions. As an example, people with genetic signs of thrombophilia are more likely to have problems when they receive anticoagulant treatment. According to recent studies, the combination of genetic and environmental factors adds another layer to this situation, highlighting the importance of personalized medicine in pharmacotherapy. Integrating genetic information into clinical practice highlights the need for a paradigm shift from traditional one-size-fits-all treatment protocols to more sophisticated, individualized methodologies that aim to improve therapeutic outcomes and reduce the incidence of adverse reactions (Dempton et al., 2011). Emerging innovations in precision medicine are transforming the way genetic predispositions are utilized in the management of cardiovascular and hematologic conditions. New developments make it possible to identify specific genetic markers, which helps doctors determine the best treatment and medications. With the advancement of treatments, doctors can now use genetic information to predict which patients are likely to have ADRs. Additionally, scientists are making progress in pharmacogenomics, which could lead to the development of new therapies tailored to each individual patient. The potential to customize treatment strategies based on genetic predispositions could vastly enhance treatment efficacy while mitigating the adverse effects that often accompany standard drug therapies (Adadzi et al., 2024) (Figure 8.4).

8.1.3. Drug Interactions Affecting Cardiovascular Function

The intricate relationship between cardiovascular well-being and medication necessitates a complete awareness of potential drug interactions and their consequent effects. Drug interactions are capable of inducing extreme alterations in hemodynamic variables, such as heart rate and blood pressure, that can have detrimental effects on already compromised patients with cardiovascular disorders. For instance, certain antihypertensive agents can interact with NSAIDs and cause additive hypertension through sodium retention. In addition, anticoagulated patients with hematologic diseases are also at higher risk for bleeding when combined with certain antiplatelet drugs, adding complexity to cardiovascular treatment. Such interactions bring into sharp focus the greatest need for HCPs to review the entire drug regimen of patients in an attempt to avoid adverse reactions that contribute to cardiotoxicity and complicating factors (Le et al., 2014). Polypharmacy, which is common among elderly patients with multiple comorbidities, significantly increases the risk of adverse cardiovascular drug interactions. Virtually all elderly patients are prescribed complex drug regimens, especially for diseases like multiple myeloma, where drugs like bortezomib produce cardiovascular problems due to interactions and side effects. In a study examining bortezomib-based therapies, the authors noted that many of the patient population presented with pre-existing cardiovascular illness, complicated even further by the concurrent use of numerous medications, averaging 13 per patient (Lee et al., 2016). These findings demonstrate the importance of attentive observation and modification of drug treatments in preventing risks associated with such interactions, thereby maintaining cardiovascular health in vulnerable patient populations. Allan S. Iglauer, FCP, FRSM. Additional responsibilities for clinicians include educating patients about the symptoms of adverse drug interactions, particularly those affecting cardiovascular function. Familiarity with signs of excessive fatigue, palpitations, or abnormal bleeding is crucial for early detection and intervention. Educating patients on the medications, their side effects, and the necessity of adherence can encourage enhanced self-management and improved health status. Frequent medication reviews and adjustment, particularly for transitions in care, are endorsed in current guidelines to assess prolonged cardiovascular risk and appropriateness of therapies. Lastly, detection and management of drug interactions are important for optimization of therapy and improvement of patient safety, whereby pharmacologic therapy of hemologic disease does not compromise cardiovascular integrity (Le et al., 2014).

8.2. Common Cardiovascular ADRs

ADRs related to cardiovascular health are a significant concern in the medical community, particularly as the prevalence of medication use increases. Among all drugs, antihypertensives, anticoagulants, and chemotherapeutic agents are known to cause cardiovascular side effects often. For example, the use of certain diuretics can lead to electrolyte imbalances, which in turn can cause arrhythmias or low blood pressure. Additionally, beta-blockers may result in a slow heart rate. These cardiovascular ADRs may cause anything from minor health issues to serious and dangerous health problems. People with heart problems should be closely watched during drug therapy since they are more likely to have adverse reactions. By being attentive in assessing patients and informing them, it becomes easier to avoid adverse effects. When healthcare providers notice the details of cardiovascular ADRs, they can provide better treatment plans for patients. Even though skin and digestive issues are the main types of irAEs, some patients may experience myocarditis and pericarditis triggered by ICIs. Autoimmune reactions that target the heart are the primary cause of these conditions, leading to inflammation and damage.

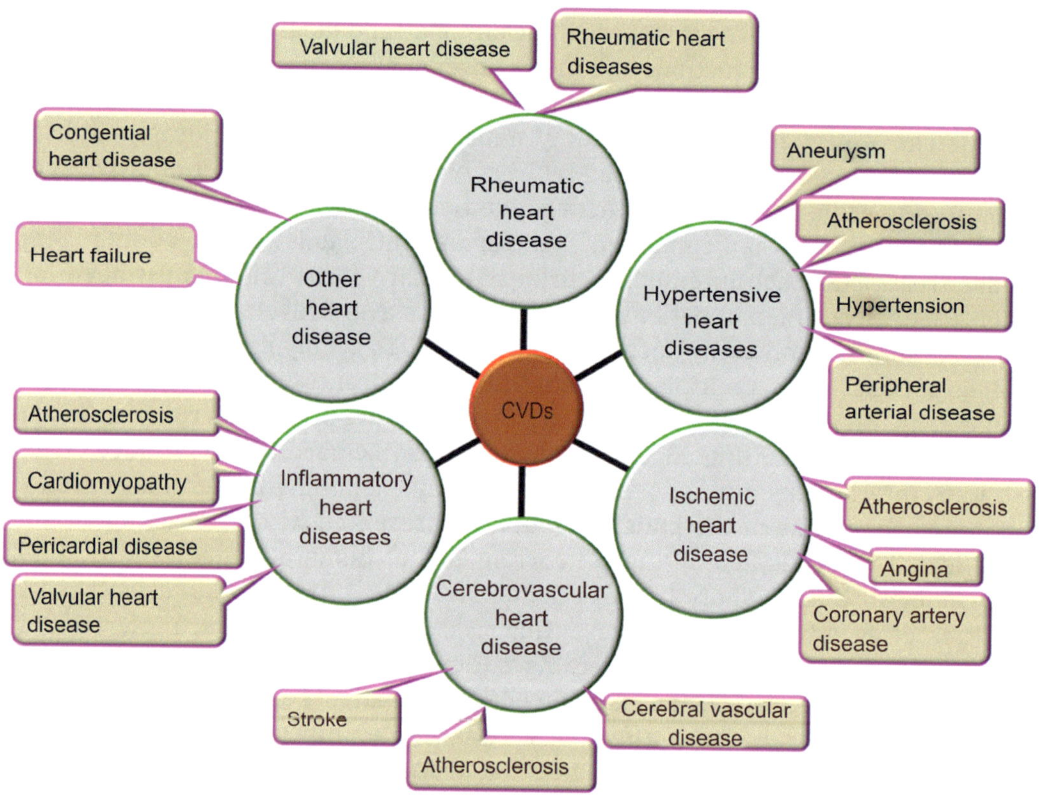

Figure 8.5. Common cardiovascular ADRs.

Source: https://www.researchgate.net/figure/Fig-1-Summary-of-common-cardiovascular-conditions_fig1_280630317.

As recent studies have shown, around 1–2% of patients on immunotherapy can develop serious cardiovascular side effects, which means that healthcare providers should watch for cardiac issues during treatment. The timing of these ADRs can be deceptive, as they may present weeks or months after initiating therapy, highlighting the importance of consistent follow-up and early intervention strategies, such as immunosuppressive therapy, to manage these complications effectively (Abdallah et al., 2017). Further complicating the landscape of cardiovascular ADRs is the interplay of concurrent therapies in patients with cancer, particularly those undergoing combination regimens. Receiving many cancer treatments can cause the patient's body to accumulate side effects, which may result in more severe heart problems if chemotherapeutic drugs are given with immunotherapies such as checkpoint inhibitors, the risk of myocardial injury and similar problems increases. Some drugs, such as anthracyclines, can cause cardiovascular problems that may work together with myocarditis to increase the overall risk for patients. This multifaceted challenge highlights the need for healthcare teams to adopt a multidisciplinary approach to monitoring and managing patients effectively (Brém et al., 2020). Including cardiovascular evaluations in standard cancer care enables doctors to select the most effective treatment plans and minimize the risk of major cardiovascular side effects that could compromise patients' well-being (Figure 8.5).

8.2.1. Arrhythmias and Their Implications

Arrhythmias constitute a significant problem in the setting of cardiovascular ADRs, usually presenting as a disabling complication of many therapeutic endeavors. These abnormal heart rhythms can develop through electrochemical imbalances and have been especially compounded in treated patients with hematologic neoplasms. The introduction of newer antineoplastic agents, while improving survival, has also raised the frequency of cardiovascular adverse events, including arrhythmias. These complications are due to the multifaceted character of such procedures, which may compromise cardiovascular integrity by inducing oxidative stress and inflammation, ultimately affecting heart rhythm and function. This intersectionality of anticancer treatment and cardiac function highlights the necessity of intensive monitoring of cardiac status in chemotherapy patients, because early intervention can minimize catastrophic outcomes and enhance the quality of life of the afflicted patients with both cancers and treatment-induced arrhythmias.

The effects of arrhythmias extend beyond immediate clinical practice, significantly influencing patient management and treatment planning. Particularly, such patients with such illnesses as light chain amyloidosis are at greater risk for arrhythmias from established cardiac dysfunction and cardiovascular toxicity of chemotherapeutic agents. Such patients are likely to have additional risk factors since both the disease process and therapy can cause arrhythmias, which diminish their overall course. In addition to this, recognition of this risk requires health practitioners to create and utilize specific management guidelines to effectively address these unpleasant reactions. In the process, doctors can maximize drug regimens, promote patient safety, and improve therapeutic efficacy while mitigating the risk of arrhythmogenic events caused by chemotherapy and other associated therapies (Barachini et al., 2024). The intricacy of arrhythmia management in the context of hematologic malignancies underscores the need for multidisciplinary care. As the recent literature demonstrates, prolonged survival rates since the advent of innovative therapeutic regimens in hematologic cancers are associated with a rise in acute and chronic cardiovascular events such as arrhythmias. Given this duality, it is the responsibility of health professionals to incorporate means for the early diagnosis and management of these ailments to prevent arrhythmogenic attacks. Patient education and patient participation are equally crucial elements that direct the treatment of drug-induced arrhythmias. Patients need to be informed about the symptoms and signs of arrhythmia so that anticipatory discussions with their care providers are made easier. Raising awareness of the cardiovascular consequences of treatment and developing collaborative care procedures will ultimately lead to improved patient outcomes and a better quality of life for malignancy patients and their associated cardiovascular complications (Blade et al., 2020) (Figure 8.6).

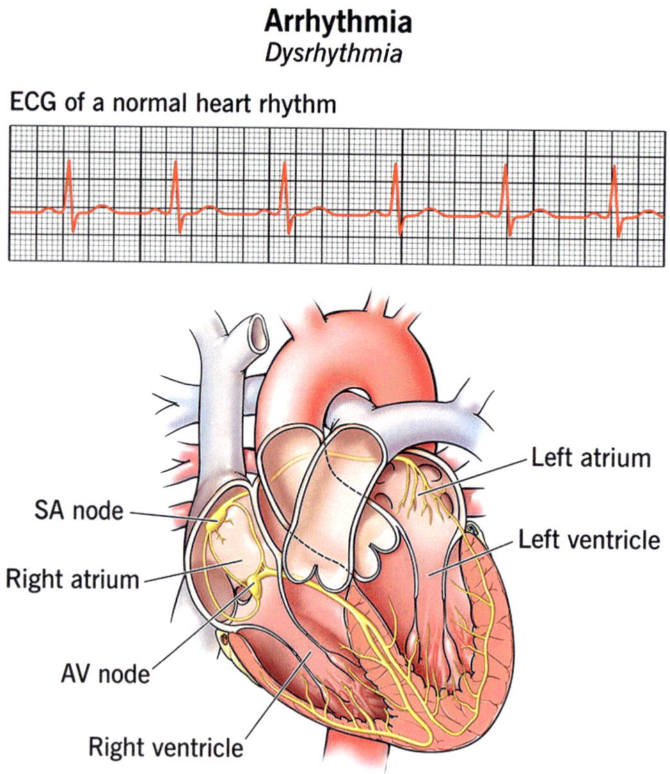

Figure 8.6. Arrhythmias and their implications.

Source: https://my.clevelandclinic.org/health/diseases/16749-arrhythmia.

8.2.2. Hypertension and Hypotension

The management of hypertension and hypotension is crucial in the context of cardiovascular health, particularly concerning the ADRs that may arise from pharmacological interventions. If blood pressure is high, or hypertension, it may cause heart disease and stroke. Antidepressants and other kinds of medications are known to increase the risk of hypertension. For instance, studies indicate that tricyclic antidepressants (TCAs) may prompt significant increases in blood pressure among certain patients, emphasizing the need for careful monitoring of cardiovascular health during treatment. This association highlights the complexities of balancing therapeutic effectiveness with potential cardiovascular risks, as evidenced by an analysis involving psychiatric inpatients, which identified severe hypertension as a notable ADR linked to specific antidepressant therapies (Agelink et al., 2015). In contrast, hypotension, characterized by abnormally low blood pressure, presents its own set of challenges and risks. Drugs from the antihypertensive and antidepressant classes may lead to adverse reactions that cause hypotension. Sometimes, the seriousness of hypotension in such situations calls for urgent medical care, mainly for those who are elderly or have heart problems. Notably, a study on adverse reactions associated with various drug therapies revealed that severe hypotension was the most frequently observed cardiovascular ADR, underscoring the importance of vigilant monitoring in clinical settings (Agelink et al., 2015). This result highlights the fine line between blood pressure medications and their potential unintended effects, prompting prescribers and caregivers to review their current practices. Examining the overall impact of these reactions is crucial for understanding their effect on patients. Some mixtures of drugs that influence the central nervous system (CNS) may either increase hypertension or lead to hypotension, making it difficult for HCPs to manage the patient's condition. It has been found that reactions to several types of drugs often cause cardiovascular ADRs, so it is important to have comprehensive monitoring. Being cautious can significantly reduce the risk of serious consequences associated with these cardiovascular complications in patients. Since these interactions are not simple, both doctors and patients need to understand how to manage the risks of hypertension and hypotension (Figure 8.7).

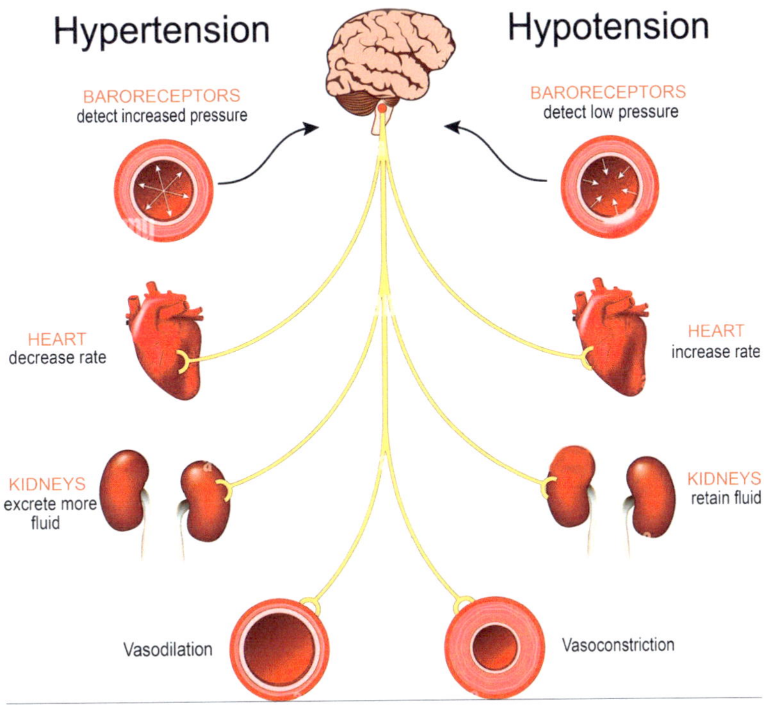

Figure 8.7. Hypertension and hypotension.

Source: https://c8.alamy.com/comp/2YC2RR5/homeostasis-for-hypotension-and-hypertension-blood-pressure-regulation-sympathetic-and-parasympathetic-nervous-system-vector-diagram-2YC2RR5.jpg.

8.2.3. Heart Failure Exacerbation

Heart failure exacerbation is a severe condition where the function of the heart in circulating blood is further compromised, typically resulting in increased morbidity and mortality. Several factors can precipitate exacerbation, including non-compliance with medication, dietary indiscretion, and underlying illness. Adverse drug interactions in patients on polypharmacy can lead to exacerbation. The potential pharmacologic interaction increases the risk of fluid overload or decreased cardiac output, exacerbating symptoms such as dyspnea, edema, and fatigue.

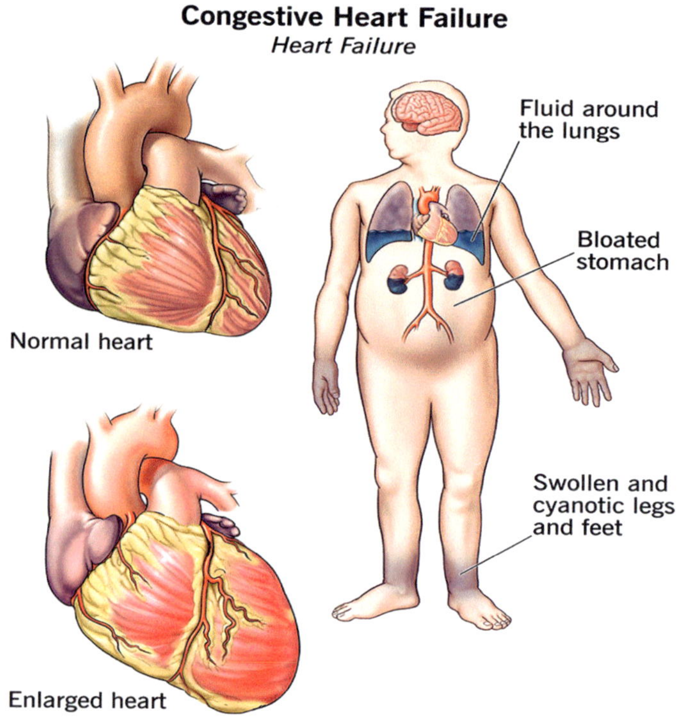

Figure 8.8. Heart failure exacerbation.

Source: https://my.clevelandclinic.org/health/diseases/17069-heart-failure-understanding-heart-failure.

The greater complexity of the treatment of heart failure requires that it should be carefully considered in the appraisal of prescribed drugs and doses. Incorporating pharmacokinetic and pharmacodynamic factors into prescribing habits minimizes such drug side effects and improves patient outcomes (Ramey et al., 2013). In the elderly population, such worsening of heart failure is also augmented by the accompanying change in PK with age, i.e., renal function and drug metabolization alterations. Such physiological alterations can cause drug toxicity and side effects in greater amounts, necessitating cautious medication management. A drug reaction can not only worsen heart function but also contribute to the clinical scenario, making it challenging for healthcare providers to determine the underlying cause of symptom exacerbation. Comprising individualized prescribing regimens that are sensitive to these variations can significantly reduce the frequency of heart failure exacerbations in the elderly, rendering therapeutic treatments both safe and effective (Ramey et al., 2013). In addition, more recent methods, such as machine learning (ML), are being used in the development of drugs to predict probable side effects and enhance drug design for cardiovascular conditions, including heart failure. With the use of advanced algorithms, researchers expect to identify compounds that minimize unwanted side effects while maximizing therapeutic efficacy. For instance, SEMTL-BERT is a future-looking prediction algorithm that employs innovative ML techniques to enhance the identification of compounds with fewer chances for ADRs. This set of computer algorithms contributes to an enhanced drug development process instrumental in forestalling heart failure exacerbation from harmful drug interactions or toxic side effects. As the scope of cardiovascular pharmacotherapy continues to evolve, even considering both therapeutic benefit and safety could redefine the treatment standard for heart failure patients (Figure 8.8).

8.3. Mechanisms of Hematologic Adverse Drug Reactions

Hematologic ADRs represent a significant concern within the broader context of pharmacotherapy, particularly for patients undergoing treatments for chronic diseases such as cancer. Such reactions may result in thrombocytopenia, hemolytic anemia, or leukopenia, worsening the patient's health and complicating their treatment. As new cancer treatments are developed, immunologic agents have brought new ways that can lead to these adverse effects. Notably, ICIs can induce hematologic irAEs through immune dysregulation, where the revival of immune surveillance inadvertently targets hematopoietic lineage cells. Since these mechanisms are quite complex, they make it harder to treat certain diseases.

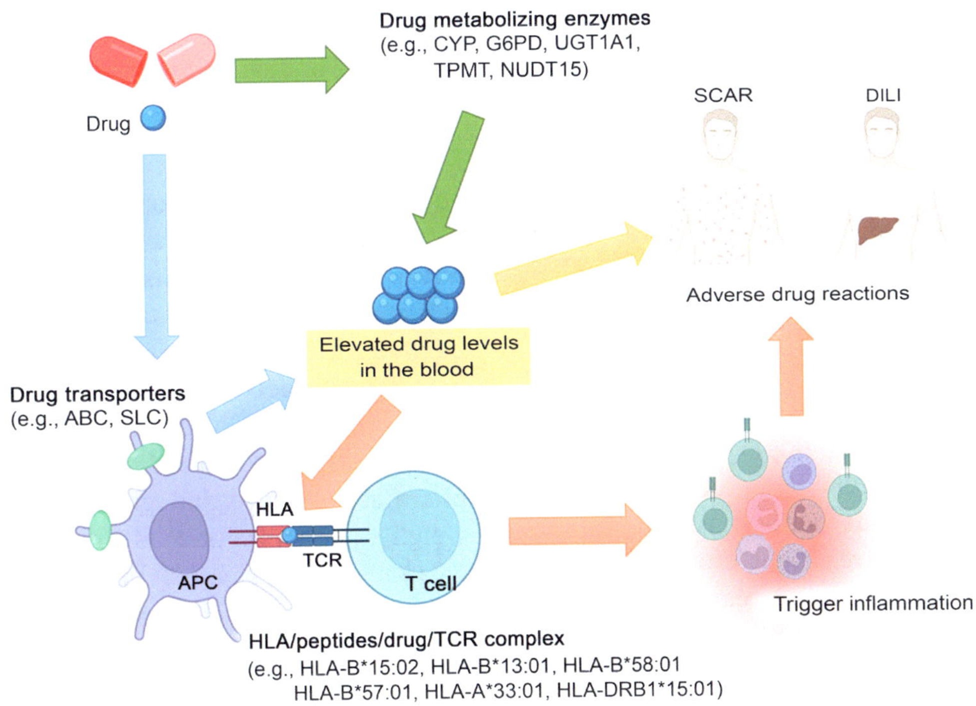

Figure 8.9. Mechanisms of hematologic adverse drug reactions.

Source: https://www.frontiersin.org/files/Articles/886377/fphar-13-886377-HTML/image_m/fphar-13-886377-g001.jpg.

Therefore, it is crucial for clinicians managing cancer treatments to recognize these mechanisms and adjust treatment plans to benefit patients. Examples of chemotherapeutic agents may lead to bone marrow suppression, resulting in a decrease in the production of blood cells and causing anemia or leukopenia. In this case, immunotherapy-related blood problems occur when T-cells are activated and begin attacking both cancer cells and hematopoietic cells. Such immune-related adverse events (irAEs) can manifest as thrombocytopenia or autoimmune hemolytic anemia, reflecting a misdirected immune response. Since reactions to chemotherapy vary significantly from one person to another, it is essential for healthcare providers to closely monitor patients' blood counts and symptoms throughout treatment. If hematologic ADRs are spotted and treated early, it can greatly help the patient's cancer treatment. It is crucial to recognize these complications early, as their symptoms can develop gradually. Doctors regularly check the complete blood counts and, if needed, use hematopoietic growth factors to lessen the effects of extreme cell count declines. Sometimes, when the disease is more serious, doctors may use corticosteroids or immunosuppressive drugs, mainly for cases of autoimmune reactions linked to ICIs. It is also important to have clear guidelines for discontinuing harmful drugs and initiating beneficial care, so that patient safety is always given top priority. Developing a clear system to detect and handle hematologic ADRs is necessary to provide better care for patients undergoing tough treatment programs and to avoid problems from such reactions affecting cancer treatment (Figure 8.9).

8.3.1. Bone Marrow Suppression

Bone marrow suppression is one of the most important concerns in the field of adverse drug effects, particularly in terms of hematologic and cardiovascular health. This is a condition in which the bone marrow is unable to produce sufficient blood cells, resulting in a shortage of red blood cells, white blood cells, and platelets. The effects of this suppression may be severe, leading to anemia, increased susceptibility to infections, and a higher risk of bleeding. Drugs, especially those with myelosuppressive activity, can cause these disorders, therefore necessitating a careful review of a patient's drug regimen. For instance, cyclophosphamide, a commonly used alkylating agent in the management of most cancers, is associated with its ability to cause bone marrow suppression, an adverse event that can complicate treatment protocols and patient outcomes, highlighting the need for monitoring and management strategies (Araújo et al., 2017). In addition to its connection to malignancies, bone marrow suppression also occurs in certain autoimmune diseases and can be exacerbated by specific pharmacological treatments. These answers can worsen underlying cardiovascular disorders, as patients with impaired perfusion are at risk of developing complications such as ischemia due to an insufficient supply of oxygen.

Further, drugs that are known to cause eosinophilia, e.g., those that have been incriminated in Drug Rash with Eosinophilia and Systemic Symptoms (DRESS), make the clinical picture more complex. The action between the cardiovascular agents and their hematologic effects can provoke severe systemic reactions, potentially leading to life-threatening conditions. These subtleties necessitate vigilant pharmacovigilance and prompt physicians to weigh the therapeutic advantages of certain treatments against their impact on the blood (Brunori et al., 2015). The best control for bone marrow suppression requires a multidimensional approach, involving frequent monitoring of blood counts and possible reductions in dose or substitution of drugs. Patient education regarding infection and signs and symptoms of bleeding is also included in the management plan, as early detection is a key factor in achieving successful outcomes. Standard protocols and guidelines for drugs like cyclophosphamide, whose recognized bone marrow depression risks are known, need to be formulated. As much as therapeutic effectiveness is encouraged by healthcare practitioners, they should be careful not to disrupt the delicate equilibrium of intervention and drug interaction. Lastly, understanding the mechanisms and actions of bone marrow suppression can guide safer prescribing and more effective patient care in at-risk individuals for both hematologic and cardiovascular adverse effects (Araújo et al., 2017) (Figure 8.10).

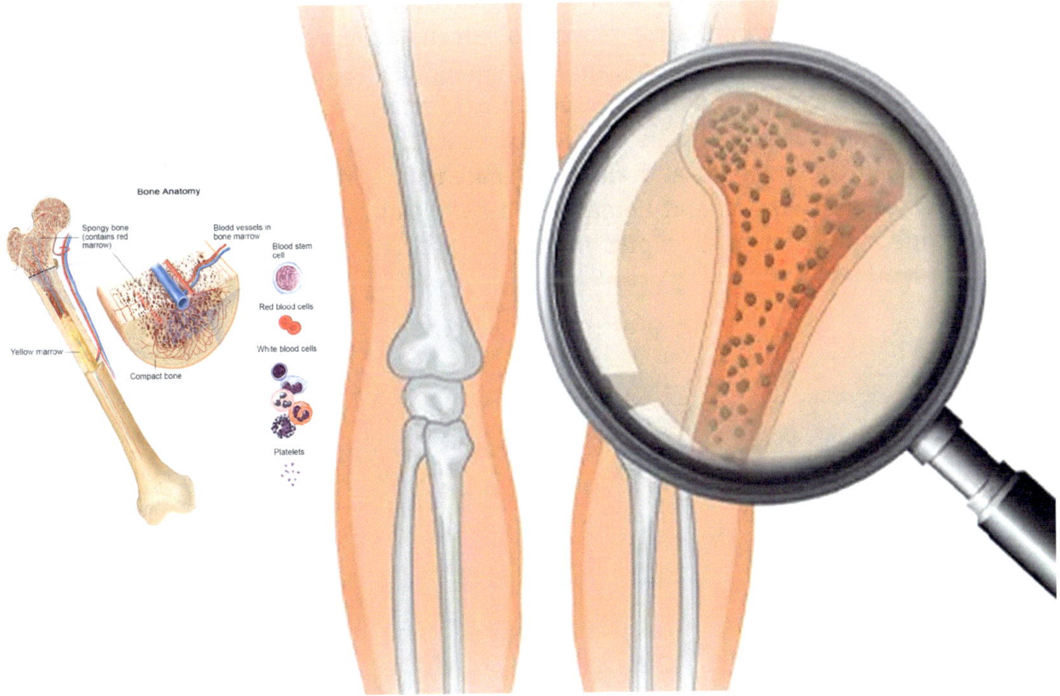

Figure 8.10. Bone marrow suppression.

Source: https://drhimanshuchaturvedi.in/inherited-bone-marrow-failure-syndromes.php.

8.3.2. Immune-Mediated Reactions

In the case of cardiovascular and hematologic ADRs, immune-mediated reactions are important because the immune system attacks the body's cells due to certain drugs. Such reactions can cause numerous health problems for those who experience them. As an example, immune-mediated myopathy can happen with atorvastatin, which is a statin commonly prescribed for heart problems. When looking back at data in the FAERS database, immune-mediated myopathy is a significant side effect of taking atorvastatin. This reinforces the necessity for clinical vigilance, as early detection and management can improve patient outcomes while minimizing the impact of such adverse reactions on long-term health, particularly in patients with existing cardiovascular vulnerabilities as outlined in recent findings (Wan et al., 2024). Further examination of immune-mediated reactions reveals their multifaceted nature, with specific incidents associated with intravenous immunoglobulin (IVIG) therapy. While IVIG is mainly prescribed for autoimmune diseases, it may still cause hematologic problems, and thrombocytopenia is a very rare example. Case reports suggest that IVIG infusion may lead to thrombocytopenia, which could be caused by the immune system damaging platelets or the formation of antibodies that depend on the drug. When treating chronic inflammatory demyelinating polyneuropathy with IVIG, it is necessary to check the patient's platelet levels to avoid complications regularly. This highlights the importance of recognizing and understanding the potential hematologic complications associated with this immunotherapy, ensuring that clinicians can adequately inform patients and adjust treatment protocols accordingly, particularly when their clinical stability is at risk (Foster et al., 2023). Moreover, immune-mediated adverse effects often complicate the management of patients with existing cardiovascular issues, as the interplay between various medications can exacerbate these reactions. For instance, when autoimmune myositis occurs in patients taking atorvastatin, it is essential to investigate the underlying immunologic causes of this condition. As we learn more about these immune responses, it becomes clear that we must continue to monitor and detect signals in medical databases. Clinicians must adopt a proactive approach in assessing the benefits and risks of pharmacotherapeutics, especially in populations already at risk for cardiovascular and hematologic conditions, thereby fostering a more informed and cautious application of such therapies in clinical practice (Wan et al., 2024) (Figure 8.11).

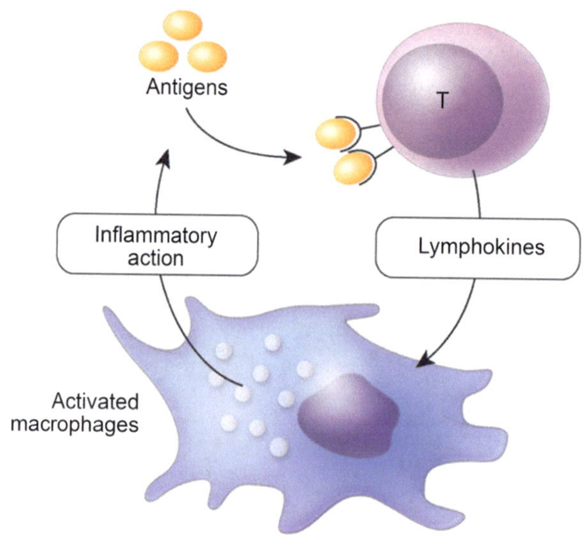

Figure 8.11. Immune-mediated reactions.

Source: https://www.dentalcare.com/en-us/ce-courses/ce537/immune-mediated-mechanisms-of-adrs.

8.3.3. Drug-Induced Coagulopathy

The phenomenon of drug-induced coagulopathy is a prime issue in the field of cardiovascular and hematologic adverse drug events. The disorder arises when drugs disrupt the delicate balance of coagulation factors and platelets within the system, to either an elevated risk of bleeding or thrombotic events. The side effect has multiple drug classes, mostly anticoagulant and antiplatelet drugs. However, even non-anticoagulant medications, such as antibiotics like quinine, are implicated in lethal coagulopathies. Ironically, quinine, generally regarded as an innocent therapy for nocturnal leg cramps, has also been linked to deadly hematologic complications, and thus careful attention to patient drug histories must be given to avoid potentially fatal repercussions (Abed et al., 2016). Therefore, understanding these mechanisms of drug interactions is crucial for safe pharmacotherapy and effective patient management in the clinical setting. Additionally, the effects of drug-induced coagulopathy have even broader implications than short-term clinical interactions, as they might result in long-term complications to health. Patients suffering from coagulopathy induced by medications can have a higher risk of chronic diseases, like recurrent thromboembolic events or chronic liver damage. For instance, studies have indicated that patients with underlying liver disease are considerably more susceptible to coagulopathy-associated severe DILI than people with no underlying disease, and their mortality is significantly higher (Barnhart et al., 2015). This has implications for the necessity of adequate patient assessment and taking their history prior to administering potentially toxic medications. In addition, patient demographic information, such as age and underlying conditions, is critical for clinicians to tailor drug regimens to the patient with the least potential for adverse coagulation interaction. Finally, recognition and management of drug-induced coagulopathy are essential to maximize drug action and protect the patient. Clinicians would be proactive, not merely educating patients about the dangers of their medications but also agitating for routine monitoring of coagulation tests in vulnerable groups, e.g., the elderly or those with comorbid disease. Accurate identification of drugs causing coagulopathy and enhanced clinical vigilance can allow clinicians to intervene promptly when adverse effects occur. By aiming this aspect of pharmacotherapy, physicians are actively countering the dangerous impact of drug-induced coagulopathy and can help in attaining better health outcomes among their patients (Barnhart et al., 2015; Abed et al., 2016).

8.4. Common Hematologic ADRs

ADRs are critical concerns in medical practice, eliciting a variety of hematologic complications that demand attention. Anemia, leukopenia, and thrombocytopenia are some of the most frequent hematologic ADRs, and they can have a significant effect on patients' health. Anemia often arises from medications such as NSAIDs and anticoagulants, leading to diminished red blood cell production or increased destruction. Similarly, leukopenia, characterized by a low count of white blood cells, can be caused by chemotherapy drugs or antibiotics, increasing the risk of infections. If platelet levels are low because of antiplatelet drugs or heparin-induced thrombocytopenia, it can be challenging to handle the risks of bleeding. Knowing about these hematologic ADRs is important for clinical practitioners to spot them early and use proper treatment. Hospitalized patients, especially those undergoing polypharmacy, face heightened risks. A study examining ADRs in hospitalized patients highlighted the alarming rate of such occurrences, which was particularly pronounced in those with chronic renal failure or prolonged hospitalization (Giavina-Bianchi et al., 2018). It shows that those who are more vulnerable need special attention when it comes to managing medications. It has also been found that cardiovascular drugs in the therapeutic group are often linked to hematologic ADRs, so clinicians need to pay closer attention and put in place more prevention methods. A proper approach to monitoring medicines helps to avoid negative effects and protect patients. As reported, only a fraction of adverse events are preventable, necessitating robust mechanisms for their detection and management (Botero et al., 2010). During the process of prescribing, HCPs should carefully review all medications to find out if they could cause hematologic reactions. It is essential to train people in healthcare on how to identify and report ADRs to promote safety.

Besides, the use of standard assessment tools and methods can help doctors identify hematologic ADRs quickly, which benefits patients and reduces their time in the hospital. Paying close attention to medications can significantly enhance patient care, particularly in the areas of cardiovascular and hematologic treatments (Figure 8.12).

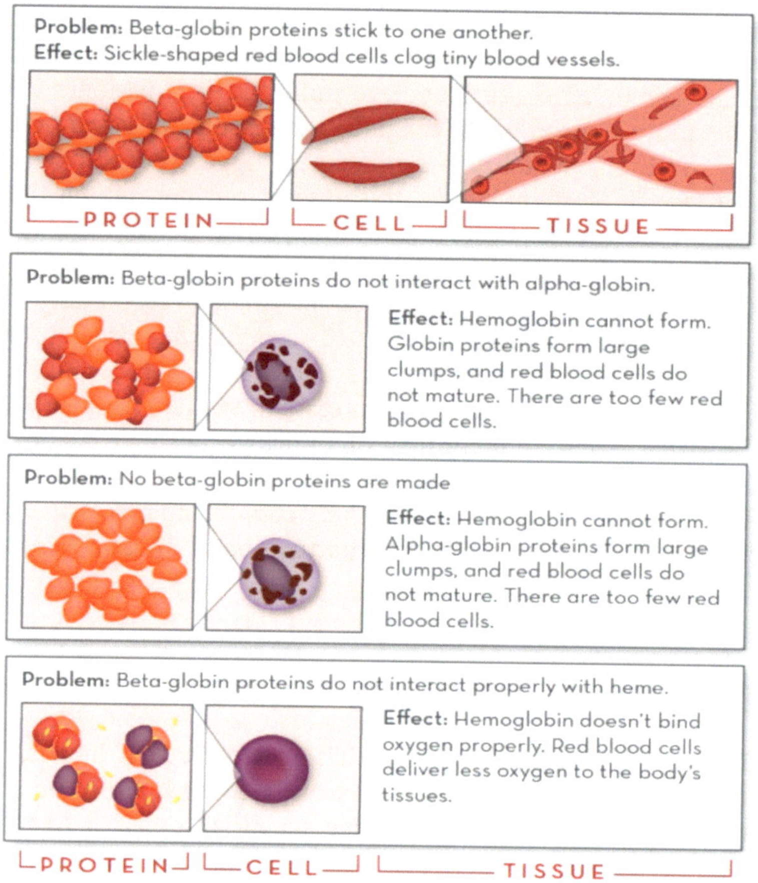

Figure 8.12. Common hematologic ADRs.

Source: https://learn.genetics.utah.edu/content/genetics/hemoglobin/.

8.4.1. Anemia and Its Causes

Anemia, or the absence of red blood cells or hemoglobin, is a significant problem in cardiovascular and hematologic drug-induced adverse reactions. There are multiple etiologies behind the development of anemia, including dietary deficiencies, chronic diseases, and drug-induced effects. The most prevalent dietary etiology is iron deficiency, typically resulting from dietary inadequacy, malabsorption, or chronic blood loss, such as gastrointestinal bleeding. Furthermore, deficiencies of vitamins B12 and folate may cause impairment of erythropoiesis, leading to megaloblastic anemia. Anemia can exacerbate underlying cardiovascular disease since the decreased oxygen-carrying capacity of blood elicits compensatory mechanisms that act to stress the heart, typically resulting in increased cardiac burden and increased risk of heart failure. Along with dietary insufficiencies, long-term conditions such as CKD and inflammatory diseases are also central to the etiology of anemia. Under such conditions, anemia may result from reduced production of erythropoietin, a hormone essential for red blood cell production, or because of secondary inflammatory reactions that suppress red blood cell production and longevity. Moreover, certain medications, especially chemotherapy drugs, will induce hemolytic anemia or bone marrow inhibition and therefore play a role in hematologic side effects. To illustrate, immune-based treatments have introduced a unique set of hematologic ADRs, a relevant consideration for those practitioners managing patients on therapy. Identification of these drug reactions is crucial to prompt intervention and management of anemia to avert deleterious cardiovascular effects. In cancer therapy, the establishment of immune-related adverse events (irAEs) contributes to the added complexity of anemia. Some hematologic side effects of ICIs include thrombocytopenia and neutropenia, aggravating anemia in predisposed patients. With the changing landscape of therapy, the impact of these therapies on hemoglobin status and overall blood health remains a continued concern for practitioners. Evidence indicates that, even though cardiovascular and hematologic ADRs are predominantly mild in nature, instances of severe anemia can emerge, necessitating a multidisciplinary therapeutic plan for the patient (Abdallah et al., 2017; Brém et al., 2020). Effective monitoring and timely intervention methods are thus needed to identify the etiology of anemia, enhance patient outcomes, and prevent cardiovascular impairment among affected populations (Figure 8.13).

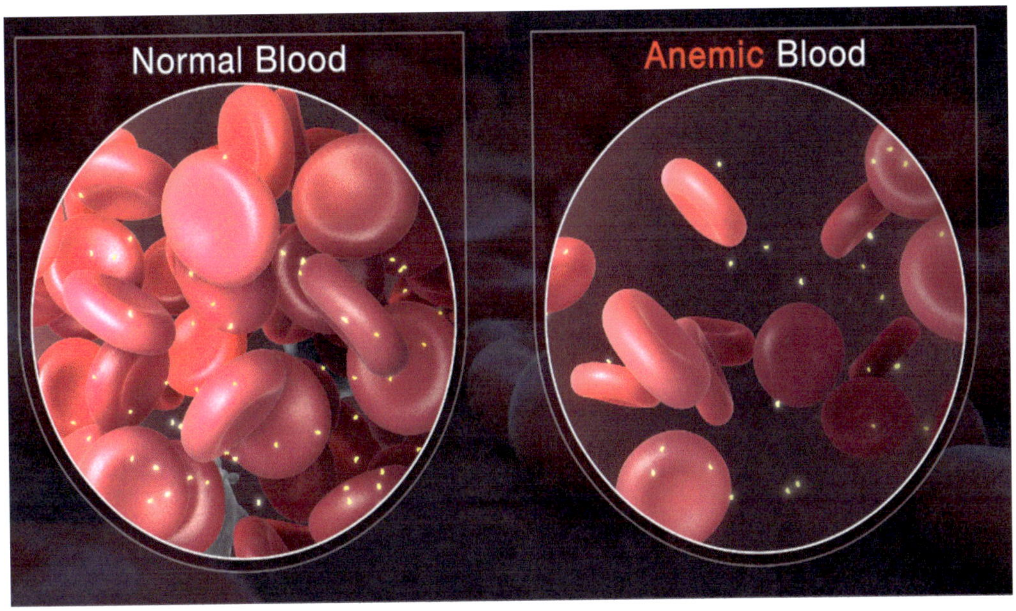

Figure 8.13. Anemia and its causes.

Source: https://www.scientificanimations.com/wp-content/uploads/2019/08/Iron-Deficiency-Anemia.jpg.

8.4.2. Thrombocytopenia and Its Risks

Having thrombocytopenia, a condition characterized by low platelet counts, can significantly impact the health of the heart and blood. Among the factors that cause the disorder are drug reactions, and these can result in severe problems such as bleeding and hematomas. In particular, intracranial hemorrhage can be severe, since it may cause lasting damage to the brain or even result in death.

In patients diagnosed with immune thrombocytopenia (ITP), the clinical manifestations often include a range of bleeding episodes, exacerbated by underlying health issues, thereby increasing hospitalization frequency. Data reveal that bleeding events occurred in over 40% of patients during a study, underscoring the critical need for vigilant monitoring and immediate interventions to mitigate these risks (Ackermann et al., 2012). The impact of thrombocytopenia extends beyond immediate health concerns, as it also deeply affects economic and healthcare resource utilization. In Germany, a study found that ITP patients who have been sick for a long time require more medical care and their expenses add up to almost double the average amount of direct medical costs for those who were recently diagnosed. Since inpatient hospital stays are the primary cause of these costs, new approaches to treating patients should be considered. Given that the average hospitalization rate in the study was around 90%, there is a pressing need for cost-effective interventions to improve patient outcomes and reduce healthcare expenditure associated with thrombocytopenia (Ackermann et al., 2012). In addition, the risks linked to thrombocytopenia, mainly when used together with two antithrombotic drugs, are very significant. According to studies, around 35% of patients who receive such therapy may suffer adverse effects, such as thrombocytopenia as well as a greater chance of digestive and kidney problems. As a result of this, patients' health problems get worse, and their treatments become more complicated. Patients with unstable angina, when treated with antithrombotic drugs, experience a dangerous mix of bleeding and thrombocytopenia, so it is important to weigh the pros and cons of their treatment. Therefore, it is necessary to continually improve monitoring and treatment plans to ensure better safety and effectiveness in caring for these individuals (Figure 8.14).

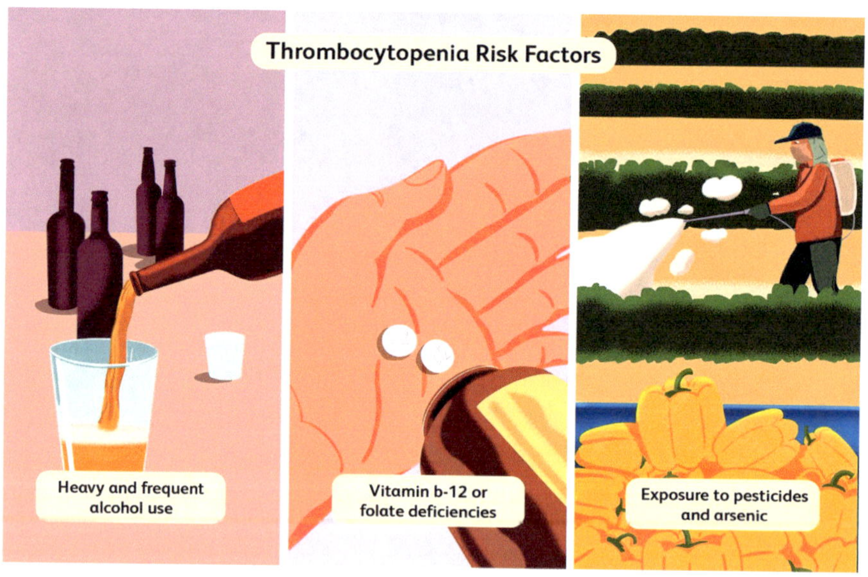

Figure 8.14. Thrombocytopenia and its risks.

Source: https://www.verywellhealth.com/thrombocytopenia-causes-and-risk-factors-5190498.

8.4.3. Leukopenia and Infection Susceptibility

Leukopenia, or a reduced white blood cell count, significantly increases the vulnerability of patients to infections. Leukopenia is caused by a variety of factors, including the effects of medications used in the treatment of cardiovascular and hematologic diseases. Some chemotherapeutic agents and immunosuppressants, for example, may inadvertently impair bone marrow function, resulting in a deficiency in leukocyte production. This is a significant area of concern because leukopenic patients have compromised immune systems, making them susceptible to bacterial, viral, and fungal infections. Therefore, opportunistic infections are much more common within this group of patients, which complicates their management as a population and necessitates close observation and preventative strategies to avoid infection arising from their compromised immunity. Furthermore, the relationship between leukopenia and vulnerability to infection is further complicated by the concurrent presence of co-morbid disease.

The majority of patients who have leukopenia that is drug-induced can also possess pre-existing cardiovascular diseases or other hematological disorders that add to their risk factors. For instance, studies on patients who are being treated, those being treated for multiple myeloma using bortezomib, have reported side effects like lymphopenia, which is associated with increased infection and other susceptibility to complications (Lee et al., 2016). These encounters emphasize the complexity of caring for leukopenic patients in which the balance of effective therapeutic regimens and risk of severe infection is paramount to patient safety and health outcomes. The effects of leukopenia extend beyond the inherent threat of infection; they influence treatment options. In the presence of leukopenia, oncologists and clinicians must balance the risk of prolonging potentially therapeutic therapy with the risk of infectious complications.

For example, infected individuals on treatment for infections such as tuberculosis (TB) must be kept under close monitoring for potential ADRs that can lead to secondary hematologic complications and drug resistance (Kurniawati et al., 2013). Hence, the relationship between leukopenia, an enhanced risk of infection, and drug reactions demands an interdisciplinary approach that not only incorporates treatment of the underlying conditions but also vigilant monitoring and supportive care to neutralize the impaired immune response that develops with leukopenia (Figure 8.15).

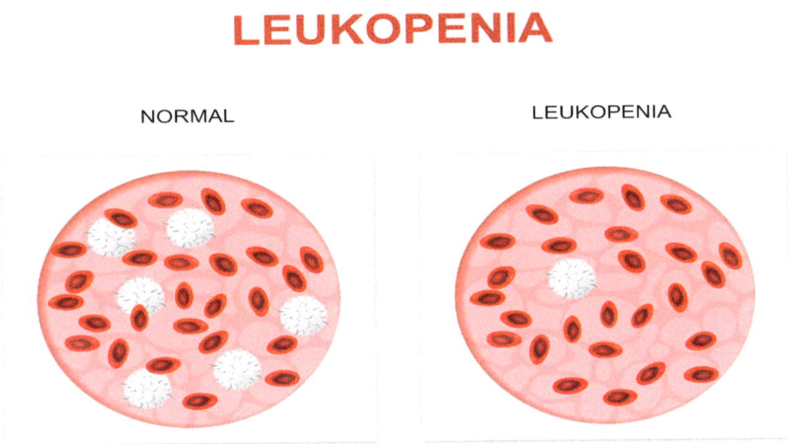

Figure 8.15. Leukopenia and infection susceptibility.

Source: https://www.netmeds.com/health-library/post/leukopenia-causes-symptoms-and-treatment.

8.5. Risk Factors for Cardiovascular and Hematologic ADRs

Understanding the risk factors contributing to cardiovascular and hematologic ADRs is crucial for improving patient safety and outcomes in pharmacotherapy. Being affected by other conditions, such as heart disease and kidney problems, increases the risk of having COVID-19. Since patients with multiple diseases usually take different medicines, they have a higher chance of experiencing drug-drug interactions and ADRs. For instance, the use of bortezomib in patients with newly diagnosed multiple myeloma reveals a substantial proportion with cardiovascular complications, as 76% of participants in a study reported such issues (Lee et al., 2016).

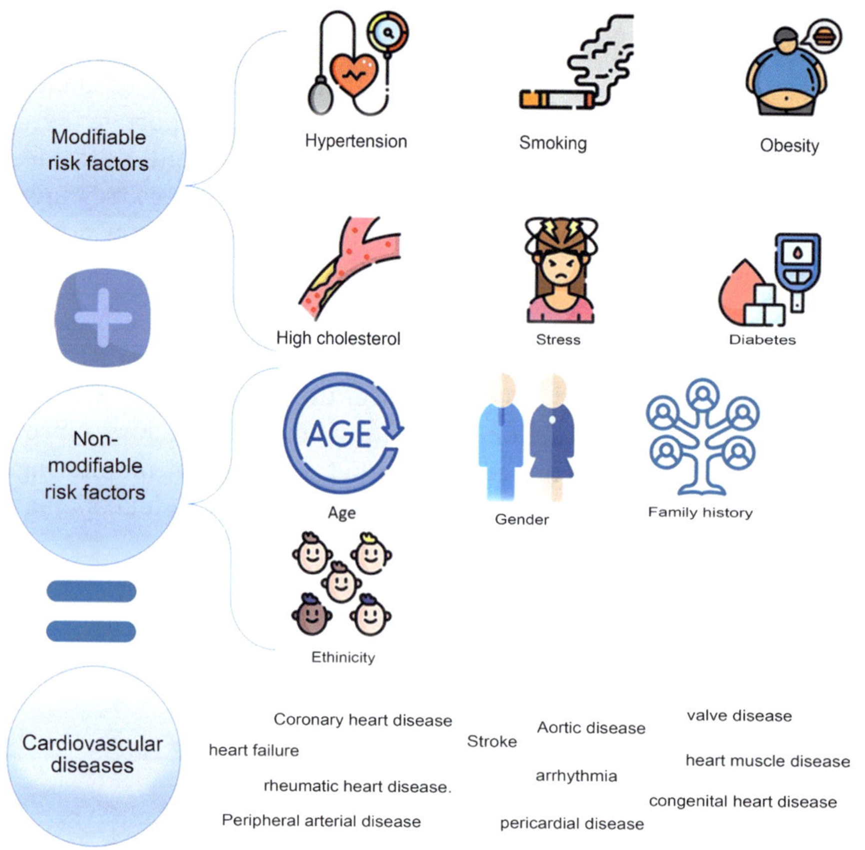

Figure 8.16. Risk factors for cardiovascular and hematologic ADRs.

Source: https://www.researchgate.net/figure/The-risk-factors-associated-with-cardiovascular-diseases-can-be-categorized-into_fig2_380068729.

Due to these pre-existing conditions, treatments may become more toxic, so patients must be carefully watched and their treatment plans adjusted to reduce the risks. For elderly patients, both aging effects and additional diseases may make it harder to predict how drugs will affect them. Studies have shown that older adults experience different adverse effects compared to younger populations, not only due to polypharmacy but also due to altered metabolism and excretion functionality (Lee et al., 2016). Therefore, doctors must pay extra attention when prescribing drugs, taking into account both the medicines' benefits and the higher chance of side effects for seniors. Such vigilance is vital for personalizing treatment and optimizing safety. Immune-related adverse events (irAEs), particularly those associated with cancer immunotherapy, further illustrate the complexity of identifying risk factors for cardiovascular and hematologic ADRs. While these therapies have transformed cancer treatment, their associated toxicities can be severe, affecting various organ systems, including cardiovascular health. Sometimes, ICIs may cause serious cardiovascular side effects, even though such events are uncommon. This phenomenon is compounded by the need for prompt recognition and management of symptoms that may emerge long after treatment initiation, often requiring multidisciplinary approaches. For this reason, being aware of these details helps clinicians choose the most suitable care for patients and prevent potential negative outcomes (Figure 8.16).

8.5.1. Patient Demographics (Age, Gender, Ethnicity)

The demographics of patient populations, i.e., age, gender, and ethnicity, form a critical part of understanding the demography of cardiovascular and hematologic ADRs. Aging influences the pharmacodynamics and PK of drugs in a significant way, particularly as it pertains to liver and kidney functions, which decline with age. Older people, especially those over 65 years, show greater susceptibility to drug-related side effects, leading to more chances of adverse reactions. Furthermore, because many patients who are elderly are treated with drugs such as ICIs, one has to define the extensive variety of adverse effects these patients have to suffer through in line with the literature available, and which is especially applicable to groups suffering from cardiovascular disease and blood disorders (Benedetti et al., 2009). Gender has also been found to play an important role in influencing the severity as well as the frequency of cardiovascular and hematologic ADRs. Research indicates that women are at greater risk when exposed to certain specific pharmacologic treatments because of the disparity in hormone levels and body composition compared to that of males. This difference can result in divergent outcomes, especially among groups undergoing drugs for cardiovascular disease, where the effectiveness and side effects cannot be universally projected. Knowledge of these gender differences is crucial in effectively customizing treatments and reducing the risks attached to drug therapy. In addition, the growing evidence identifies that women given treatments for immune reaction-related diseases may exhibit profoundly different rates and profiles of adverse drug effects from men, and hence, gender-sensitive approaches in clinics become imminent (Benedetti et al., 2009). Ethnicity is also a key demographic factor in addressing the complexities of ADRs. Genetic heterogeneity and environmental factors among different ethnic populations can influence drug metabolism and drug response, thus influencing the rate and intensity of drug adverse reactions. It has been found that some ethnic populations are disproportionately affected by certain cardiovascular conditions, which may have an aggregate synergistic effect of aggravating the impact of ADRs when pharmacotherapy is administered. For instance, Asian patients are reported to be more susceptible to drug-induced hematologic adverse effects, which necessitates a critical reappraisal of monitoring patterns and prescribing behavior in such populations. By recognizing and addressing these ethnic variations in the healthcare system, practitioners can make evidence-based, patient-specific drug therapy decisions based on evidence that is tailored to the specific demographic composition of their patients (Rong et al., 2022).

8.5.2. Pre-Existing Health Conditions

Pre-existing health conditions significantly complicate the landscape of ADRs, particularly within the realms of cardiovascular and hematologic health. People who have long-term health problems such as hypertension, diabetes, or hematologic disorders usually react differently to medicines. When these conditions and medications are used together, there is a greater risk of ADRs that healthcare providers may not be ready for. Patients who use antipsychotic drugs may be at greater risk of heart problems, especially if they also have other health issues. Therefore, it is essential for managers to understand how various health conditions can affect the efficacy of drugs, which means that each patient's treatment should be tailored to their specific needs. When the body changes medications due to PK, older people with other health problems can experience unpredictable results. Elderly people with schizophrenia may have heart problems as well, so they are more likely to suffer from side effects of antipsychotic drugs, such as blood clots or abnormal heart rhythms. It is necessary to carefully evaluate patients and check their health regularly, especially when using drugs like phenothiazines, because the different factors can easily interact. Although antipsychotic drugs are helpful in treating mental illnesses, they may pose more risks if a patient has other health problems. For instance, Anderson et al. (2022) highlight how high-potency phenothiazines can effectively address acute psychotic episodes but may also lead to significant cardiovascular complications in patients with pre-existing hypertension or heart disease. The analysis of literature on medication management in this group shows that there is a strong need for guidelines that address both their mental and physical health at the same time. This is particularly important in light of findings, such as those summarized by Brown et al. (2014), which emphasize the need for a comprehensive approach to medication management among older adults, facilitating safer and more effective treatment pathways that mitigate the risks associated with both cardiovascular and hematologic ADRs (Figure 8.17).

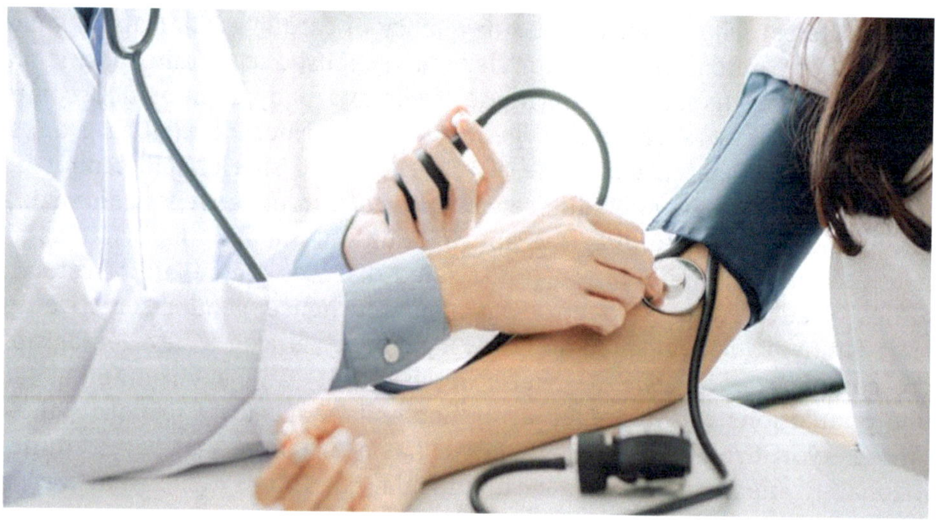

Figure 8.17. Pre-existing health conditions.

Source: https://www.careinsurance.com/upload_master/media/posts/August2020/YAE8yzDZ1DKFDJ2DGpR7.jpg.

8.5.3. Polypharmacy and Its Implications

Polypharmacy, or the concomitant administration of two or more drugs, is a significant problem in the management of cardiovascular and hematologic illnesses. As patients typically have complex medical history that requires multifaceted pharmacologic treatments, the potential for ADRs is greatly amplified. It is stated in the research that the elderly, in whom polypharmacy is traditionally utilized, are particularly vulnerable because changes in physiological states associated with aging affect drug metabolism and pharmacodynamics. These alterations can synergize the effect of drugs, leading to cardiovascular adverse effects of hypotension, arrhythmias, and even heart failure. Also, when drugs interact, it can heighten unwanted effects, which, if not closely monitored, can result in serious health consequences and reduced quality of life. The scenario of polypharmacy is further exacerbated by the higher prevalence of comorbidities in patients with cardiovascular disease, wherein additional drugs may need to treat secondary conditions.

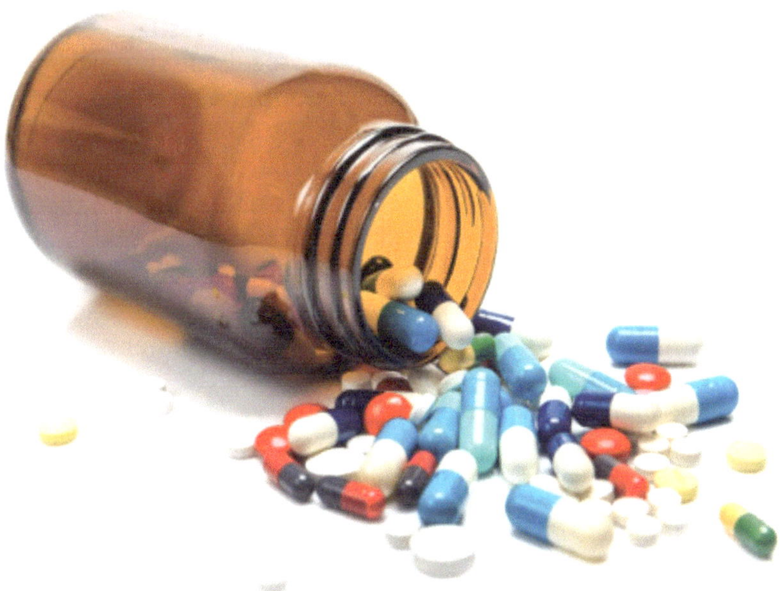

Figure 8.18. Polypharmacy.

Source: https://pharmaceutical-journal.com/article/ld/polypharmacy-a-framework-for-theory-and-practice.

Therefore, HCPs face the dilemma of balancing effective treatment schedules with the prevention of risk for adverse events. Studies documenting the incidence of ADRs indicate that serious complications resulting from polypharmacy are accountable for increasing admissions and longer length of stay, and hence, the total burden to the healthcare system is increased. Surprisingly, the majority of the adverse effects relate to well-established drug classes, i.e., anticoagulants and antiplatelet agents, which are essential in the management of cardiovascular disease but risk hematologic side effects like thrombocytopenia and bleeding. Acceptance of the dual character of such drugs is important in minimizing the dangers of polypharmacy and optimizing patient care. Besides, the effects of polypharmacy are not merely confined to short-term clinical outcomes but also reach as far as long-term management of cardiovascular and hematologic disease. Inefficient monitoring of drug interactions, dose adjustment, and patient education can lead to non-adherence, elevating the dangers of side effects. Evidence suggests that the rate of medication errors increases significantly in polypharmacy environments, which indicates the necessity of interprofessional coordination between HCPs for ensuring patient safety. Hence, implementing comprehensive medication reviews and protocolized programs for assessing the appropriateness of drug treatments can significantly contribute to reducing the frequency of ADRs. The bedrock for early strategy, tailored interventions, and communication between healthcare teams is paramount to safeguarding patients from the adverse effects of polypharmacy, optimizing therapeutic outcomes while minimizing harm (Ayalew et al., 2016; Moirana et al., 2023) (Figure 8.18).

8.6. Strategies for Prevention and Management

Effective management of cardiovascular and hematologic ADRs necessitates a multifaceted approach, integrating both prevention strategies and treatment protocols. It is very important to monitor patients who are taking high-risk medications regularly to find and deal with any possible issues. It is essential to undergo regular blood tests to detect any signs of hematological toxicity, such as myelodysplastic syndrome or acute myeloid leukemia. This method of monitoring ensures that patients are quickly referred to hematology specialists and also reminds them to be vigilant for early symptoms. It is necessary to come up with a complete management plan that covers lifestyle changes, regular doctor visits, and consultations with different HCPs, mainly for patients whose drug regimen may be causing early cardiovascular issues. By following such a strategy, the number and severity of ADRs are reduced, which helps keep patients safe. At the same time, monitoring and making changes to food and habits significantly help prevent gastrointestinal toxicity in patients receiving chemotherapy or PARP inhibitors. Taking medicine at the right time, eating a light meal, and staying hydrated are believed to significantly reduce gastrointestinal issues such as nausea and vomiting. It is also essential to provide prompt symptomatic care to alleviate pain and enhance a patient's well-being during treatment. According to the information, psychological care can help patients manage their fatigue, which in turn enables them to take care of themselves and maintain a positive home environment. Taking care of the gut microbiota is now considered a promising method to avoid major complications that may occur after ADRs. The gut microbiome supports the immune system and can influence the risk of infections, particularly in patients taking immunosuppressive drugs. Taking care of the gut microbiota may make it easier for people with weak immune systems to fight off pathogenic bacteria. Taking care of gut health means using antibiotics only when necessary, monitoring their impact on the gut's microorganisms, and using probiotics when needed. Since gut health influences the effectiveness of treatment, efforts to support the microbiome may provide additional protection against gastrointestinal side effects following chemotherapy. Because the healthcare field is advancing, using these preventative methods shows why it is important to use whole approaches to help patients with cardiovascular and hematologic ADRs.

8.6.1. Monitoring and Early Detection

Early detection and monitoring of cardiovascular and hematologic ADRs are essential to enhance the outcomes of patients in clinical practice. With the changing dynamics of the practice of medicine as a result of the growing practice of immunotherapies and targeted therapies, it becomes essential to explore the spectrum of possible adverse effects. For instance, the use of ICIs has been linked with a range of immune-related adverse events (irAEs), including those affecting cardiovascular health. Early diagnosis of such conditions, such as arrhythmias or myocarditis, is important since it can decrease complications as well as potentially salvage the patient's quality of life. Moreover, the complexity of immunologic mechanisms that underlie ADRs necessitates rigorous monitoring systems to identify subtle clinical changes indicative of cardiovascular toxicity, thereby emphasizing the importance of regulation in healthcare to ensure patient safety. In hematology, early warning systems are equally important, particularly in patients undergoing therapy for diseases such as B-cell acute lymphoblastic leukemia (B-ALL).

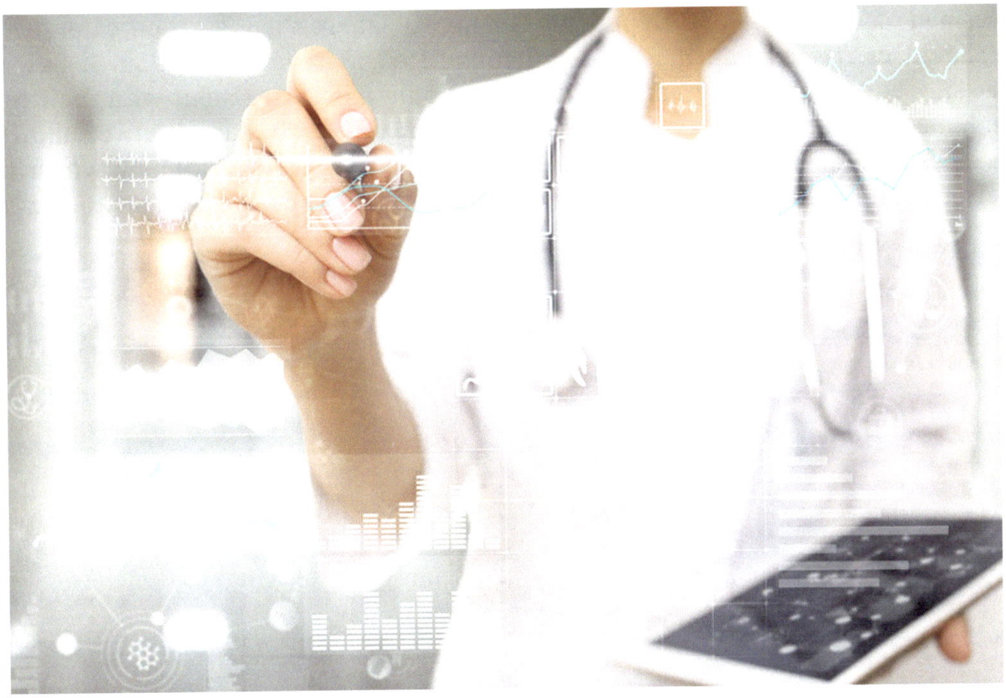

Figure 8.19. Monitoring and early detection.

Source: https://www.cosinuss.com/en/2023/01/01/sepsis-early-detection-aftercare/.

The routine therapies have had suboptimal long-term results in the past, to which newer immunologic therapies such as blinatumomab and CAR-T cell therapy may be applied. These newer therapies can be watched for their capacity to detect adverse effects that can arise as a consequence, including the risk of febrile neutropenia or graft-versus-host disease after hematopoietic cell transplantation (HCT). Patient response monitoring through blood analysis and clinical assessment enables clinicians to gain a better understanding of treatment efficacy while simultaneously predicting and preempting potential adverse effects, thereby improving patient management outcomes. Moreover, multidisciplinary monitoring and early detection is pivotal in dealing with the complexity involved in cardiovascular and hematologic ADRs. Multidisciplinary activities among oncologists, cardiologists, and hematologists help create a comprehensive monitoring system that emphasizes the early detection of key signs. The formation of standard treatments, promoted by groups such as the Society for Immunotherapy of Cancer, encourages HCPs to detect, report, and manage organ-specific toxicities. As has been documented in the literature, without early detection and intervention, serious complications such as treatment-related mortality may occur in up to 2% of patients who have undergone immunotherapy (Abdallah et al., 2017). Thus, a coordinated strategy for monitoring enhances both the quality of patient care and the overall safety profile of new therapeutic approaches to managing complex diseases (Figure 8.19).

8.6.2. Patient Education and Adherence

Teaching patients effectively helps them adhere to their medication schedules, which is crucial for managing cardiovascular and hematologic diseases. If patients are informed about their condition, the available treatments, and the potential negative effects of their medications, they tend to adhere to the prescribed plan. Because of this, patients can participate in choosing their care, so healthcare providers should clearly explain the pros and cons of each treatment option. It has also been found that using educational programs can help people be more consistent with their medication adherence. Educating patients and offering support through educational initiatives allows HCPs to build a partnership that increases the patient's commitment to their treatment, which eventually leads to better health and fewer serious problems from cardiovascular and hematologic reactions.

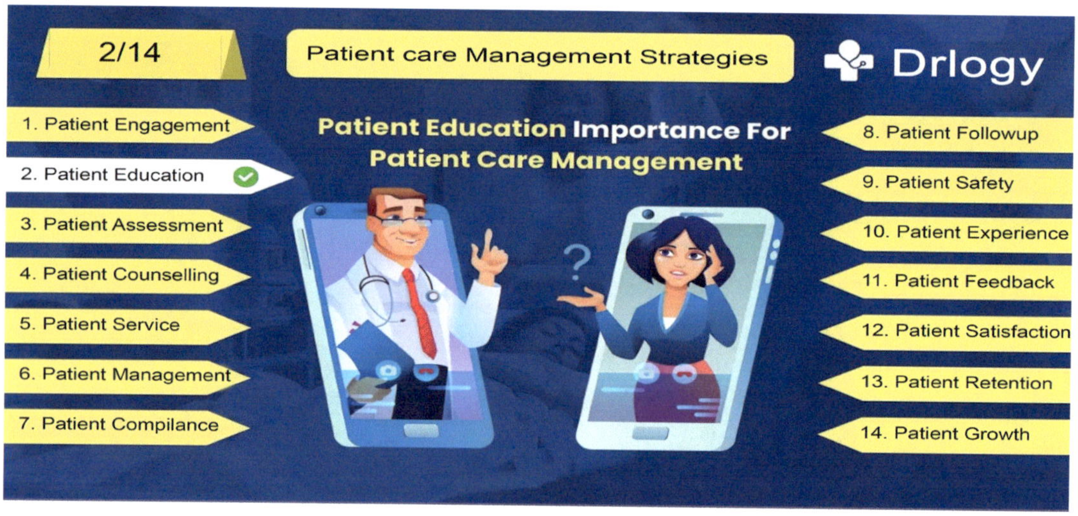
2/14
Patient care Management Strategies
Drlogy
Patient Education Importance For Patient Care Management
1. Patient Engagement
2. Patient Education
3. Patient Assessment
4. Patient Counselling
5. Patient Service
6. Patient Management
7. Patient Compilance
8. Patient Followup
9. Patient Safety
10. Patient Experience
11. Patient Feedback
12. Patient Satisfaction
13. Patient Retention
14. Patient Growth

Figure 8.20. Patient education and adherence.

Source: https://images.drlogy.com/assets/uploads/img/admin/blog/patient-education.webp.

Factors such as a person's income, education, and having someone to support them can significantly impact their ability to take their medications as directed. For some patients, not understanding their diseases well can make it difficult to see why they should take all the medications they are given. In addition, real-world evidence suggests that more educated and engaged patients are more likely to adhere to their medication plans, as seen in the Fingolimod Patient Support Program (F-PSP). This program demonstrates that patient characteristics, including education and living situation, directly influence medication adherence, highlighting the need for tailored educational interventions (EIs) to effectively navigate these variables (Berger et al., 2021). Besides teaching patients at the start, HCPs should offer continuous help to maintain their adherence. Seeing the doctor regularly, either in person or through telehealth, helps patients stick to their treatment and makes it possible to change the plan when needed. It is also necessary to help patients overcome problems such as side effects from their medicines or not understanding how to take them. Involving patients in choosing their treatment and giving them the opportunity to share their views helps them learn more and feel more responsible for their health. Ultimately, when patients feel supported and informed, they are more likely to adhere to their treatments, thus reducing the incidence of cardiovascular and hematologic ADRs and improving overall patient safety (Le et al., 2014) (Figure 8.20).

8.6.3. Pharmacovigilance and Reporting Systems

Pharmacovigilance, the rigorous science for detecting, assessing, understanding, and preventing adverse reactions to drugs (ADRs), is critical in the interest of safeguarding patient safety, particularly in the event of cardiovascular and hematologic adverse reactions. Effective pharmacovigilance systems are crucial in identifying and managing drug risks.

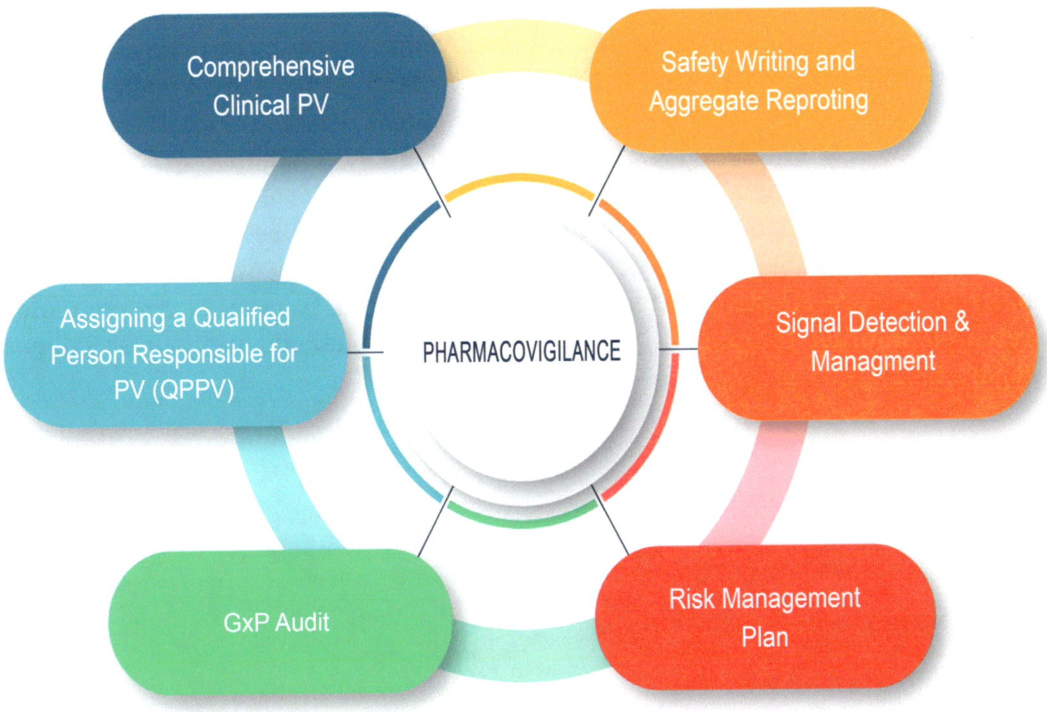

Figure 8.21. Pharmacovigilance and reporting systems.

Source: https://www.freyrsolutions.com/blog/pharmacovigilance-a-regulatory-synopsis.

These systems rely on voluntary reporting schemes, where HCPs and patients report ADRs suspected by regulatory agencies. Not only do these reports enhance the knowledge base of drug safety, but they also facilitate lifecycle management of the drug, resulting in timely action when the issues are potential. The problem is to improve these reporting systems so that they are sufficient to capture valuable information without being complicated for the ones who report them. Ultimately, effective pharmacovigilance can inform regulatory action, including drug withdrawal where necessary, as in specific well-known examples in the past. Analysis of information collected on pharmacovigilance systems has revealed valuable insights into the relationship between drug safety and adverse effects, particularly those affecting the cardiovascular and hematologic systems. Evidence has shown that certain drugs, particularly those in the management of cardiovascular diseases, have been frequently linked with serious side effects such as arrhythmias or hematologic conditions such as thrombocytopenia and anemia. For instance, researchers cited instances of drug withdrawals based on drug-related deaths, which would help to support the argument that strong and swift action would be called for when corroboratory evidence exists. Such data aligns with findings that indicated a high percentage of justification (96%) for drug withdrawals when associated with lethal outcomes and reiterates the importance of scientific scrutiny and supporting studies in pharmacovigilance. The employment of formal methodologies is pivotal in informing future regulatory practice and enhancing patient safety. The addition of international reporting systems such as the WHO Vigibase and the US FDA Adverse Event Reporting System (FAERS) significantly enhances the pharmacovigilance landscape by providing one universal data repository. This global coverage provides for the possibility to have a better comprehension of drug adverse events in different populations and therefore make a finer interpretation of the risk of various therapeutics. Recent pharmacovigilance reports have focused on immune-mediated drug adverse effects from new therapies, with stress on the necessity for an adaptive understanding of drug complications, especially in those with underlying cardiovascular and hematologic conditions. The fluid nature of such reports enables oncologists and prescribing practitioners to revise their prescribing practices in advance, becoming mindful of risks recently uncovered, thus instigating an active response to the possibility of adverse effects. Greater education about such systems is required, along with constant research, in order to optimize patient management methods and deliver safety in drug therapy (Figure 8.21).

Summary

In examining the implications of cardiovascular and hematologic ADRs, it becomes evident that the complexities involved necessitate a nuanced understanding of patient populations and their unique responses to various pharmacological treatments. Studying the data from a long time revealed that combination therapies for cardiovascular conditions can result in many side effects. Particularly, some drug interactions, like amlodipine and atorvastatin, led to jaundice, showing how important it is to oversee patients in clinical settings. As shown in the findings, the combination therapy approaches adopted may not uniformly benefit all patients and can precipitate increased risks, particularly among different demographics, thus emphasizing the necessity for tailored therapeutic strategies in treating cardiovascular conditions (Wang et al., 2025). Moreover, the findings underscore the importance of pharmacovigilance in protecting patient health amid complex medication regimens. The high number of ADRs in people with chronic rheumatoid heart disease shows that healthcare settings should have better monitoring systems. The study at Netaji Subhash Chandra Bose Medical College proved that some combinations of drugs, such as Digoxin with Clopidogrel, can cause serious side effects for patients with chronic illnesses. This serves as a crucial reminder of the potential for drugs to interact in unforeseen ways, which can exacerbate existing health issues, highlighting the importance of thorough patient education and awareness regarding the risks associated with combination drug therapies (Izhar et al., 2024). In conclusion, addressing cardiovascular and hematologic ADRs is paramount for enhancing patient safety and improving therapeutic outcomes. Because of the evidence, scientists can explore the reasons behind these reactions, which allows healthcare providers to design treatments that are safer for each patient. The advancement of personalized medicine in the future will depend significantly on understanding how different drug combinations affect various patient groups. When the healthcare community utilizes better data and enhances the delivery of treatments, it can prevent and manage adverse reactions, benefiting those at risk of heart and blood diseases. These strategies play a crucial role in reducing the number of ADRs and ensuring that patients benefit the most with the least possible harm.

The exploration of cardiovascular ADRs unveils critical findings, particularly in relation to selective cyclooxygenase inhibitors such as rofecoxib. The agent was first used to decrease the risk of colorectal cancer coming back, but it was found to increase the number of cardiovascular thrombotic events in patients. In a randomized, placebo-controlled trial documented in a comprehensive analysis, patients receiving rofecoxib experienced a relative risk of 2.66 for cardiovascular events during or shortly after treatment (Stanley et al., 2007). It shows that serious cardiovascular problems can outweigh the positive effects of a drug when it comes to therapy. why HCPs must consider the pros and cons of these drugs, particularly in patients with heart problems. In addition, the effects of rofecoxib on the heart were closely examined, and it was found that cardiovascular events still appeared after patients stopped using the drug. Although the risk of blood clots went down during the follow-up period, the medication still had a significant risk factor, proving that concerns about its safety were still valid. In total, the analysis documented 23 confirmed cardiovascular thrombotic events, of which 16 occurred within the treatment window, indicating a temporal correlation between the drug administration and adverse outcomes (Stanley et al., 2007). Therefore, researchers and clinicians should pay attention to both the quick and lasting effects of drugs on patients who have had heart problems in the past. The guidelines in the V-FIT study serve as a reference to ensure that participants are safe and the correct clinical data is obtained.

Therefore, having a strict trial design and monitoring is crucial because it ensures the safety of participants and enhances the quality of drug safety assessments. Since the field of pharmaceutical interventions keeps developing, it is important for medical professionals to regularly review and update their practices using the latest evidence on cardiovascular and hematologic ADRs, helping patients achieve better results throughout their care.

CLOSER LOOK

GENE POLYMORPHISMS CAN INFLUENCE METABOLISM

Gene polymorphisms, which are variations in DNA sequence that occur commonly within a population, can significantly influence individual differences in metabolism. These genetic variations can affect the expression or function of enzymes, transporters, and receptors involved in metabolic pathways, thereby altering how the body processes nutrients, drugs, and toxins. One well-studied example involves polymorphisms in cytochrome P450 enzymes, such as CYP2D6, CYP2C19, and CYP3A4, which play key roles in drug metabolism. Depending on the variant, individuals may be classified as poor, intermediate, extensive, or ultra-rapid metabolizers, impacting drug efficacy and risk of adverse reactions.

In addition to drug metabolism, gene polymorphisms can influence nutrient metabolism. For instance, variations in the MTHFR gene can affect folate metabolism and homocysteine levels, which are linked to cardiovascular health and neural development. Similarly, polymorphisms in genes like FTO and MC4R are associated with differences in fat metabolism and susceptibility to obesity. These genetic differences can contribute to inter-individual variability in dietary response and disease risk, making them a central focus in the emerging field of nutrigenomics.

Understanding how gene polymorphisms affect metabolism has important clinical implications. In pharmacogenomics, this knowledge helps guide personalized medicine by tailoring drug type and dosage to an individual's genetic profile. In nutrition science, it informs the development of personalized dietary recommendations to prevent or manage metabolic diseases. However, translating genetic information into clinical practice remains complex due to gene-environment interactions and the influence of multiple genes on metabolic outcomes. Nevertheless, as research progresses and genetic testing becomes more accessible, gene polymorphism analysis is expected to become a key tool in optimizing health outcomes through individualized care.

References

1. Puzanov, I., Diab, A., Abdallah, K., Bingham, C. O., Brogdon, C., Dadu, R., Hamad, L., Kim, S., Lacouture, M. E., LeBoeuf, N. R., Lenihan, D., Onofrei, C., Shannon, V., Sharma, R., Silk, A. W., Skondra, D., Suarez-Almazor, M. E., Wang, Y., Wiley, K., . . . Ernstoff, M. S. (2017). Managing toxicities associated with immune checkpoint inhibitors: consensus recommendations from the Society for Immunotherapy of Cancer (SITC) Toxicity Management Working Group. *Journal for ImmunoTherapy of Cancer*, *5*(1). https://doi.org/10.1186/s40425-017-0300-zAbed, F., Bachuwa, G., & Baniya, R. (2016). Quinine-induced disseminated intravascular coagulation. https://core.ac.uk/download/235680200.pdf (accessed on 9 June 2025).
2. Ackermann, B., Bauer, M., Baumann, A., Berger, U., et al. (2012). A retrospective observational single-centre study on the burden of immune thrombocytopenia (ITP). https://core.ac.uk/download/16432314.pdf (accessed on 9 June 2025).
3. Adadzi, J., Alozie, U. G., Anderson II, J., Azi, M., et al. (2024). Current strategies and future directions in multiple myeloma: Disease overview and pathophysiology, conventional treatments and emerging therapies, challenges and innovations in management. https://core.ac.uk/download/621451768.pdf (accessed on 9 June 2025).
4. Adhikari, P., Padmaja, U., & Pereira, P. (2009). A prospective analysis of adverse drug reactions in a South Indian hospital. https://core.ac.uk/download/pdf/87416.pdf.
5. Agelink, M. W., Bleich, S., Engel, R., Greil, W., et al. (2015). Cardiovascular adverse reactions during antidepressant treatment: A drug surveillance report of German-speaking countries between 1993 and 2010. https://core.ac.uk/download/216471244.pdf (accessed on 9 June 2025).
6. Anderson, A., Armistead, G., Cornett, E. M., Edinoff, A. N., et al. (2022). Phenothiazines and their evolving roles in clinical practice: A narrative review. https://core.ac.uk/download/554057814.pdf (accessed on 9 June 2025).
7. Araújo, B. G. de, Lima, F. A. C., Lima, R. A. C., et al. (2017). Rotina de administração de ciclofosfamida em doenças autoimunes reumáticas: Uma revisão. https://core.ac.uk/download/154231178.pdf (accessed on 9 June 2025).
8. Ardizzoni, A., De Ponti, F., Gatti, M., Gelsomino, F., Poluzzi, E., & Raschi, E. (2020). Lessons to be learnt from real-world studies on immune-related adverse events with checkpoint inhibitors: A clinical perspective from pharmacovigilance. https://core.ac.uk/download/385957945.pdf.
9. Aronson, J. K., Heneghan, C., & Onakpoya, I. (2017). Post-marketing regulation of medicines withdrawn from the market because of drug-attributed deaths: An analysis of justification. https://core.ac.uk/download/346498850.pdf.
10. Arpino, G., Bianchini, G., Curigliano, G., Danesi, R., De Laurentiis, M., Del Mastro, L., Dri, A., et al. (2024). Breaking barriers in triple-negative breast cancer (TNBC)–Unleashing the power of antibody-drug conjugates (ADCs). https://core.ac.uk/download/614046780.pdf (accessed on 9 June 2025).
11. Ayalew, E., Teka, F., Teklay, G., & Teshome, T. (2016). Potential drug–drug interactions among elderly patients admitted to the medical ward of Aider Referral Hospital, Northern Ethiopia: A cross-sectional study. https://core.ac.uk/download/pdf/81594378.pdf (accessed on 9 June 2025).

12. Barachini, S., Buda, G., & Petrini, I. (2024). Cardiovascular toxicity of antineoplastic treatments in hematological diseases: Focus on molecular mechanisms to improve therapeutic management. https://core.ac.uk/download/638795249.pdf (accessed on 9 June 2025).

13. Barnhart, H., Bonkovsky, H. L., Chalasani, N., et al. (2015). Features and outcomes of 899 patients with drug-induced liver injury: The DILIN prospective study. https://core.ac.uk/download/81634421.pdf (accessed on 9 June 2025).

14. Benedetti, E., Edison, M., Gehm, L., et al. (2009). A descriptive analysis of 1251 solid organ transplant visits to the emergency department. https://core.ac.uk/download/pdf/8280523.pdf.

15. Berger, J., Bourdin, A., Bugnon, O., et al. (2021). Longitudinal analysis of safety and medication adherence of patients in the fingolimod patient support program: A real-world observational study. https://core.ac.uk/download/389866046.pdf (accessed on 9 June 2025).

16. Bladé, J., Cibeira, M. T., Dimopoulos, M. A., et al. (2020). Challenges in the management of patients with systemic light chain (AL) amyloidosis during the COVID-19 pandemic. https://core.ac.uk/download/341794895.pdf (accessed on 9 June 2025).

17. Botero, M., López, L. C., Palacios, M., & Pino, et al. (2010). Reacciones adversas a medicamentos en salas de medicina interna de un hospital universitario: Estudio descriptivo piloto. https://core.ac.uk/download/11863075.pdf (accessed on 9 June 2025).

18. Brém, E., Koyfman, A., & Long, B. J. (2020). Oncologic emergencies: Immune-based cancer therapies and complications. https://core.ac.uk/download/305124082.pdf (accessed on 9 June 2025).

19. Brown, E. M. (2014). Best practice for antipsychotic medication management in community-dwelling older adults with schizophrenia. https://core.ac.uk/download/217670135.pdf.

20. Brunori, G., Di Lorenzo, G., Florena, A. M., et al. (2015). A case of fatal drug rash eosinophilia and systemic symptoms from allopurinol. https://core.ac.uk/download/53305999.pdf (accessed on 9 June 2025).

21. Chen, E., & Xi, L. (2024). Cardiovascular adverse effects of antiviral therapies for COVID-19: Evidence and plausible mechanisms. *Acta Pharmacological Sinica, 46*, 554–564. https://www.semanticscholar.org/paper/2828976af7bbf714b91437a832c5b8fa01c94cc2 (accessed on 9 June 2025).

22. Cox, S., Halcox, J., Kamala, B. A., et al. (2014). Vascular function intervention trial in sickle cell disease (V-FIT): Trial protocol. https://core.ac.uk/download/77514046.pdf (accessed on 9 June 2025).

23. Dawson Foster, E. O., Evbayekha, J., & Sokhn, J. (2023). A paradoxal reaction from intravenous immunoglobulin. *Blood*. https://www.semanticscholar.org/paper/b0bff99e57284d4e6262c89ace011117f5ecd7c2 (accessed on 9 June 2025).

24. Dempton, J. L. (2011). Genetic intervention as a lifestyle approach: An analysis of disease and treatment. https://core.ac.uk/download/236291395.pdf (accessed on 9 June 2025).

25. Giavina-Bianchi, P., Kalil-Filho, J., Marcondes-Fonseca, L. A., et al. (2018). Increase of 10% in the rate of adverse drug reactions for each drug administered in hospitalized patients. https://core.ac.uk/download/268270050.pdf (accessed on 9 June 2025).

26. Grantham, K. (2023). AI-enabled drug design and side effect prediction powered by

multi-objective evolutionary algorithms & transformer models. https://core.ac.uk/download/589235752.pdf (accessed on 9 June 2025).

27. Jacobs, I. A., Lichtman, S. M., & Reske, T. (2016). Biosimilars and cancer treatment of older patients. https://core.ac.uk/download/pdf/81942988.pdf.

28. Jallorina, A. G., Vij, K., Wan, L. S., Thomas, J., Drum, D. L., Glick, S. A., & Lee-Wong, M. F. (2024). A decadal exploration of cutaneous adverse effects of FDA-approved cardiovascular medications: Insights from 2013 to 2023. *Journal of Cardiovascular Pharmacology, 85*, 97–107. https://www.semanticscholar.org/paper/3422289df6bff7a6e5ce95e9bdf92fe15cc70470 (accessed on 9 June 2025).

29. Kurniawati, F. (2013). Explorative study of adverse drug reactions and drug-resistant tuberculosis among tuberculosis patients in Hospital Pulau Pinang, Malaysia. https://core.ac.uk/download/199246298.pdf (accessed on 9 June 2025).

30. Lanza, F., Maffini, E., & Saraceni, F. (2019). Treatment of adult patients with relapsed/refractory B-cell Philadelphia-negative acute lymphoblastic leukemia. https://core.ac.uk/download/287849316.pdf (accessed on 9 June 2025).

31. Le, H., Pham, T., & Tsu, L. (2014). Bipolar disorder: A pharmacotherapy management overview. https://core.ac.uk/download/215741464.pdf (accessed on 9 June 2025).

32. Lee, S. (2016). Efficacy and safety of bortezomib with dexamethasone regimen in elderly newly diagnosed multiple myeloma patients with co-morbidities. https://open.bu.edu/bitstream/2144/14373/9/Lee_bu_0017N_10435.pdf (accessed on 9 June 2025).

33. Mansoori, I., Kumar, P., Rai, G., & Dave, S. (2024). Adverse drug reactions and safety profiles in cardiovascular drug therapy: A pharmacovigilance analysis. *Journal of Pharmaceutical Research International*. https://www.semanticscholar.org/paper/c6c7d2db1d7dd45cafa9762524a122f697234465 (accessed on 9 June 2025).

34. Moirana, E. L. (2023). The prevalence of antiretroviral-therapy-related adverse reactions, hospitalization, and mortality among people living with HIV in Africa—A systematic review and meta-analysis. https://core.ac.uk/download/590318230.pdf (accessed on 9 June 2025).

35. N/A. (2021). Recent advances in gout. https://core.ac.uk/download/478126595.pdf (accessed on 9 June 2025).

36. Perwitasari, D. A. (2009). Monitoring of antithrombotic' adverse effect on unstable angina pectoris patients in a public hospital of Yogyakarta, Indonesia. https://core.ac.uk/download/42900544.pdf (accessed on 9 June 2025).

37. Ramey, C., & Saum, L. M. (2013). Geriatric medication therapy: Weighing the evidence versus best practice. https://core.ac.uk/download/62436341.pdf (accessed on 9 June 2025).

38. Rong, Y. (2022). Immune-related adverse events of immune checkpoint inhibitors: Incidence, risk factors, clinical outcomes, and economic burden in older adults with non-small cell lung cancer. https://core.ac.uk/download/588485720.pdf (accessed on 9 June 2025).

39. Society of Obstetrics and Gynecology of Zhejiang Medical Association, Society of Urology of Zhejiang Medical Association, Committee of Breast Cancer of Zhejiang Anticancer Association, Committee of Clinical Pharmacy on Oncology of Zhejiang Anticancer Association, & Committee of Urology of Zhejiang Society for Mathematical Medicine. (2022). Guidance on the management of adverse reactions induced by poly(ADP-ribose) polymerase inhibitors. *Zhejiang da xue xue*

bao. Yi xue ban = Journal of Zhejiang University. Medical Sciences, 51(6), 765–774. https://www.semanticscholar.org/paper/784035e215c7773bf2c4521cc063cefd9f697b92 (accessed on 9 June 2025).

40. Stanley, A., McConkey, C. C., Iveson, C., Kerr, D. J., Giovannucci, E., Dunn, J. A., Stokes, J. C., et al. (2007). Rofecoxib and cardiovascular adverse events in adjuvant treatment of colorectal cancer. https://core.ac.uk/download/105271.pdf (accessed on 9 June 2025).
41. Wan, H., Xu, X., Yi, D., & Shuai, K. (2024). Real-world safety evaluation of atorvastatin: Insights from the US FDA adverse event reporting system (FAERS). *Expert Opinion on Drug Safety, 24*, 305–314. https://www.semanticscholar.org/paper/d3264d86ee8088cdacf0d8ecb8e8b916696be02e (accessed on 9 June 2025).
42. Wang, J., Liang, J., He, M., Xie, Q., Wu, Q., Shen, G., Zhu, B., et al. (2022). Chinese expert consensus on intestinal microecology and management of digestive tract complications related to tumor treatment (version 2022). *Journal of Cancer Research and Therapeutics, 18*, 1835–1844. https://www.semanticscholar.org/paper/cfceb7a5b7820877fc2228979de94e00be8ecbc6 (accessed on 9 June 2025).
43. Wang, J., Zhao, Y., Chen, Z., & Huang, R. (2025). Safety of combined drug use in patients with cardiovascular and cerebrovascular diseases: An analysis based on the spontaneous reporting database of adverse drug reactions in Hubei Province. *Frontiers in Pharmacology, 15*. https://www.semanticscholar.org/paper/35bb2d4bcbe5728bc5c055be4435878792c34304 (accessed on 9 June 2025).

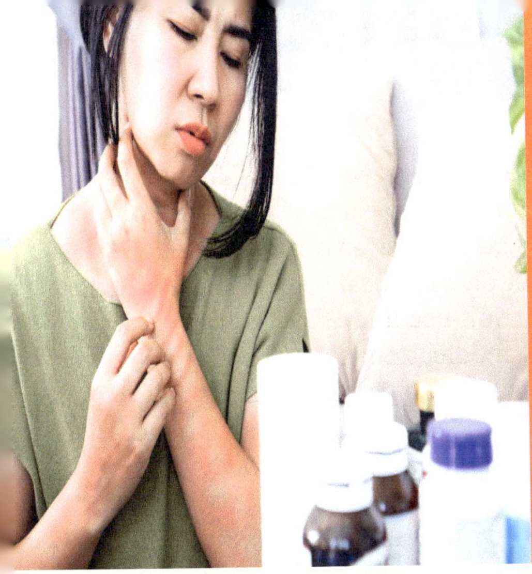

Chapter 9

NEUROLOGICAL AND PSYCHIATRIC ADVERSE DRUG REACTIONS (ADRS)

Contents

Introduction

In the case of pharmacotherapy, the use of psychotropic medication, particularly antidepressants and antipsychotics, has significantly increased among different patient populations. While these medications are crucial in the management of mental diseases, they are not devoid of risks. Neurological and psychiatric adverse drug reactions (ADRs) are a particular issue for treating doctors who prescribe such treatments. ADRs can encompass a wide range of effects, from sedation and mental disturbances to more severe effects such as suicidal thoughts. Understanding the prevalence and nature of these reactions is crucial in efforts to enhance patient care and safety in mental health settings. Research like the therapeutic drug monitoring (TDM)-VIGIL study is significant because it evaluates severe ADRs in children and adolescents undergoing treatment, bringing out the evolving correlation between treatment intake and patient impact (Antony et al., 2022). The complexity of drug-drug interactions (DDIs) makes the landscape of psychiatric therapy even more challenging, particularly among patients who require being put on polypharmacy. Assessment of potential DDIs is necessary as they are the primary reason for treatment failure, as well as preventable medical adverse effects. According to reports, the majority of psychiatric inpatients are exposed to one or more potential DDIs, thus monitoring and scrutiny of medication regimens are required. Certain combinations of psychotropic drugs have a high tendency to increase neurological symptoms or induce adverse psychiatric effects. By adopting a mechanistic conceptualization of these interactions, medical professionals can more effectively mitigate risks associated with concomitant medication use and thereby maximize therapeutic effectiveness (Deore et al., 2021). Increasing off-label medication usage among child and adult psychiatric patients provides additional concerns regarding psychotropic drug safety and efficacy. In the TDM-VIGIL study context, it was revealed that there was a high rate of off-label prescriptions for antidepressants and antipsychotics, with an existing gap in clinical evidence supporting their use. Although most prescriptions were for off-label purposes, data showed that severe adverse drug events were expressed at comparable rates for off-label and on-label use, prompting a further review of how these drugs are applied in everyday practice. While the study suggests that off-label prescribing would not necessarily pose an additional risk, it emphasizes the need for holistic assessment practices in healthcare to ensure patients' well-being is maintained (Antony et al., 2022). As such, understanding both ADRs and DDIs remains crucial for practitioners who intend to optimize treatment planning and deliver better results in psychiatry (Figure 9.1).

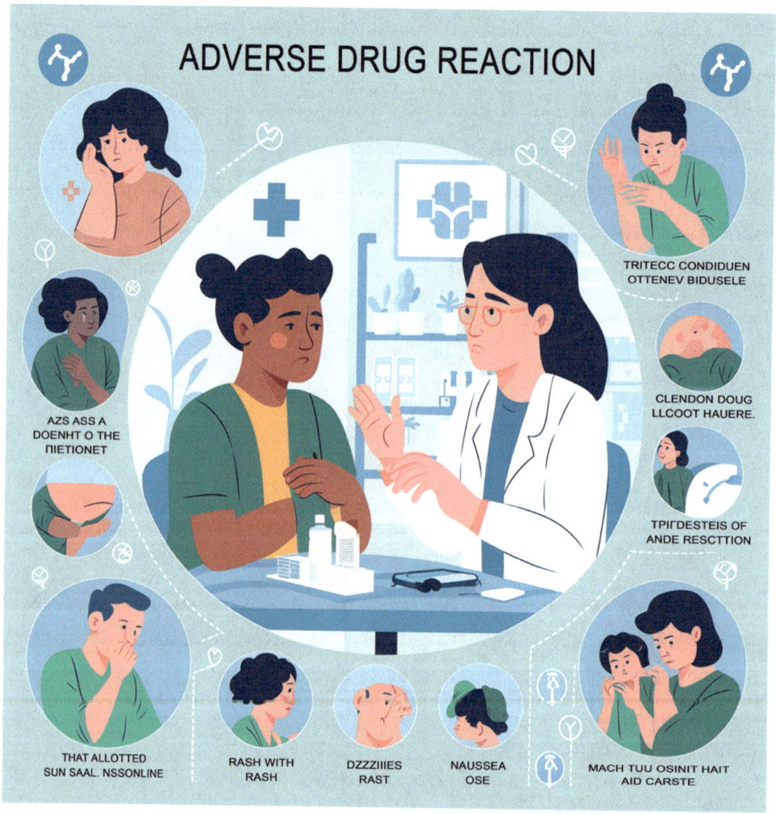

Figure 9.1. Neurological and psychiatric adverse drug reactions.

Source: https://thepharmadaily.com/media/uploads/admin/2024/05/06/image-20240506131352-1.png.

Definition of Adverse Drug Reactions (ADRs)

ADRs are defined as harmful or unintended responses that arise due to the administration of pharmaceutical agents. Some of these reactions are only mild, such as nausea, while others can be severe, for example, anaphylaxis. ADRs harm patients and also make drugs less effective, which leads to treatment being stopped and more expenses for healthcare. The definition of ADRs highlights the relationship between drug therapy and unexpected results, making it crucial to monitor these reactions using effective pharmacovigilance systems in real-time. In medicine, it is very important to understand ADRs, especially when assessing the benefits and risks of drugs used in the treatment of neurological and psychiatric disorders, since the effects of ADRs can be severe. The way ADRs are classified typically depends on their cause, when they occur, and the symptoms they exhibit.

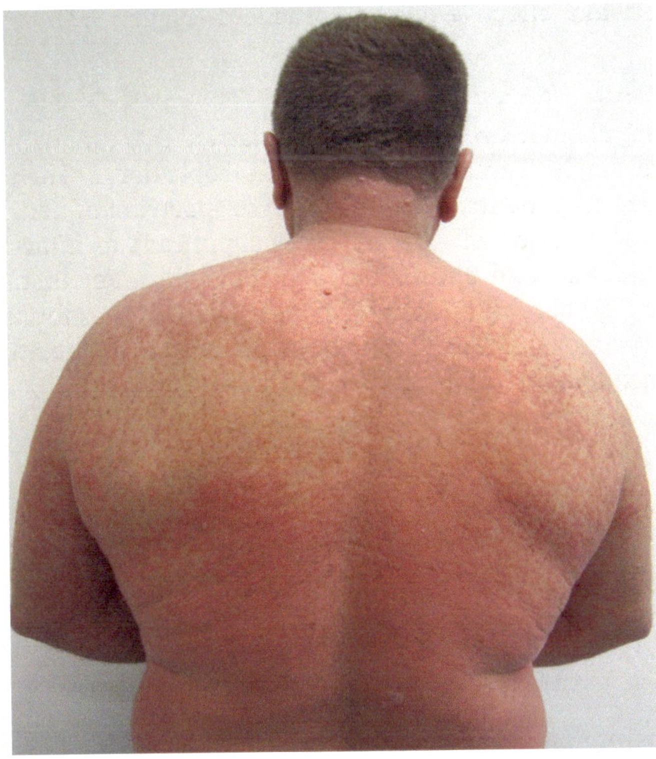

Figure 9.2. Definition of adverse drug reactions.

Source: https://www.healthcare-treatment.com/wp-content/uploads/2024/01/adverse-drug-reactions2.jpg.

They are often categorized into two primary types: Type A (augmented) and Type B (bizarre) reactions. Type A reactions occur in a way that can be predicted, since their cause is well-known, but Type B reactions are not related to drug dosing and are hard to predict. An example is that some psychotropics may bring on neurological symptoms (Type A), and allergic reactions are considered Type B. It helps healthcare providers prepare for potential reactions and respond to them appropriately. Furthermore, the pharmacovigilance framework aims to streamline the detection and reporting of ADRs, ensuring that clinicians are aware of serious reactions associated with particular therapies, especially where innovative drugs are concerned, as emphasized by recent regulatory adjustments to pharmacovigilance practices in the EU (Aislaitner et al., 2015). ADRs can affect vulnerable groups, such as children and the elderly, more often since they have a greater chance of having neurological and psychiatric side effects from drugs. For example, recent studies have reported a higher incidence of nervous system disorders among pediatric patients when compared to adults, underlining the importance of rigorous monitoring in these age groups (Domènech et al., 2021). Administering medications for unapproved uses going against the usual guidelines for the drug makes the situation more complicated as it can increase the risk of severe side effects. For this reason, healthcare providers should continue their education, patients should be involved through informed consent, and strong systems for reporting ADRs are necessary to protect the health of these patients. Those working in the field should constantly analyze ADR data to help ensure safety and effective medical practices (Figure 9.2).

Importance of Studying Neurological and Psychiatric ADRs

The significance of knowing about neurological and psychiatric ADRs cannot be overstated, particularly in a medical setting increasingly characterized by psychotropic drugs. The effect of these drugs can have a significant influence on patients, eliciting a diverse spectrum of neurological and psychiatric signs and symptoms. Interpretation of ADR trends is significant to inform prescribing practices, identify vulnerable populations, and optimize patient outcomes. For instance, in a population of psychiatry outpatients, a high observed rate of incidence of ADRs was found, with somnolence and tremors being common reactions. These observations are crucial for healthcare providers seeking to minimize risks and maximize treatment efficacy (Gawali et al., 2017).

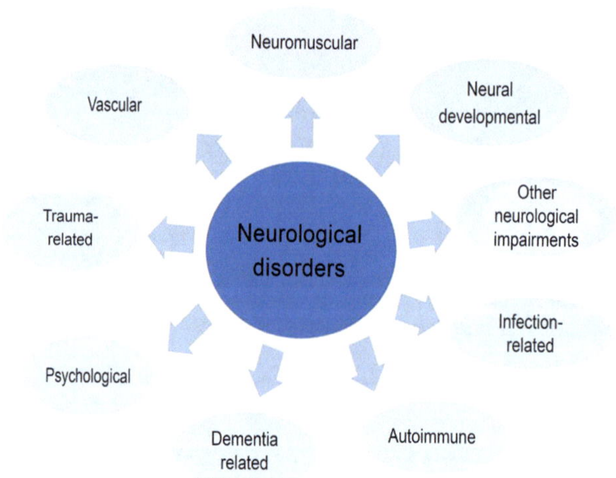

Figure 9.3. Importance of studying neurological and psychiatric adverse drug reaction.

Source: https://www.intechopen.com/chapters/76045.

Monitoring and understanding these ADRs facilitate better-informed decisions and tailored patient management, such that the therapeutic benefits of drugs outweigh the risks. Moreover, the significance of neurological and psychiatric ADRs is also recognized beyond the care of individual patients to encompass overall public health concerns. With aging populations on the rise and mental illness becoming more prevalent, psychotropic drug use is sure to become more prevalent.

Consequently, there is also an enhanced risk of developing ADRs, emphasizing the need for continuous monitoring and research. The need for rigorous research is reflected in methods such as those involved in nondrug therapies; for example, the addition of nonpharmacological treatments, such as exercise or art therapy, can decrease undesirable effects while providing symptomatic relief. This integrated approach not only enhances therapeutic outcomes but also fosters a richer, more complex understanding of patient health, closing knowledge gaps regarding drug-to-drug interactions and side effects (Erakhtin et al., 2018). In addition, education concerning ADRs can play an important part in developing education programs for patients and HCPs. Awareness of potential side effects of psychiatric and neurological drugs empowers patients to detect and report ADRs in time, embracing a participatory care culture. Findings from studies like the ones featured in ADR pattern studies can serve as the foundation for training healthcare practitioners. With this, they are better prepared with the tools necessary to identify, manage, and advise against ADRs. This complex understanding thus enhances the safety of treatment and patient adherence to regimens. Only by maintaining the study of neurological and psychiatric ADRs as a priority are the health professionals able to work towards limiting drug-related morbidity while optimizing health outcomes in vulnerable groups (Gawali et al., 2017; Erakhtin et al., 2018) (Figure 9.3).

9.1. Types of Neurological ADRs

Neurological ADRs encompass a range of symptoms resulting from medication intervention that impact the nervous system. Seizures are a particular concern since they may be caused by several drugs, for example, antiepileptics and anesthetics. A significant example includes local anesthetic systemic toxicity (LAST), which primarily affects pediatric populations during surgical procedures. In many of the cases, neurological problems were observed, which underlines how widespread and serious these reactions are for children. Factors such as the type of local anesthetic and the dosing regimen significantly influenced the likelihood of developing life-threatening outcomes, highlighting the critical need for careful monitoring and dosing adherence in clinical settings to mitigate risks associated with neurological ADRs (Schweitzer-Chaput et al., 2023). Another category of neurological ADRs involves the cognitive and psychiatric effects of certain medications, particularly in the context of novel therapies such as proprotein convertase subtilisin/kexin type 9 inhibitors (PCSK9Is). According to what has been reported, these agents might lead to headaches, sleeping difficulties, and depression. A systematic analysis of individual case safety reports (ICSRs) for alirocumab and evolocumab highlighted that up to 22.7% of reports featured neuropsychiatric reactions, raising concerns about the broader implications of these drugs on mental health. Interestingly, while no significant differences were found in the reporting rates of these ADRs between PCSK9Is and statins, the former's higher reporting likelihood for neurological disorders suggests that ongoing surveillance and patient education about potential cognitive side effects are essential (Gabriella et al., 2020). Besides, drug-induced movement disorders are a significant group of neurological ADRs and are commonly caused by drugs that work on dopamine, antipsychotics, and certain antidepressants. Some of these disorders are tardive dyskinesia and akathisia, which can significantly impact a person's health and make it difficult to control their main psychiatric illnesses. Typically, these reactions occur due to dopaminergic pathways, which cause movements that are beyond the person's control. Since patients may experience these side effects when taking the drugs for an extended period, it is essential to recognize them and inform the patients. That is why doctors and nurses should consider the benefits of using drugs and the risk of neurological side effects, and plan how to manage and monitor these side effects.

9.1.1. Central Nervous System (CNS) Effects

ADRs of the central nervous system (CNS) are a significant problem in neurological and psychiatric practice. The diversity of CNS effects that various drugs can produce can lead to a range of symptoms from impairment of cognition to severe neurological illness. For instance, psychotropic drugs aimed at psychiatric disorders, such as antidepressants and antipsychotics, have been linked to a range of CNS effects, including, sedation, insomnia, and extrapyramidal symptoms. Of specific interest, the growing evidence would indicate that the incidence of such untoward reactions might be substantial, since the said studies mentioned incidence rates of up to 15.06% among psychiatric patients who experience ADRs from medication they are given. Awareness of these effects is important for the clinician to construct treatments that reduce risk with optimal therapeutic gain.

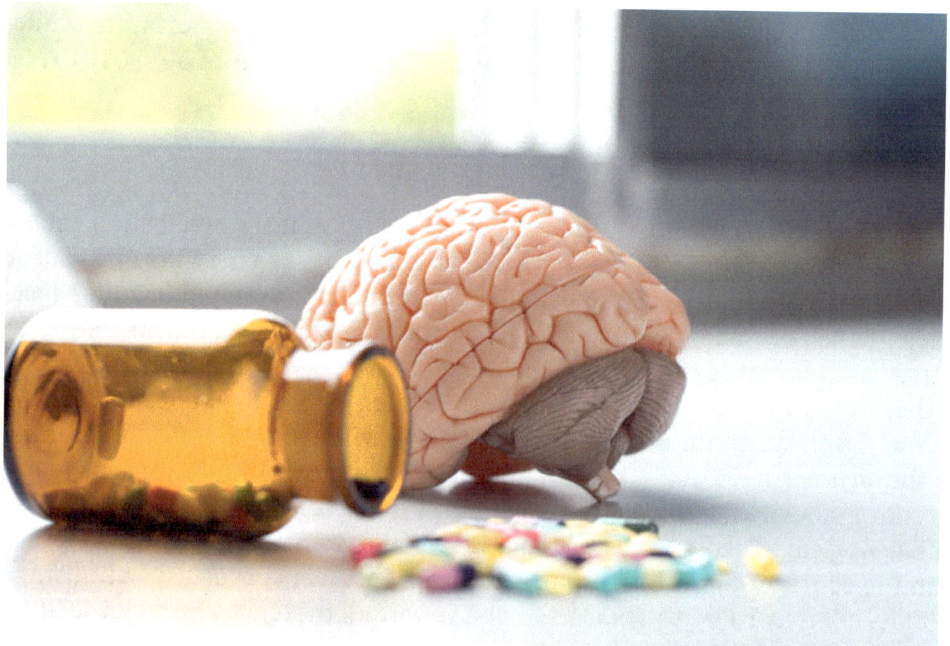

Figure 9.4. Central nervous system (CNS) effects.

Source: https://addictionresource.com/wp-content/uploads/2022/01/The-Brain-layout-and-some-pills-on-the-table.jpg.

CNS-related ADRs have polyfactorial etiologies consisting of complex interactions between pharmacologic agents and neurological processes. Antidepressants, particularly SSRIs, have been reported to have a propensity to influence neurotransmitter systems with desired as well as undesired effects. Additionally, the neurochemical actions of such drugs may even aggravate underlying conditions or provoke new psychiatric pathology, such as mania in susceptible individuals. It should be remembered that the cumulative effect of treatment is often the case because long-term administration of psychotropic medication may lead to chronic CNS action affecting the quality of life of a patient. Besides, the enhanced vulnerability of the CNS to drug effects accentuates the role of pharmacotherapy specifically designed for vulnerable populations in a way that maximizes the advantage of therapy and minimizes the risks involved. The implications of CNS ADRs extend beyond the instance of a single patient to influence public health programs and clinical practice guidelines. A growing recognition of the incidence of CNS effects has encouraged increased emphasis on monitoring regimens to identify and manage such ADRs. It has been found through research that the majority of ADRs in psychiatric practice were inevitable and had a tendency to occur following extremely lengthy treatment periods, reaffirming once more that there has to be active pharmacovigilance (Stanghellini et al., 2012). With the advent of new therapies, such as combination therapies like the nifurtimox-eflornithine treatment for conditions like sleeping sickness, ongoing observation of the safety profile in heterogeneous populations becomes a priority (Stanghellini et al., 2012). Last but not least, enhanced awareness and knowledge regarding CNS effects of ADRs will result in safer prescribing and improved patient management outcomes in psychiatric and neurological practices (Figure 9.4).

9.1.2. Peripheral Nervous System (PNS) Effects

The peripheral nervous system (PNS) plays a crucial role in transmitting sensory and motor information between the CNS and the rest of the body. However, the interaction of pharmacological agents with the PNS can lead to substantial ADRs, causing a spectrum of neurological and psychiatric symptoms. As an illustration, chemotherapy drugs may result in neuropathy, which is linked to pain, weakness, or problems with sensations. For this reason, patients using these drugs should be monitored regularly. It is helpful to learn how these agents affect the PNS. The immune-mediated pathogenesis of conditions like paraneoplastic neurological syndromes (PNSs) highlights the complexity of these interactions, suggesting that immune responses may modulate neurotoxic effects induced by medications (Desestret et al., 2020). Neuroimmunology research also examines how drugs might change the immune system and the well-being of the PNS. In some cases, drugs may bring about inflammation that can harm the myelin sheath or nerves, and this effect might be worse for patients who already have PNS issues. Conditions such as Guillain-Barré syndrome and chronic inflammatory demyelinating polyneuropathy can lead to more severe reactions, making it more challenging to help the patient. Also, when a person's genetic traits and the drugs they take interact, it may cause abnormal symptoms in the PNS. Noticing these interactions can help improve how HCPs handle risk and give treatment to patients. The evolving field of neuroimmunology offers insights into these mechanisms, providing valuable information for healthcare providers dealing with patients who experience ADRs related to PNS (Amor et al., 2019). Some drug interventions may result in psychiatric symptoms that are a significant worry for medical professionals. Patients with drug-induced peripheral neuropathy may suffer from constant pain and also feel anxiety and depression, since the condition affects their nervous system and quality of life. Although there is limited research available on the mental aspects of persistent PNS, it appears that the CNS is also involved. Hence, when patients have these conditions, doctors are required to give them thorough care. Taking care of these additional conditions is necessary to achieve better outcomes and maintain the patient's health. Future studies must investigate the neuropsychological dimensions of ADRs, as understanding the full impact of drugs on both PNS function and mental health can lead to more effective management strategies (Desestret et al., 2020) (Figure 9.5).

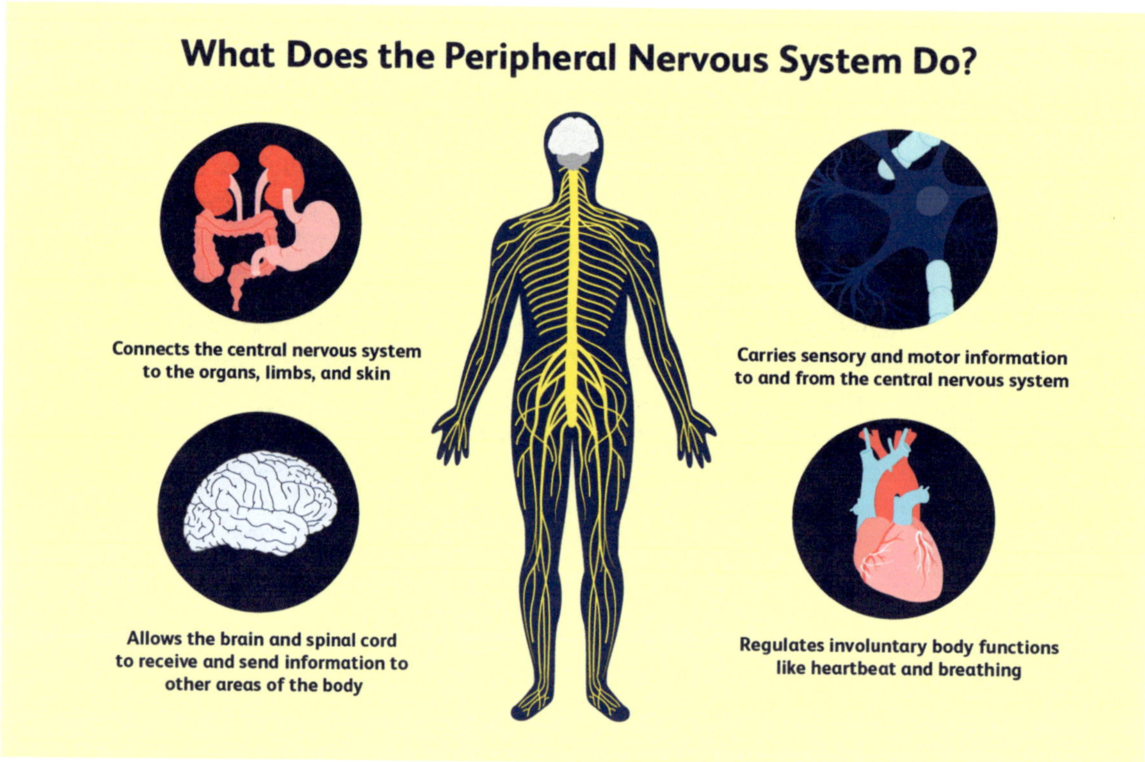

Figure 9.5. Peripheral nervous system (PNS) effects.

Source: https://www.verywellmind.com/thmb/S6e2zuErsAfYKwHcrd1yKL2iLt8=/1500x0/filters:no_upscale():max_bytes(150000):strip_icc()/what-is-the-peripheral-nervous-system-2795465-FINAL-b69e1bb803654212a83d9e68eb4847d0.png.

9.1.3. Examples of Drugs Causing Neurological ADRs

The branch of pharmacotherapy frequently intersects with the nervous system, leading to neurological adverse drug effects (ADRs) with a bearing on outcomes in patients. Certain antibacterial medications, for instance, are perpetrators of neuropsychiatric effects, albeit not commonly discussed, but of central importance in clinical practice. These adverse effects range from seizures to acute psychotic conditions in approximately 30% of patients with no history of psychiatric disorders. This alarming statistic brings focus to the imperative of greater vigilance on the part of medical professionals to the potential neurotoxicity of such drugs. Furthermore, the diagnostic challenge of such ADRs, due to their often subtle presentation, underscores the importance of ongoing monitoring of neurological function in patients taking these medications (Cyriac et al., 2021). Aside from antibiotics, numerous other classes of medications exhibit a striking propensity to produce neurological ADRs. Antidepressants operating on the cytochrome P450 (CYP) enzymes are implicated in potentiating or catalyzing their adverse neurological effects. To illustrate, patients who suffer from genetic variations within their CYP2D6 genotypes are susceptible to therapeutic failure and increased risk of ADRs after being treated with drugs that are metabolized by this enzyme. In a population of bipolar disorder patients, significant correlations between specific CYP2D6 metabolizer phenotypes and the induction of extrapyramidal symptoms have been reported, illustrating the significance of genetic variation in response to drugs. Such findings not only affirm the utility of pharmacogenetic screening in individualized medicine but also underscore the principle that knowledge of drug interactions is essential in minimizing health risks associated with psychiatric medications (Bellomo et al., 2018). In all, the category of drugs with the possibility of causing neurological ADRs is wide-ranging. It includes numerous categories of therapeutics, highlighting the multidisciplinary aspect of pharmaceutical practice. The interplay between drug effects, individual genetic makeup, and individual characteristics of neurological response presents a complex dilemma for practitioners. In order to avoid risks posed by neurological ADRs, physicians need to be constantly on guard to monitor patients for neurotoxicity and change treatment regimens as needed. Through the development of an open discussion culture surrounding potential side effects, healthcare professionals can facilitate their patients' informed understanding of the risks and benefits of their medication, thereby facilitating safer pharmacological treatments for both neurological and psychiatric disorders (Bellomo et al., 2018; Cyriac et al., 2021).

9.2. Types of Psychiatric ADRs

In the context of psychiatric ADRs, the interplay between pharmacological interventions and mental health presents a complex landscape deserving of thorough exploration. Among all types of psychiatric ADRs, mood changes are especially noticeable, involving symptoms such as depression, mania, and a lack of feeling. Corticosteroids, antidepressants, and antipsychotics can occasionally induce mood swings. These mood swings can exacerbate a patient's mental health issues, make it more difficult for patients to follow their treatment plans, and make it more difficult for clinicians to manage the illness.

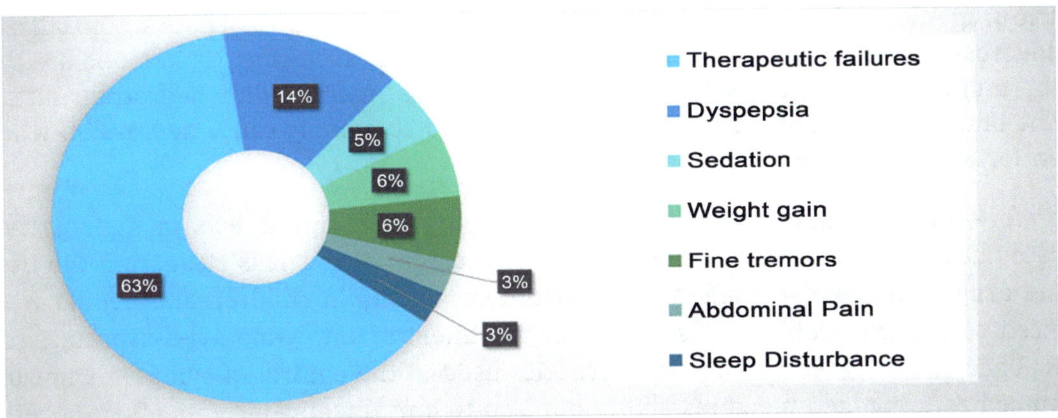

Graph 2: Distribution of Adverse Drug Reactions seen in psychiatry OPD

Figure 9.6. Types of psychiatric adverse drug reactions.

Source: https://biomedpharmajournal.org/wp-content/uploads/2022/06/Vol15No2_Adv_Mit_gra2.jpg.

For example, some people may experience anxiety or depression after taking antidepressants, proving how carefully psychiatric drugs should be prescribed. It is essential to understand these mood-related side effects to improve how patients with psychiatric disorders are treated. Many psychiatric ADRs are related to cognitive problems, which include memory loss, problems focusing, and a general decline in thinking abilities. Such cognitive-related side effects are particularly prevalent with medications used to treat conditions like schizophrenia, bipolar disorder, and attention-deficit/hyperactivity disorder (ADHD). Antipsychotic drugs, and especially the atypical type, could result in cognitive problems, making it hard for the patient to take part in daily activities or keep up social ties. Noticing cognitive ADRs is important for safe medication use over time and might require a full review of the drug's effects on both the body and mind. By analyzing the results, clinicians can design customized treatment plans that reduce the risk of memory problems and help patients manage psychiatric issues, enabling them to recover successfully. The presence of psychotic symptoms in psychiatric ADR demonstrates how some medicines can significantly affect a person's mental health. Antidepressants and stimulants are among the drug classes that may cause psychosis in people who are susceptible or when the dosage is increased. If someone develops psychosis, it may result in hallucinations, delusions, or severe restlessness that calls for urgent care. Pharmacovigilance research keeps revealing how psychotic ADRs occur and what factors increase the risk, which helps update guidelines for prescribing drugs. Because drug-induced psychosis might look like other psychiatric problems, doctors should be careful when assessing the onset of symptoms in patients using drugs. Understanding these side effects well is important for healthcare providers to protect patients and maintain the effectiveness of medicines for mental health (Figure 9.6).

9.2.1. Mood Disorders Induced by Medications

The status of drug-induced mood disorders is a significant concern in the area of neurological and psychiatric drug ADRs. It has been found that many drugs, including antipsychotics, benzodiazepines, and antidepressants can cause depressive or manic symptoms. Such changes in mood are typically caused by multiple factors, often linked to the way drugs interact with neurotransmitters and impact the brain. Antipsychotic drugs have been found to commonly cause depression when they are taken for a certain amount of time.

Therefore, doctors should be vigilant in identifying such side effects in their patients, as timely recognition can help prevent lasting psychological problems. It is clear from the literature that some drugs can negatively affect mood disorders, mainly in children and people who have experienced psychiatric problems. A study of the treatment of anti-N-methyl-d-aspartate receptor (NMDAR) encephalitis revealed that antipsychotics used in the control of symptoms not only led to heightened agitation and mood instability but also to a frightening adverse effect-benefit ratio. The study once again showed that antipsychotics may be helpful, but they can also cause serious psychiatric problems, so it is important to use them carefully. Effective management, therefore, entails not only the wise selection of pharmacologic drugs but also constant monitoring of the patient's mental state for prevention of mood disorder development during treatment. Also, since people react differently to drugs, it is important to create individual care plans. What benefits one patient may cause a serious mood disorder in another, demonstrating that all parties should be involved in the decision-making process regarding treatment. When giving treatment advice for tics such as Tourette Syndrome, efforts are made to consider any additional conditions and how medicines can affect a person's mood. The interplay between various health determinants necessitates a process that balances symptom control with the patient's psychological state in a bid to mitigate the incidence of ADRs, which include mood disorders induced by drugs like antipsychotic or other psychotropic drugs, as part of comprehensive therapeutic practice (Brilot et al., 2016; Cavanna et al., 2019) (Figure 9.7).

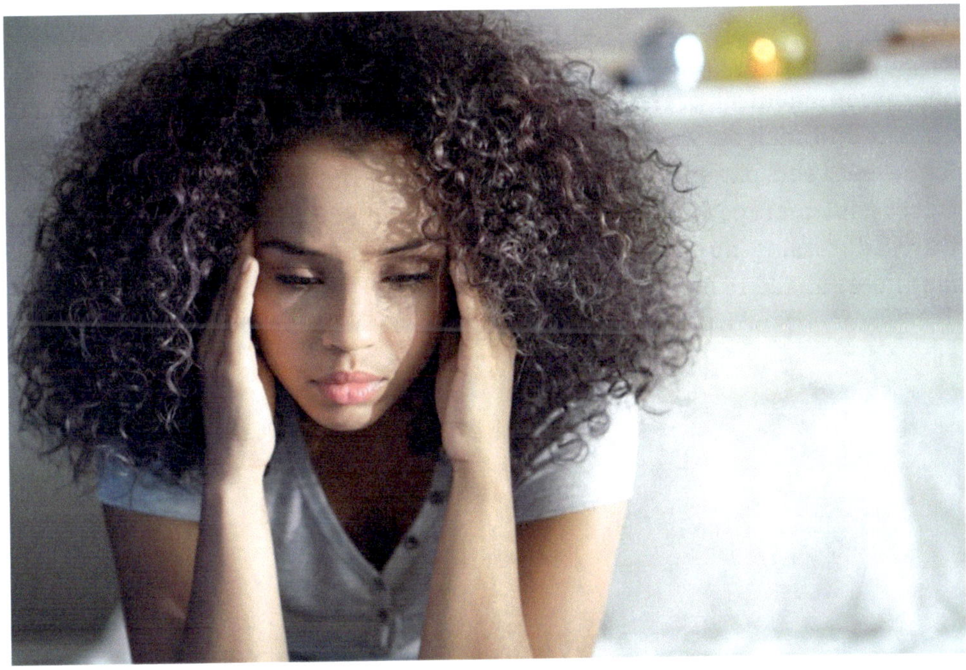

Figure 9.7. Mood disorders induced by medications.

Source: https://www.beachesrecovery.com/wp-content/uploads/2019/07/Substance-Induced-Mood-Disorder.jpeg.

9.2.2. Anxiety and Agitation as ADRs

In the larger framework of the neurological and psychological consequences connected to medication, the appearance of anxiety and agitation as adverse drug reactions (ADRs) is a significant topic of concern. Antidepressants and antipsychotics might occasionally cause these symptoms. They must remember that some of these symptoms may happen because of the medicine, not because of a disease. Because anxiety usually involves feeling tense and fearful, it can seriously affect a patient's life and make it harder to treat the condition. For this reason, patients should be closely monitored, especially during the initial or when changing the use of medicines that can cause these side effects. Certain medications, particularly selective serotonin reuptake inhibitors (SSRIs) and classic antipsychotics, have been documented to exacerbate anxiety and agitation in vulnerable populations. At the start, SSRIs can make anxiety worse, since they tend to increase the intensity of risk factors for suicide, such as feeling down and acting on impulses. This reaction highlights the importance for patients to understand that the early stages of treatment can actually increase their anxiety, rather than alleviate it. Moreover, classic antipsychotics can result in extrapyramidal side effects that may indirectly make people with psychiatric disorders feel more anxious and agitated. This interplay emphasizes the need for careful assessment and management strategies to mitigate these ADRs throughout the treatment process (Ore et al., 2010).

Additionally, agitation and anxiety as adverse drug reactions (ADRs) might affect a patient's willingness to continue taking the medication as well as the overall outcome of treatment. Patients may quit taking their medicine if it causes them to feel more agitated or nervous, which could lead to improper treatment of their mental health issues. As a result, non-following treatment guidelines can make mental health symptoms worse and lead to more interventions that could cause similar ADRs. For this reason, medical professionals should know about these possible reactions to give the best treatment and include ways to manage anxiety and agitation in each patient's plan. The ongoing dialogue between patient and clinician is critical in navigating these complex dynamics to promote successful therapeutic outcomes while minimizing adverse effects, as highlighted in recent literature addressing novel psychoactive substances (NPS) and their complex psychiatric profiles (Chiappini et al., 2019) (Figure 9.8).

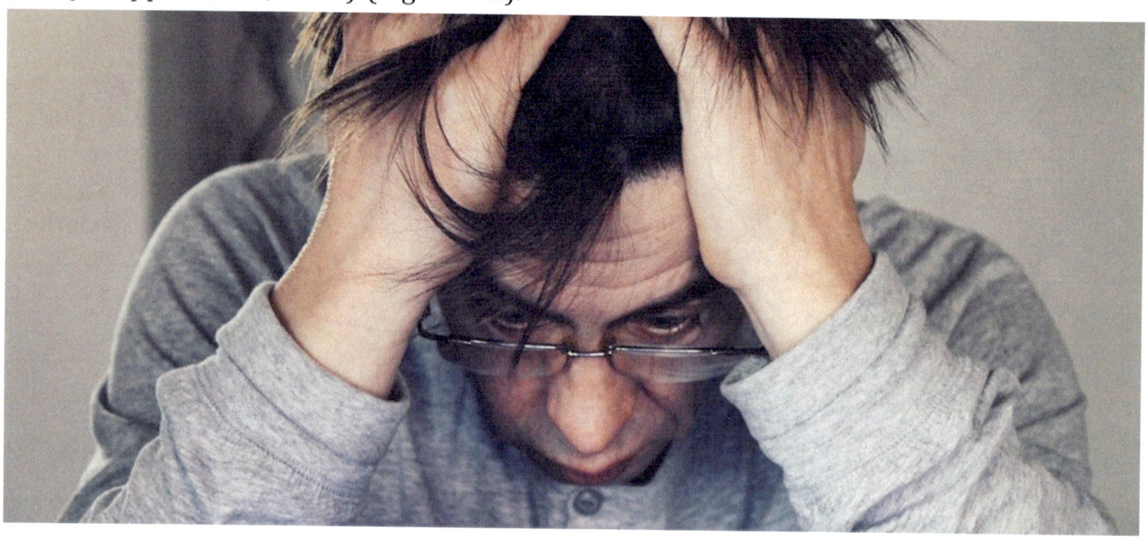

Figure 9.8. Anxiety and agitation as adverse drug reactions.

Source: https://www.anxietycenter.com/wp-content/uploads/2020/07/agitation-anxiety-l.jpg.

9.2.3. Psychotic Symptoms Related to Drug Use

The onset of psychotic symptoms related to drug consumption is a serious concern against the backdrop of Neurological and Psychiatric ADRs. The symptoms are usually identified in instances of substance use disorders, such that the patient may experience hallucinations, delusions, or even extreme changes in behavior. The impact of such symptoms extends beyond the individual level of the patient and affects interpersonal relationships and societal functioning. A significant concern has been the engagement of several drugs, including stimulants like cocaine and methamphetamine, with acute paranoid psychosis production, making the treatment challenge for clinicians greater. It is critical to know which precise mechanisms the drugs employ to induce psychotic states so that treatment protocols can be designed to address the psychological as well as the neurological components of drug-induced psychosis. The intricacy of psychotic presentation has been brought to light by recent research, especially when a history of substance addiction and mental illness is involved. For instance, psychotic symptoms are frequently seen in Parkinson's disease patients, especially when they are using specific atypical antipsychotic drugs that can result in adverse drug reactions on their own.. In one study involving patients with idiopathic Parkinson's disease (iPD), the prevalence of psychotic presentation was about 22.2%, the most frequent of which was hallucinations. These signs can occur years after primary diagnosis, reflecting a chronic interaction between substance-induced phenomena and the underlying neurologic disorder. The findings suggest that a thorough understanding of personal risks and prudent management of pharmacological interventions is required to combat the adverse influences on mental welfare and overall quality of life (Bizzarri et al., 2017). Also, the rise of NPS added more complexity in drug-induced psychosis. The drugs, usually sensationalized for having unpredictable effects, have been found to produce novel psychopathological patterns other than the usual psychoses. Clinicians must be vigilant and familiar with such new psychoses, as the presentation of the signs differs extensively based on the nature of the involved compounds, i.e., synthetic cannabinoids and cathinones. Research has indicated that the clinical presentation of NPS-induced psychoses may demand a different therapeutic strategy than what is employed in traditional presentations of psychosis. With evolving drug-use patterns, an urgent need exists for clinicians to remain abreast of new trends, underlying neurochemistry, and evidence-based approaches to management in order to confidently tackle the psychotic symptomatology related to drug use (Chiappini et al., 2019) (Figure 9.9).

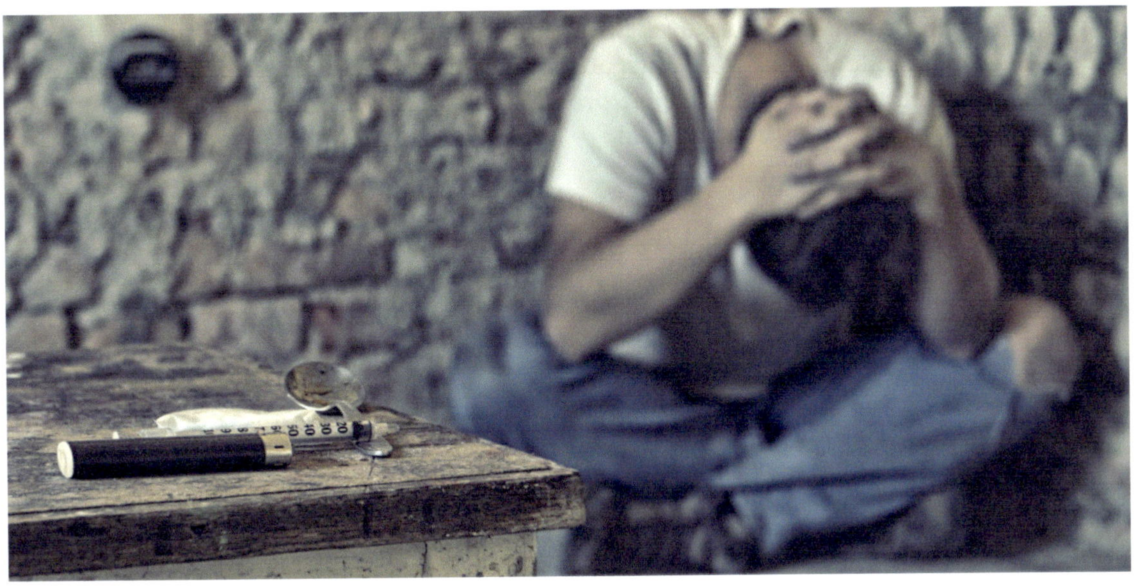

Figure 9.9. Psychotic symptoms related to drug use.

Source: https://www.cadabamshospitals.com/wp-content/uploads/2018/06/pasted-image-0-3.png.

9.3. Mechanisms of Neurological ADRs

Understanding the mechanisms underlying neurological ADRs is crucial for improving patient outcomes and optimizing therapeutic interventions. An important point is that drug PK and pharmacodynamics can sometimes cause unexpected problems in the brain. As an illustration, some drugs have the potential to change the levels of neurotransmitters or the way receptors work, which can disrupt CNS functions. Some of the symptoms include problems with thinking and with movement. Because of how complicated neurological pathways are, drugs prescribed for different conditions can still cause ADRs. For this reason, clinicians should always be vigilant for the possibility of ADRs and regularly review and adjust their patients' medication plans to minimize the risks. Neuroinflammation is another important aspect of neurological ADRs because it is now seen as a primary reason for adverse reactions. The immune reaction of the CNS is known as neuroinflammation and it involves the participation of microglia and astrocytes. When drugs are used to trigger the immune system, it can go out of control and cause more cellular changes that worsen neurological disorders. It has been suggested that ongoing neuroinflammation is related to several neurological diseases, like Alzheimer's and Parkinson's, so ADRs could affect the brain for a long time. The modulation of neuroinflammatory pathways represents a promising direction for mitigating these ADRs, allowing for the development of therapeutic strategies that target these pathways while considering the risk of neuroinflammatory responses induced by specific drugs (Berwian et al., 2020). It is essential to reduce the impact of neurological ADRs, especially in people who are old or have neurological problems before taking the drug. Many studies indicate that dance therapy can greatly enhance balance and walking in patients with Parkinson's disease by focusing on both their physical and mental health. They stimulate the brain's motor circuits and may help mitigate the negative effects of drugs that impact executive functions. The combination of exercise and medication improves quality of life and offers new ideas for rehabilitation that can be used in conjunction with standard drug treatment. By exploring multifaceted treatment models, healthcare providers can better navigate the intricate landscape of neurological ADRs and personalize care based on individual patient profiles, ultimately leading to improved therapeutic outcomes (Agnetti et al., 2012) (Figure 9.10).

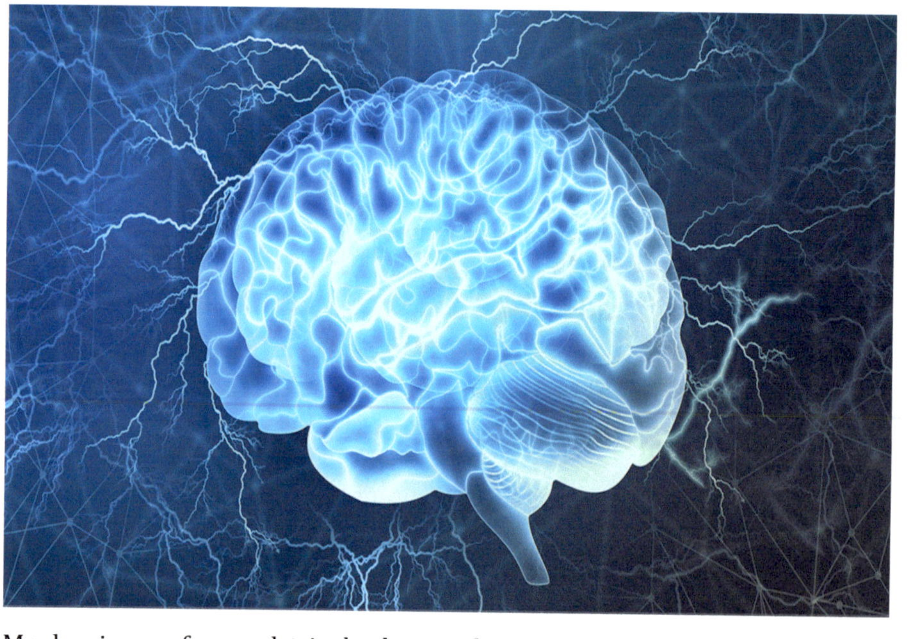

Figure 9.10. Mechanisms of neurological adverse drug reactions.

Source: https://regionalneurological.com/wp-content/uploads/2019/11/AdobeStock_172813720.

jpeg.

9.3.1. Pharmacological Mechanisms

The pharmacological processes of neurological and psychiatric drug-induced ADRs are complex and multifactorial. On a molecular level, interaction between drugs and neurotransmitter systems can lead to dysregulation, resulting in drug side effects. A case in point is the application of atypical antipsychotics to treat a condition such as Parkinson's disease psychosis (PDP), leading to side effects due to their action as dopamine and serotonin receptor antagonists. While these drugs decrease psychotic symptoms, their pharmacodynamic effect is often followed by side effects such as sedation, cognitive impairment, and extrapyramidal effects. According to studies, 70% of people with PDP have hallucinations, which get worse after taking these drugs. This suggests that a thorough evaluation of the drugs' pharmacological effects and the associated adverse drug reactions is necessary. (Bizzarri et al., 2017). Other than receptor interactions, the pharmacology of a drug can have receptor-independent mechanisms that also contribute to ADRs. Modulation of endocannabinoid systems or other new targets in pain medicine, like palmitoyl ethanolamide (PEA), is but one. Studies have shown that PEA holds promise for safety and effectiveness in migraine relief through non-canonical mechanisms. This medication has activity on several cell and tissue targets that can modulate nociceptive transmission, with the absence of the significant side effects typically associated with NSAIDs. As impressive as its benefits in migraine treatment are, the intricate interplay among its biological activities makes it challenging to predict the outcome of patients; thus, the necessity for profound knowledge of its pharmacology compared to other drugs (Caroleo et al., 2018). The identification of pharmacologic mechanisms is important in the regimen optimization process to minimize ADR risk to an absolute minimum and maximize therapeutic benefit. Evaluation of these mechanisms promotes evidence-based practice of medication selection, dosing, and monitoring of adverse effects by practitioners. The time profile and dose-response relationship of drug action, for example, must be considered in patients with complicated comorbidities. As personalized medicine advances, more emphasis is placed on pharmacogenomics to understand better how genetic variations influence drug metabolism and receptor interactions. This knowledge has the potential to lead to individualized treatments that reduce the risk of neurological and psychiatric ADRs, ultimately leading to enhanced patient outcomes in various clinical contexts.

9.3.2. Genetic Predispositions

Genetic predispositions play a significant role in the manifestation of neurological and psychiatric ADRs, influencing how individuals metabolize and respond to various pharmacological agents. Unequal drug effects and side effects among people can happen if the genes responsible for metabolizing drugs are not the same. As an example, individuals who have some genetic differences may react more severely to certain drugs, causing more problems. Since these drugs target brain chemicals, looking at a person's genes can show why some are strongly affected by them and others are not. Additionally, learning about genetic factors that increase the risk of ADRs enables doctors to provide more personalized drug treatments tailored to each patient's unique genetic profile. As an example, those using D-penicillamine for Wilson's disease may experience side effects since their genes make it hard for them to process and eliminate copper. Studies have indicated that approximately 30% of patients on this medication experience neurological complications, including tremors and mood disturbances, underlining the need for genetic screening to predict potential adverse reactions (Svetlana et al., 2025). By using this approach, doctors can reduce the risk of drug interactions and get better outcomes for patients, especially those who may be affected negatively.

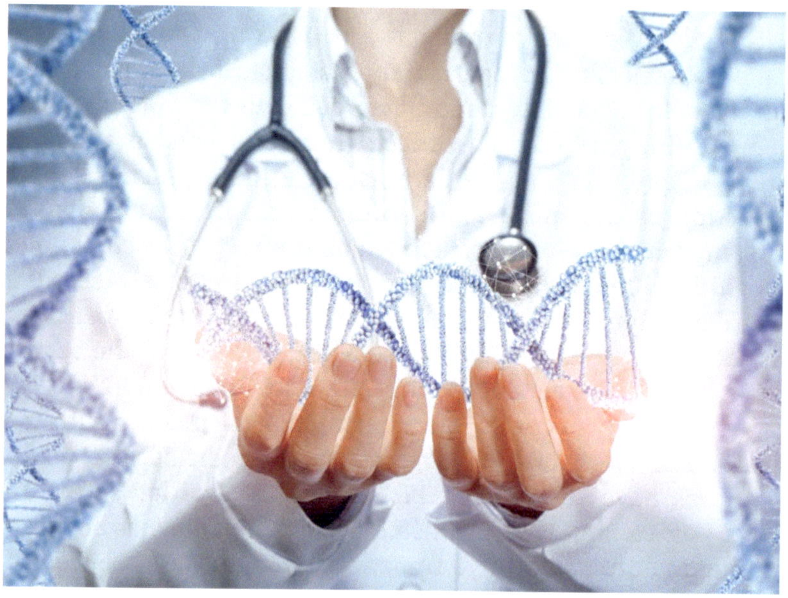

Figure 9.11. Genetic predispositions.

Source: https://www.verywellhealth.com/thmb/9ocWbniWGh4MP6OqRjVyVbSZ7TI=/2000x1500/filters:fill(87E3EF,1)/DNA1-b5956a41a92044f7ad1e0fd2bdcfe47e.jpg.

Additionally, specific genetic variants are implicated in severe conditions like Stevens-Johnson syndrome (SJS), which can occur following the administration of commonly used medications such as lamotrigine. The pathophysiology of SJS involves complex immune mechanisms that may be influenced by an individual's genomic makeup, highlighting the importance of genetic predispositions in drug reactions (Shingala et al., 2025). They demonstrate the need for caution while performing pharmacogenetic testing, particularly whenthere have been serious drug reactions in the past. All in all, using genetic information in healthcare will reduce the risk of neurological and psychiatric ADRs and make sure mental health treatments are safer (Figure 9.11).

9.3.3. Environmental Factors Influencing ADRs

Understanding the environmental determinants of ADRs is crucial in neurological and psychiatric care. Environmental determinants like socioeconomic status, access to healthcare, and exposure to toxicants can have the ability to affect patients' responses to drugs quite significantly. Socioeconomic disparities have been discovered to have an impact on patients' adherence to prescribed therapies and, therefore, the success of therapies as well as the incidence of ADRs. For instance, lower socioeconomic individuals may not be exposed to good-quality health care services, which can impact the surveillance and management of possible drug-drug interactions, particularly in individuals who are on polypharmacy. Thereafter, these deficits may worsen neurological and psychiatric illnesses, which call for a comprehensive approach towards handling ADRs in at-risk populations. Environmental exposures can also impact the PK and pharmacodynamics of drugs. Diet, lifestyle, and environmental toxin exposure also modify drug activity and metabolism, thus enhancing ADRs to the nervous system and psychiatric disease. For example, certain foods have been observed to inhibit or enhance the effect of drugs by altering their absorption and excretion. Environmental toxins are also known to induce neurodevelopmental and psychiatric illness, and these can allegedly enhance the susceptibility of patients to ADRs to commonly utilized antiepileptics and antidepressants. This refinement highlights the need for ongoing research into the interactions between environmental factors and pharmacological agents, thereby filling knowledge gaps that facilitate the interpretation of their implications for treatment protocols. Interactions at the pharmacodynamic level between antidepressants and antiepileptics can thus become clinically meaningful, as investigated in studies that underscore the imperative for greater knowledge and observation within treatment algorithms (de Leon et al., 2014). In addition, ethnic and regional variation in response to medicines should be noted when managing the environmental factors of ADRs. Others will possess genetic tendencies that interact with the environment to yield different responses to medication. Prescriptions for treating epilepsy, as outlined in the Malaysian guidelines, emphasize the importance of cross-cultural management (N/A, 2024). These guidelines reflect the importance of local knowledge in understanding the role that environmental determinants like access to healthcare and local disease epidemiology play in influencing neurology and psychiatry practices. By incorporating these guidelines in clinical practice, healthcare providers are better equipped to manage and minimize the risk of ADRs more effectively, resulting in safer and more effective care for diverse groups of patients (Figure 9.12).

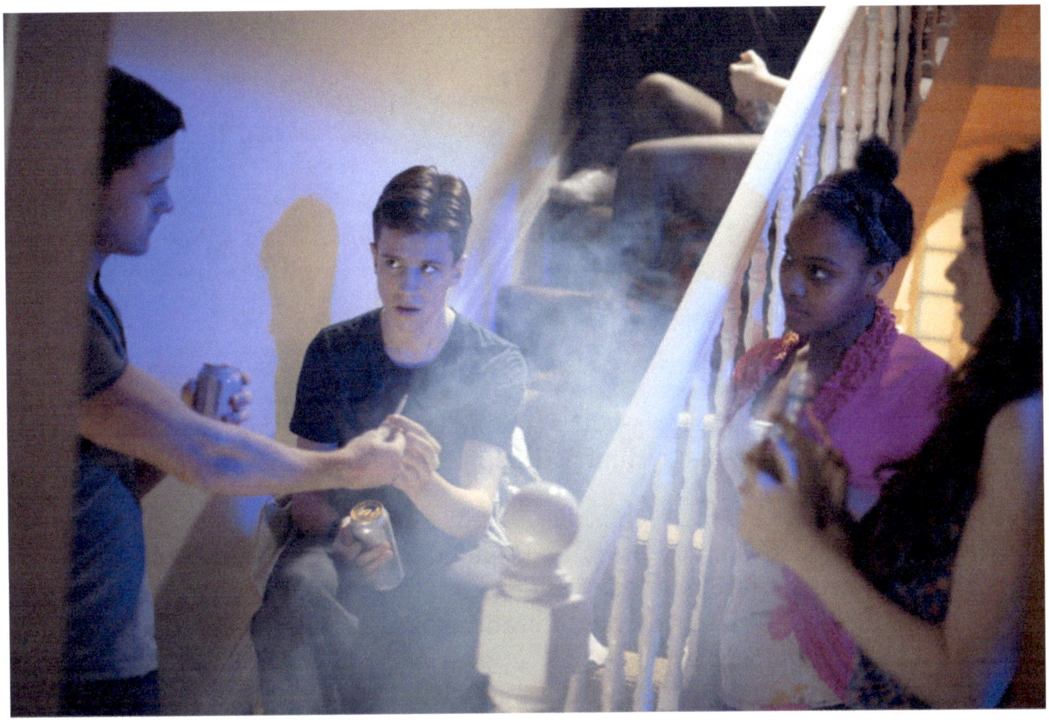

Figure 9.12. Environmental factors influencing adverse drug reactions.

Source: https://cyclesofchangerecovery.com/wp-content/uploads/2021/11/How-Environmental-Influences-Affect-Drug-Addiction.png.

9.4. Mechanisms of Psychiatric ADRs

The mechanisms underlying psychiatric ADRs are complex and multifaceted, often involving both pharmacological and genetic factors. Antipsychotic drugs belong to psychiatric medicines that mainly alter the activities of dopamine and serotonin in the brain. If these systems are disrupted, it can lead to metabolic syndrome, movement issues, and changes in a person's mood or thought patterns. As an example, people who are easily affected by drugs may experience increased symptoms or develop additional mental health problems. Researchers have discovered that high levels of hydrogen sulfide in the body might be related to schizophrenia, which means that metabolic issues could play a significant role in psychiatric symptoms. Investigating these pathways enables a more informed approach to drug selection and monitoring in vulnerable populations, ultimately improving therapeutic outcomes and minimizing the detriments associated with these treatments (Ide et al., 2019).

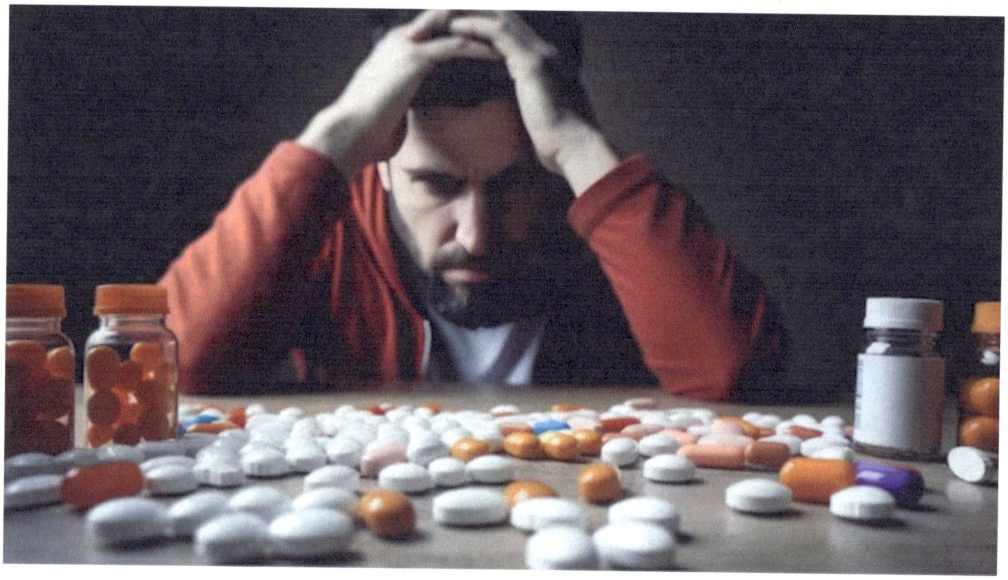

Figure 9.13. Mechanisms of psychiatric adverse drug reactions.

Source: https://safetherapeutics.com/wp-content/uploads/2023/12/Managing-Medication-Risks-Tackling-Adverse-Drug-Reactions-in-Psychiatric-Hospitals-Safe-Therapeutics.jpg.

Certain people may be more prone to psychiatric ADRs due to their genes. If patients have changes in genes that control drug metabolism, receptors, and signaling pathways, their reactions to psychiatric medications may be altered. There is a lot of evidence that genes play a part in triggering ADRs. Some research indicates that certain genetic differences may influence how various ethnic groups respond to medical treatments. Therefore, new approaches to prescribing and treating mental health are being created by using genetic tests and biomarkers to prevent ADRs. This ensures that therapy is tailored to meet the unique needs of patients, thereby addressing critical safety concerns during treatment (McClellan et al., 2013). Besides, particular environmental situations and personal experiences can make it more likely for psychiatric ADRs to occur with the use of medicines. Issues that appear when a child is young, pressure from social and emotional concerns, and health problems can have a major impact on treatment. Using stressors and drugs at the same time could result in new issues or make current health problems more serious. For instance, early-onset schizophrenia is often associated with an increasesd incidence of adverse events from treatment, indicating that developmental factors play a crucial role in drug efficacy and safety. The most recent studies indicate that both the actions of doctors and the patient's surroundings should be taken into account when evaluating a case. A holistic assessment of these elements can significantly contribute to more effective and safer management of psychiatric disorders, thereby enhancing overall patient care and well-being (Ide et al., 2019) (Figure 9.13).

9.4.1. Neurotransmitter Imbalances

Control of neurotransmitters in the brain is at the root of complete psychological and neurological balance. Unbalances in neurotransmitter levels have been recognized to produce a range of psychiatric diseases, most prominently depression and anxiety, all too prevalent nowadays. ADRs occur most severely in this context by psychotropic drug abuse. For example, SSRIs are widely used to treat depression, but long-term use has been linked to alterations in brain chemistry that potentially worsen the very symptoms they are used to treat. This demonstrates how pharmacological treatment can result in neurotransmitter imbalances, which can set off a vicious cycle in mental health treatment that needs careful monitoring and management to avoid detrimental long-term effects. In looking at the impact of drug-induced disturbances in neurotransmitters, it is important to address sleep disturbances, a significant component of most psychiatric conditions. Drugs used to induce sleep are hypnotic drugs such as benzodiazepines and newer drugs referred to as Z drugs.

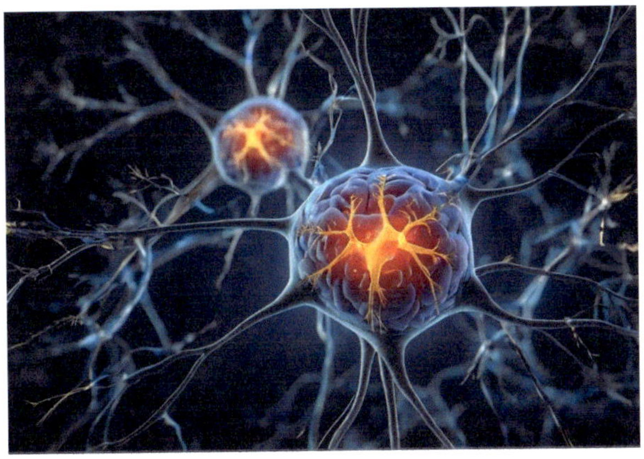

Figure 9.14. Neurotransmitter imbalances.

Source: https://magnifymind.com/wp-content/uploads/2024/08/symptoms-of-neurotransmitter-imbalance-1024x680.jpg

Such drugs develop tolerance and addiction, which means that disturbances in neurotransmitter systems such as gamma-aminobutyric acid (GABA) become worse with time. Evidence is such that, while some antidepressants are employed for easing insomnia, their efficacy is questionable. It might be a cause of additional dissatisfaction with sleep quality, giving rise to a complex dynamic of interference of neurotransmitters. Insomnia, in turn, then adversely affects an individual's overall mental health and pattern of recovery, indicative of the necessity of a more nuanced approach towards treatment that takes into consideration such chemical dynamics (Adam et al.,

2018). In addition, major depressive disorder (MDD) is a classic case of the absolute importance of being familiar with neurotransmitter actions in psychiatric disorder etiology and the dangers of pharmacotherapy.

Since SSRIs are stated to be effective in reducing depressive symptoms, their long-term use is worrisome due to potential undesirable consequences such as tachyphylaxis and tardive dysphoria. These side effects suggest that neurotransmitter balancing is not merely a matter of replenishing the quantity, but rather a process of stabilizing them in the long run. Such intricacy highlights the dilemma under which the drugs could, over time, worsen symptoms or new neurological problems, rendering the treatment less potent than initially imagined (Giblin et al., 2018). This calls for prolonged evaluation and examination of the neurochemical processes that are influenced by conventional psychiatric treatments, guiding practitioners to optimize therapeutic interventions, closely monitoring and addressing these transmitter imbalances (Figure 9.14).

9.4.2. Inflammatory Responses in the Brain

Inflammatory responses in the brain are critical mechanisms that can profoundly influence neural function and behavior, particularly in the context of neurological and psychiatric ADRs. Neuroinflammation, which is triggered by the activation of microglia and astrocytes, plays a crucial role in protecting the brain. However, excessive or prolonged inflammation can be detrimental. A lot of research suggests that neuroinflammation is linked to both depression and schizophrenia, showing that it is a common factor in many psychiatric conditions. As drug reactions can provoke or exacerbate inflammatory processes, understanding the nuances of neuroinflammatory responses is vital for developing safer therapeutic interventions and improving patient outcomes in the realm of psychiatry and neurology (Berwian et al., 2020). When studying the brain's inflammatory responses and their relationship to ADRs, the kynurenine pathway for tryptophan degradation is also a significant focus of interest. For a long time, research concentrated on serotonin, but it has recently been shown that kynurenine metabolites play a role in neurotransmitters and brain activities. When stress or infection are present with ADRs, they may change the kynurenine pathway and cause more harmful chemicals to be made. Because of this, psychiatric disorders may develop, and the side effects of some medications may become worse. As insights into the kynurenine pathway continue to evolve, it is imperative for future research to explore these metabolic changes in depth to identify potential novel therapeutic targets (Schwarcz et al., 2017). With a deeper understanding of neuroinflammation, treating inflammation in the brain has become increasingly important in the pharmaceutical field. Limiting the overactivity of the immune system may help control some of the side effects caused by antipsychotics and antidepressants. Therapies that target microglia or cytokines may help alleviate symptoms of neurological and psychiatric disorders, and also make medications more effective and safer. As research continues to address neuroinflammation and its effects on new drugs, it is necessary to establish a detailed system for evaluating the advantages and disadvantages of using these drugs. This integrative approach might redefine therapeutic paradigms, ultimately steering the field toward more effective and safer interventions for patients facing neurological and psychiatric challenges (Berwian et al., 2020).

9.4.3. Drug Interactions Affecting Mental Health

When treating neurological and psychiatric disorders, the problem of drug interactions is significant.

Mixing antidepressants, antipsychotics, and mood stabilizers with other drugs can lead to different results and more possible side effects. TB drugs have been shown to cause depression and other psychiatric conditions that make it harder for patients to follow the treatment plan and improve their health. Good management needs to be aware of drug interactions, since not handling them can make the patient's mental state worse and increase neurological problems. It is tough for healthcare practitioners to improve treatment plans when the use of multiple drugs can cause both effectiveness and safety issues. Since psychiatric comorbidity is usual in chronic diseases, it is necessary to consider that drug interactions may have a significant effect on patients' mental health and quality of life. A review of the literature points out that depression is often made more complicated by drugs that are commonly used. In the case of epilepsy, the drug used to control seizures may also cause adverse psychological effects. It is found from research that seizures are mainly considered in dog epilepsy, while the general effect on a dog's life, mental state, and brain function, as well as comorbidities, are often ignored. The need for a multidimensional intervention becomes imperative in managing the impact of drug interactions on mental health among such patients (Packer et al., 2025). These complications from drugs also affect how patients stick to their treatments and take their medications as prescribed. The review of TB patients reveals that having a psychiatric disorder, especially depression, makes it harder for patients to follow treatment. Applying mental health strategies and giving medication can help healthcare workers enhance both drug-taking habits and treatment results. The implications are considerable, suggesting that full treatments need to be utilized in order to treat neurology and psychiatry's complicated treatment topographies, especially where ADRs instill a destructive health cycle. Therefore, inter-professional practice between HCPs is necessary to offer complete care that involves both physical and mental dimensions of health (Bratis et al., 2013) (Figure 9.15).

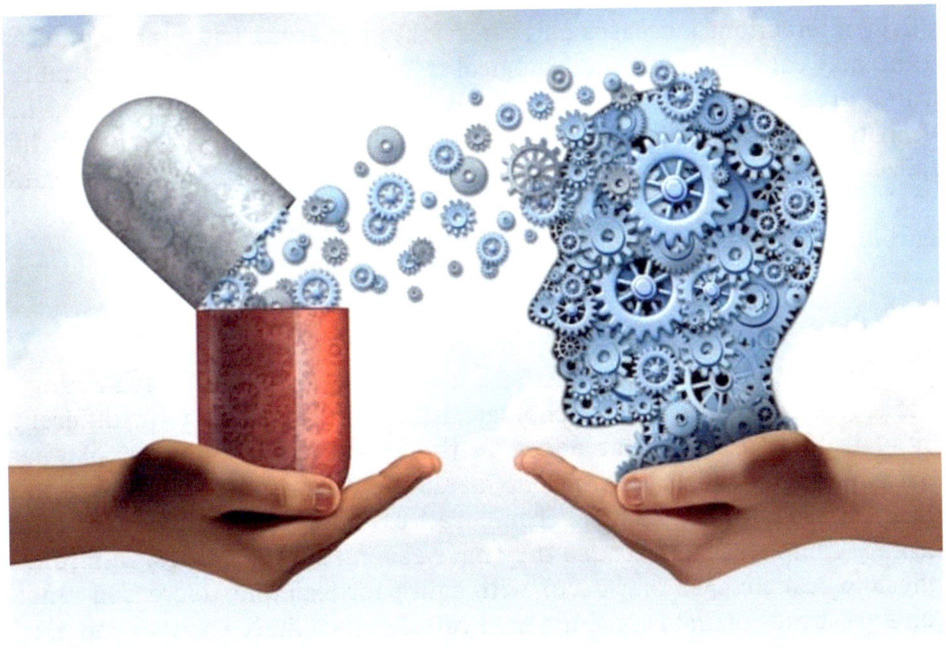

Figure 9.15. Drug interactions affecting mental health.

Source: https://www.wphealthcarenews.com/wp-content/uploads/2019/10/download-1.jpeg.

9.5. Risk Factors for Neurological and Psychiatric ADRs

The relationship between age and the occurrence of neurological and psychiatric ADRs is a critical area of study, especially regarding quinolone antibiotics. It has been found that older people are at greater risk of these ADRs, mainly when they take ciprofloxacin. The literature indicates that people under the age of 70 do not experience neurological adverse drug reactions. Drug side effects may be more common in older adults due to changes that occur with aging. Consequently, clinicians must exercise heightened caution when prescribing such medications to older adults, given their altered PK and potential pre-existing neurological conditions, as highlighted in a recent observational study that revealed a 3.6% incidence of neurological ADRs among older patients treated with ciprofloxacin (Hartinger et al., 2023). If someone has a previous neurological or psychiatric problem, they are at a higher risk of experiencing quinolone-related ADRs. Taking ciprofloxacin may result in more side effects for patients who have depression, anxiety, or epilepsy. As a result, any pre-existing conditions in a person can affect their responses to medications, making them stronger or last longer. It was discovered after studying quinolone cases that these patients had a higher risk of experiencing neurological and psychiatric problems. As the management of these patients requires careful consideration, healthcare providers should prioritize thorough patient histories to assess these risks and potentially adjust treatment plans accordingly, ensuring that the benefits of antibiotic therapy outweigh the risks posed by their mental health histories (Scavone et al., 2020). Besides, when other medications are taken at the same time, neurological and psychiatric ADRs may be harder to manage. When quinolone antibiotics are combined with anticonvulsants and corticosteroids, the risk of side effects increases. If a patient takes many medicines, the possibility of drug interactions increases and can result in neurotoxicity. Taking multiple therapies at the same time may cause patients' neurological issues to worsen and lead to more potent side effects. According to statistical analysis, these relevant risk variables were present in over half of reported ADR instances associated with quinolones, highlighting the need for careful monitoring and individualized pharmacotherapy, particularly in patients with complex medication regimens (Hartinger et al., 2023). It helps to know the patient's condition well to prevent the problems caused by neurological and psychiatric ADRs.

9.5.1. Patient Demographics (Age, Gender, etc.)

Patient demographics, in terms of age and sex, are vital knowledge in evaluating neurological and psychiatric ADRs. Biological and psychological factors associated with different age groups have been found to have a significant effect on the efficacy and tolerance of pharmacological treatment. Younger groups can have different metabolic rates and organ development that can shift drug PK and trigger different ADRs compared to older individuals, who tend to present with polypharmacy complications because they have several comorbidities. Different studies have shown that physiological changes that occur with aging, for example, decreased renal and hepatic function, require great caution in prescribing medications since these changes can heighten the risk of ADRs, thus having a significant influence on clinical outcomes. Similarly, the influence of gender differences is considerable in the presentation and occurrence of ADRs. Research highlights that women are apt to have a contrasted side effect profile compared to men, and this can be attributed to psychosocial problems, body composition, and endocrinological changes. For instance, there was a focus on the relationship between impulsivity characteristics and psychiatric disorders, stating that the former could be moderated by seizure characteristics in Juvenile Myoclonic Epilepsy (JME) patients (Andrade et al., 2020). Additionally, the frequency of typical adverse reactions may vary significantly with gender; hence, awareness of such variations is important for the customization of drug regimens. Such a demographic indicator is dealt with in order to enable health professionals to make evidence-based decisions that suit individual patient profiles, optimizing therapeutic effectiveness while maintaining ADR risks at a low level. Moreover, the geographic and socio-economic implications inherent in patient demographics cannot be overstated. In the majority of low- and middle-income countries (LMICs), mental healthcare is provided by non-specialist health workers (NSHWs) who are bound to encounter diverse patient groups with heterogeneous ADR profiles (Altman et al., 2011). Demographic contexts would thus need to be determined so that the efficacy of mental healthcare interventions can be measured across various settings. It then becomes vital to evaluate how age and sex interact with socio-economic status and regional health infrastructure, which may affect access to and compliance with medicine. A combined approach in which demographics are brought into the analysis of ADRs not only makes our understanding of their occurrence more robust but also aids better resource allocation and customization of health interventions to better outcomes within various population segments (Figure 9.16).

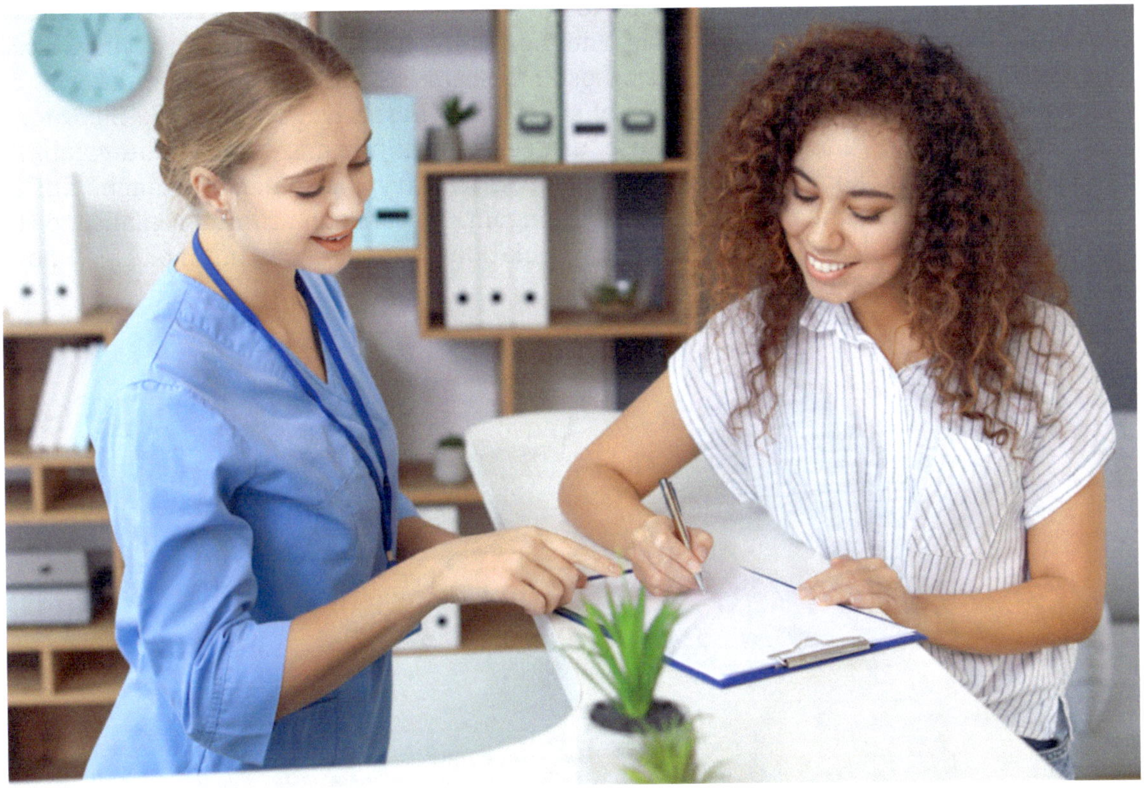

Figure 9.16. Patient demographics (age, gender, etc.).

Source: https://appliedmedicalsystems.com/wp-content/uploads/2016/10/AMS_Patient-Demographics-Blog.jpeg.

9.5.2. Pre-Existing Medical Conditions

Pre-existing medical conditions play a critical role in the development and severity of neurological and psychiatric ADRs. People who have diabetes or heart-related problems may have weaker neurological systems, so they are more likely to experience drug side effects. As an example, taking certain medicines for these diseases with psychotropic drugs may increase the severity of symptoms. It is important to keep an eye on these pre-existing conditions and the medications taken together, since using several drugs at once may cause serious mental health issues. Therefore, reviewing a patient's medical history is necessary for healthcare providers to plan treatments that are best for that person and safe for them. Besides chronic diseases, psychiatric disorders can also play a significant role in increasing the risk of ADRs. Those who have had depression or anxiety before are usually treated with medicines that may not have been tested on people with both conditions. The absence of clinical trials specifically designed for individual drugs raises concerns, as the actual incidence of neurological side effects is often not reported. Besides, people in this group might react strongly to some drugs, causing more potent effects on their minds and brains. For this reason, clinicians should carefully check for previous psychiatric problems when prescribing drugs and use a thorough assessment to avoid adverse reactions. The proper use of drugs in patients with pre-existing conditions requires knowing how drugs interact and how each person's metabolism works. Differences in genes can cause patients to have problems metabolizing certain medications, which can lead to more severe adverse effects. Therefore, pharmacogenomic research plays a crucial role in selecting treatments for individuals whose medical histories can influence the way drugs are metabolized. Moreover, the development of safer drug alternatives, such as the incorporation of combination therapies, has shown promise, as seen with nifurtimox-eflornithine combination therapy in treating complex conditions like Human African trypanosomiasis (Stanghellini et al., 2012). Such advancements underscore the need for ongoing research and clinical vigilance to ensure optimal drug safety, particularly in vulnerable populations with pre-existing medical conditions (Altman et al., 2011) (Figure 9.17).

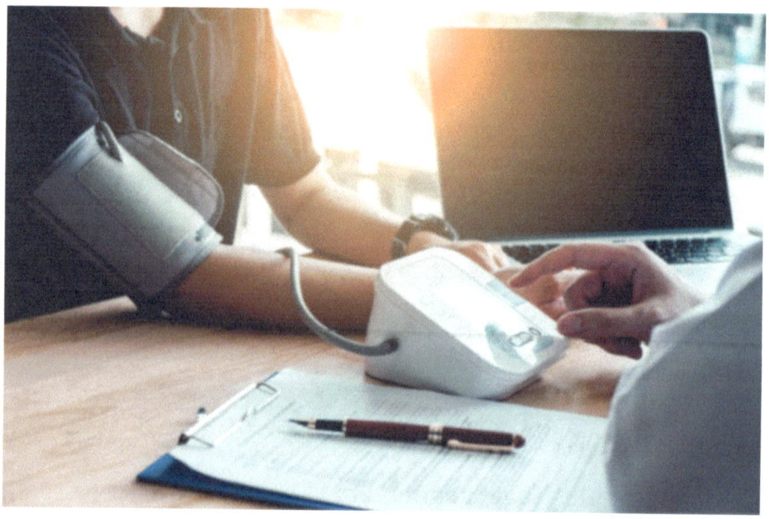

Figure 9.17. Pre-existing medical conditions.

Source: https://www.insurewithpetra.com/wp-content/uploads/2021/04/pre-existing-conditions-and-medical-insurance-in-dubai.jpg.

9.5.3. Polypharmacy and Its Implications

It is now a significant issue in psychiatric and neurological care that patients are given several medications at the same time. Patients who are elderly and have several chronic conditions are usually the ones who receive the preventive practice. Polypharmacy has profound effects, with the rate of ADRs elevating exponentially as more medicines are added. Besides affecting the results of therapy, drug-drug metabolic interaction also leads to mental issues, such as increased anxiety or confusion, that are hard to distinguish from worsening psychiatric disease.

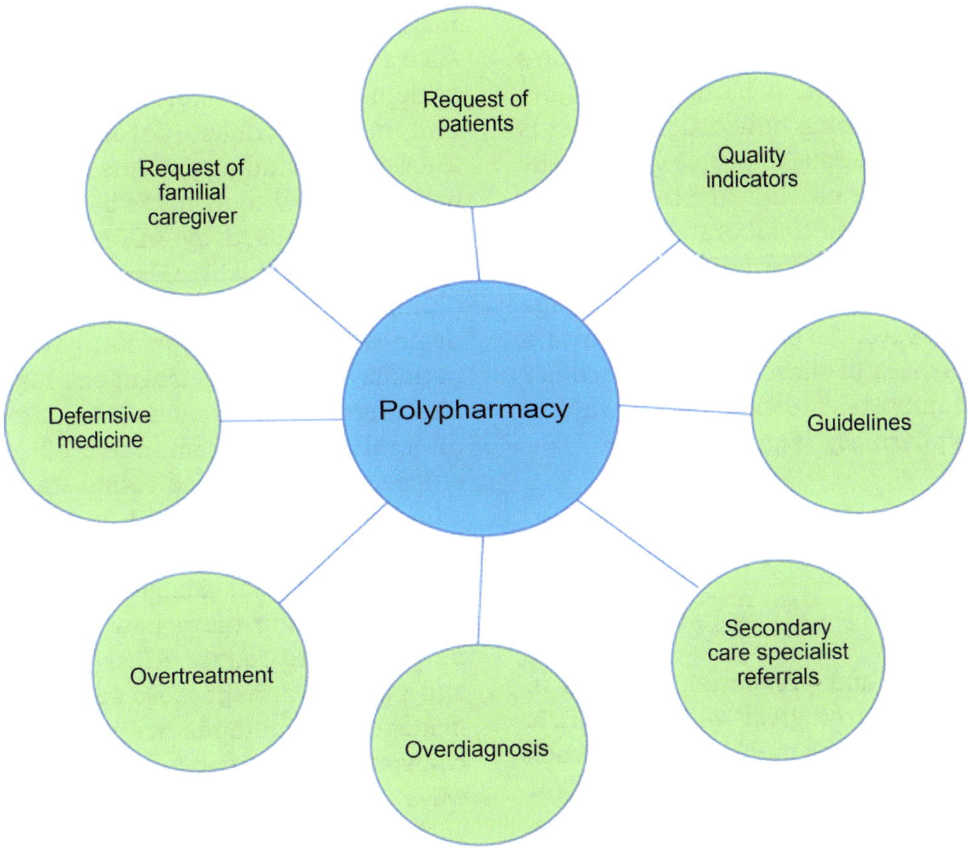

Figure 9.18. Polypharmacy and its implications.

Source: https://media.springernature.com/lw685/springer-static/image/art%3A10.1186%2Fs12880-024-01349-7/MediaObjects/12880_2024_1349_Fig1_HTML.png.

Doctors then address these issues by reviewing all the medications a patient is taking to ensure that the benefits of the therapy outweigh the risks associated with taking multiple medications. Besides, because there are not many clear guidelines for handling polypharmacy, the risk of ADRs is higher in psychiatric and neurological medicines. The updated British Association for Psychopharmacology guidelines capture an optimism about addressing the complexities of pharmacotherapy for disorders like schizophrenia, as they acknowledge the necessity of weighing risk-benefit profiles for various mixtures of drugs (Thomas et al., 2019). When doctors employ a careful prescription approach, they can minimize many side effects, as they are encouraged to use evidence-based treatments tailored to each patient's needs. It is essential to consider this viewpoint because polypharmacy may cause mental confusion, worsen psychiatric problems, and result in more medication that does not work for patients. In addition, recent findings point out that the effects of polypharmacy can be seen in various neurological and skin-related problems. For instance, certain medications might trigger pruritus, wrongly diagnosed as a sign of underlying disease due to drug interaction (Wei et al., 2019). This symptom may significantly affect a person's quality of life and make it harder for doctors to diagnose, so knowing how drugs interact is very important, especially in people who already have neurological or psychiatric problems. It is essential for doctors to collaborate and develop personalized treatment plans for patients that prioritize safety and effectively manage their health issues. As people become aware of the seriousness of these issues, it becomes increasingly important to find simple ways to manage polypharmacy (Figure 9.18).

9.6. Management and Prevention of ADRs

The management and prevention of ADRs in the context of neurological and psychiatric treatments necessitates a multifaceted approach that integrates careful monitoring, patient education, and tailored intervention strategies. The first thing to do in effective management is to find patients at risk, mostly those who take many medications or are hospitalized for a long period, as the study reveals that ADRs are common and can be very dangerous in neurology departments. Clinicians should regularly review the treatments they administer to these patients to prevent any adverse outcomes. Additionally, performing routine assessments, such as using standard scales to evaluate the cause and severity of ADRs, helps ensure drug safety and improve treatment outcomes. It is necessary in ADR prevention to explain to patients the risks that may come with their neurological or psychiatric medicines. If healthcare providers communicate effectively with each other, it helps them work as a team and makes patients feel comfortable sharing their concerns right away. Furthermore, clinical decision support systems (CDSS) enable healthcare workers to identify potential drug interactions or conditions that should not be used for each patient. For instance, knowledge of specific ADR patterns, such as skin reactions commonly associated with antiepileptics, can inform prescribing practices and mitigate risks (Caroleo et al., 2018). Therefore, including patients in their treatment and using new tools helps both parties handle the issues caused by ADRs. Exploring novel therapeutic alternatives, such as ultramicronized palmitoylethanolamide (umPEA), presents promising avenues for mitigating ADRs in patients undergoing treatment for conditions like migraine with aura. The administration of umPEA has demonstrated significant efficacy and safety, indicating its potential as a beneficial adjunct in pain management while minimizing unwanted effects commonly linked with conventional analgesics (Caroleo et al., 2018). By using these new therapies, it may be possible to reduce ADRs in at-risk people and make treatment more successful. Because management methods are constantly shifting, clinicians should keep learning and adjust their ways of working to protect and help patients with neurological and psychiatric conditions.

9.6.1. Monitoring and Reporting ADRs

The proper reporting and surveillance of ADRs are central points in guaranteeing the safety of patients, particularly in the management of neurological and psychiatric diseases. Because pharmacological treatments in these fields are complex, physicians must be careful when prescribing medication that is usually associated with a vast array of ADRs. The importance of systematic reporting was underscored by a comprehensive review comparing ADRs in psychiatric patients, which indicated a high incidence of reactions that were directly associated with antidepressants and antipsychotics (Barvaliya et al., 2019). The evidence revealed that among the overall 4368 ADRs reported, 658 cases were from psychiatric patients, emphasizing the importance of effective monitoring systems for the detection and management of these treatment-induced side effects at the earliest. In addition to collecting baseline information on the incidence of ADRs, there should be measures in monitoring systems to establish causality and assess the severity of reported effects. By utilizing standardized tools such as the WHO-UMC criteria and Naranjo's score, it is now possible to make a more accurate identification of the drug-adverse effect relationship.

This approach could enhance the quality of reporting and facilitate a more accurate evaluation of risks associated with specific drugs in neurological and psychiatric disorders (Barvaliya et al., 2019). Such rigorous evaluation also helps in supporting safer therapeutic regimens and provides valuable information to regulatory bodies that want to establish guidelines for the safe use of psychiatric drugs. Increased awareness of ADR reporting systems is crucial for enhancing patient management outcomes and minimizing the risks associated with drug therapy. The findings of the population of psychiatric patients, in which the majority of ADRs were observed to be mild but non-preventable, highlight the need for constant surveillance and best communication among health professionals (Barvaliya et al., 2019). At the global health strategy level, for example, the addition of novel therapies, such as the nifurtimox-eflornithine combination therapy in the treatment of Human African trypanosomiasis, can support ongoing surveillance of safety profiles in diverse populations, leading to more informed drug development and clinical practices. Thus, instilling a culture of ADR monitoring and reporting in both research and clinical environments is essential to building patient safety and therapeutic efficacy.

9.6.2. Strategies for Minimizing Risk

In the context of minimizing the risks associated with Neurological and Psychiatric ADRs, the adoption of personalized medicine emerges as a pivotal strategy. Doctors use personalized medicine to select treatments that match each patient's unique genetic profile, other health issues, and primary psychiatric diagnosis. Using this method helps make more accurate predictions about ADRs and their seriousness, especially when patients take several drugs at once. Research underscores that polypharmacy can significantly heighten the incidence of adverse reactions, with severe effects potentially arising from various drug combinations, particularly in vulnerable patients (Bachmann et al., 2022). Suppose healthcare providers consider each patient's particular needs before starting treatment. In that case, they can avoid ADRs and improve the effectiveness of the treatment, thereby avoiding the common approach in pharmacotherapy today. It is important to educate people and keep an eye on them to help avoid problems from ADRs in neurological and psychiatric treatments. HCPS need to teach patients about possible side effects and why it is important to stick to the prescribed treatment plan. As a result, patients can notice any adverse reactions promptly and can seek help as soon as possible. In addition, frequent follow-up visits enable doctors to track patients' progress, make adjustments to the treatment plan as needed, and identify any new side effects. Using the same evaluation instruments during consultations helps to monitor treatment more effectively; they make it easier to assess the treatment's effectiveness and safety, allowing for prompt action to be taken when any side effects appear. This way of acting helps healthcare providers and patients team up, which reduces the chances of severe ADRs. Using non-pharmacological methods in treatment plans is a key approach to prevent the risks caused by ADRs. Psychotherapy, cognitive-behavioral therapy (CBT), and making changes to a person's lifestyle are effective ways to treat mild to moderate psychiatric conditions. Emphasizing non-pharmacological therapies not only lessens dependence on pharmacological agents but also mitigates potential drug interactions and adverse effects (Nanjegowda et al., 2009). Physical activity is often recommended as an additional therapy because it helps improve mental health and sometimes lowers the need for drugs. If healthcare providers use a holistic approach to patient care, they can handle the challenges of treatment and only give drugs when truly required, which helps reduce the risk of ADRs.

9.6.3. Role of Healthcare Professionals in Patient Education

The role of the healthcare provider in patient education is crucial when it comes to neurological and psychiatric ADRs. Patients are more likely to be obedient and actively involved in their health management when they are informed about potential ADRs. As antipsychotic drugs have complex components, patients can be subjected to more than one side effect, which induces distress and non-compliance with prescribed medications. Healthcare providers are not only medication dispensers but also key information providers, with an understanding that can empower patients to identify and report adverse reactions.

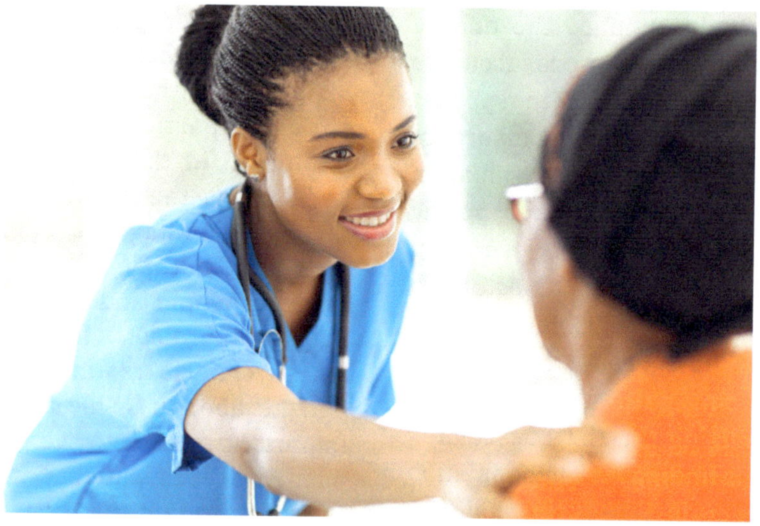

Figure 9.19. Role of healthcare professionals in patient education.

Source: https://assets.contenthub.wolterskluwer.com/api/public/content/9664e3098ab147ce977cf897548fdaf6.

Such empowerment turns the patient from a passive recipient of care to an active participant in the health process, leading to better health outcomes and fewer ADRs. Furthermore, the EIs performed by medical professionals, particularly on mental health issues, are of special significance in the prevention of ADRs. Evidence has confirmed that the implementation of certain education interventions has improved the level of knowledge amongst HCPs and patients as well. Documentation and discussion of documentation-based ADRs regarding antipsychotic medications, for instance, are at the heart of optimizing patient outcomes. Research identifies that training healthcare practitioners on proper reporting procedures for ADRs, such as recording the nature of reactions and providing necessary counseling, significantly improves the quantity and quality of reporting. By fostering a sense of responsibility for monitoring patient reactions, HCPs can provide a tighter safety net that maximizes the monitoring and management of ADRs, ultimately building a stronger healthcare system. Furthermore, some training programs aimed at providing improved knowledge and skills to NSHWs and other healthcare personnel will have a long-term impact on the delivery of mental health care, particularly in low- and middle-income nations (LMICs). They are often the first point of contact for patients, and their ability to advise patients about the outcomes of mental healthcare therapies—like the identification and notification of ADRs—is crucial. By prioritizing education for NSHWs and integrating them into the broader healthcare system, it is straightforward to significantly improve the outcomes of disease management. This patient-based model of education by a team of HCPs not only ensures integrative care but also reduces the overall workload of specialist services, recognizing the contributing role of every healthcare professional towards the prevention of the challenges posed by neurological and psychiatric ADRs (Altman et al., 2011; Purcell et al., 2014) (Figure 9.19).

Summary

The exploration of neurological and psychiatric ADRs underscores the complexity of drug interactions within the CNS. Taking drugs that target neurotransmitters can cause various neurological problems such as tremors, mental impairments, and trouble with movements. In some cases, antipsychotics have been associated with severe motor problems that lower the patient's quality of life. It is crucial to understand these interactions, particularly in clinical settings, as adjusting medications can lead to improved outcomes. Since monitoring ADRs properly is crucial for patients and their treatment, it is now especially important to use a comprehensive approach that combines clinical evaluations and pharmacogenomics. Research should continue in the field of ADRs, especially for psychiatric medications, since it is essential. Analysis of genetic factors related to haloperidol-induced side effects gives important information about people's responses, suggesting that precision medicine should be used in psychiatry. According to recent studies, differences in the CYP3A4 gene may cause drugs to be processed differently and could predict the outcomes of treatment. Therefore, clinicians need to include genetic screening in their regular psychiatric assessments to help them foresee and control any adverse outcomes. As a result, these new developments may guide doctors in creating personalized treatments that keep patients safe and enable them to gain the most from their therapies. Moreover, using dance therapy and other non-pharmacological methods may be a creative way to handle neurological problems caused by medicines. A study that shows dance therapy can help people with Parkinson's Disease improve their walking proves that combining alternative methods with standard medication may be beneficial. Working on both motor and cognitive skills using a well-planned approach helps patients and also reduces the risks of ADR. When such strategies are used, healthcare providers can help patients recover for longer and achieve better results, which proves the importance of using a mix of approaches to treat neurological and psychiatric ADRs.

A comprehensive examination of neurological and psychiatric ADRs reveals significant insights crucial for HCPs. A main worry is whether the medications used on patients with psychiatric disorders are both practical and safe. Studies show that the right medications and their proper use are important for successful mental health care. Evidence shows that NSHWs and other professionals with health roles (OPHRs) have potential in delivering acute mental health interventions in LMICs (Altman et al., 2011). Therefore, it is essential for these professionals to understand how these frameworks can benefit or harm patients and how they can achieve the best possible results. The ability of drugs to quickly calm a patient is also essential when dealing with ADRs. Reviewing existing guidelines shows that there is not much agreement on the best treatment for agitation and aggression in psychiatric facilities. Research compiled by the National Institute for Health and Care Excellence (NICE) has identified critical gaps in high-quality clinical trial evidence, making it challenging to recommend a definitive medication regime for rapid tranquillisation (Branford et al., 2008). As best practices keep changing, it becomes clear that healthcare providers need to pay close attention to their treatment methods since ADRs may present as worsened psychiatric symptoms or physical health problems. To handle neurological and psychiatric ADRs, it is important to analyze the current guidelines for treating patients. The use of evidence-based practices and the involvement of NSHWs in mental health care can positively affect patients' outcomes now and in the future. With more research available, doctors should change their prescribing habits to lower the risk of adverse reactions and keep patients safe. There is an urgent need for further research that offers a hierarchy of clinical options, thereby equipping practitioners with the necessary tools to effectively navigate the complexities of psychiatric pharmacotherapy while managing the adverse effects associated with these medications (Altman et al., 2011). Besides, increasing the education of health workers in handling ADRs can enhance mental health care services.

CLOSER LOOK

SELECTIVE SEROTONIN REUPTAKE INHIBITORS (SSRIS)

Selective serotonin reuptake inhibitors (SSRIs) are a class of antidepressant medications widely used to treat mood disorders such as depression, anxiety disorders, obsessive-compulsive disorder (OCD), and post-traumatic stress disorder (PTSD). SSRIs work by increasing the level of serotonin, a key neurotransmitter involved in regulating mood, emotion, and sleep. They achieve this by blocking the reabsorption (reuptake) of serotonin into neurons, making more of it available in the brain. Common SSRIs include fluoxetine, sertraline, paroxetine, citalopram, and escitalopram. Compared to older antidepressants like tricyclics and monoamine oxidase inhibitors (MAOIs), SSRIs are preferred due to their more favorable side effect profile and greater safety in overdose situations.

Despite their efficacy, SSRIs are not universally effective and can take several weeks to show noticeable benefits. Side effects may include nausea, insomnia, sexual dysfunction, and weight changes, although these often lessen over time. In some cases, particularly in young adults and adolescents, SSRIs may increase the risk of suicidal thoughts during the initial stages of treatment, necessitating close monitoring. Additionally, abrupt discontinuation can lead to withdrawal-like symptoms, known as SSRI discontinuation syndrome, which can include dizziness, irritability, and flu-like symptoms.

SSRIs are often considered the first-line pharmacological treatment for depression and related disorders, and they are frequently used in combination with psychotherapy for more comprehensive care. Ongoing research explores the genetic and biological factors that influence individual response to SSRIs, aiming to personalize treatment and minimize adverse effects. While not a cure for mental illness, SSRIs have significantly improved the quality of life for many individuals by stabilizing mood and enabling functional recovery. As understanding of brain chemistry and personalized medicine advances, SSRI use may become more precisely targeted, maximizing benefits while minimizing risks.

References

1. Agnetti, V., Aiello, E., De Natale, E., et al. (2012). Effects of dance therapy on balance, gait and neuro-psychological performances in patients with Parkinson's disease and postural instability. https://core.ac.uk/download/16749566.pdf (accessed on 9 June 2025).
2. Borg, J. J., Tanti, A., Kouvelas, D., Lungu, C., Pirozynski, M., Serracino-Inglott, A., & Aislaitner, G. (2015). European Union pharmacovigilance capabilities: potential for the new legislation. *Therapeutic Advances in Drug Safety*, *6*(4), 120–140. https://doi.org/10.1177/2042098615591802Amor, S., Martino, G., Nutma, E., et al. (2019). Neuroimmunology–the past, present and future. https://core.ac.uk/download/237397381.pdf.
3. Andrade, D. M., Beier, C. P., Crudgington, H., et al. (2020). Trait impulsivity in juvenile myoclonic epilepsy. https://core.ac.uk/download/478090975.pdf (accessed on 9 June 2025).
4. Antony, G., Briegel, W., Correll, C. U., et al. (2022). Serious adverse drug reactions in children and adolescents treated on- and off-label with antidepressants and antipsychotics in clinical practice. https://core.ac.uk/download/552136397.pdf (accessed on 9 June 2025).
5. Arulsamy, A. (2024). *Consensus Guidelines on The Management of Epilepsy 2024*. https://core.ac.uk/download/622492633.pdf (accessed on 9 June 2025).
6. Bachmann, S., Bridler, R., Cattapan, K., et al. (2022). Detailing the effects of polypharmacy in psychiatry: Longitudinal study of 320 patients hospitalized for depression or schizophrenia. https://core.ac.uk/download/551536593.pdf (accessed on 9 June 2025).
7. Barnes, T. R. E., Drake, R., Paton, C., Cooper, S., Deakin, J. F. W., Ferrier, I. N., Gregory, C. J., et al. (2019). Evidence-based guidelines for the pharmacological treatment of schizophrenia: Updated recommendations from the British Association for Psychopharmacology. *Journal of Psychopharmacology, 34*, 3–78. https://doi.org/10.1177/0269881119889296.
8. Barvaliya, S., Desai, M. K., Panchal, J. R., et al. (2019). Pattern of adverse drug reactions in psychiatric patients. https://core.ac.uk/download/539896551.pdf (accessed on 9 June 2025).
9. Bellomo, A., Daniele, A., di Mauro, L., et al. (2018). CYP2D6 genotypes in revolving door patients with bipolar disorders: A case series. https://core.ac.uk/download/199256441.pdf (accessed on 9 June 2025).
10. Berwian, B., Brites, D., Campbell, I., Heneka, M. T., Heras-Sandoval, D., Kenis, G., Müller, N., et al. (2020). Neuroinflammation and its resolution: From molecular mechanisms to therapeutic perspectives. https://core.ac.uk/download/305118427.pdf (accessed on 9 June 2025).
11. Bevinahalli Nanjegowda, R., Muthugaduru Shivarudrappa, N. K., Mysore Nagaraj, A., Anil Kumar, Pai, et al. (2009). Etiology and management of sexual dysfunction. https://core.ac.uk/download/pdf/87259.pdf.
12. Bizzarri, C., Cummings, J. L., Fernandez, H. H., Fernandez, H., Fénelon, G., Gama, R. L., Goldman, J. G., et al. (2017). Atypical antipsychotic therapy in Parkinson's disease psychosis: A retrospective study. https://core.ac.uk/download/323069922.pdf.
13. Branford, D., Chandler-Oatts, J., Johnston, S., et al. (2008). Establishing gold standard approaches to rapid tranquillization: A review and discussion of the evidence on the safety and efficacy of medications currently used. https://core.ac.uk/download/48632.pdf (accessed on 9 June 2025).

14. Bratis, D., Moussas, G., Pachi, A., et al. (2013). Psychiatric morbidity and other factors affecting treatment adherence in pulmonary tuberculosis patients. https://core.ac.uk/download/205350310.pdf (accessed on 9 June 2025).
15. Brilot, F., Dale, R. C., Hong, M., et al. (2016). Symptomatic treatment of children with anti-NMDAR encephalitis. https://core.ac.uk/download/154325198.pdf (accessed on 9 June 2025).
16. Caroleo, M. C., Chirchiglia, D., Cione, E., et al. (2018). Effects of add-on ultra micronized n-palmitoylethanolamide in patients suffering from migraine with aura: A pilot study. https://core.ac.uk/download/188825458.pdf (accessed on 9 June 2025).
17. Cavanna, A. E., Holler-Managan, Y., Jankovic, J., et al. (2019). Practice guideline recommendations summary: Treatment of tics in people with Tourette syndrome and chronic tic disorders. https://core.ac.uk/download/322826139.pdf (accessed on 9 June 2025).
18. Chiappini, S., Corkery, J. M., De Berardis, D., et al. (2019). The bridge between classical and 'synthetic'/chemical psychoses: Towards a clinical, psychopathological and therapeutic perspective. https://core.ac.uk/download/287582435.pdf (accessed on 9 June 2025).
19. Cyriac, S. T., & Iype, D. S. (2021). Neuropsychiatric adverse effects of antibacterial agents. https://core.ac.uk/download/482241775.pdf (accessed on 9 June 2025).
20. de Leon, J., Italiano, D., & Spina, E. (2014). Pharmacokinetic and pharmacodynamic interactions between antiepileptics and antidepressants. https://core.ac.uk/download/232567273.pdf (accessed on 9 June 2025).
21. De Ronchi, D., Drago, A., Giegling, I., et al. (2012). No association of a set of candidate genes on haloperidol side effects. https://core.ac.uk/download/12175449.pdf (accessed on 9 June 2025).
22. Deore, A., Deshpande, P., Jacob, A., et al. (2021). Appraisal and discernment of prevalent drug-drug interactions in patients with psychiatric disorders. https://core.ac.uk/download/543134071.pdf (accessed on 9 June 2025).
23. Desestret, V., Honnorat, J., Joubert, B., Muniz-Castrillo, S., & Vogrig, A. (2020). Pathophysiology of paraneoplastic and autoimmune encephalitis: Genes, infections, and checkpoint inhibitors. https://core.ac.uk/download/576927694.pdf (accessed on 9 June 2025).
24. Di Mauro, G., Zinzi, A., Scavone, C., Mascolo, A., Gaio, M., Sportiello, L., Ferrajolo, C., et al. (2020). PCSK9 inhibitors and neurocognitive adverse drug reactions: Analysis of individual case safety reports from the Eudravigilance database. *Drug Safety, 44*, 337–349. https://www.semanticscholar.org/paper/0e57a37f837b1319916c454a9d326e4a818f7690 (accessed on 9 June 2025).
25. Domènech, È., Farré, M., Gich, I., López Valverde, M., et al. (2021). Spontaneous reporting of adverse drug reactions in a pediatric population in a tertiary hospital. https://core.ac.uk/download/541736890.pdf (accessed on 9 June 2025).
26. Erakhtin, E., Narodov, A., Narodova, E., et al. (2018). The role of nondrug treatment methods in the management of epilepsy. https://core.ac.uk/download/322439899.pdf (accessed on 9 June 2025).
27. Everitt, H., Baldwin, D. S., Stuart, B., Lipinska, G., Mayers, A., Malizia, A. L., Manson, C. C. F., & Wilson, S. (2018). *Antidepressants for Insomnia in Adults*. https://core.ac.uk/download/157860236.pdf (accessed on 9 June 2025).

28. Gawali, U. P., Gawand, K. S., & Kesari, H. V. (2017). Adverse drug reaction profile at psychiatry outpatient department of a tertiary care center. https://core.ac.uk/download/539896693.pdf (accessed on 9 June 2025).

29. Giblin, S. (2018). *Ambiguities in the Efficacy of Selective Serotonin Reuptake Inhibitors in The Treatment of Depression*. https://core.ac.uk/download/231068077.pdf (accessed on 9 June 2025).

30. Hartinger, J., Dvořáčková, E., Mysliveček, M., Hrušková, Z., Satny, M., Zlatohlavek, L., Krizova, J., et al. (2023). The frequency of, and predisposing risk factors for, ciprofloxacin-induced neuropsychiatric adverse drug reactions. *Bratislavské Lekárske Listy, 124*(10), 779–782. https://www.semanticscholar.org/paper/9fa0af78f67b1ce410bb91fb7ec999b9edf55dd5 (accessed on 9 June 2025).

31. Ide, M., Ohnishi, T., Toyoshima, M., Balan, S., Maekawa, M., Shimamoto-Mitsuyama, C., Iwayama, Y., et al. (2019). Excess hydrogen sulfide and polysulfides production underlies a schizophrenia pathophysiology. *EMBO Molecular Medicine, 11*. https://doi.org/10.15252/emmm.201910695.

32. Lee, D. W., Santomasso, B., Locke, F. L., Ghobadi, A., Turtle, C. J., Brudno, J. N., Maus, M. V., et al. (2018). ASTCT consensus grading for cytokine release syndrome and neurologic toxicity associated with immune effector cells. *Biology of Blood and Marrow Transplantation, 25*, 625–638. https://doi.org/10.1016/j.bbmt.2018.12.758.

33. Maheswari, E., Grace, J. R., Srinivasa, R., Saina, S., et al. (2018). Assessment of adverse drug reactions occurring at Department of Neurology of a tertiary care hospital in India. https://core.ac.uk/download/477854727.pdf (accessed on 9 June 2025).

34. McClellan, J., & Stock, S. (2013). Practice parameter for the assessment and treatment of children and adolescents with schizophrenia. *Journal of the American Academy of Child & Adolescent Psychiatry, 52*, 976–990. https://doi.org/10.1016/j.jaac.2013.02.008.

35. Orešković, A., Restek-Petrović, B., Bodor, D., Mihanović, M., Presečki, P., & Molnar, S. (2010). Suicidality and side effects of antidepressants and antipsychotics. https://core.ac.uk/download/14419902.pdf (accessed on 9 June 2025).

36. Packer, R. M. A., & Volk, H. A. (2025). Epilepsy beyond seizures: A review of the impact of epilepsy and its comorbidities on health-related quality of life in dogs. https://core.ac.uk/download/36778816.pdf (accessed on 9 June 2025).

37. Paunova, S. S., Labutina, N. V., Zubavina, M. N., Shibilova, M. M., Skvortsova, T., Strokova, T. V., Bagaeva, M., et al. (2025). Drug-associated nephrotic syndrome in a child with Wilson–Konovalov disease. *Russian Medicine*. https://www.semanticscholar.org/paper/e85cf7522d316b42b1d94fe327276ce26115a072 (accessed on 9 June 2025).

38. Purcell, G. M. (2014). *Intervention to Improve the Level of Documentation of Antipsychotic-Related Adverse Drug Reactions*. https://core.ac.uk/download/145036001.pdf.

39. Scavone, C., Mascolo, A., Ruggiero, R., Sportiello, L., Rafaniello, C., Berrino, L., & Capuano, A. (2020). Quinolones-induced musculoskeletal, neurological, and psychiatric ADRs: A pharmacovigilance study based on data from the Italian spontaneous reporting system. *Frontiers in Pharmacology, 11*. https://www.semanticscholar.org/paper/b980a3c8bfbb971dbae1f95a3f0a3ea01656a92c (accessed on 9 June 2025).

40. Schwarcz, R., & Stone, T. W. (2017). The kynurenine pathway and the brain: Challenges, controversies and promises. https://core.ac.uk/download/46559921.pdf.

41. Schweitzer-Chaput, A., Callot, D., Bouazza, N., Lesage, F., Oualha, M., Paret, N., Boyer-Gervoise, M., et al. (2023). Local anesthetics systemic toxicity in children: Analysis of the French pharmacovigilance database. *BMC Pediatrics, 23.* https://www.semanticscholar.org/paper/c44c7c4f5ef51aaf396e49fbb8cdc5df99cf3918 (accessed on 9 June 2025).

42. Shingala, K., & Nariya, D. (2025). Severe cutaneous adverse reaction to lamotrigine: A case of Stevens-Johnson syndrome in a psychiatric patient. *Cureus, 17.* https://www.semanticscholar.org/paper/a5ae4f0f4c46c35621757e694a5d15bcac034d17 (accessed on 9 June 2025).

43. Stanghellini, A., Kuemmerle, A., Burri, C., Schmid, C., Schmid, C., Tete, D., Matovu, E., et al. (2012). In-hospital safety in field conditions of Nifurtimox Eflornithine Combination Therapy (NECT) for T. B. gambiense sleeping sickness. https://core.ac.uk/download/pdf/10674384.pdf (accessed on 9 June 2025).

44. van Gerven, J., & Bonelli, M. (2018). Commentary on the EMA guideline on strategies to identify and mitigate risks for first-in-human and early clinical trials with investigational medicinal products. *British Journal of Clinical Pharmacology, 84*, 1401–1409. https://doi.org/10.1111/bcp.13550.

45. van Ginneken, N., Tharyan, P., Lewin, S., Rao, G. N., Romeo, R., & Patel, V. (2011). Non-specialist health worker interventions for mental health care in low- and middle-income countries. https://core.ac.uk/download/13113977.pdf (accessed on 9 June 2025).

46. Weißhaar, E., Szepietowski, J. C., Dalgard, F., Garcovich, S., Gieler, U., Giménez-Arnau, A. M., Lambert, J., et al. (2019). European S2k guideline on chronic pruritus. *Acta Dermato-Venereologica, 99*, 469–506. https://doi.org/10.2340/00015555-3164.

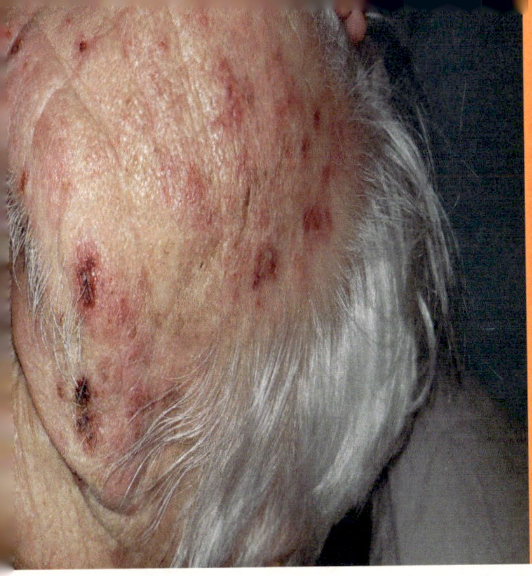

Chapter 10

DERMATOLOGICAL REACTIONS TO DRUGS

Contents

Introduction

Over the past two decades, the fact that skin reactions have become a central problem in drug safety has been of significant interest. The reaction may manifest in various ways, ranging from mild rashes to severe infections, such as SJS. The polymorphic character of the skin reactions poses a challenge to clinicians and drug researchers. Clarification of the mechanisms responsible for such reactions is imperative for effective patient management and the avoidance of morbidity due to ADRs. As the clinician is faced with a variety of drugs and patient types, recognition of the broad array of dermatologic reactions is essential. The significance of the topic is underscored by the increasing complexity of pharmacotherapy that necessitates meticulous monitoring and reporting of ADRs to inform future prescribing practice and improve the outcomes of patients (Adhikari et al., 2009). Furthermore, the surveillance of dermatological reactions becomes particularly relevant in light of the expanding drug armamentarium introduced into clinical practice. In particular, the role of antimicrobial medications and psychotropic drugs has been emphasized in numerous research studies, revealing that these agents have often been associated with a significant proportion of ADRs. According to a study, it was found that antimicrobials were a significant share of observed adverse events, alluding to the need for better surveillance and reporting mechanisms of ADRs in various clinical environments (Adhikari et al., 2009). Such findings not only indicate a requirement for vigilant close observation but also point to how such responses can impact drug treatment protocols and overall healthcare delivery. Since patient treatment is increasingly reliant on multi-drug regimens, how drugs interact with cutaneous systems remains important to understand. The requirement for strict ADR monitoring extends beyond mere detection to encompass a sustainable method for patient safety, which includes active assessment and management by healthcare professionals (HCPs). Initiatives aimed at educating HCPs regarding the risk for dermatological reactions, especially in vulnerable populations, can actually enhance the quality of care and improve patient outcomes. The prevalence of infections like Chagas disease, which requires specific drug treatment with documented side effects, constitutes the best example of the need for these educational measures. As an illustration, the benznidazole experience with the treatment of Chagas disease revealed a high frequency of minor side effects, highlighting the need for education of patients and monitoring during treatment. Thus, a thorough understanding of drug safety and the ability to anticipate and manage potential dermatologic effects are crucial for achieving optimal therapeutic benefits and ensuring patient safety in the clinic (Figure 10.1).

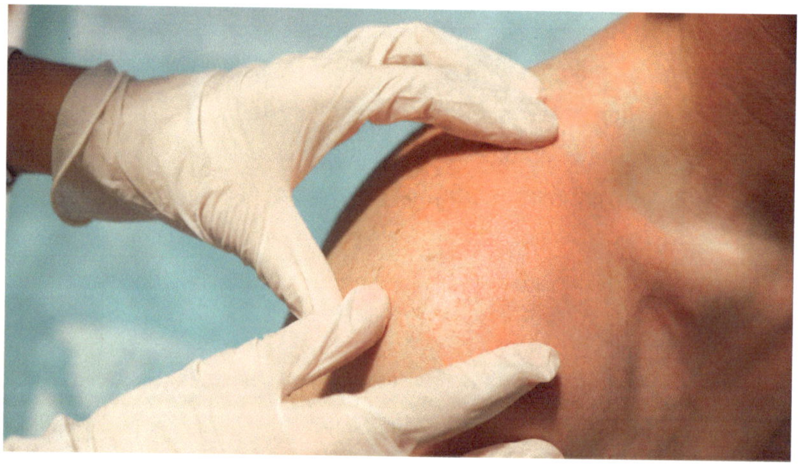

Figure 10.1. Dermatological reactions to drugs.

Source: https://images.ctfassets.net/4f3rgqwzdznj/18uwruYkfW9LLF2pYvpTJO/4ca55097f0ba97970b37cb90d9aaa176/closeup_man_shoulder_rash_1327181307.jpg.

Definition of Dermatological Reactions

It is necessary to define what dermatological reactions to drugs involve before discussing them. Typically, dermatological reactions are skin problems that occur as a result of pharmacological treatment. Some reactions are only mild, while others are very serious, such as drug-induced dermatitis, which might cause rashes, urticaria, and eczema. A widely accepted definition of adverse drug reactions (ADRs) comes from the World Health Organization (WHO), describing them as any harmful and unintended response that occurs at doses typically used in humans. This definition highlights the importance of recognizing the diverse manifestations that dermatological reactions can present, as they not only affect the skin but also significantly impact a patient's quality of life and treatment compliance, particularly in chronic conditions (Gupta et al., 2021). When dealing with these reactions, it is necessary to tell apart the different types. For instance, some dermatological reactions fall under the category of cutaneous adverse drug reactions (CADRs), which may be classified into several types based on their pathophysiology, ranging from immunological reactions to pharmacological toxicity. Sometimes, psoriasis can appear or worsen while undergoing drug treatment, pointing to how complicated and surprising these reactions can be. Many studies have pointed out that dermatological ADRs are common and make up a significant portion of all reported adverse reactions in different areas of medicine. For example, in an observational study on individuals undergoing antiretroviral therapy (ART), dermatological reactions were identified in 12.8% of cases, indicating the need for ongoing surveillance in clinical practice (Gupta et al., 2021). Additionally, there are cases where patients develop new or more severe skin problems due to the treatment, which introduces a new aspect to dermatological reactions. The literature documents instances where patients undergoing treatment for psoriasis with biologics developed psoriatic lesions at different anatomical sites, often categorized as paradoxical adverse events (PAEs). Such cases can alter the way treatment is administered, prompting doctors to reconsider the benefits and drawbacks for patients. Such reactions must be addressed by acting promptly and by employing long-term strategies that include reevaluation and, if necessary, modification of the treatment plan. For the best results and patient safety in drug therapy, it is necessary to fully understand what dermatological reactions mean and how they can affect treatment.

Importance of Studying Drug Reactions

Study of drug reactions, particularly cutaneous reactions, is vital to both therapeutic effectiveness and patient safety. Cutaneous adverse reactions can range from benign rashes to morbid, even life-threatening conditions like SJS. Understanding the mechanisms by which drugs induce such reactions allows clinicians to recognize at-risk populations, tailor treatments, and prevent adverse consequences. With the pharmaceutical environment consistently evolving, new drugs being introduced to the market at regular intervals, close monitoring of these responses becomes increasingly essential. In this regard, the importance of an efficient pharmacovigilance system that identifies and analyzes information on drug reactions becomes increasingly essential in enabling clinical guidelines and policy formulations for safe consumption of drugs. These systems not only protect the patients but also allow for the overall progress of medical treatments such that the drug interventions' advantages are greater than the risk incurred. Over the last few decades, advances in therapies such as targeted therapies, specifically therapeutic monoclonal antibodies (mAbs), have revolutionized the treatment of numerous diseases, including cancer. However, the new skin reactions of these drugs require stern consideration and understanding. The heightened application of monoclonal antibody treatments has placed a strain on targeted dermatologic research, as some patients can develop hypersensitivity or allergic reactions that, if poorly managed, can lead to treatment discontinuation or even severe complications (Ruei-Lu et al., 2020). This is an evolving situation where healthcare providers must build a strong knowledge base of cutaneous side effects associated with new therapeutics, embracing evidence-based practice to mitigate such adverse effects. By monitoring drug reactions closely, clinicians can maximize patient care, maximize compliance with treatment, and maximize therapeutic strategies to minimize the dangers of drug-induced skin reactions. In addition to providing individualized care for patients, understanding the clinical significance of drug reactions has broader implications that extend into public health. Cutaneous expressions of drug reactions can have a disproportionate impact on drug development and regulation. For instance, the pattern recognition of a reaction to a skin irritant can prompt regulatory agencies to revise labeling requirements, incorporate risk communication methods, and initiate monitoring programs for a new medication (Daniel et al., 2018). This leads to enhanced transparency within the healthcare system, promoting informed decision-making by both patients and providers. Additionally, continuous learning about drug reactions is crucial for healthcare professionals to enhance their diagnostic skills and achieve better patient outcomes. Since cutaneous reactions have a tendency to be the first sign of systemic disease, their examination not only boosts patient safety but also provides insight into the general effectiveness of therapy (Figure 10.2).

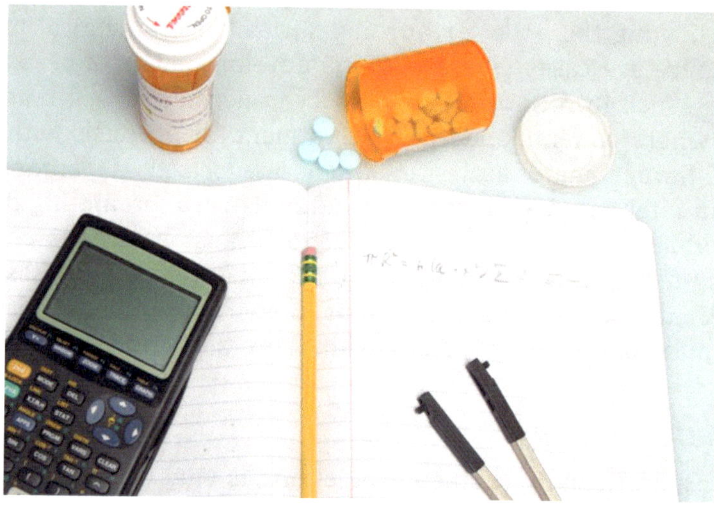

Figure 10.2. Importance of studying drug reactions.

Source: https://ranchatdovetree.com/wp-content/uploads/2016/04/study-drugs-college.jpg.

10.1. Types of Dermatological Reactions

There are many ways dermatological problems can develop from taking medicines, and these are mainly divided into allergic and non-allergic reactions. An allergic reaction typically occurs when a person is overly sensitive to a substance, causing the immune system to react and resulting in symptoms such as urticaria, eczema, and contact dermatitis. In some cases, non-allergic reactions occur due to toxic effects or the direct impact of medications, even when the immune system is not involved. Common examples include fixed drug eruptions and drug-induced photosensitivity. It is crucial to distinguish between these two categories because the treatment and diagnostic strategies differ for each one. Within the realm of allergic dermatoses, drug reaction with eosinophilia and systemic symptoms (DRESS) syndrome presents a severe manifestation, characterized by fever, lymphadenopathy, and skin rash, accompanied by eosinophilia and internal organ involvement. Since DRESS syndrome can be life-threatening, it is important to identify it and take the offending drug out of the patient's system right away. It is essential to utilize various areas of expertise when managing a condition that affects the entire body, as demonstrated in numerous clinical studies. In some serious cases, doctors may have to give certain treatments to reduce the effects of severe inflammation, which shows how important it is for HCPs to watch for major drug-induced allergies. Apart from hypersensitivity reactions (HSRs) and DRESS, other skin reactions to drugs consist of fixed drug eruptions and lichenoid drug reactions. If a fixed drug eruption occurs, it appears as one or more slightly raised patches that come back in the same place when the drug is taken again, so it should be recognized early to avoid further problems. Because lichenoid drug reactions look like lichen planus, it is important to tell them apart from other skin problems. In most cases, the offending drug needs to be stopped and, in some cases, topical corticosteroids are used to reduce the symptoms. With this knowledge, doctors can better handle their patients and lower the risk of serious complications from drugs that affect the skin.

10.1.1. Allergic Reactions

Drug allergic reactions are characterized as a significant issue in dermatological practice because they can cause a range of skin manifestations. Allergic drug reactions tend to be more grouped under the category of HSRs, i.e., types I to IV, characterized by unique immune mechanisms. Dermatological reactions are typically characterized by urticaria, eczema, and, in more severe cases, anaphylaxis, which may present in severe forms as skin symptoms such as pruritus and erythema. Their research is needed as they can cause serious health issues if not treated immediately. Pruritus, for instance, or severe itching, is one of the most prevalent symptoms that also plagues patients, affecting their quality of life quite significantly. Use of kandugna medicines has been found to relieve this disturbing symptom, testifying to the usefulness of information regarding drug interactions in the successful treatment of dermatologic allergic manifestations (Vd. Chipkar et al., 2024).

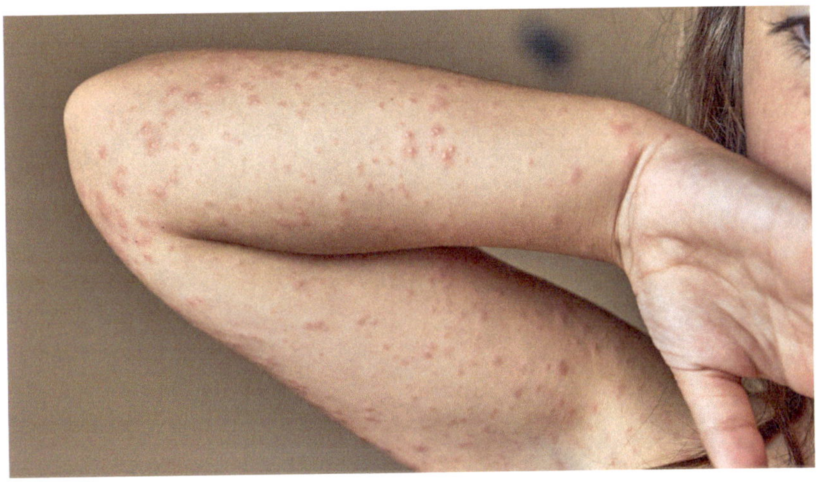

Figure 10.3. Allergic reactions.

Source: https://images.ctfassets.net/4f3rgqwzdznj/2TaXFCCvvdpN2MdWVmTpoE/4e3d68bea6db1eb537556cd181db8a14/cropped_womans_arm_allergic_rash-1337085512.jpg.

Drug allergic reactions are also made more challenging due to their varied presentation, which may often mimic dermatologic conditions due to infections or systemic illnesses. Allergic reactions can lead to skin diseases such as acanthosis nigricans, which is a symptom that may be a precursor to occult malignancies and must therefore be assessed for the patient. An example is Sweet syndrome, a drug reaction and malignancy-associated neutrophilic dermatosis, characterized by erythematous papules with pain on examination and evidence of systemic involvement, such as fever. The coexistence of these cutaneous manifestations and severe systemic diseases emphasizes the importance of a paradigm of differential diagnosis. Recognition of the etiology of skin reactions will lead clinicians to the appropriate therapeutic strategies for managing skin manifestations and precipitating disorders (Syed et al., 2023). Treatment of allergic reactions in clinical practice is multidimensional with identification of the etiological factors and symptom management. Selection of the appropriate antihistamines and corticosteroids is crucial for preventing skin eruptions and associated discomfort. Additionally, physicians must closely monitor patients for potential recurrences or exacerbations of symptoms upon re-exposure to allergens. The need for individualized treatment protocols is still more essential when one considers the vast range of drug reactions that may manifest in the same dermatologic presentations. Physicians must educate patients on how to recognize early warning signs of allergic reactions and the importance of seeking medical care promptly. This patient education concern, coupled with critical clinical assessment, forms the basis of effective management practices in drug-induced allergic dermatological reactions (Figure 10.3).

10.1.2. Irritant Reactions

Irritant reactions are an important type of drug-induced skin reaction, caused by direct harm to the skin's barrier and not by the immune system. Common reactions can occur when people use corticosteroids or other medications that contain cleansers or irritants. Allergic reactions require the immune system to be involved, whereas irritant reactions can occur in anyone exposed to a high concentration of the irritant, making them non-selective. Both clinicians and patients should fully understand this distinction, as it guides both the prevention and management of these reactions. In most cases, irritant reactions are assessed based on the patient's history and the appearance of lesions, rather than through numerous tests.

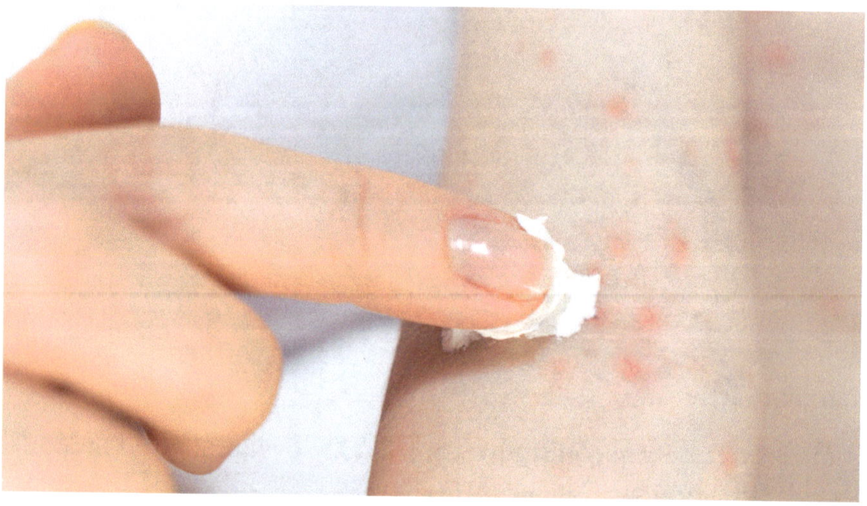

Figure 10.4. Irritant reactions.

Source: https://images.ctfassets.net/4f3rgqwzdznj/3xy8qGciMu5fpQ3uPqwuYP/9c8c7efad9e1ffcacb1552af838e12d4/applying_cream_on_rash_1166704810.jpg.

For example, if eyeglass frames cause irritant contact dermatitis, it is necessary to examine the materials, including metals and plastics, as they can irritate the skin at the points of contact. It has been observed recently that certain eyeglass frame materials, including plasticizers and nickel, may trigger irritation in individuals who are sensitive. Clinicians use patch testing to determine the cause of the problem, which enables them to provide the appropriate treatment. Because of this, it is essential to select eyewear materials that prevent skin irritation and ensure patients feel comfortable. Sometimes, the use of topical corticosteroids for skin problems can lead to irritant reactions. Although they are effective in reducing inflammation in skin conditions, using them excessively or incorrectly can lead to skin atrophy in the affected area, which can exacerbate the irritation. A study on how topical steroids are prescribed pointed out that hypopigmentation and acne are common side effects. However, they can be mistaken for different skin conditions instead of being linked to the medicine. According to the study, checking and reviewing steroid prescriptions is very important to control these risks. Stressing the importance of both the effectiveness of a drug and its potential for irritation enables doctors to enhance patient care and reduce dermatological issues associated with medications, thereby facilitating the selection of the most suitable topical agents (Figure 10.4).

10.1.3. Photosensitivity Reactions

Photosensitivity reactions are a significant problem in the arena of drug dermatologic reactions, manifesting most frequently as an abnormal sensitivity of the skin to light after being given certain drugs. The hypersensitive response can vary wildly in its presentation and potentially result in such concerns as rashes, hives, or even life-threatening conditions such as toxic epidermal necrolysis (TEN). Patients also exhibit erythema, pruritus, and lesions in sun-exposed areas, indicating a direct relationship between the photoreactive character of the drugs and sun exposure. Interestingly, drugs such as dapsone have been noted to induce such reactions, and the presented cases placed a stress on being cautious when starting medications known to cause photosensitivity. Understanding the mechanisms and clinical presentations of photosensitivity will enable healthcare workers to manage and diagnose these skin reactions effectively, thereby reducing patient morbidity. Photosensitivity reaction mechanisms are usually intricate biochemical interactions between specific medications and ultraviolet (UV) light. Some medications can adsorb UV light, with resultant reactive species causing damage to cells or inducing an inflammatory response in the skin. For instance, photodegradation of surface agents has the potential to alter their structure, with the potential to generate toxic by-products or enhance their dermatological activity. The process is particularly significant in the case of dermatological preparations, where local application is the standard. As mentioned in the literature, the susceptibility of surface materials to photodegradation is of utmost significance in understanding the therapeutic activity and safety of compounds in sun-exposed areas. Other variables that may influence the severity of such reactions include light intensity, chemical structure, and environmental factors (Kryczyk-Poprawa et al., 2019). Knowledge of such a process is crucial in making informed decisions about drug prescriptions and patient education regarding sun protection. The management of photosensitivity reactions encompasses both preventive and therapeutic actions. Physicians must educate patients regarding risk factors related to specific drugs, especially drugs with known phototoxic or photoallergic potential. Practical advice includes avoiding sunlight during peak hours, using protective clothing, and applying broad-spectrum sunscreens. In cases of photosensitivity, withdrawal of the offending drug is generally necessary on an immediate basis, as evident in examples of patients developing adverse reactions to drugs like dapsone; the symptoms tend to improve on withdrawal and recur on re-exposure (Garg et al., 2017). Moreover, monitoring of patients with close observation for cutaneous reactions during the commencement of therapy will be helpful in minimizing adverse outcomes. Lastly, understanding and management of photosensitivity reactions are crucial in the therapeutic application of dermatologic medications, thereby ensuring therapeutic efficacy while prioritizing patient safety (Figure 10.5).

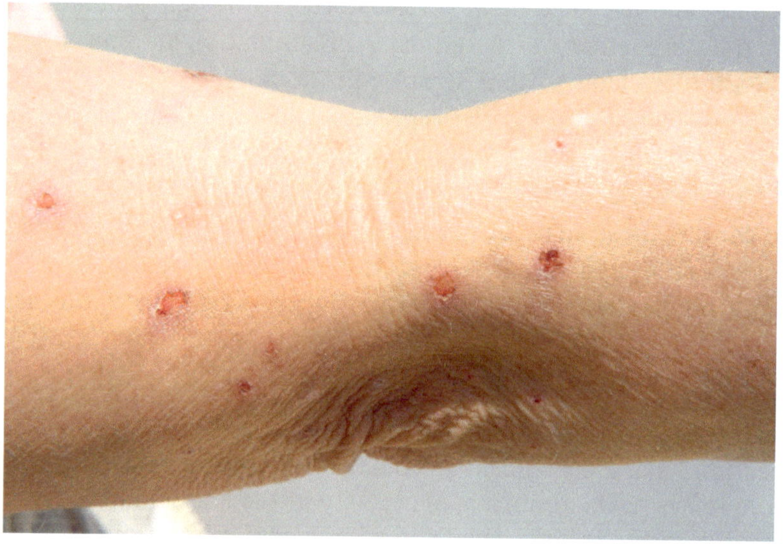

Figure 10.5. Photosensitivity reactions.

Source: https://www.verywellhealth.com/thmb/5-C38gQPeD8GHYZLFeIkpTddNmA=/2107x1423/filters:fill(87E3EF,1)/GettyImages-182025759-588702ff5f9b58bdb3966315.jpg.

10.2. Mechanisms of Drug-Induced Skin Reactions

The ways drugs can cause skin reactions are complex and typically involve the immune system. A common way it works is by binding to proteins in the skin and making new antigenic complexes. As a result of this process, a person may develop contact dermatitis. If an allergen is encountered, the immune system gets sensitized first and then, on subsequent exposures, it causes erythema, edema, and itching. The effects of such responses depend on things like a person's genetic background and how much they have been exposed to the offending substance. It is essential to understand both the way a drug is metabolized in the body and the state of the person's immune system to predict potential skin reactions. The effects of drugs on skin can also be caused by their ability to harm cells directly. Skin damage caused by certain drugs occurs when oxidative stress leads to the death of keratinocytes and disrupts the skin barrier. Such a reaction is noticeable with antineoplastic agents, as these drugs harm both cancerous and rapidly dividing cells, including those in the skin. Besides, drugs can start inflammatory processes involving cytokines and chemokines, which can lead to dermatological problems such as erythema nodosum or pemphigus. For instance, the use of certain antibiotics or non-steroidal anti-inflammatory drugs (NSAIDs) has been associated with an increased risk of skin conditions that exhibit these inflammatory responses. When these mechanisms are understood, scientists can anticipate and manage the dermatological effects of various treatments. Also, when drug metabolites come into contact with skin cells, it can cause serious reactions on the skin. Certain drugs are changed by the liver or skin, forming active metabolites that can show different effects than the original drug. Such a change in metabolism can, at times, increase the allergy-causing ability of drugs or alter how they bind to skin proteins, causing the immune system to react more strongly. Telaprevir used for hepatitis C has been linked to several skin side effects in patients who take it. During clinical studies, half of the patients experienced a rash, indicating that the drug can elicit immune reactions when it is activated in the body. Understanding these pathways is crucial for doctors and scientists to develop more effective strategies for preventing drug-related skin problems and promoting patients' overall health.

10.2.1. Immune-Mediated Mechanisms

The role of immune-mediated mechanisms in cutaneous drug reactions is at the heart of understanding the nature and scope of such drug reactions. Drug-induced skin reactions typically follow an interaction between the pharmacologic profile of the drug and the host's complex immune response. For instance, if a foreign substance is introduced by way of medication, it may trigger an inappropriate immune response leading to conditions such as drug rashes, urticaria, or even dangerous ones such as SJS. Advances in melanocyte biology and the immune system suggest that alterations in melanocyte function also play a role in the causation of such reactions, necessitating ongoing research in the field of dermatological sciences to elucidate the specific pathways through which the phenotype of these responses is expressed (Birlea et al., 2018).

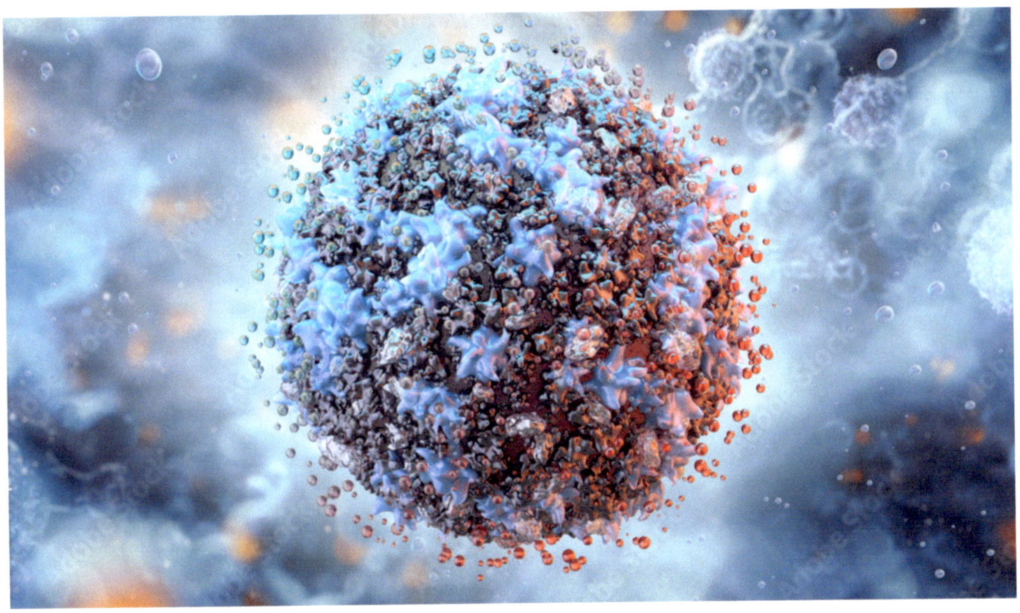

Figure 10.6. Immune-mediated mechanisms.

Source: https://as1.ftcdn.net/v2/jpg/09/56/47/24/1000_F_956472487_KCuOIY8Od0Uy9ANN1SwjFcq7R4MfnRNb.jpg.

Therapeutic medications used in treating dermatological conditions tend to consist of immunomodulatory drugs, whose immune-mediated pathways become more intricate. Medications such as TNF-α inhibitors have also been used in conditions such as psoriasis and psoriatic arthritis in a widespread manner, presenting a contrasting picture of immune mediation. A research paper on various anti-TNF medications, such as adalimumab and infliximab, detailed their efficacy and survival in treating these conditions. The findings showed that adalimumab had a higher likelihood of patient responses, as indicated by the reduction in psoriasis severity scores (PASI) compared to other TNF inhibitors (Berardesca et al., 2018). Such findings underscore the importance of selecting therapeutic drugs that strike a balance between efficacy and the risk of immune-mediated skin reactions. Apart from biologic agents, other systemic medications have been linked to immune-mediated cutaneous drug reactions, highlighting the need for heightened clinical awareness. Commonly prescribed drugs like antibiotics, anticonvulsants, and NSAIDs may cause HSRs in the pattern of drug eruptions. Pathogenic processes rely on the activation of immune cells such as T lymphocytes and B cells, which recognize drug metabolite complexes as foreign antigens. These immune reactions can cause cytotoxicity and inflammation, which are manifested as dermatological manifestations from mild rashes to severe systemic reactions. It is essential for clinicians to understand these immune-mediated pathways so that they can effectively manage drug reactions and tailor their treatment strategies, thereby maximizing patient safety and achieving optimal therapeutic effects (Birlea et al., 2018) (Figure 10.6).

10.2.2. Non-Immune-Mediated Mechanisms

Besides immune reactions, non-immune processes are also important in the range of drug-related skin problems. They consist of various biochemical and physiological pathways that lead to drug-related skin problems, but do not involve the immune system. For example, some medicines can harm the skin by being toxic or by changing how cells grow and change.

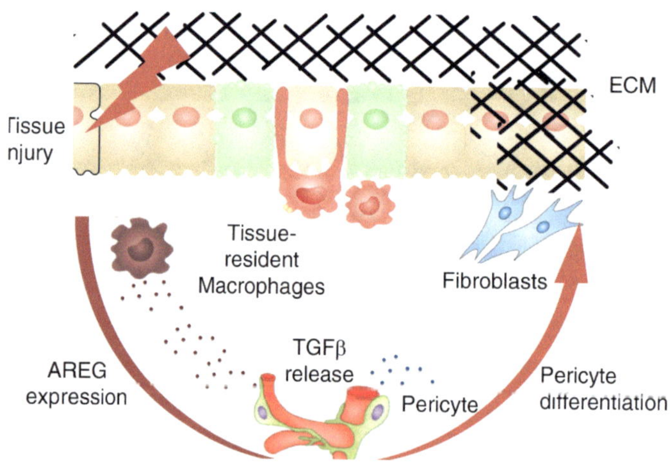

Figure 10.7. Non-immune-mediated mechanisms.

Source: https://onlinelibrary.wiley.com/cms/asset/bfc939ba-a8c6-4ec2-934b-07c6081787a3/imm13057-fig-0002-m.jpg.

As an example, some antiepileptic drugs (AEDs) can cause keratinocytes to grow too much, which may result in drug-induced psoriasis or other inflammatory skin diseases. With this knowledge, clinicians can more easily spot, predict, and handle dermatological issues that may occur due to certain drugs. Sometimes, drugs can cause reactions on the skin by directly affecting skin cells, rather than triggering the immune system. Certain drugs, when activated by UV light, can produce ROS, leading to oxidative stress and subsequent cellular damage. Often, this reaction is referred to as photodermatitis and presents as red, blistered skin lesions. Other mechanisms occur when the skin becomes more permeable or when certain metabolic pathways are triggered, resulting in more cutaneous adverse reactions. With new information, it becomes clear that clinicians should be well-informed about the dermatological side effects that can result from using different drugs. In addition, the effects of non-immune-mediated mechanisms are notable in the context of specific drug classes, such as tumor necrosis factor (TNF) inhibitors used in the treatment of psoriasis and psoriatic arthritis. Biologics may affect the skin and its cells, even without directly impacting the immune system. It is worth noting that recent studies have highlighted the significant differences in drug survival rates and responses among patients treated with various anti-TNF agents. Specifically, adalimumab has demonstrated greater effectiveness than etanercept and infliximab in maintaining therapeutic responses, as reported in the literature. Understanding these pharmacological differences informs the choice of therapy, benefiting patient management in dermatological disorders where non-immune-mediated mechanisms contribute to drug reactions (Berardesca et al., 2018). By continuing research, it will become vital to integrate knowledge from immune and non-immune pathways to improve the safety and effectiveness of dermatological therapies (Figure 10.7).

10.2.3. Genetic Predisposition

Genetic propensity is at the heart of understanding cutaneous drug reactions, particularly in evaluating an individual's reaction to pharmacological drugs. The genetic inclination towards side effects is present in some individuals and leads to dermatitis caused by drugs or some forms of alopecia. Research indicates that polymorphisms in immune response genes, such as IL-17, significantly influence the severity of cutaneous reactions and the effectiveness of therapeutic interventions in skin disorders. Variation in the expression of these genes can dictate how a patient's skin responds to drugs and thereby necessitate individualized therapy in dermatology. Genetically predisposed patients may occasionally require intensive monitoring and other interventions to mitigate skin side effects triggered by drug therapy, highlighting the importance of incorporating genetic information into clinical decision-making (Frioui et al., 2021). Beyond the direct genetic impacts, environmental factors often act in an interactive fashion with a person's genetic makeup to further complicate drug response. For instance, certain irritants or allergens may predispose individuals with a specific genetic background to a dermatological reaction.

Research has established that the heterogeneity of environmental stimuli, combined with genetic susceptibility, is central to the etiopathogenesis of skin disorders. Such dualism is characteristic of dermatological problems, as they necessitate multifactorial management that considers both genetic backgrounds and environmental interactions. It then becomes imperative for drug prescribers to keep these overlapping factors in mind while prescribing drugs, especially in patients with mixed responses to medication, thereby maximizing therapeutic effectiveness and avoiding the risk of drug-related dermatologic adverse effects (Boda et al., 2019). Lastly, knowledge of genetic susceptibility maximizes the discussion on the pathogenesis of drug dermatologic reactions. This intersection of genetics, immunology, and the environment invites further studies to demystify drug response variability. By establishing genetic markers for side effects, dermatologists are better equipped to tailor treatments, potentially through methods such as pharmacogenomic testing. These advances can advance on targeted therapies that not only minimize risks for dermatological reactions but enhance patient quality of life. The genetic role in this context underscores the necessity of developing a multidisciplinary practice, including dermatology, genetics, and pharmacology, to optimize patient care and establish the discipline of dermatological medicine (Frioui et al., 2021) (Figure 10.8).

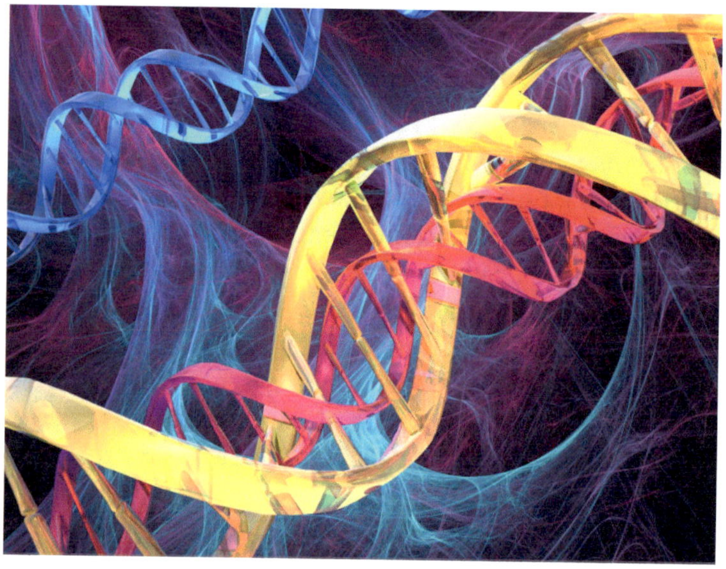

Figure 10.8. Genetic predisposition.

Source: https://www.verywellhealth.com/thmb/9ocWbniWGh4MP6OqRjVyVbSZ7TI=/2000x1500/filters:fill(87E3EF,1)/DNA1-b5956a41a92044f7ad1e0fd2bdcfe47e.jpg.

10.3. Common Drugs Associated with Skin Reactions

Many medications can cause skin side effects, which may impact a person's overall well-being. Antiretroviral medications used for HIV are some of the drugs most often related to this condition. Studies have indicated that patients undergoing ART often experience skin-related ADRs. Notably, the TLE regimen has been associated with a high incidence of dermatological side effects, accounting for approximately 27.4% of reported cases in clinical studies, with skin rash being the most prevalent reaction observed in 28.3% of these cases (Datta et al., 2022). Therefore, it is essential to monitor these patients closely and, in some cases, intervene with treatment, particularly for those with severe forms of the skin conditions. Knowing the side effects of these reactions is crucial for clinicians when selecting ART. Apart from antiretrovirals, different types of drugs may cause severe reactions on the skin. NSAIDs and antibiotics are common offenders. Antibiotics, including penicillin and sulfonamides, are known to cause skin problems that range from simple rashes to more serious reactions, such as Stevens-Johnson syndrome (SJS). Besides, the use of NSAIDs has been linked to urticarial reactions that may appear like other skin diseases, making it difficult for doctors to diagnose correctly. A particular challenge arises with acute urticarial lesions, which can take on forms that resemble erythema multiforme or urticarial vasculitis (Daronat et al., 2011). This confusion highlights the importance of a comprehensive medical and physical examination in determining the most effective treatment for patients experiencing these reactions. Besides the physical side, these drug-related skin reactions can also harm a patient's mental health. People with skin conditions that are noticeable may develop anxiety, depression, or a low sense of self-worth. Since some dermatological reactions require long-term care, doctors and patients must communicate effectively to ensure empathy throughout the care process. Additionally, using strategies tailored to each patient's drug regimen can help improve their outcomes. The high number of severe skin reactions caused by medicines highlights the need for better monitoring and education on how to manage such serious reactions.

10.3.1. Antibiotics

The widespread use of antibiotics has significantly altered the dermatologic landscape, primarily in terms of treating skin infections and inflammatory conditions, such as acne vulgaris. Topical and systemic antibiotics are commonly applied to treat the pathogenic proliferation of disease-causing agents in dermatologic disorders. However, their efficacy is increasingly being made more challenging through the mechanism of antimicrobial resistance (AMR)—a consequence of overuse and, in some instances, unwise application. Studies reveal that among the patients with drug adverse reactions (ADRs), antibiotics are usually implicated and cause a vast majority of reported cases. This highlights the importance of vigilant monitoring of ADRs, especially in dermatological disorders, as most of these cutaneous drug reactions may not be reported or classified under other pathologies and thus obscure optimal treatment modalities (Adhikari et al., 2009).

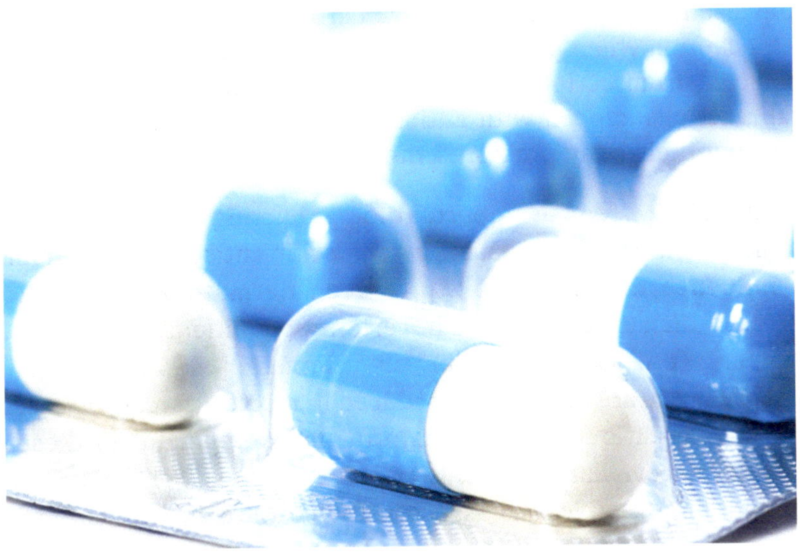

Figure 10.9. Antibiotics.

Source: https://medlineplus.gov/images/AntibioticsAndAbscess_share.jpg.

Although antibiotics are effective against most bacterial infections, they can also cause dermatological reactions that complicate patient prognosis. Antibiotic therapy, for instance, has been associated with diseases such as drug-induced hypersensitivity that can present as erythema multiforme or even SJS. Such reactions can significantly worsen an individual's quality of life, accompanied by psychological disturbances that are as severe as the dermatological condition itself. Additionally, the occurrence of such side effects underscores the necessity for physicians to counterbalance antibiotic application in dermatology against the benefits and risks. Unfortunately, antibiotic side effects often lead to the withdrawal of the treatment, aggravating the initial skin condition and promoting an alarming cycle (Patton et al., 2016). The interconnectedness of antibiotics and dermatologic side effects underscores a pressing need for stringent protocols in prescription practice. Recent research indicates that careful selection of patients and scrutiny of specific treatment plans are critical to minimizing the risk of ADRs. Educating HCPs and patients regarding the risks of antibiotic therapy may promote a more conservative practice. Lastly, educating the public about possible drug reactions, in addition to monitoring, can deter adverse effects and improve therapeutic effects among patients who have dermatological disorders requiring antibiotic medication. Continued investigation of the risks associated with antibiotics is imperative in developing dermatological treatment techniques and patient safety in clinics (Adhikari et al., 2009) (Figure 10.9).

10.3.2. Anticonvulsants

Anticonvulsants are mainly prescribed to treat seizures, and they commonly result in dermatological side effects. These medications, including phenytoin, carbamazepine, and lamotrigine, can trigger various skin manifestations ranging from mild rashes to severe conditions such as SJS. Since these drug reactions are unusual, they make it hard for clinicians, as they might occur suddenly, even when the drug has been used for a long time without any problems. Because dermatological reactions to anticonvulsants can lead to more serious problems in the body, healthcare providers should exercise extra caution when prescribing them. If skin adverse effects are spotted early, the patient can be protected from serious conditions by discontinuing the medication quickly. The way dermatological reactions happen with anticonvulsants can be due to several factors, such as a person's genes or how their body processes the drugs.

Pharmacogenomics is now seen as important for predicting bad reactions to drugs, especially among people who have had a previous reaction to specific anticonvulsants. Moreover, the patient demographic can influence the susceptibility to such dermatological reactions; studies have highlighted an increased incidence of CADRs in certain populations. The latest evidence suggests that the overall number of CADRs linked to anticonvulsants requires us to remain vigilant, as new types and doses of these drugs are regularly introduced in medical care. Awareness among clinicians is crucial for enhancing patient outcomes and improving the reporting of these adverse reactions through structured pharmacovigilance systems (Vedavathi et al., 2016). SJS and TEN are some of the most severe dermatological reactions associated with anticonvulsants. Since these conditions involve much tissue death and separation of the epidermis, it is necessary to treat them right away to prevent serious harm and death. Many cases have confirmed that SJS is linked to anticonvulsants, and a case of SJS from co-trimoxazole shows why these drugs should be prescribed with caution for kids. Clinicians must maintain a high index of suspicion for SJS in patients presenting with mucosal lesions accompanied by fever and widespread rash after initiating anticonvulsant therapy (Bhosale et al., 2017). It is essential to identify the risk factors, diagnose these reactions promptly, and employ effective management methods to prevent them from worsening. Since the safety of anticonvulsants keeps changing, it is important to keep educating both HCPs and patients about them.

10.3.3. Non-Steroidal Anti-Inflammatory Drugs (NSAIDs)

Non-steroidal anti-inflammatory drugs (NSAIDs) are commonly used for their analgesic, anti-inflammatory, and antipyretic properties. While their therapeutic effect is beneficial, they are recognized to have many side effects, the most significant being dermatological reactions. Skin reaction rates are likely to vary considerably depending on the specific NSAID used, the course of treatment, as well as the patient's personal susceptibility. Dermatological presentations range from rashes, urticaria to, in severe cases, SJS.

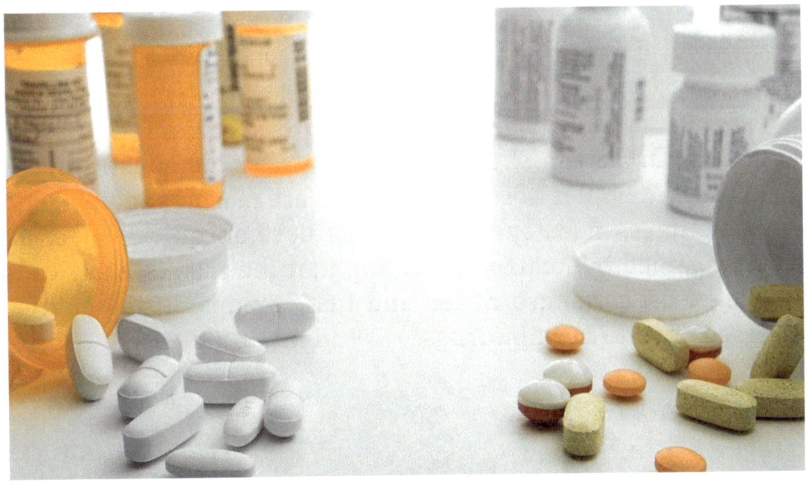

Figure 10.10. Non-steroidal anti-inflammatory drugs (NSAIDs).

Source: https://embed.widencdn.net/img/veritas/davc9dlv8c/1200x630px/prescription-non-prescription-pill-bottles.jpg?u=at8tiu&use=d502n&k=c.

Awareness of these risks is important, as a few patients can develop immediate HSRs that require urgent medical intervention. Additionally, cross-reactivity between various NSAIDs complicates the management of patients with established drug allergy, highlighting the need for proper patient history and monitoring during NSAID treatment. More recent epidemiological studies have elucidated the incidence of drug hypersensitivity reactions (DHRs), especially with NSAIDs. Research indicates that NSAIDs contribute to a high percentage of these side effects, causing both morbidity and higher healthcare costs. Among university students, research indicated that NSAIDs caused 45.9% of self-reported hypersensitivity drug cases, highlighting the severe health consequences of the drug. Dermatological symptoms were the majority in most reports, and most of the patients had immediate type reactions. These findings highlight the importance of medical professionals being aware of the risk of NSAID-induced cutaneous reactions, as early identification and intervention are crucial for maximizing patient outcomes and preventing the risk of severe complications, as suggested by Amigo et al. (2010). The rationale for NSAID administration, particularly in those with chronic diseases, must be critically evaluated against their potential side effects. This becomes especially relevant when the use of adjunct therapy, such as misoprostol, is considered, for the intention of preventing NSAID-induced gastric damage. However, evidence suggests that a consensus does not exist regarding the costing of such co-therapies, and calls for further research. The synergism between the administration of NSAIDs and their dermal effects is crucial in questioning patient safety, in addition to the efficacy of these treatment combinations. With the possibility of serious NSAID-associated adverse effects, clinicians should engage in open dialogue with their patients regarding the therapeutic modalities, discussing the balance between efficacy and risk. In the absence of definitive proof for the efficacy of such adjuvant therapies in clinical settings, as described by Johannesson et al. (1994), healthcare practitioners should exercise care when prescribing NSAIDs to susceptible groups (Figure 10.10).

10.4. Clinical Presentation of Dermatological Reactions

Dermatological reactions to drugs can show up in many ways, demonstrating that each person's response to drugs is unique. Examples of common rashes are maculopapular, urticaria, and in some cases SJS and TEN. Sometimes, maculopapular rashes develop quickly after taking medication, and they are often accompanied by itching, indicating that the rash is likely caused by an allergic reaction. Hives, also called urticaria, are raised and itchy bumps on the skin, and could suggest that a person is hypersensitive to certain drugs.

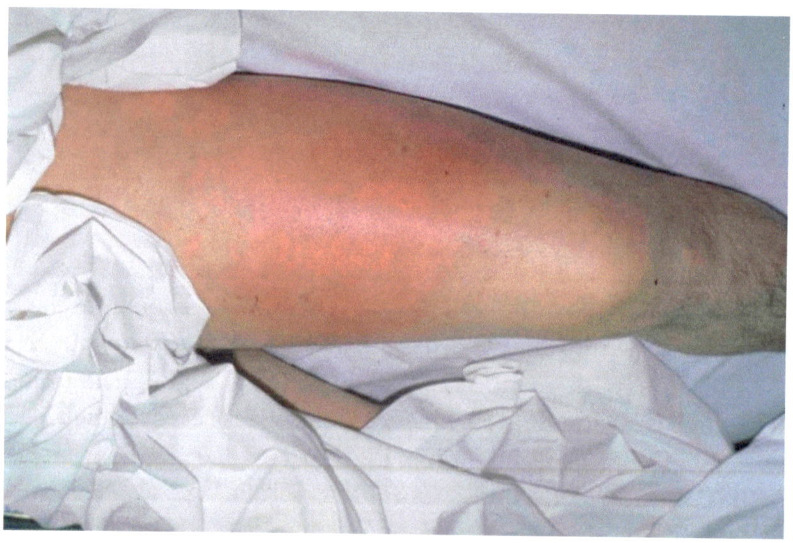

Figure 10.11. Clinical presentation of dermatological reactions.

Source: https://storage.googleapis.com/dl.dentistrykey.com/clinical/ DermatologicPresentations/ 3_3s20B9780323757898001079.jpg.

Knowing the main clinical features enables healthcare providers to identify and treat drug-induced skin reactions safely and effectively, thereby supporting the safe and proper use of medicines in patients. Several studies underlining the prevalence of CADRs reveal that these reactions can significantly hamper the treatment process, particularly in patients undergoing therapies such as epidermal growth factor receptor inhibitors (EGFRIs). In a recent observational study, a high incidence of dermatological adverse events (dAEs) was reported, with manifestations like papulopustular rashes and nail lesions being prevalent among patients receiving EGFRIs. The study highlighted the importance of recognizing these reactions to prevent them from impacting patients' adherence to their treatment. Moreover, the median incubation time for dAEs was identified as a critical factor, suggesting that certain demographics, such as ethnicity and occupation, might influence the onset and severity of these reactions (Qu et al., 2024). The information from this data guides treatment and also calls for regular monitoring while the patient is on drugs. Additionally, it is crucial to educate both healthcare providers and patients on the effective management of CADRs. Several studies emphasize the importance of recognizing early symptoms, such as erythematous rashes, edema, and erosions of the mucous membranes, for prompt treatment. In a retrospective analysis conducted at an Adverse Drug Reaction Monitoring Center, antimicrobials emerged as the most common culprits for CADRs, with serious outcomes observed in certain cases, such as SJS (Chindhalore et al., 2024). Thus, it is essential to ensure that the therapy plan includes educating patients about potential skin reactions, monitoring them during the initial stages of treatment, and employing flexible strategies to manage any adverse effects. Knowing how dermatological reactions appear is vital for helping patients and reducing the risk of serious drug-related complications (Figure 10.11).

10.4.1. Rashes and Eruptions

Drug rashes and eruptions constitute a significant class of CADRs that can take various forms and severity levels following exposure to drugs. The cutaneous drug reactions present in the form of erythematous maculopapular rashes, vesicular lesions, or even in more severe forms, such as SJS. The presentation of these rashes varies depending on patient-specific considerations and the drugs involved. Worthy of mention are drug-induced acneiform eruptions and fixed drug eruptions among the most commonly reported CADR subtypes, alluding to the heterogeneity in clinical presentations due to pharmaceuticals. It is therefore critical for clinicians to suspect CADRs with new rashes with a high index of suspicion, particularly in patients with a history of sensitivity to drugs, as early diagnosis and treatment are critical in guaranteeing patient safety and recovery. Research has shown that a significant proportion of CADRs is attributed to the administration of antibiotics, and in one study, this accounted for a substantial percentage of reported reactions. Antimicrobials were implicated in approximately 32% of the reactions, ranking them as the leading therapeutic class in terms of risk factor.

Other commonly implicated agents are corticosteroids, anticancer drugs, and NSAIDs. Studies on CADRs have revealed population patterns, with the middle-aged individuals most affected. Studies have indicated that advancing age is linked with a higher risk of severe CADRs. This population data calls for the use of caution among healthcare workers in the administration of drugs to older adults, since they are more sensitive to drugs and need personalized care when prescribing and monitoring them. The CADR management relies heavily on early detection, accurate causality assessment, and the withdrawal of implicated drugs. Process is significant, since evidence demonstrates that early suspect drug withdrawal plays a pivotal role in recovery in involved patients. For instance, in one Indian study, over 76% of CADR cases reported implicated drug withdrawal to encourage better patient outcomes. Furthermore, identification of rashes as a reaction to drugs is of utmost importance due to the danger posed by the severe complications. Erythematous maculopapular rashes were identified as the most common presentation of cases involving CADRs, but clinicians should also be aware of indicators of allergic reactions. The intricate relationship between drug exposure and skin manifestations necessitates ongoing education for clinicians to ensure efficient management of this preventable health condition, ultimately simplifying the burden on healthcare systems (Panigrahy et al., 2024; Surekha et al., 2025) (Figure 10.12).

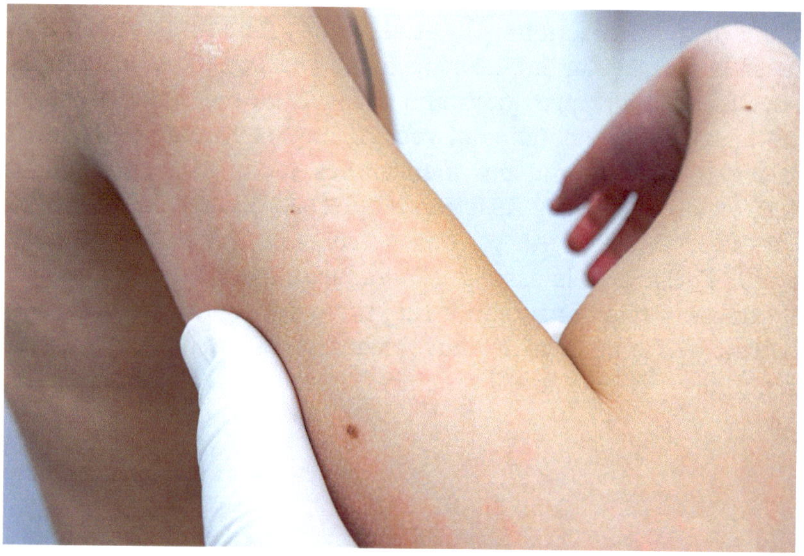

Figure 10.12. Rashes and eruptions.

Source: https://www.parents.com/thmb/s6yX76yd4FGXJxqbBg953-uloAA=/1500x0/filters:no_upscale():max_bytes(150000):strip_icc()/GettyImages-1464134307-c15360b842ad4b1d93073cfa451a1621.jpg.

10.4.2. Urticaria and Angioedema

Many things can lead to urticaria and angioedema, and one of them is medication. Acute urticaria is characterized by hives that may affect a small area or the entire body, and it is typically accompanied by itching. Angioedema appears as swelling of the skin and mucous membranes. Many of these diseases occur when histamine is released from mast cells, leading to the widening of blood vessels and increased permeability of the blood vessels. There are many cases where the cause of acute urticaria is difficult to determine. Studies reveal that idiopathic cases constitute more than 50% of presentations, leaving clinicians to navigate a nuanced landscape of diagnosis and treatment (Faisal et al., 2024). Since some medicines can cause strong allergic reactions, it is important to accurately assess when drug-induced urticaria is suspected. Many types of drugs can trigger urticaria and angioedema, as shown by medical studies. Among these, beta-lactam antibiotics, NSAIDs, and certain antihypertensives have been implicated in numerous cases. For instance, a clinical case study highlighted a 23-year-old patient who developed severe urticaria and angioedema after commencing treatment with bupropion for major depressive disorder and attention deficit hyperactivity disorder (Faisal et al., 2024). After stopping the previous medication and starting antihistamines and corticosteroids, the patient's symptoms improved and disappeared in two weeks. This case demonstrates the importance of healthcare workers identifying and treating drug-related skin reactions, as prompt action can significantly improve patient outcomes. Typically, antihistamines, corticosteroids, and avoiding triggers are the primary treatments for urticaria and angioedema. In cases of acute allergies, doctors usually prefer second-generation antihistamines because they are safer and have less sedative effects than the first-generation drugs. For those whose standard treatment does not work, especially in chronic urticaria, other options such as omalizumab or immunosuppressants may be used. The aim is to alleviate symptoms and improve the patient's quality of life. Furthermore, education regarding potential drug interactions and the avoidance of known allergens is crucial for long-term management (Dom et al., 2024). All in all, although urticaria and angioedema are serious issues, especially when they occur due to drugs, a planned method of diagnosis and treatment can lead to good results.

10.4.3. Severe Reactions: Stevens-Johnson Syndrome and Toxic Epidermal Necrolysis

The development of severe dermatologic reactions to medication includes two especially hazardous conditions: TEN and SJS. These syndromes, which are more of a continuum in severity, present with widespread peeling of the epidermis and can be fatal. SJS involves less than 10% body surface area, manifesting as blisters over erythematous macules and target lesions. Conversely, TEN is associated with more widespread skin peeling, involving over 30% of the body surface area, and, in most instances, resulting in considerable fluid loss, sepsis, and multi-organ failure. Prompt diagnosis and treatment of these disorders are paramount, considering that they have the potential to rapidly progress and cause significant morbidity, making them pertinent areas of study and clinical focus in dermatology and pharmacology (Andrews et al., 2019).

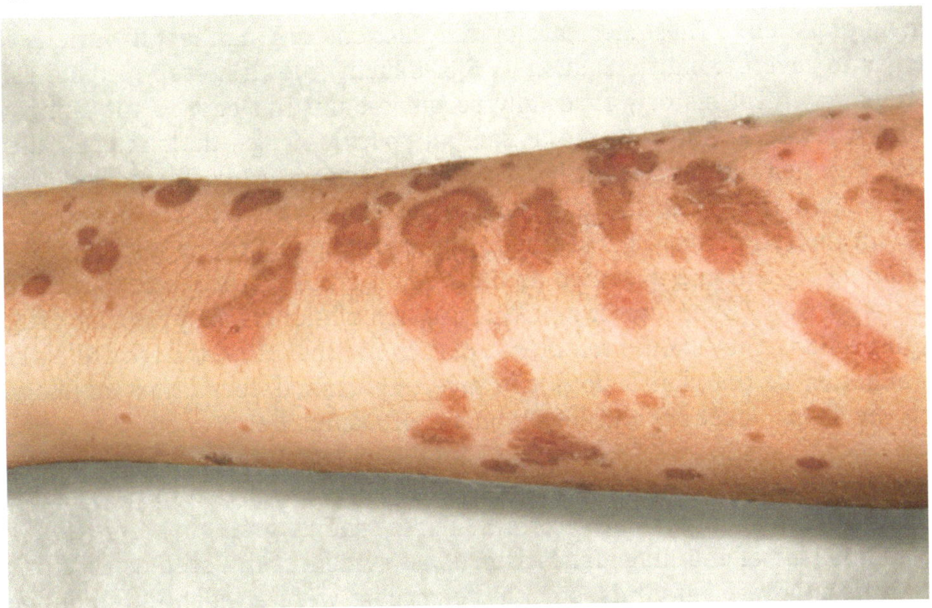

Figure 10.13. Severe reactions: Stevens-Johnson syndrome and toxic epidermal necrolysis.

Source: https://pharmaceutical-journal.com/wp-content/uploads/2021/01/LEAD-PIC_Stevens-_Johnson_syndrome-SPL-1456x967.png.

Pathophysiologically, SJS and TEN involve complex immunological mechanisms triggered by certain drugs. The key role is the activation of cytotoxic T cells and macrophages by cytokines such as IL-2 and interferon gamma. The involvement of eosinophils and B lymphocytes in the immune response underscores the multifactorial etiology of these reactions. A clear understanding of such mechanisms is crucial in designing strategies to identify vulnerable individuals and establishing a framework for prevention. Despite many drugs that may trigger such reactions, antibiotics, anticonvulsants, and NSAIDs are the most frequently implicated. This highlights the most critical importance of pharmacovigilance and meticulous patient history taking at the time of prescribing drugs, particularly to patients who are already known to have sensitivities or prior ADRs (Casha et al., 2012). Treatment of SJS and TEN patients requires a holistic approach, sometimes mirroring the care strategy employed for burn patients. Due to the risk of developing serious complications like infection and organ failure, these patients need to be hospitalized, usually in intensive or specialty burn treatment units. Treatment is primarily supportive, focusing on fluid and electrolyte resuscitation, wound care, and pain management. Corticosteroids and other immunosuppressive therapies can be used judiciously according to patient status, but their utility is disputed. Most importantly, multidisciplinary teamwork among dermatologists, intensivists, and pharmacists is crucial for optimizing patient outcomes. Effective management of SJS and TEN relies heavily on timely diagnosis, careful therapeutic management, and ongoing monitoring of treatment efficacy in response to changing patient needs (Andrews et al., 2019) (Figure 10.13).

10.5. Diagnosis of Drug-Induced Skin Reactions

It is important to identify and diagnose drug-related skin reactions to guarantee the safety and proper treatment of patients. These dermatological reactions can manifest in various ways, ranging from mild rashes to severe conditions such as SJS. Usually, the first step in diagnosis is to learn about the patient's medical history, especially recent medication use, as the timing of exposure can help identify the cause. Knowing the actions of specific drugs, their effects, and how rashes typically appear can help doctors identify the cause of a rash. It is noted in the literature that for some drug-related reactions, the drug should be stopped right away, and care should be given to help with the symptoms. This strategic approach highlights the importance of healthcare providers remaining vigilant and informed about the numerous medications that can elicit adverse dermatological responses (Bourlière et al., 2011). When clinicians suspect that drugs may cause dermatological reactions, they should tell these apart from other similar dermatological conditions. A careful examination of the skin lesions can give important information for diagnosis. In this way, assessing the shape, location, and development of lesions helps doctors distinguish between different types of drug eruptions, such as maculopapular eruptions or urticaria. We should also pay attention to the patient's demographics, especially if they have atopic dermatitis, since this may impact the skin's response to medications. Furthermore, grading the severity of reactions forms a core component of the diagnostic criteria, as evidenced by studies indicating that most rashes resulting from newer antivirals, such as telaprevir, were either mild or moderate, raising concerns about severe cutaneous adverse reactions (SCARs) that warrant different management strategies (Bourlière et al., 2011). When treating drug-induced skin reactions, the treatment should be adapted to the patient's condition and the drug that caused it. First, you should remove the medicine that caused the problem; however, you may also need additional treatment to alleviate the symptoms. Topical corticosteroids and emollients are often used to control mild dermatitis and its related symptoms. Fluticasone propionate, a potent anti-inflammatory corticosteroid, is considered a suitable option for treating various types of dermatitis due to its safety in sensitive areas. Sometimes, a severe reaction requires more serious actions, such as hospitalization or treatments that affect the entire body. Thus, a multifaceted approach encompassing accurate diagnosis, diligent management, and patient education is crucial in addressing drug-induced skin reactions effectively and safely (Bourlière et al., 2011).

10.5.1. Patient History and Medication Review

Patient history and review of medication are critical elements in both dermatologic drug reaction diagnosis and treatment. A patient's entire medical history is significant because it provides critical information on previous drug reactions, underlying dermatological conditions, and other relevant health issues that could potentially affect the choice of treatment. Notably, acute urticarial lesions can also present as a variety of dermatological diseases, such as erythema multiforme and urticarial vasculitis; therefore, it is essential that clinicians record accurate histories and conduct meticulous physical examinations. Clinical evaluation should also address potential risk factors, for example, age, gender, co-morbidities, and prior drug exposure, which can inform the likelihood of individual drug reactions. A directed history not only facilitates differentiation of acute urticaria from its mimics, as exemplified in the case evidence for a 20-month-old child, but also informs subsequent diagnostic investigation and management strategies that optimize patient outcomes (Daronat et al., 2011). Paralleling the utility of accurate patient histories, reviewing medications prescribed is an orderly way to ascertain which drugs are likely to trigger adverse dermatologic effects. Prescribing doctors should go over previous and current drug regimens and consider the timing of drug administration in the development of dermatologic signs. Certain drugs, such as Imatinib Mesylate, are associated with some dermatological findings, i.e., mucosal pigmentation in otherwise asymptomatic patients. Such side effects need to be monitored closely, particularly in chronic therapy, where prolonged exposure puts patients at higher risk for cutaneous reactions. By integrating medication review elements into day-to-day practice, doctors can more effectively identify and treat any drug-induced conditions, thereby enabling appropriate interventions in patients while avoiding harm (Bosco et al., 2015). Additionally, patient open communication with doctors can also make the patient history and medication review processes more effective. Patients can give important insights into their own experiences with drugs, including recollections of previous reactions that would not be immediately evident from medical history. Such discussions can lead to more individualized treatment strategies, potentially influencing the selection of alternative medications when appropriate. Furthermore, patient education on recognizing the initial symptoms of dermatitis or other reactions empowers them to access prompt medical care promptly, which ensures improved health outcomes. With advancing dermatology, incorporation of comprehensive patient histories and in-depth reviews of drugs into practice continues to be paramount to the effective management of skin reactions to drugs.

10.5.2. Skin Tests and Patch Testing

Identifying skin reactions to drugs is possible with the help of skin tests and patch testing. Using these methods, doctors can assess a person's sensitivity to specific allergens or medications. To find out about immediate HSRs, doctors often use skin tests such as prick and intradermal testing. In this case, patch testing is used to spot delayed hypersensitivity, which usually appears after someone is exposed to a drug. When allergens are applied to the skin and the reaction is checked after a set period, dermatologists can determine what is causing the allergy. The tests are useful because they show how a patient's skin will react to usual situations. The usefulness of skin tests and patch testing is very high, particularly in cases of drug allergies. Because ADRs are happening more often, it is very important to find out which drugs cause them accurately. If a patient shows a good response to a drug during patch testing, doctors can choose different medicines to prevent possible severe skin reactions. Moreover, these tests play a crucial role in determining how to treat patients, as a negative patch test can confirm that a drug is safe for them. Additionally, educating patients about the process is crucial for the success of skin and patch tests. If patients understand the reason and steps for the test, they may feel less anxious and work more effectively with the team. It is essential for clinicians to remind patients to avoid known allergens and follow all instructions provided before the test to ensure accurate results. It is necessary to discuss potential outcomes and next steps, as some patients may experience delayed reactions after a negative patch test. Overall, the integration of skin tests and patch testing into clinical practice not only facilitates the diagnosis of dermatological reactions but also contributes to improving patient safety and treatment efficacy in drug therapy (Calvieri et al., 2014; Dunn et al., 2020) (Figure 10.14).

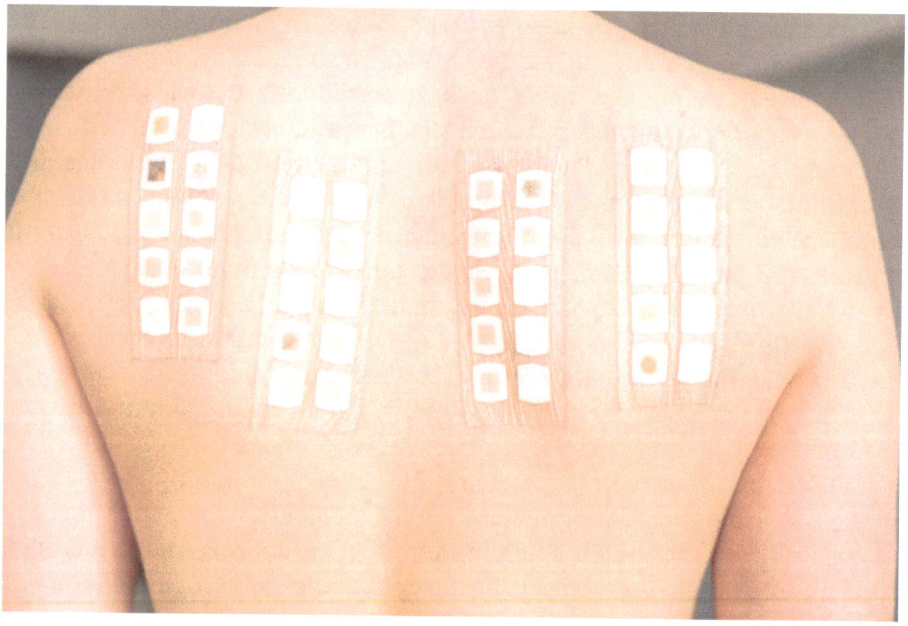

Figure 10.14. Skin tests and patch testing.

Source: https://brisbaneskin.com.au/wp-content/uploads/patch-testing-1-1.webp.

10.5.3. Differential Diagnosis

Differential diagnosis of drug dermatological reactions is based on a thorough understanding of various skin reactions that pharmacologic agents can cause. Drugs may cause as mild a reaction as rash or a perilous reaction like SJS or TEN. To establish the correct underlying cause, clinicians must have an excellent patient history that encompasses a detailed drug history, the chronology of symptom onset, and any previous allergies. A thorough physical examination ideally focuses on the morphology and distribution of lesions, which can provide key pointers. Since the overlapping nature of dermatological disorders, it is essential to differentiate drug eruptions from viral exanthems and other dermatologic diseases to prevent incorrect diagnosis and subsequent inappropriate management, ultimately harming the patient.

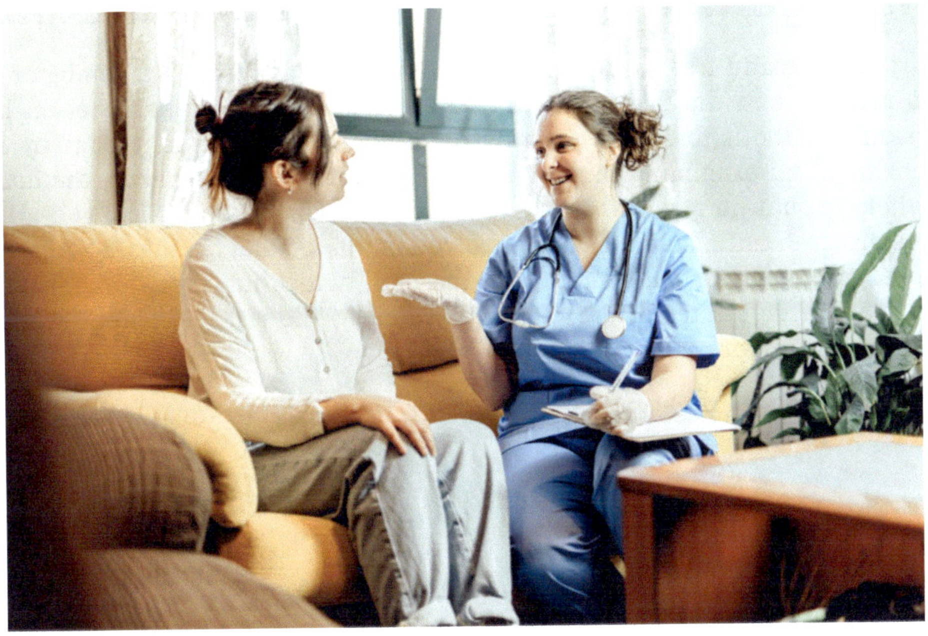

Figure 10.15. Differential diagnosis.

Source: https://gentwenty.com/wp-content/uploads/2025/05/a-c-2BwUmyRmywA-unsplash-scaled.jpg.

In cases of suspected drug-induced skin reactions, diagnosis may also depend on performing diagnostic tests. Although skin biopsy and laboratory analysis are helpful, they are not necessarily diagnostic, as drug reactions may be multifactorial. Clinical grading scales, such as the Naranjo algorithm, can help assess how likely a drug is to be the cause of a given case. The patient population and comorbidities should also be carefully considered. For instance, elderly patients and those with multiple comorbid conditions may not only develop heterogeneous cutaneous reactions but also are more vulnerable to drug side effects, as seen in the examples, particularly with increased age and compromised immunity, when differential diagnosis is more complex (Tairova et al., 2020). Additionally, the development of novel dermatologic presentations associated with recent health emergencies, including the COVID-19 pandemic, illustrates the evolving dynamic of differential diagnosis in drug reactions. During SARS-CoV-2 infections, patients have also presented with diverse cutaneous manifestations, further complicating the differential diagnosis. Although some dermatologic manifestations may immediately be a consequence of the viral infection itself, others may ensue as a result of coincidental drug therapies administered to control COVID-19-related complications. For instance, macular rashes in patients treated for COVID-19 can be an indicator of HSRs to antibiotics or anticoagulants used (Ridolo et al., 2021). It is thus best to obtain the proper differential diagnosis through a multidisciplinary approach, involving cooperation among dermatologists, primary healthcare workers, and specialists, to address both the infection and potential Dermatological impacts of drug therapy (Figure 10.15).

10.6. Management and Treatment Strategies

The best way to handle and treat drug-related skin problems is through a combined effort, since each person's reaction and the drug used can be quite different. The first step in handling any drug-related skin reaction is to quickly identify the cause, which is usually done by asking about the patient's history and examining them. When the condition is recognized, the drug should be stopped, and help should be given to ease the symptoms. For this purpose, you might be given topical corticosteroids or antihistamines to control inflammation and itching. In addition, healthcare providers should watch for serious reactions in the body, which may get worse if the drug is not stopped on time. If these strategies are put in place early, the risk of complications is reduced, and patients' outcomes improve.

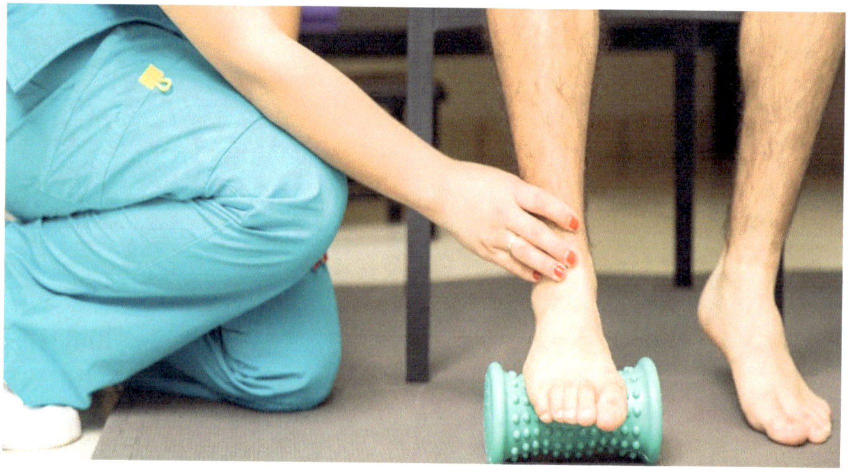

Figure 10.16. Management and treatment strategies.

Source: https://www.neurolutions.com/wp-content/uploads/2024/10/Claw-Toe-Effective-Strategies-for-Management-and-Treatment-of-Related-Toe-Conditions.jpg.

If patients suffer from SJS or TEN due to drugs, a more serious approach to care may be needed. Most of these conditions require hospitalization because they can be very dangerous. The patient receives care through the administration of fluids via a vein, specialized nutrition, and specialized wound care. Additionally, treating the immune system with specialized drugs may be recommended, depending on the severity of the reactions. It is essential for healthcare providers to collaborate with dermatologists, allergists, and pharmacists to develop the most effective treatment plan for each patient. Therefore, it is essential for patients and clinicians to be aware of potential drug reactions so that they can be identified as soon as possible. Managing severe drug allergies for the long term means being cautious about the medicines given to the patient. Patients who have had drug reactions should be told about their allergies and might want to wear medical identification. In the future, using medications from different drug groups that do not cause the same skin reactions would be wise. Sometimes, desensitization is used in a closely supervised manner, primarily when there are no other options for emergency medications. Patients must be always informed about the signs and symptoms of drug reactions, so they can seek help fast and avoid more risks if exposed to the same drugs again. When these strategies are employed, the effects of dermatological reactions are significantly reduced, ensuring patients receive safe and uninterrupted care (Figure 10.16).

10.6.1. Discontinuation of the Offending Drug

Withdrawing the offending drug is a critical aspect of the treatment of cutaneous drug reactions to medications. Cutaneous drug reactions range from mild irritations to life-threatening illnesses like SJS and TEN, which have dire implications for the health of patients. Identification and withdrawal of the offending drug alleviate symptoms promptly and prevent further sequelae. The initial step is most often patient assessment that includes the drugs recently administered, following which a knowledgeable decision regarding what drug needs to be stopped is made. In interesting contrast, prompt withdrawal can lead to the reversal of symptoms so that the patients regain their initial state earlier, as observed in studies on the commonness of cutaneous drug reactions among patients undergoing specific treatments, e.g., ART (Era et al., 2017). Additionally, the clinicians must also be thoroughly conversant with the necessity of observing the patients after cessation to note any residual effects or drug withdrawal complications. The array of reactions, ranging from morbilliform eruptions to fixed drug eruptions, justifies the necessity for close observation on the part of healthcare practitioners. One should be able to understand that even though discontinuation of the causative agent most often leads to an improvement in the symptoms, patients may still require support throughout this period. Identification of effective alternative therapies becomes crucial to manage the underlying condition without subjecting the patient to similar ADRs. The mounting bulk of evidence for drug class-specific association with specific cutaneous reactions underlines the importance of monitoring and assessment alertness following drug withdrawal (Kalola et al., 2024). The therapeutic significance of stopping the offending drug extends beyond the short-term treatment strategy to symptom relief; long-term patient safety precautions and drug adherence measures are also involved. HCPs must engage in comprehensive consultations with patients, outlining why drug withdrawal is necessary and emphasizing compliance with alternative treatments. Patients are likely to have a fear of altering their drugs in anticipation of experiencing further side effects, and thus, empathetic counseling and education are essential. Evidence-based, patient-centered care empowers patients to take charge of their dermatological health and increases the likelihood of achieving long-term treatment outcomes. By encouraging awareness of the drugs that have a greater tendency to cause cutaneous reactions and also developing safe drug handling guidelines, healthcare practitioners can reduce the incidence of ADRs and improve overall patient satisfaction in dermatology clinics (Era et al., 2017).

10.6.2. Symptomatic Treatment Options

Managing dermatological drug reactions primarily involves prescribing medications to alleviate symptoms and prevent further complications. Many ADRs manifest as skin conditions such as rashes, urticaria, or more severe syndromes like SJS and TEN. The first step in treating the symptoms is to stop using the agent that caused the reaction, as this is crucial for halting the reaction. After that, clinicians tend to treat itching and inflammation with antihistamines or corticosteroids. They can make patients feel much better by reducing their pain as they wait for their skin to heal. In addition, applying emollients and topical corticosteroids can protect the skin and aid in its healing, which underscores the importance of using specific symptomatic management plans in dermatological drug reactions. Certain drug-related conditions may require additional care and specialized treatments for their symptoms. In the case of Erythema Nodosum Leprosum, an intense immune reaction associated with leprosy treatment, patients require powerful treatments to control the inflammation. Giving high-dose corticosteroids is the usual choice, but these drugs may harm a person's quality of life, so other options should be considered. Case studies have pointed out that using tofacitinib, a non-selective Janus kinase inhibitor, can help patients with rheumatoid arthritis who do not respond to corticosteroids. The new developments in treatment highlight how dermatology is evolving and the importance of creating therapy regimens tailored to each patient's needs and well-being. Although there are many benefits, we should still pay attention to the possible adverse effects of drugs used in treatment. Typically, acetaminophen is used to help with pain in drug-related skin problems, but its connection to severe conditions like SJS and TEN is confusing. These life-threatening reactions necessitate a thorough understanding of individual patient factors, including genetic predispositions related to human leukocyte antigens (HLA), to mitigate risks. Those who are treating patients with symptomatic drugs should regularly check that the drugs are helping more than causing harm. Both healthcare providers and patients should be aware of the signs of serious adverse reactions, as this enables them to actively manage drug-related skin problems and emphasizes the need for a team approach to enhance patient outcomes (Figure 10.17).

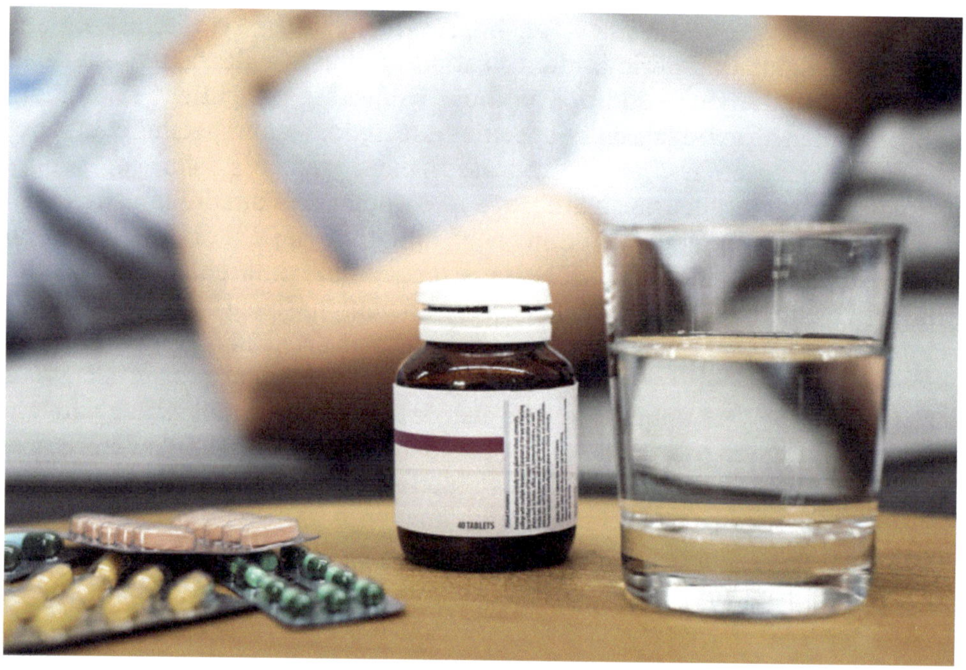

Figure 10.17. Symptomatic treatment options.

Source: https://userfiles.steadyhealth.com/userfiles/23630/articles/Feb%202016/Approved-And-Symptomatic-Treatment-Options-For-ALS-And-Non-drug-Therapies.jpg.

10.6.3. Referral to Dermatology Specialists

Among the complex network of drug-induced cutaneous reactions, the referral to dermatologists takes a central position in offering effective treatment and management. Primary care physicians are often the first doctors for patients reporting adverse cutaneous reactions following medication intake. As highlighted by Alfuraih et al. (2023), the ability of general practitioners to detect potentially severe dermatologic conditions is critical because they might encounter cases that require urgent treatment, such as SJS or TEN.

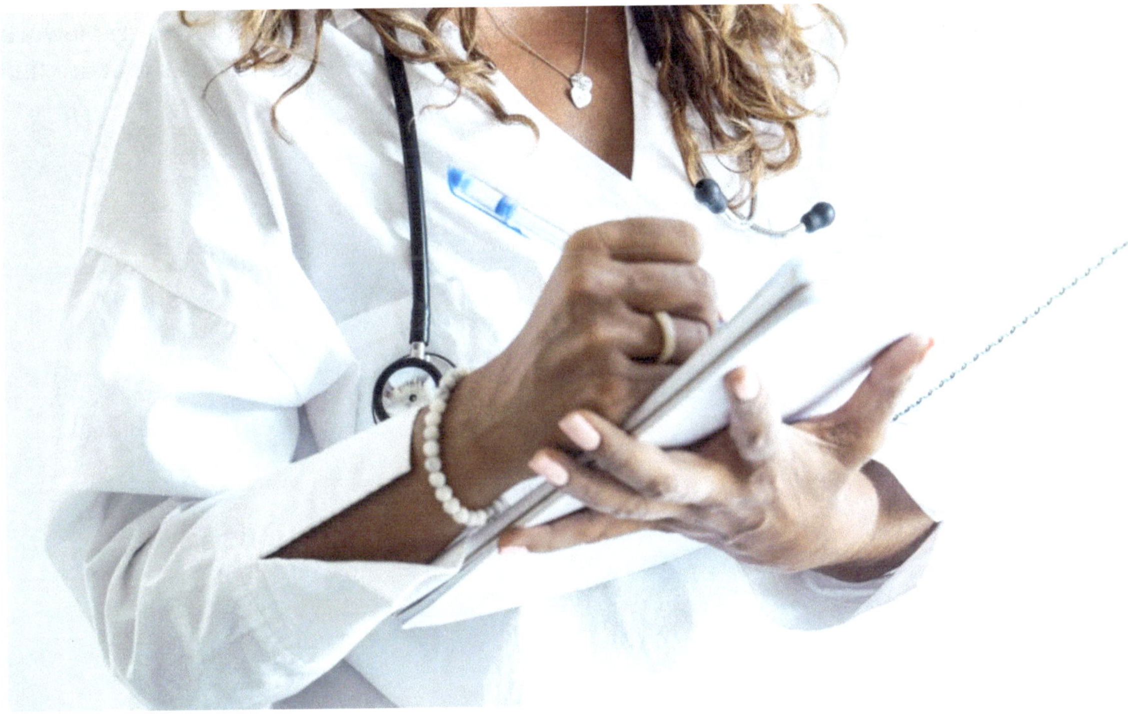

Figure 10.18. Referral to dermatology specialists.

Source: https://rivercityderm.com/wp-content/uploads/pexels-anna-tarazevich-7904454-1920x1143.webp.

These are conditions that require rapid referral of patients to dermatologists because they possess the skills required to implement individualized treatment protocols and avoid side effects. The referral process not only optimizes patient care but also maximizes the expertise of drug reactions among clinicians for better prevention and management tactics. Dermatologists possess the skill sets needed to perform extensive assessments and interventions of drug-induced skin reactions, from benign rashes to life-threatening events. As observed in renal transplant recipient cases, where infection was a frequent referral cause for dermatologic reasons, the intricate interplay between immunosuppressed states and dermatologic conditions indicates the necessity of specialty care (Borges-Costa et al., 2017). Referrals in such cases can lead to the early detection of precancerous lesions and enhance the chances of controlling skin cancers. The dermatologist's subtle observation of variable presentations of drug reactions allows the taking over of individualized treatment protocols that account for acute as well as chronic patient requirements. Moreover, the interprofessional collaboration between primary care physicians and dermatology specialists ensures a holistic approach to treating dermatological drug reactions. Such collaboration allows for the sharing of information regarding the clinical presentation of drug-induced adverse effects, ensuring that family physicians can appropriately assess and refer patients who present with severe symptoms to specialists. Identification of dermatologic emergencies not only requires clinician know-how but also patient history acumen in terms of prior drug exposure and concomitant comorbidities. By integrating referrals to dermatology experts into their everyday practice, healthcare practitioners are strengthening an active healthcare system that emphasizes patient safety and effective disease control, as highlighted in the cases (Alfuraih et al., 2023). Thus, a robust referral framework is crucial in optimizing patient outcomes for individuals with dermatological diseases that are linked to pharmacotherapy (Figure 10.18).

Summary

In concluding the discussion on dermatological reactions to drugs, it is essential to recognize the complexity and prevalence of ADRs affecting the skin. The data indicate that ADRs occur frequently among hospitalized patients, so healthcare workers must carefully monitor and document them. For instance, a study outlined that of 1250 patients admitted, 250 reported adverse events, with 66% classified as severe and leading to extensive medical intervention (Adhikari et al., 2009). As a result, it is important to spot these reactions quickly and to do more research on how they happen to improve patient care and reduce the risks of using drugs. It is also clear from the data that different body systems and drugs can cause dermatological reactions. As the analysis indicated, antimicrobials accounted for a notable percentage of ADRs, while the CNS drugs exhibited particularly concerning side effects (Adhikari et al., 2009). Due to this difference, it is necessary to employ customized approaches for administering medications and educating patients about potential skin-related issues. Understanding the drugs and systems involved can help healthcare workers prevent serious problems and improve patients' health. To achieve this, it is essential for staff to continue learning and for strong reporting to be encouraged. Ultimately, dermatological reactions to drugs should be evaluated in several ways, one of which is to assess skin tolerance to various treatments. Various studies on advanced wound dressings have pointed out that adhesion and skin comfort are vital for preventing more problems. It is essential to monitor patients' reactions to both medications and other therapies to minimize the risk of skin problems. The integration of research findings will be necessary for clinicians and researchers to improve the safety of patients who take drugs.

Dermatological reactions to drugs show that there is a complicated relationship between drugs and changes in the skin. Drug-induced dermatological adverse events (AEs) are particularly concerning in the context of treatments for chronic conditions, such as hepatitis C virus (HCV) infection. In this group, peginterferon and ribavirin may cause many kinds of dermatitis. In addition, new direct-acting antivirals have shown better results in clinical studies; however, they have also caused a rise in skin-related side effects compared to previous treatments. For instance, telaprevir has been associated with significant rates of rash. However, the majority of these events are mild to moderate, underscoring the need for continuous monitoring and effective management strategies to prevent potential complications during treatment (Bourlière et al., 2011). It is crucial to classify drug reactions for both diagnosis and management. Distinct dermatological reactions, such as xerosis, pruritus, and eczema, may emerge from drug therapies, with a subset falling under the category of SCAR. It is very important to tell apart routine rashes caused by drugs from potentially deadly SCAR. The guidelines explain that telaprevir should be stopped immediately if a patient develops severe rashes; however, mild cases can be controlled by applying topical treatments. This delineation underlines the importance of healthcare providers being vigilant in assessing skin reactions thoroughly to prevent adverse outcomes, which can significantly impact patient adherence to therapy (Bourlière et al., 2011). Aside from medicines, what we eat has proven to be a significant contributor to acne vulgaris and similar skin conditions. It appears that consuming dairy products may impact acne by altering hormone levels in the body, which in turn leads to increased sebaceous gland activity and swelling. This demonstrates that dermatology and nutrition are closely related, as more practitioners now look at patients' diets when treating skin problems. Although observational research suggests these connections, there are still no randomized controlled trials to confirm that they are the cause. Addressing these research gaps could help doctors develop more effective treatments for acne vulgaris by incorporating dietary advice into their plans, ultimately benefiting patients.

CLOSER LOOK

GENETICALLY PREDISPOSED PATIENTS

Genetically predisposed patients are individuals who inherit specific genetic variations that increase their susceptibility to certain diseases or health conditions. These predispositions do not guarantee the development of a disorder but significantly elevate the risk when combined with environmental or lifestyle factors. Common examples include BRCA1 and BRCA2 mutations, which are strongly associated with breast and ovarian cancer, and mutations in the APC gene linked to familial adenomatous polyposis and colorectal cancer. Similarly, genetic predispositions are also seen in chronic diseases such as diabetes, cardiovascular disease, and autoimmune conditions, where multiple genes contribute to disease risk in a polygenic manner.

Identifying genetically predisposed patients through genetic testing allows for early intervention, personalized prevention strategies, and targeted monitoring. For instance, individuals with a strong family history of cancer can undergo more frequent screenings or consider prophylactic treatments. In pharmacogenomics, understanding a patient's genetic makeup can help predict their response to medications, such as the risk of adverse reactions or likelihood of treatment success. This is particularly relevant for drugs metabolized by enzymes with known gene variants, such as those in the cytochrome P450 family.

However, genetic predisposition also presents ethical and psychological challenges. Patients may face anxiety over their future health, concerns about discrimination, or dilemmas regarding family planning. Genetic counseling plays a crucial role in helping individuals understand their risk and make informed decisions. Moreover, advances in gene editing and personalized medicine continue to evolve, offering future hope for modifying or managing genetic risks more effectively. Overall, recognizing genetically predisposed patients is a critical step toward precision medicine, where prevention and treatment are tailored not just to symptoms but to the underlying genetic blueprint of the individual, potentially transforming healthcare outcomes for at-risk populations.

References

1. Padmaja, U., Adhikari, P., & Pereira, P. (2009). A prospective analysis of adverse drug reactions in a South Indian hospital. *Online Journal of Health and Allied Sciences*, *8*(3). http://cogprints.org/6959/Agata Kryczyk-Poprawa, Kwiecień, A., & Opoka, W. (2019). Photostability of topical agents applied to the skin: A review. https://core.ac.uk/download/361286448.pdf (accessed on 9 June 2025).
2. Alfuraih, A. A., Alotaibi, A. A. B., Asiri, A. A., Albrahem, A. A., Hamdi, A. M., Alabdulaziz, A. A. M., Al-Doaan, D. H., et al. (2023). *Dermatological Emergencies in Family Medicine: Recognition, Management, And Referral Considerations*. https://core.ac.uk/download/603897626.pdf.
3. Amigo, M. H. L., Ensina, L. F. C., Guzman, E., Koch, M., et al. (2010). *Drug Hypersensitivity in Students from São Paulo, Brazil*. https://core.ac.uk/download/pdf/8476438.pdf.
4. Andrews, L. P., Dhanalakshmi, K., Kavitha, R., et al. (2019). Assessment of prescribing pattern and cost analysis of topical steroids for skin disorders in dermatological outpatient department of a tertiary care hospital. https://core.ac.uk/download/539897491.pdf (accessed on 9 June 2025).
5. Ankita Panigrahy, Begum, A., Pingali, U., Padmaja, M., & Sajeev, A. (2024). Evaluation of cutaneous adverse drug reactions in a tertiary care hospital in southern India: A retrospective analysis. *Asian Journal of Pharmaceutical and Clinical Research*. https://www.semanticscholar.org/paper/7dca3435b93f2363be4c8316a8020f7fcff22956 (accessed on 9 June 2025).
6. Atsuta, J., Boner, A. L., Bridgman, A., Callen, J., Delescluse, J., Dooms-Goossens, A. E., Dykes, P. J., et al. (2005). Safety and efficacy of fluticasone propionate in the topical treatment of skin diseases. https://core.ac.uk/download/16432247.pdf (accessed on 9 June 2025).
7. Avvaru Surekha, Babu, M. N., Thejaswini, K., Vishnupriya, A., Vishnupriya, B., Yugesh, S., & Kushma, T. (2025). A prospective study of clinical patterns and assessment of causality and severity of cutaneous adverse drug reactions in a tertiary care hospital. *Journal of Clinical and Scientific Research*. https://www.semanticscholar.org/paper/d5f8754d14d571a79050881eef575e868a97bb88 (accessed on 9 June 2025).
8. Banegas Ruiz, R., Valderrama Treviño, A. I., Gómez Mendoza, F. F., Baca Domínguez, C. R., Campos Angulo, G., Alejo Fuentes, L. F., Jiménez Nateras, C. N., Ramos Lojero, V. M., Espejel Blancas, J. A., & Baltazar Barrera Mera, M. (2019). Stevens-Johnson syndrome and toxic epidermal necrolysis: A review. https://core.ac.uk/download/539910118.pdf (accessed on 9 June 2025).
9. Berardesca, E., Bernardini, N., Bianchi, L., Chimenti, S., et al. (2018). Use of biological drugs in patients with psoriasis and psoriatic arthritis in Italy: Results from the PSONG survey. https://core.ac.uk/download/154948747.pdf (accessed on 9 June 2025).
10. Bhosale, R. R., Mokase, Y. G., & Patil, A. V. (2017). *Co-Trimoxazole Induced Stevens-Johnson Syndrome in Pediatric Age Group*. https://core.ac.uk/download/544390242.pdf.
11. Bielfeldt, S., Rippon, M., & Waring, M. (2015). *An Evaluation of Properties Related to Wear Time of Four Dressings During a Five-Day Period*. https://core.ac.uk/download/30734135.pdf (accessed on 9 June 2025).
12. Birlea, S., Bosenberg, M. W., Box, N. F., Brash, D. E., et al. (2018). *Frontiers in Pigment Cell and Melanoma Research*. http://arxiv.org/abs/1808.01869 (accessed on 9 June 2025).

13. Boda, D., & Dehelean, C. (2019). Immuno-dermatological processes involved in chronic skin diseases: Highlights of the Second Conference of the Romanian Society for Immuno-Dermatology, Bucharest, September, 2018. *Experimental and Therapeutic Medicine, 18*, 873–874. https://www.semanticscholar.org/paper/c0a044ef033de561e536bd7ddfcda992d2f766a1 (accessed on 9 June 2025).

14. Borges-Costa, J., & Garrido, P. (2017). *Skin Disorders in Renal Transplant Recipients: A Retrospective Study*. https://core.ac.uk/download/534005199.pdf.

15. Bosco, D., Fantozzi, P. J., Palaia, G., Romeo, G., et al. (2015). A rare case of melanosis of the hard palate mucosa in a patient with chronic myeloid leukemia. https://core.ac.uk/download/98339063.pdf (accessed on 9 June 2025).

16. Bourlière, M., Buggisch, P., Cacoub, P., Dupin, C., et al. (2011). Dermatological side effects of hepatitis C and its treatment: Patient management in the era of direct-acting antivirals. https://core.ac.uk/download/pdf/82383033.pdf.

17. Božo Vojniković, Toth, I., Lugović-Mihić, L., Šitum, M., Martinis, M., Peternel, R., & Bulat, V. (2013). Dermatological aspects of contact dermatitis from eyeglass frames and optical materials. https://core.ac.uk/download/14466225.pdf (accessed on 9 June 2025).

18. Calvieri, S., Cantisani, C., D'Andrea, V., Frascani, F., et al. (2014). New patents on topical anesthetics. https://core.ac.uk/download/54511696.pdf.

19. Calvieri, S., Didona, D., Macrì, G., Mercuri, S., et al. (2018). Nasopharyngeal melanoma. https://core.ac.uk/download/159269626.pdf.

20. Casha, J., Elnikety, S., Kamal, T., Mashaly, M., et al. (2012). Acute compartment syndrome of the forearm as a rare complication of toxic epidermal necrolysis: A case report. https://core.ac.uk/download/pdf/8718355.pdf.

21. Chindhalore, C., Gupta, A. V., Dakhale, G., & Srivastava, A. (2024). Analysis of cutaneous adverse drug reactions (ADR) reported at an ADR monitoring center of a tertiary care teaching institute in Central India. *Cureus, 16*. https://www.semanticscholar.org/paper/cf85cd63a9ac8e629333b829a37f2be2e3380066 (accessed on 9 June 2025).

22. Chipkar, V. B., & Chondikar, V. S. (2024). Perception of Kandu and critical review of Kandugna Mahakshaya. *International Journal of Pharmaceutical Research and Applications*. https://www.semanticscholar.org/paper/a91d42a2c0f98f526025c9c5c87244078bd7bb14 (accessed on 9 June 2025).

23. Daniel, W. L., Santomasso, B., Locke, F. L., Ghobadi, A., Turtle, C. J., Brudno, J. N., Maus, M. V., et al. (2018). ASTCT consensus grading for cytokine release syndrome and neurologic toxicity associated with immune effector cells. *Biology of Blood and Marrow Transplantation, 25*, 625–638. https://doi.org/10.1016/j.bbmt.2018.12.758.

24. Daronat, J. M., Deltour, R., & Guerrier, G. (2011). Unusual presentation of acute annular urticaria: A case report. https://core.ac.uk/download/pdf/9418220.pdf.

25. Datta, S., Gunindro, N., Meena, D. N., Nameirakpam, S., et al. (2022). Adverse drug reaction patterns of anti-retroviral drugs: A study in a tertiary care teaching institute of North East India. https://core.ac.uk/download/524962465.pdf.

26. Domínguez, E. D. M., & Muñoz Estrada, V. F. (2024). Urticaria aguda. *Revita Alegria México*. https://www.semanticscholar.org/paper/c324b5618f873f28b715a74d654333ee9409a1e2 (accessed on 9 June 2025).

27. Dunn, S. (2020). Development and management of canine adverse food reactions and its connections to the grain-free dog food movement. https://core.ac.uk/download/304169066.pdf (accessed on 9 June 2025).

28. Elali, F. R., & Grant, A. C. (2024). Tolerance of bupropion SR after delayed-onset urticaria and angioedema associated with bupropion XL. *Case Reports in Psychiatry, 2024.* https://www.semanticscholar.org/paper/28e599b2dd8a6df67754752c0e51f03ad46e0437 (accessed on 9 June 2025).

29. Era, N., Mukherjee, S., Saha, B., Tripathi, K., et al. (2017). Monitoring cutaneous adverse drug reactions in patients on TDF+3TC+EFV: A single center experience. https://core.ac.uk/download/539895908.pdf (accessed on 9 June 2025).

30. Faulkner, M. A., & Tolman, J. A. (2011). Treatment options for refractory and difficult to treat seizures: Focus on vigabatrin. https://core.ac.uk/download/pdf/8618198.pdf.

31. Frioui, R., Mokni, S., Tabka, M., Belajouza, C., & Denguezli, M. (2021). Frontal fibrosing alopecia following beta blocker injectable mesotherapy: Is it more than a simple coincidence? *Dermatologic Therapy, 35.* https://www.semanticscholar.org/paper/e401dad861b9e7e293cec572d19037cd5157463a (accessed on 9 June 2025).

32. Garg, Y., Gore, R., Jain, S., Kumar, R., et al. (2017). Dapsone induced photosensitivity in Indian women: A rare case. https://core.ac.uk/download/543134423.pdf (accessed on 9 June 2025).

33. Gupta, V., & Agarwal, A. (2021). A study on adverse drug reactions in patients on antiretroviral therapy in a tertiary care hospital at Jaipur, Rajasthan. *International Journal of Medical and Biomedical Studies.* https://www.semanticscholar.org/paper/cc3c4b092b9bbc83a98b288ee36115221f27418f (accessed on 9 June 2025).

34. Johannesson, M., Liang, M. H., & Stucki, G. (1994). Is misoprostol cost-effective in the prevention of nonsteroidal anti-inflammatory drug–induced gastropathy in patients with chronic arthritis? https://core.ac.uk/download/12171041.pdf (accessed on 9 June 2025).

35. Kalola, A. S., Mistry, C. B., & Shah, S. M. (2024). A study of cutaneous adverse drug reactions in the dermatology department of a tertiary care teaching hospital in Gujarat. https://core.ac.uk/download/603896206.pdf (accessed on 9 June 2025).

36. Lee, R. M., Hwang, Y. C., Liu, I. J., Lee, C. C., Tsai, H. Z., Li, H. J., & Wu, H. C. (2020). Development of therapeutic antibodies for the treatment of diseases. *Journal of Biomedical Science, 27.* https://doi.org/10.1186/s12929-019-0592-z.

37. Patton, E. E. (2016). Nutritional factors associated with acne vulgaris. https://open.bu.edu/bitstream/2144/19444/1/Patton_bu_0017N_12304.pdf (accessed on 9 June 2025).

38. Pirro, F., Caldarola, G., De Simone, C., Moretta, G., Giovanardi, G., & Peris, K. (2019). Multiple paradoxical reactions during ixekizumab therapy. *Dermatologic Therapy, 32.* https://www.semanticscholar.org/paper/acfb1fcf50b7b2ca4a7924c559ac397e2fff8f84 (accessed on 9 June 2025).

39. Qu, J. M., Wen, S. J., Lin, Y. K., Lu, H. X., Huang, K. Q., Maansson, C. T., Lee, C. S., et al. (2024). Retrospective clinical study analysis of skin adverse reactions related to epidermal growth factor receptor inhibitors. *Translational Cancer Research, 13*, 3016–3030. https://www.semanticscholar.org/paper/d61dbb901bc4f5fabe5c3f78ba443fb04dcb3126 (accessed on 9 June 2025).

40. Ridolo, E., Pucciarini, F., Barone, A., Nouvenne, A., Meschi, T., Peveri, S., & Incorvaia, C. (2021). Dermatological manifestations during COVID-19 infection: A case series and discussion on the problem of differential diagnosis. *Acta Bio Medica: Atenei Parmensis, 92*. https://www.semanticscholar.org/paper/8290e1cf29a8b08691a8c72266ee175d27509362 (accessed on 9 June 2025).

41. Spillers, N. J., Luther, P. M., Talbot, N. C., Ly, G. H., Downs, E., Lavespere, G., Pavlickova, D., et al. (2023). Association of acetaminophen with Stevens–Johnson syndrome and toxic epidermal necrolysis: Pharmacologic considerations and treatment options. *Cureus, 15*. https://www.semanticscholar.org/paper/43449904b1c4c789ea1ea12c2dc3f9c7d1e20bff (accessed on 9 June 2025).

42. Stabile, A., Kiviranta, A. M., Shukralla, A. A., Chauvet, A. E., Cook, A. K., Nash, A. S., Dayrell-Hart, B., et al. (2016). Antiepileptic drugs' tolerability and safety–A systematic review and meta-analysis of adverse effects in dogs. https://core.ac.uk/download/45467661.pdf (accessed on 9 June 2025).

43. Suresh, B., Reshmi, P. R., Jaipal, J., Pise, G. A., Prasad, S. S., & Manohar, N. (2024). Tofacitinib in leprosy: A novel therapeutic approach in chronic recalcitrant type II reactions. *Cureus, 16*. https://www.semanticscholar.org/paper/b9eddf72c6184f8fd3197684f1669c372a8fa86f (accessed on 9 June 2025).

44. Syed, Z. S., Abbas, S. W., & Shaikh, U. (2023). P14 Bullous Sweet syndrome as a presentation of chronic myelogenous leukaemia. *British Journal of Dermatology*. https://www.semanticscholar.org/paper/d9c999e9cbfbd4bb337ef367a0eaaad3a8dee53e (accessed on 9 June 2025).

45. Tairova, R., Gaydina, T., Dvornikov, A. S., Tazartukova, A. D., & Lyang, O. (2020). Difficulties in differential diagnosis of cutaneous manifestations in patients with coronavirus infection. Innate antiviral immunity. https://www.semanticscholar.org/paper/533ff0d15c985e503f38faee4ffc655293384b11 (accessed on 9 June 2025).

46. Valencia, A., Schijman, A. G., de Andrade, A. L., Luquetti, A. O., Fernandes, C. D., Segura, E., Guhl, F., et al. (2009). Feasibility, drug safety, and effectiveness of etiological treatment programs for Chagas disease in Honduras, Guatemala, and Bolivia: 10-year experience of Médecins Sans Frontières. https://core.ac.uk/download/pdf/9417445.pdf (accessed on 9 June 2025).

47. Vedavathi, H., Dadapeer, H. J., Lourdes, J. M., Prasad, B., et al. (2016). A study on cutaneous adverse drug reactions at district McGann teaching hospital, Shimoga Institute of Medical Sciences, Shivamogga, Karnataka, India. https://core.ac.uk/download/539896187.pdf (accessed on 9 June 2025).

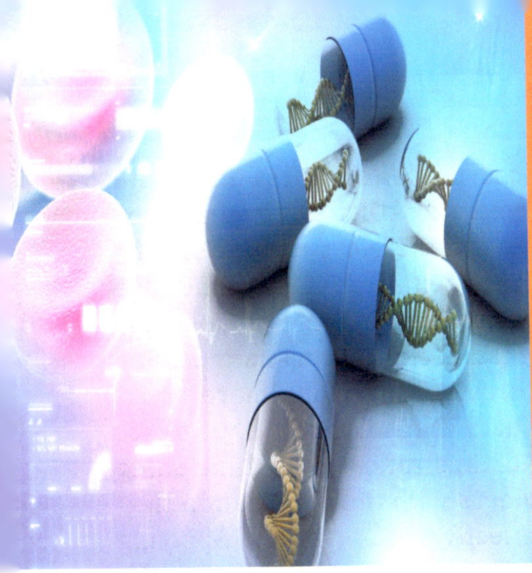

Chapter 11

PHARMACOGENOMICS AND ADRS

Contents

Introduction

The field of pharmacogenomics is an innovative intersection of genetics and drug studies, aiming to develop personalized drug therapies based on an individual's genetic profile. It is important to pharmacogenomics to understand how differences in genes, especially those involved in drug metabolism, affect the patient's response to drugs. Since ADRs are a significant health concern, knowing a person's genetic factors might help reduce risks and increase the effectiveness of drugs. Pharmacogenomic testing is now recognized in recent studies as a means to transition from treating all patients the same to treating them individually, leading to better results and fewer side effects. The change is significant in handling the issue of different drug responses in various patient groups, which helps explain how drugs interact and act based on each person's genes. All over the world, health care systems face many challenges due to ADRs of all levels of severity. Since idiosyncratic

ADRs are unpredictable, they prove difficult to manage and may cause a lot of illness and death in some cases. Research has confirmed that the majority of idiosyncratic ADRs are mediated by genetic influences, specifically alleles associated with the HLA gene, and therefore underscore the importance of the application of pharmacogenomic principles in the identification of vulnerable individuals. Since some genetic markers are associated with ADRs, pharmacogenomics enables the development of preventive measures that ensure patient safety. Because pharmacogenetic testing can be helpful in clinical practice, it is essential for healthcare providers to learn more about how to maximize its benefits. The move to use pharmacogenomic data in clinical care shows that more people value personalized medicines. The Food and Drug Administration is now including pharmacogenomic details in drug labels, providing healthcare providers with the information they need about how an individual's genes can affect the safety and effectiveness of drugs. Applying pharmacogenomics in pediatric medicine enables doctors to prescribe treatments tailored to the genetic makeup of each individual child. When healthcare providers have a deeper understanding of pharmacogenomics, they will be better equipped to utilize test results to inform treatment decisions. Also, the pharmacist's role changes in the new model, as they can handle complex information on pharmacogenomics and guide patients on the right drug treatments based on genetic testing. Besides improving clinical effectiveness, this new approach is necessary to avoid ADRs and build a better and more flexible healthcare system (Figure 11.1).

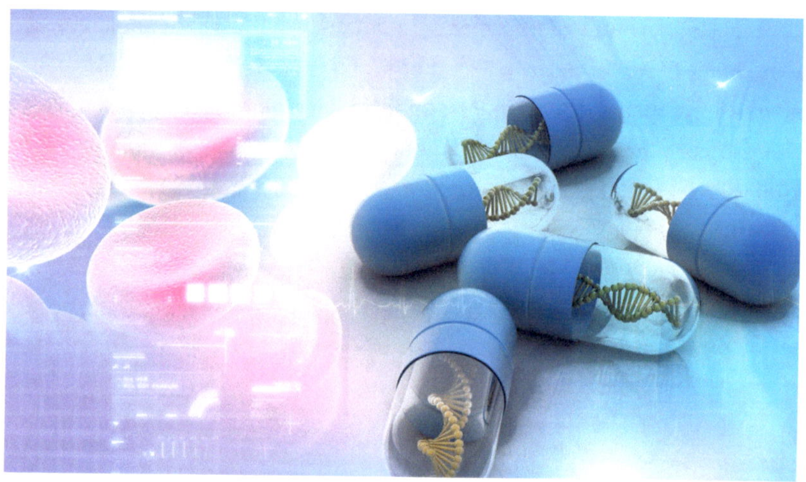

Figure 11.1. Pharmacogenomics and ADRs.

Source: https://www.genomebc.ca/wp-content/uploads/2019/08/107.008_Pharmacogenomics_DP4537834_ds.jpg.

Definition of Pharmacogenomics

Pharmacogenomics combines pharmacology and genomics to determine how genes affect a person's response to medications. This branch of personalized medicine examines the impact of genetic variations on drug metabolism, efficacy, and the potential for ADRs. Pharmacogenomics helps predict how drugs will work in patients and select the most effective medications for them. Since ADRs cause many cases of illness and death, using pharmacogenomic information in medical care helps reduce the risks of pharmacotherapy. The predictive power of this field not only enhances the safety profile of medications but also advances the development of targeted therapies that correspond to unique genetic profiles, thereby improving overall healthcare outcomes (Sad et al., 2023). The shift from pharmacogenetics to pharmacogenomics has led to a significant improvement in understanding how genes influence drug interactions and reactions. With this change, it becomes possible to examine genetic variations that affect how drugs are metabolized, transported, and work in various populations. Alterations in genes that code for drug-metabolizing enzymes, transporters, and receptors may result in either an increased likelihood of side effects or a failure of the drug to work properly. Consequently, integrating pharmacogenomics into pharmacovigilance strategies can optimize drug safety monitoring by providing insights into patient-specific factors that contribute to ADRs, further reinforcing the importance of personalized medicine in mitigating drug-related risks (Bate et al., 2021). Moreover, the use of pharmacogenomics helps create guidelines for doctors to predict, prevent, and manage potential side effects of drugs. Healthcare providers can determine the most effective medicines and doses for patients by utilizing genetic testing. This approach to prescribing drugs is especially important for managing complex diseases, as multiple medications may be required. With the improvement of pharmacogenomic technologies, real-time data can soon help doctors make decisions, which may decrease or eliminate ADRs by using customized therapies. Ultimately, pharmacogenomics represents a paradigm shift in the relationship between genetics and drug therapy, making it a critical component of modern medicine aimed at improving patient safety and efficacy (Sad et al., 2023) (Figure 11.2).

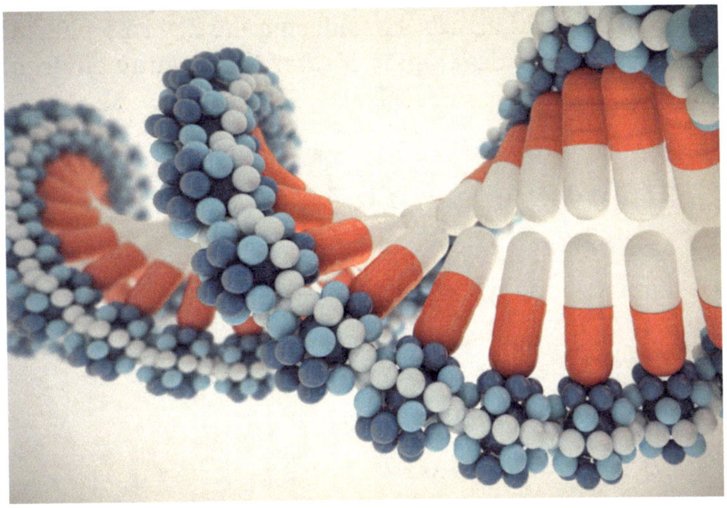

Figure 11.2. Definition of pharmacogenomics.

Source: https://pharmaceutical-journal.com/wp-content/uploads/2021/01/pharmacogenomics-concept-ss-17-927x617.png.

Importance of Understanding ADRs (Adverse Drug Reactions)

It is essential to study ADRs in pharmacogenomics because it makes it possible for healthcare practitioners to tailor the drug regimens to their patients based on their genetic makeup. Pharmacogenomics reveals that variations in genes can alter how drugs are metabolized and increase the likelihood of side effects. As a result, practitioners can utilize this area of science to assist patients by selecting the appropriate drug and administering the correct dosage. If physicians learn about the genetic causes of ADRs, they can identify those at risk and therefore improve patient care and cut down on the costs of drug therapy errors. When healthcare professionals are informed about the risks of ADRs, they can easily discuss a patient's genetic data and treatment options, resulting in better personalized care. In addition, enhanced awareness of pharmacovigilance as mandated by institutions such as India's Central Drugs Standard Control Organisation (CDSCO) emphasizes the importance of surveillance of ADRs throughout the drug lifecycle. Regular monitoring of ADRs through good pharmacovigilance systems keeps dangerous effects away, making it possible to fix mistakes in medicine use quickly. It helps patients and also encourages medical professionals to work safely. The data gathered by pharmacovigilance programs is helpful in enhancing drug safety and making well-informed decisions in the field of health policy. Conceptualization of ADRs in this respect emphasizes the necessity for collective responsibility on the part of stakeholders like HCPs, drug regulatory agencies, and pharmaceutical companies in promotion of safe drug practice and public health advantages (Suke et al., 2015). Additionally, ADRs have implications that extend beyond the patient's experience to encompass broader public health concerns. Since a large number of ADRs are responsible for both sickness and death among populations, more awareness is needed. In India, ADRs are often not appropriately reported, which makes it harder to examine their occurrence and consequences. If a structured training program is implemented to educate healthcare workers about ADR strategies and ADR awareness, they will be able to identify and report them accurately. Besides, it is essential to apply pharmacogenomics in daily medical practice to reduce the risks of ADRs. For future directions in individualized medicine, it is essential to understand and mitigate ADR risk hazards, considering the key role pharmacogenomics plays in reversing drug-induced diseases and developing a safer therapeutic environment for all patients (Adithan et al., 2015) (Figure 11.3).

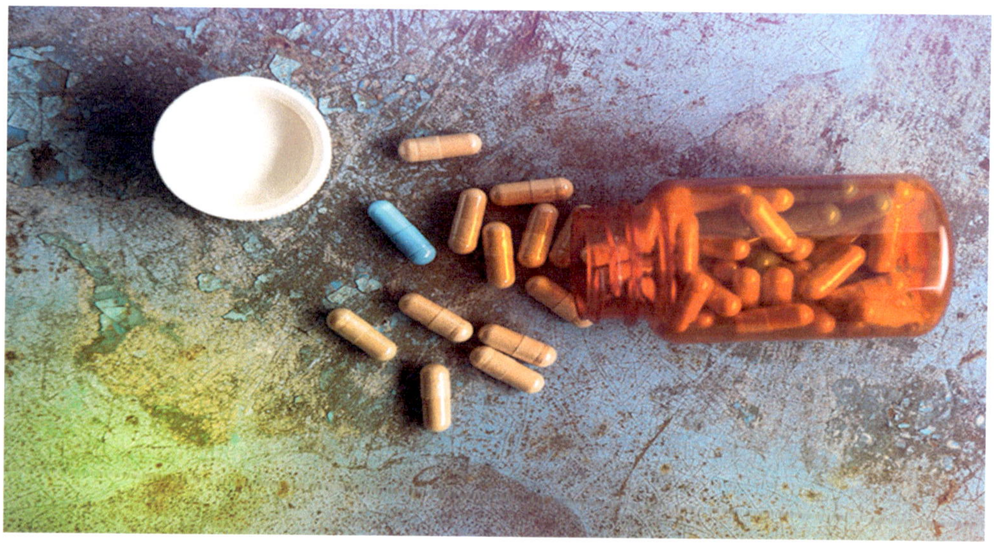

Figure 11.3. Importance of understanding ADRs (adverse drug reactions).

Source: https://hospitalpharmacyeurope.com/wp-content/uploads/2004/03/ADR-1.jpg.

Overview of the Relationship Between Pharmacogenomics and ADRs

The relationship between pharmacogenomics and ADRs has gained increasing attention in recent years as the medical community seeks to understand how genetic variations influence drug responses.

Pharmacogenomics looks at how someone's genes can change their reaction to drugs, and ADRs refer to adverse and unexpected effects caused by taking medications. Learning more about these interactions can help treatments work better and, at the same time, reduce the risk of serious side effects. Evidence indicates that many ADRs are linked to genetic causes, which is why people are urging the use of genomic data in healthcare. With the help of advanced tools, such as DGANet, it is now possible to predict ADRs based on both pharmacogenomics and drug data, which opens the door to personalized medicine. When examining the predictive aspect of pharmacogenomics, it is evident that the numerous genetic differences among patients can significantly impact how drugs are metabolized, their efficacy, and safety. It is crucial in this relationship to identify the specific gene variants that alter how drugs interact with the body. Polymorphisms in genes responsible for drug metabolism may cause differences in drug elimination, which can result in more cases of ADRs. For this reason, learning about genetics can help doctors find the best treatment plans for each patient. As highlighted in recent studies, leveraging pharmacogenomics can significantly enhance the understanding of drug-gene interactions, aiding HCPs in selecting appropriate medications and dosages for individual patients (He et al., 2025). In addition, including pharmacogenomic data in healthcare routines is a significant step forward in reducing ADRs and improving how patients do. Using machine learning (ML) and biomedical text mining, researchers can analyze drug interactions, patient reviews, and genetic data to identify risks associated with certain drugs. Using this approach, drug development becomes more efficient and monitoring ADRs after the drug is approved is also improved by watching for them in various groups of people. As underscored by recent literature, the synergistic relationship between pharmacogenomics, drug reviews, and sentiment analysis contributes to a comprehensive understanding of ADRs, empowering clinicians to make informed decisions regarding medication choices that align with individual genetic dispositions (Nafea et al., 2024). Pharmacogenomics plays a crucial role in ensuring the safer and more effective use of drugs.

11.1. Historical Background of Pharmacogenomics

Pharmacogenomics began as a field when scientists first discovered a link between genetics and how drugs are metabolized. During the 1950s, scientists in molecular biology proposed that genetic coding could affect a person's reaction to drugs. It was when scientists discovered certain genetic markers that showed links to the effectiveness and safety of drugs that this field began to progress. A major study at that time showed that how genes produce enzymes can affect a person's reaction to medications, forming the basis for pharmacogenomics. As researchers continued to study the human genome, it became clear that tailored medicine was not only possible but also inevitable, making it a key part of today's medical practices. These studies made it possible to add pharmacogenomics to regular clinical examinations. Pharmacogenomics made significant progress during the late 20th and early 21st centuries due to the development of new genomic technologies. In 2003, scientists completed the Human Genome Project, gaining a comprehensive map of the human genome and its variants. This monumental achievement encouraged further investigation of genetic polymorphisms' effects on drug response, so that more was learned about ADRs. The introduction of pharmacogenomic testing made clinicians appreciate the benefits these tests could bring to choosing the proper treatment for each patient. Still, some challenges stood in the way, for example, the difficulty of interpreting genetic information and the requirement for the same testing methods to be used for all groups of people. Because of these efforts, it has become easier to use precision medicine, as the value of linking genetics and drugs has been recognized. Even though technology was advancing, bringing pharmacogenomics to clinical practice has been a challenging task, primarily due to the need for population-specific adjustments. Although developed nations are now offering pharmacogenomic testing as part of their healthcare, it remains challenging for emerging economies due to a lack of resources. Qatar is an example of a country that wants to apply pharmacogenomics in practice for its varied immigrant population. Currently, efforts are underway to educate healthcare providers about pharmacogenomics and incorporate it into medical training programs. Still, there are issues such as ethical matters, the importance of strong policies, and the chance that health inequality will increase that must be handled. As pharmacogenomics develops, it can only help improve drug safety and effectiveness by conducting more research and utilizing advanced technology to address current issues and achieve the highest level of patient care in this field (Figure 11.4).

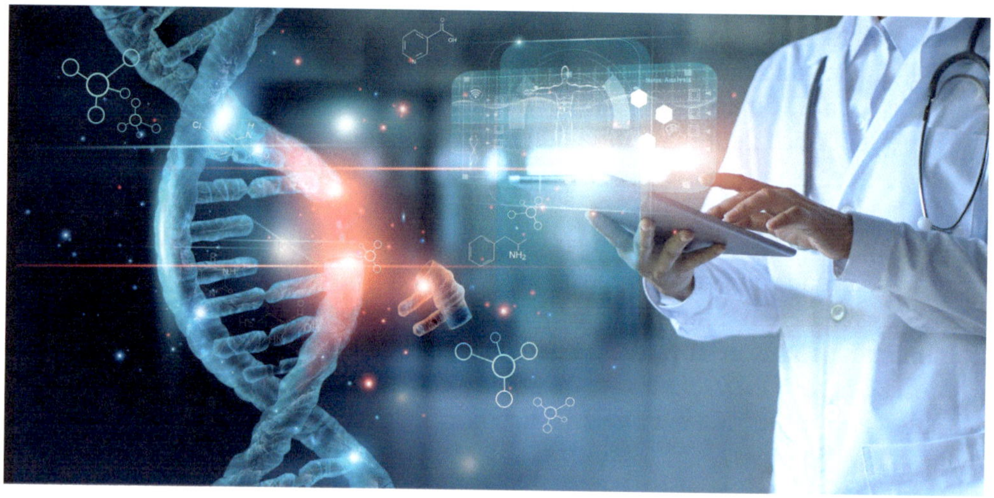

Figure 11.4. Historical background of pharmacogenomics.

Source: https://www.omnipgx.com/blog/wp-content/uploads/2020/02/AdobeStock_268793354-scaled.jpeg.

11.1.1. Early Discoveries in Genetic Variability

Discoveries about genetic variability in the past helped build the basis for understanding how different people react to drugs. Initially, scientists observed that certain traits are passed down through generations and decided to investigate the genes that control drug metabolism and their effectiveness. It became clear that these insights were significant, as research revealed that small changes in a single gene could impact the way many drugs are processed and utilized in the body. Therefore, this knowledge about genetic variability played a key role in making personalized medicine possible. Recognizing these genetic differences not only illuminated the complex interactions between drugs and biological systems but also set the stage for evolving therapeutic strategies aimed at minimizing ADRs and enhancing treatment outcomes. Additionally, early studies by geneticists highlighted the significance of changes in key enzymes involved in drug metabolism. It has been shown that variations in genes, such as those encoding cytochrome P450 enzymes, can lead to people reacting differently to drugs due to their genetic makeup. Because such variability often leads to ADRs, it is important to include genetic testing in medical care. According to studies, some people do not have the enzymes needed to properly activate or deactivate drugs, which can bring about either poor treatment results or harmful side effects.

As a result, the early findings in genetics were immediately applied in medicine, changing how drugs are prescribed by recommending a method that considers each patient's genetic profile. As the study of pharmacogenomics advanced, new studies showed that genetic differences have a significant effect on drug safety and how well they work. It was difficult for genetic findings to be used in medicine because laws and regulations were not able to keep up with the rapid progress in science. The lack of standardized rules and insufficient knowledge among healthcare workers made it hard for many to use pharmacogenomic approaches to reduce ADRs. Despite these difficulties, the basic research conducted by geneticists was crucial in forming today's pharmacological approaches. Since it was clear that a single way of treating everyone was not enough to handle the complexities of drug reactions, it is still necessary to keep improving these discoveries and apply them in clinical settings to support personalized medicine and reduce the number of ADRs in patients (Figure 11.5).

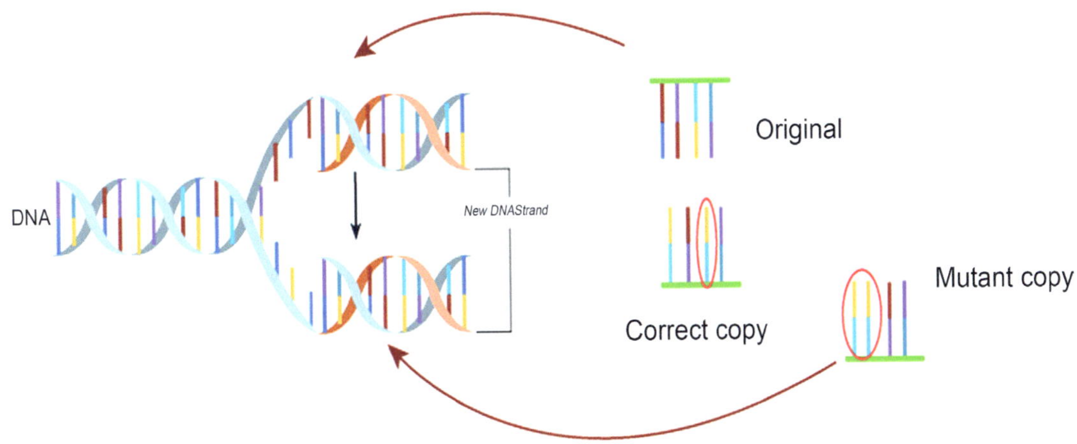

Figure 11.5. Early discoveries in genetic variability.

Source: https://media.geeksforgeeks.org/wp-content/uploads/20240119101553/Genetic-Variation.png.

11.1.2. Development of Pharmacogenomic Testing

Significant progress in genetic science and technology has played a big role in the development of pharmacogenomic testing. Pharmacogenomics is a branch of pharmacogenetics, which looks at how genetics affects a person's response to drugs. While research on such novel genetic markers, such as single-nucleotide polymorphisms (SNPs), continued to improve, researchers began linking the variations to drug efficacy and the risk of ADRs. Various studies have demonstrated that inherited genetic differences can impact drug metabolism, potentially leading to treatment failure or an increased risk of side effects, underscoring the need for personalized medicine. Public awareness of the influence of genetics on drug response remains limited, despite growing recognition of interindividual variation in therapeutic response (Magavern et al., 2025). It is also challenging to introduce pharmacogenomic testing into clinical care because unified guidelines and more education are needed for physicians. Although pharmacogenomic data offers considerable potential, doctors are not very familiar with genetic testing or understanding its outcomes. Present-day technologies, such as next-generation sequencing (NGS), provide detailed information about an individual's genomic signature, enabling more effective drug selection and dosing regimens. Even so, some issues such as the cost of genetic testing, changes in insurance policies, and ethical matters with genetic data still prevent its wider use. Continuous growth of pharmacogenomics in nursing practice serves to heighten the need for more education to bridge the knowledge divide and eventually equip healthcare providers with the tools to effectively reduce ADRs while optimizing pharmacotherapy (Alanazi et al., 2019). In addition, recent surveys show that many people are interested in pharmacogenomic testing, prompting healthcare systems to respond to these changes. According to the survey in the UK, most patients are eager to try pharmacogenomic testing and support its inclusion in everyday healthcare routines. This interest is mainly sparked by the observation that standard treatments often do not help or cause unpleasant side effects. Most of the respondents wished for easy access to pharmacogenomic data and also wanted healthcare providers to offer this testing. The intersection of public demand and clinical promise evokes a reconsideration of health infrastructure to include pharmacogenomics, thereby enhancing patient outcomes and lessening ADRs on a greater scale (Magavern et al., 2025) (Figure 11.6).

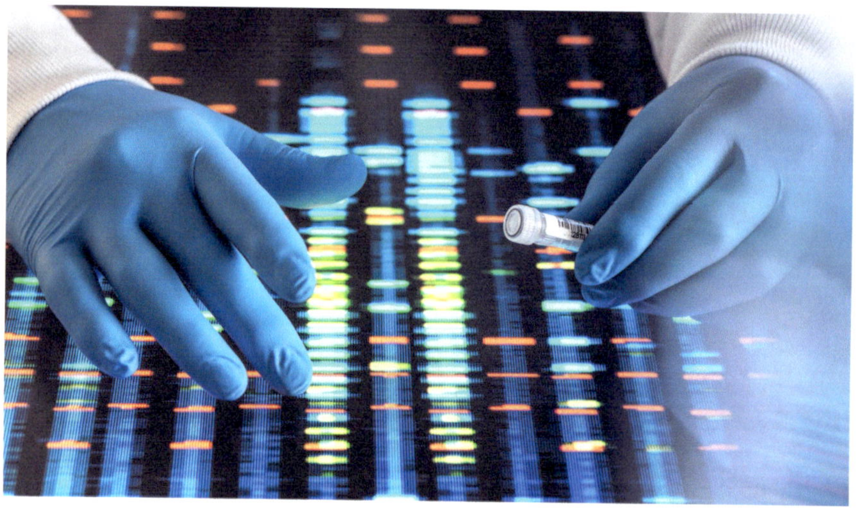

Figure 11.6. Development of pharmacogenomic testing.

Source: https://www.cvshealth.com/news/pharmacy/the-role-of-pharmacogenomic-testing-in-precision-medicine.html.

11.1.3. Milestones in the Study of ADRs

The study of ADRs has undergone significant milestones that have enhanced our understanding of patient safety in pharmacotherapy. Since ADRs were first recognized as a serious problem in the early 20th century and new regulations were introduced, the field of pharmacology has undergone significant changes. The WHO played a pivotal role in this evolution by launching global initiatives in the 1960s to collect and analyze ADR data. Thanks to this effort, it became clear that monitoring the safety of drugs after they are released is important. Therefore, healthcare systems everywhere have started using reporting systems and sharing data to spot and address ADRs, which helps create a safer environment for patients. Pharmacogenomics is now being utilized in ADR research to elucidate how individuals' genes can influence their reactions to medications. After the Human Genome Project was completed in the late 20th century, researchers began to understand the role of genes in how drugs are metabolized and how they work. Thanks to pharmacogenomic testing, doctors can now find out which patients are likely to have ADRs and choose the proper treatment for each person. This approach to treating patients has helped medicine work more effectively and reduced the likelihood of adverse events. However, despite significant progress, genetic diversity alone accounts for only a limited proportion of individual variability in drug responses, highlighting the need for further research to explore additional factors that might contribute to ADRs (Zhao et al., 2023). It is now known that the gut microbiota can influence how well drugs work and their safety, a concept known as pharmacomicrobiomics. Recent studies have demonstrated how gut microbiota can modulate the absorption, distribution, metabolism, and excretion (ADME) of therapeutic agents, leading to variations in patient response. How microbiota and drugs interact can lead to significant changes in the microbiome, which can worsen or lessen the risk of ADRs. The new field highlights the need to employ multi-omics methods to accurately study these interactions. By integrating genomic data from both human hosts and their microbiomes, researchers can enhance the precision of drug therapies, thereby paving the way for improved patient outcomes and personalized medicine (Zhao et al., 2023). Looking into these connections confirms that pharmaceutical sciences are always progressing and that it is essential to handle ADRs properly.

11.2. Mechanisms of Adverse Drug Reactions

Mechanisms of ADRs should be understood to maximize patient safety and therapeutic effectiveness. ADRs can be caused by several factors, including genetic variability that affects drug metabolism, which leads to unexpected therapeutic failures or toxicities. Pharmacogenomics—information on how genes affect an individual's response to drugs—is the core of understanding these mechanisms. For instance, drug-metabolizing enzyme-encoding polymorphisms could significantly influence the PK of drugs and result in subtherapeutic efficacy or toxic side effects.

Hence, the detection of individuals prone to ADRs through genetic screening could be used to inform prescribing and individualize drug regimens, thereby minimizing adverse effects and enhancing drug efficacy. The financial burden of ADRs is another crucial sector to address, as evidenced by research that estimates hospitalization expenses associated with such reactions. For example, it has been well documented that the hospitalization cost of ADRs can be staggering, and thus, there needs to be some preventative intervention in clinical practice. A promising approach is the application of preemptive pharmacogenetic testing, which could potentially identify patients who are genetically susceptible to ADRs before treatment is administered. The issue is how to estimate the breakeven cost of testing, as in one study where the cost of preventable hospitalization was assessed to justify investments in pharmacogenomics. Through the successful implementation of this testing as part of routine care, health systems may be able to eliminate the incidence and economic burden of ADRs, improving both clinical practice and health policy decision-making (Brunham et al., 2019). Personalized medicine advancements are the future of overcoming ADRs by using alternative approaches that include elements of network pharmacology principles. This approach emphasizes the interconnectivity of biological networks and drug interactions within them that dictate their safety and efficacy. Clinicians, by applying network pharmacology concepts to pharmacogenomic data, can not only predict but also tailor treatments for ADR prevention to a patient's specific profile. This advancement will yield safer and more efficient therapies. Additionally, this drug design paradigm change requires the reassessment of traditional practices within chemistry and pharmacology, ultimately culminating in a more comprehensive conceptualization of medication interactions and variabilities (Marsh et al., 2010). Through these collaborative efforts, the field can move towards preventing the occurrence of ADRs and enhancing patient outcomes (Figure 11.7).

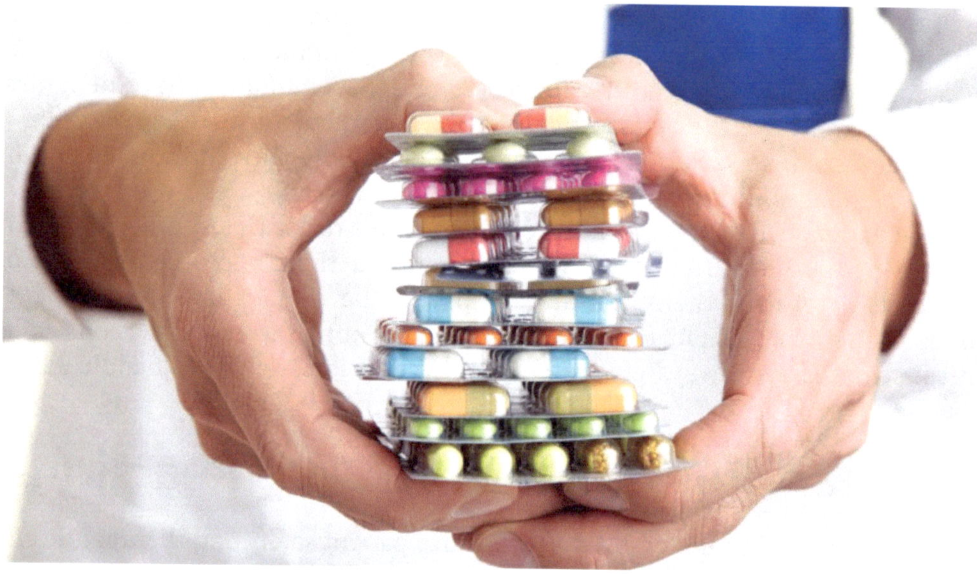

Figure 11.7. Mechanisms of adverse drug reactions.

Source: https://healthvision.in/wp-content/uploads/2018/03/Adverse-Drugs_1.jpg.

11.2.1. Genetic Factors Influencing Drug Metabolism

The way a person metabolizes drugs is largely affected by their genes, which is a main concern in pharmacogenomics. Drug metabolism is primarily mediated by enzymes, which are often subject to genetic variations, notably single-nucleotide polymorphisms (SNPs). These genetic variations can significantly affect the enzymatic activity that dictates how drugs are metabolized, leading to inter-individual differences in therapeutic outcomes and susceptibility to ADRs. If there are polymorphisms in genes for cytochrome P450 enzymes, which are important for phase I metabolism, people may be categorized as poor, intermediate, extensive, or ultra-rapid metabolizers. Because of this classification, a poor metabolizer may be exposed to too much of the drug and could suffer from its side effects. In contrast, an ultra-rapid metabolizer may not get the full benefits of the treatment. Furthermore, genetic factors interacting with drug transporters also play a critical role in drug metabolism, a concept explored in studies focusing on the ATP-binding cassette (ABC) transporters. Changes in ABCB1 and ABCC2 genes are related to differences in drug reactions and the number of ADRs. It has been shown that some genetic variants connected to these transporters can indicate the risk of gastrointestinal side effects in patients receiving carboplatin and paclitaxel for non-small cell lung cancer. This connection between genotypes and clinical outcomes demonstrates that incorporating genetic testing into drug treatment helps predict potential problems and enhances drug effectiveness. Individualizing drug therapy based on genetic markers not only maximizes treatment benefits but also minimizes the risks associated with ADRs, thereby improving patient safety and treatment outcomes (Cecília et al., 2025). Based on these results, the application of pharmacogenomic principles could significantly impact the practice of medicine. As genetics advances, it is now easier for clinicians to utilize this information to select the most effective treatments and minimize the risk of drug side effects. The increased awareness of how genes affect drug metabolism proves that personalized medicine should be based on each patient's genetic information. Many studies have pointed out that studying genetic markers related to ADRs is essential for improving how safe and effective drugs are. This research trajectory promises not only to refine existing therapeutic strategies but also to foster the development of new, targeted pharmacological agents designed with the patient's genetic makeup in mind (Anunobi, 2024) (Figure 11.8).

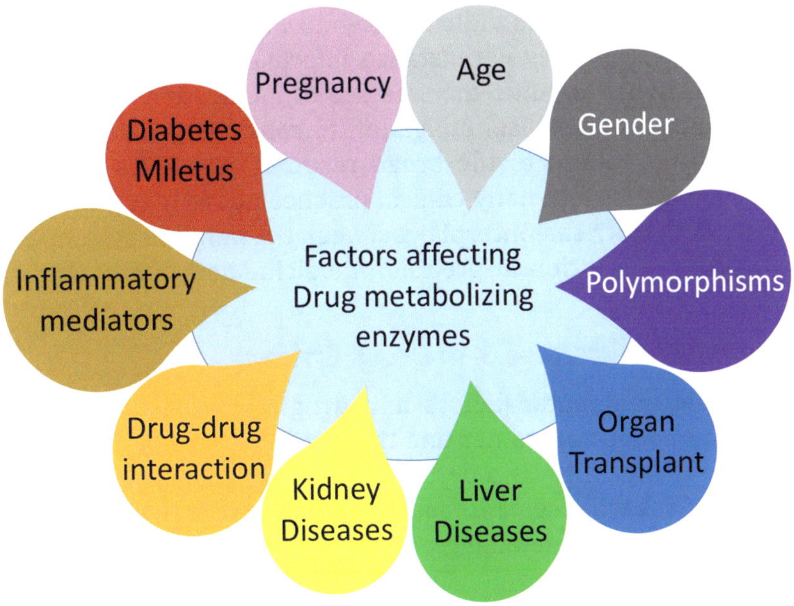

Figure 11.8. Genetic factors influencing drug metabolism.

Source: https://duckduckgo.com/?q=Genetic+Factors+Influencing+Drug+Metabolism&t=h_&iar=images&iaf=size%3ALarge&iai=https%3A%2F%2Fd3i71xaburhd42.cloudfront.net%2F175820a5fa750f9f9de9e4253cc356f3a23f1b4f%2F12-Figure4-1.png.

11.2.2. Immune System Responses to Medications

The immune system's reaction to drugs can have a range of consequences, primarily ADRs, which are founded mainly on an individual's genetic makeup. Pharmacogenomics explores the way genes influence the response to drugs and is thus highly important in the context of ADRs. Certain populations, for instance, have typical genetic profiles which determine their vulnerability to experiencing side effects from frequently prescribed drugs such as statins. In the Asian population, research has indicated that specific genetic variations related to drug transport and metabolism can affect the safety and efficacy of statin treatment (Yow et al., 2023). This is because it demonstrates the necessity for personalized medicine. After all, the understanding of genetic susceptibility in patients can direct personalized therapeutic management and balance the risk of ADRs with drugs like atorvastatin and rosuvastatin. Also, SCARs exhibit a complex immune response to drugs. Delayed and T cell-mediated reactions that are generally induced by genetic variance, particularly in the HLA genes, are possible. Certain gene polymorphisms can modify antigen processing and presentation in a way that results in severe and even lethal hypersensitivity. SCAR patients may require prolonged hospitalization and aggressive medical management, which account for high healthcare costs and morbidity among patients. The unpredictable nature of the onset and clinical presentation of SCARs also renders their association with drug exposure less predictable, requiring more knowledge on genetic and immunological determinants. Pharmacogenomic strategies are built into predicting susceptibility to SCARs and improving patient outcomes through tailored therapy (Tempark et al., 2022). Furthermore, expanding the understanding of the immune response to drugs has the potential to enhance the options for pharmacogenomic applications in clinical practice. The discovery of genetic markers associated with ADRs enables health practitioners to personalize medicine selection and dosage for individual patients, minimizing toxic adverse effects while achieving maximum therapeutic efficacy. For instance, information regarding polymorphisms of drug metabolism can provide insights to guide the safe use of medication among various populations. This tailored approach imposes an ethical obligation to consider genetic variation when creating treatment plans, especially in regard to the broad range of responses observed. Ultimately, the integration of pharmacogenomics into daily clinical practice not only enhances medication efficacy and safety but also reveals the intricate interplay between the immune system and pharmacological therapy, paving the way for innovation in precision medicine and improved patient care.

11.2.3. Environmental Influences on Drug Efficacy

The interplay between environmental factors and drug efficacy is complex and multifaceted, significantly impacting therapeutic outcomes and the incidence of ADRs. Things like diet, exposure to toxins, and lifestyle can change the way a person's body processes drugs and affect their response to medications. For example, having certain foods or pollutants in the body can either slow down or speed up the activity of drug-metabolizing enzymes, thereby altering drug levels in the body.

Pharmacogenomics allows us to understand how environmental factors can affect the way people respond to medications and the chances of developing ADRs due to their genetics. Recognizing environmental factors helps healthcare providers develop the most effective treatment plans for each patient. Additionally, genetic differences can significantly contribute to variations in drug responses, but they are not the only factor involved. As Anunobi (2024) indicates, genetic factors alone might explain 15–30% of the variability observed in drug efficacy and the occurrence of ADRs. This highlights the importance of considering the environment in pharmacogenomic strategies. Factors such as geographical location, lifestyle choices, and socioeconomic status can impact the absorption, distribution, metabolism, and excretion (ADME) of drugs, further complicating the relationship between genetic factors and drug response. Implementing comprehensive pre-emptive pharmacogenetic testing, as emphasized by Chenchula et al. (2024), could help identify individuals at risk for ADRs while taking into account the environmental contexts that modify drug efficacy. It is essential for this approach to ensure that medicine is tailored to each patient and that they receive safe and effective treatment. Given these observations, it is clear that understanding environmental factors is crucial for the success of drug treatment in patients. When pharmacogenomics and environmental risks are combined, it becomes easier to provide personalized treatment tailored to each patient's needs.

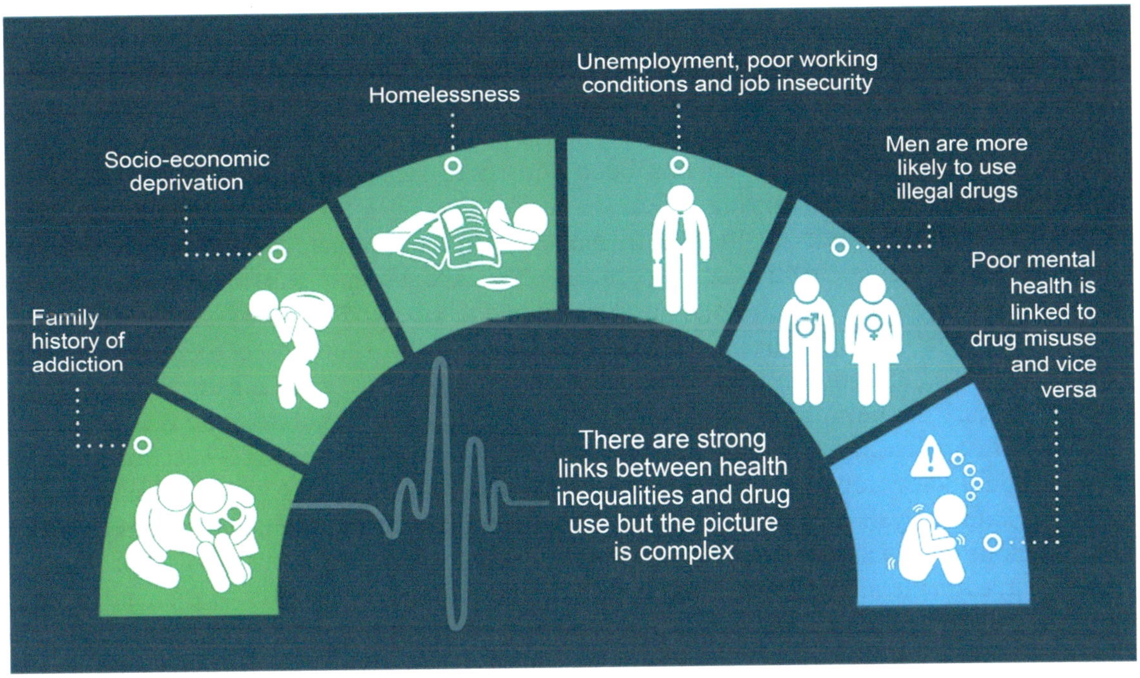

Figure 11.9. Environmental influences on drug efficacy.

Source: https://3.bp.blogspot.com/-tIhnldjgm4s/WTFOml1Vy7I/AAAAAAAAAHs/fuGAX9degasrnTbZgg7iGSIdDFZU4wiJACLcB/s1600/Risk%2BFactors%2Bof%2BAddiction.jpg.

As Chenchula et al. (2024) highlights, employing pre-emptive pharmacogenetic testing can not only enhance patient compliance but also mitigate serious ADRs that lead to hospitalization or emergency treatment. When clinicians consider genetic and environmental factors, they can choose the best drug and its proper dose. Looking at the whole picture is important for making patients safer, lowering healthcare expenses, and ensuring good health outcomes for many people. Giving more importance to this integration in pharmacology will eventually result in a better understanding of how both genes and the environment affect drug results (Figure 11.9).

11.3. Role of Pharmacogenomics in Personalized Medicine

The rise of pharmacogenomics has significantly altered the landscape of personalized medicine, primarily by providing insights into genetic variations that influence drug responses. This field of genomics introduces a system for exploring the interaction between a patient's genomic content and their response to a given pharmaceutical, especially with regard to ADRs. Importantly, research has established that variations in DNA can dramatically influence the efficacy of drugs as well as the frequency of ADRs. However, despite such promising results, its clinical translation has been slow to materialize, with public awareness and education about its application still lagging behind. As demonstrated by recent public opinion surveys, while there is a general willingness to undergo pharmacogenomic testing, there is a lack of knowledge of the critical role played by genetics in predicting therapeutic efficacy and susceptibility to ADRs (Magavern et al., 2025). Further, a high degree of knowledge of pharmacogenomics is fundamental in optimizing treatment regimens and minimizing ADRs. Pharmacogenetic variation exploits genetic testing to tailor drug choice and dose according to individualized genetic profiles, thereby increasing the accuracy of treatment. Pharmacogenetic variation has been shown to result in different drug metabolisms among individuals, leading to varying efficacy and toxicity. With increasing recognition of these factors, clinicians stand better positioned to make precise decisions, thereby improving patient safety and increasing treatment success. Integrating pharmacogenomic information into clinical care not only promises to reduce harmful reactions but also enhance patient compliance with treatment protocols, as patients will be more satisfied with therapeutics tailored to their genetic profiles (Leonova, 2024). The integration of pharmacogenomics into health systems emphasizes the need for interdisciplinary cooperation among scientists, clinicians, and regulatory bodies to ensure the safe and efficient application of genetic data. Advances in pharmacovigilance—according to recent literature—should allow for ADR detection and drug-drug interactions to be streamlined through the use of big data analysis and ML technology. These innovations are the keys to better preventing adverse reactions by healthcare providers prior to their occurrence, enabling proactive rather than reactive treatment alternatives. Hence, building enhanced awareness of pharmacogenomics among both the medical community and the general public is critical to maximizing the benefits of tailored medicine and mitigating the pharmacological risks of drug therapies (Leonova, 2024) (Figure 11.10).

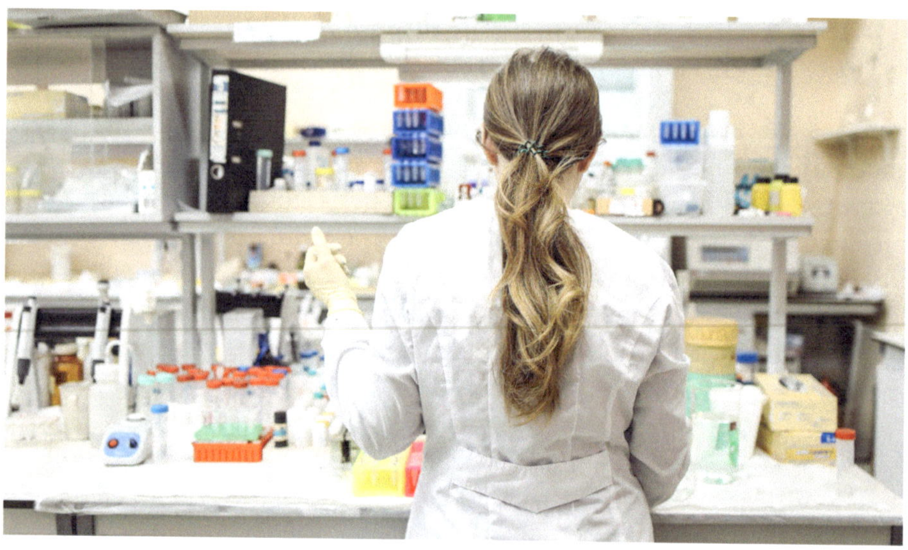

Figure 11.10. Role of pharmacogenomics in personalized medicine.

Source: https://www.thedailydispatches.com/wp-content/uploads/2023/05/Pharmacogenomics.jpg.

11.3.1. Tailoring Drug Therapy Based on Genetic Profiles

Pharmacogenomics offers the possibility of selecting treatments based on an individual's genes, which can significantly enhance both the safety and effectiveness of medication. By understanding a patient's genetic makeup, healthcare providers can identify the most appropriate medications and dosages, drastically reducing the risk of ADRs. It changes the previous all-in-one approach to medicine, which is now more tailored to each patient. For example, changes in genes that encode drug-metabolizing enzymes can lead to varying reactions to drugs in patients, with some individuals benefiting from the effects and others experiencing adverse side effects. As a result, pharmacogenomic testing serves as a crucial tool in personalizing medicine, providing clinicians with valuable insights that go beyond traditional prescribing practices, ultimately improving patient outcomes and promoting safer healthcare practices (Meurer et al., 2003). In addition, pharmacogenomic testing is expected to bring both advantages and challenges, primarily in the areas of drug development and the marketing of drugs. Because drug patent owners are rewarded for creating ADR-predicting genetic tests, they begin focusing on making medicines that are both effective and safe for specific patients.

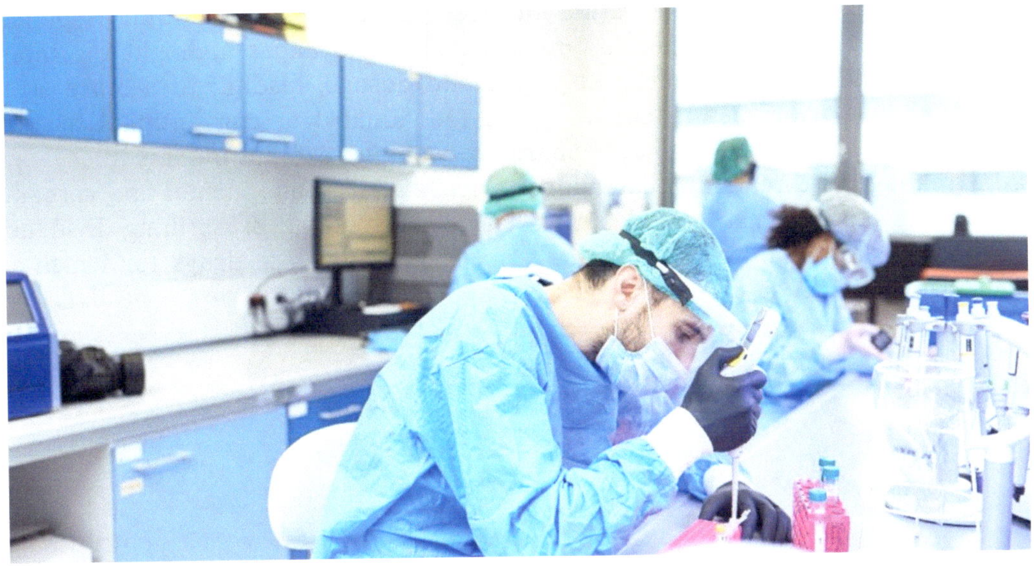

Figure 11.11. Tailoring drug therapy based on genetic profiles.

Source: https://mapdrug.com/wp-content/uploads/2024/01/Pharmaceuticals-1024x533.jpg.

This creates a complex interplay between public and private sector involvement in pharmacogenomic research and development (R&D). Although private businesses want to profit from tests that go with their patented drugs, the public sector has to spot where genetic testing is not available enough. Such gaps are often caused by tests not providing people with sufficient personal benefits, despite their being highly beneficial to society. Thus, careful consideration of research funding and incentives is essential to ensure the comprehensive adoption and development of pharmacogenomic solutions in clinical practice (Hulot et al., 2010). The benefits of tailoring drugs to a patient's genes extend beyond helping one person and encompass various aspects of healthcare. Pharmacogenomic methods can help cut healthcare costs by avoiding the use of ineffective treatment plans that result in ADRs. Early detection of genetic risks helps healthcare systems save resources and improve patient safety, as well as the system's sustainability. As genetics and biotechnology continue to advance, healthcare providers should stay current with the latest discoveries in pharmacogenomics to incorporate them into their daily practice. As a result, ongoing education and interdisciplinary collaboration will be pivotal in harnessing the full potential of pharmacogenomics, ensuring that therapies are both safe and effective for diverse patient populations (Meurer et al., 2003) (Figure 11.11).

11.3.2. Case Studies Demonstrating Successful Outcomes

In exploring the realm of pharmacogenomics, specific case studies illustrate the vast scope for reducing ADRs through the use of personalized medicine. One such case is abacavir hypersensitivity syndrome, for which genetic screening for the HLA-B*5701 allele has dramatically reduced the incidence of this life-threatening reaction. This case illustrates the successful integration of pharmacogenomic data into clinical practice, enabling clinicians to avoid prescribing abacavir to individuals at risk. With genetic screening, practitioners can proactively minimize the risk of adverse reactions to medications, illustrating how personalized therapy optimizes patient safety and simultaneously enhances therapeutic outcomes. These advances highlight the integral role of pharmacogenomics in directing drug selection and dosage, leading to a more streamlined healthcare model that prioritizes response by the individual over conventional trial-and-error methodologies. The revolutionary impact of pharmacogenomics extends outside idiosyncratic drug reactions. In treating life-threatening cutaneous ADRs related to allopurinol and carbamazepine, pharmacogenomics research has provided useful evidence guiding prescribing. Evidence shows that certain HLA alleles significantly enhance susceptibility to these drugs for which screening prior to their use has been advised.

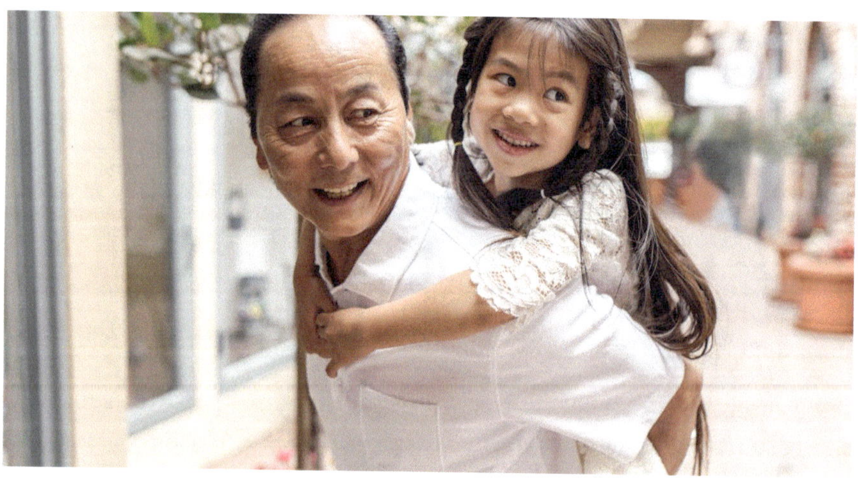

Figure 11.12. Case studies demonstrating successful outcomes.

Source: https://paediatricspeechtherapy.com/case-studies-of-successful-treatment-of-phonological-disorders-300486.jpg?key=mPOv9y.

This safety measure not only saves patients from fatal diseases but also enhances the confidence in therapy as health professionals advocate for individualized therapy. By offering concrete evidence of improved patient outcomes by genetic screening, these case studies support the contention for the blanket use of pharmacogenomic approaches in clinical practice, eventually creating an enormous reduction in ADRs and enhancing overall treatment effectiveness. However, with hopeful results being testified by several case studies, there still exist challenges for the universal implementation of pharmacogenomics in the pharmaceutical industry. Such challenges as high research costs and judicial liabilities deter companies from investing in pharmacogenomic research. Though it can help personalize drug development and patient treatment, pharmacogenomics is not a silver bullet. The complexities involved in drug approvals, drug regulation, and market dynamics can make it challenging to integrate into daily clinical practice. These challenges must be addressed through a concerted effort from regulators, healthcare professionals, and pharmaceutical companies to develop systems that foster innovation while protecting patient interests. This debate on the pharmacogenomics not only emphasizes the need for further research but also sets the theme of debate on the ethical and practical use of this evolving science, so that maximum medical benefit is made accessible to all the patients and harm due to ADRs is prevented to the extent possible (Koch et al., 2012; Becquemont et al., 2017) (Figure 11.12).

11.3.3. Challenges in Implementing Personalized Approaches

The primary challenge in applying personalized approaches in pharmacogenomics is that people's genes are not identical. A person's genetic makeup is different so that they may react differently to the same medication. Therefore, it is essential to conduct comprehensive genetic testing; however, this practice remains uncommon in most clinics. It is necessary to identify important genetic markers and then interpret them in relation to a person's overall health, other health issues, and environmental factors. Genetic information should be more effectively incorporated into treatment plans, as most healthcare providers are currently unable to utilize it effectively. Furthermore, disparities in access to genetic testing can exacerbate health inequalities, limiting the benefits of pharmacogenomics to those who are already privileged within the healthcare system (Youssef, 2025).

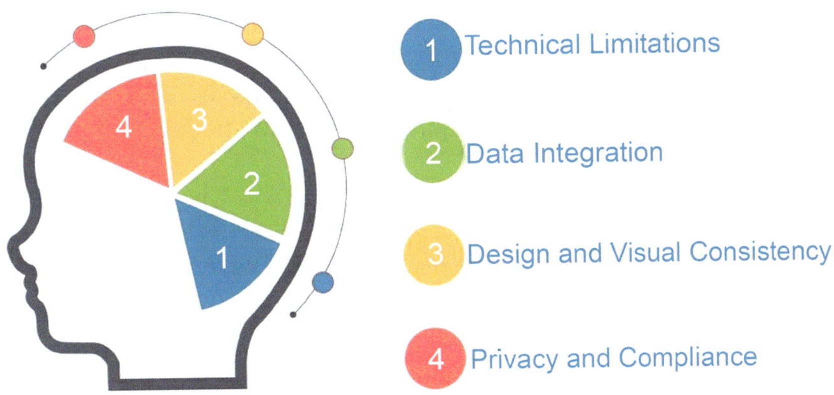

Figure 11.13. Challenges in implementing personalized approaches.

Source: https://fastercapital.co/i/Personalized-Images--Visual-Storytelling--Elevating-Email-Personalization-with-Personalized-Images--Overcoming-Challenges-in-Implementing-Personalized-Images-in-Email-Marketing.webp.

It is also challenging to ensure that pharmacogenomic data is effectively utilized in current medical practices. Healthcare practitioners regularly deal with excessive genetic information that they must integrate with their usual clinical data. It is necessary to develop user-friendly interfaces and decision-support systems that transfer the necessary genetic information about treatments to healthcare providers. Additionally, since policies on pharmacogenomic testing are not always uniform, patients may end up paying more than they should. Unless healthcare systems have detailed information and clear guidelines on the cost-effectiveness of pharmacogenomics, they may not be prepared to utilize these approaches. Standardizing pharmacogenomic protocols across institutions could alleviate some of these challenges but requires significant collaboration and investment in both technical infrastructure and professional education (Kayani et al., 2025). There are significant ethical issues that make it hard to use pharmacogenomics in personalized medicine. When genetics is involved in drug selection, the primary concerns are privacy, informed consent, and the safety of patients' data. Some patients are hesitant to get genetic testing because they are afraid their information could be used against them. Additionally, the possibility of discovering something unexpected during tests presents another challenge to the process of explaining and obtaining consent. To address these ethical concerns, there should be robust frameworks that prioritize patient autonomy and safeguard the security of genetic information. Policymakers and healthcare providers must work collaboratively to establish clear ethical guidelines that reflect the nuances of pharmacogenomics, as failing to address these issues could hinder the broader acceptance and success of personalized medicine strategies in clinical practice (Youssef, 2025) (Figure 11.13).

11.4. Current Technologies in Pharmacogenomic Testing

Advancements of current technologies in pharmacogenomic testing have revolutionized the field of personalized medicine. With the advent of high-throughput sequencing and microarray technologies, researchers are now capable of analyzing genetic variations at a previously unimaginable scale. Such technologies allow one to test single-nucleotide polymorphisms (SNPs) and other genetic markers involved in influencing drug metabolism, drug response, and the potential for ADRs. Therefore, clinical practitioners can now tailor drug therapy to the individual characteristics of the patient, thereby optimizing treatment benefits while minimizing harm. Not only does this finding approach optimizing pharmacotherapy, but it also aligns with growing recognition of population genetic heterogeneity, which is imperative for planning treatment regimens universally (Ozdemir et al., 2008).

In addition to high-throughput sequencing, advances in bioinformatics have also made considerable contributions toward understanding pharmacogenomics. With advancements in computational capabilities, it is now feasible to process complex genetic information more accurately and efficiently. Bioinformatics platforms enable the integration of genetic and clinical data to recognize gene-drug interactions that are vital to predicting ADRs. Also, the sites enable the creation of databases that compile pharmacogenomic information, which can be utilized by clinicians so that they can make evidence-based prescribing choices. Not only does the predictability of patient responses to medications improve with this use of technology, but it also provides an evidence-based system to pharmacogenomic analysis, thus making a contribution to improved development in the area (Koch et al., 2012). While holding out the promise of current technology in pharmacogenomic testing, several challenges remain to be overcome before it can be widely used. Industry reluctance and regulatory concerns stem from research and development financial costs and legal liability considerations that may be factors in ADR due to pharmacogenomic profiles. The urgency of addressing these challenges, however, is at the top of the list. Keeping that FDA rule in step with scientific advancements is crucial to make the transformation of pharmacogenomics research into practice possible. Additionally, evolution toward an optimal regulatory environment can facilitate innovation while safeguarding the rights of patients and allowing them to receive the optimal medical treatment. As a result, resolving these issues will facilitate a more seamless integration of pharmacogenomic technology into healthcare, leading to the prescription of personalized medicine that mitigates the risks of ADRs (Koch et al., 2012) (Figure 11.14).

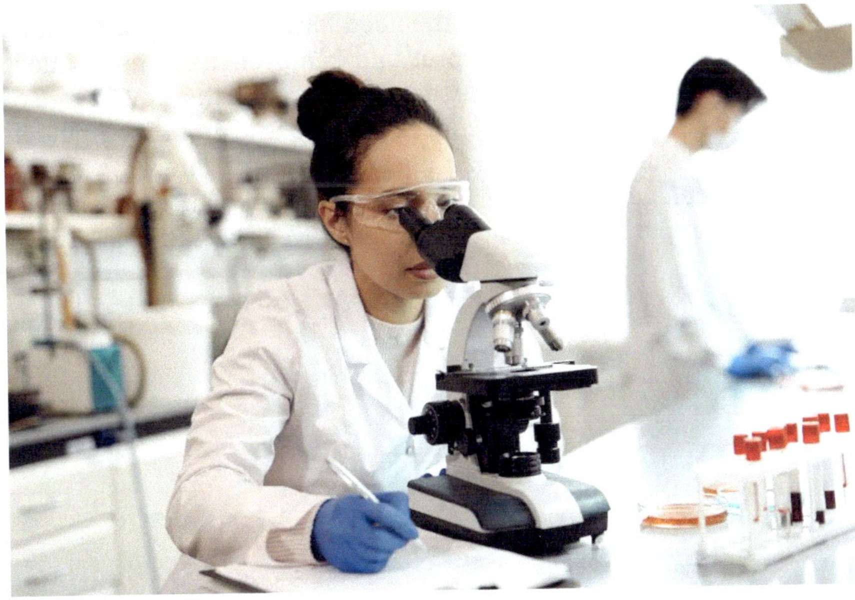

Figure 11.14. Current technologies in pharmacogenomic testing.

Source: https://lifetentcare.com/wp-content/uploads/2023/04/genetic-testing-for-psychotropic-medication.jpg.

11.4.1. Next-Generation Sequencing Techniques

The advent of next-generation sequencing (NGS) techniques has revolutionized the field of pharmacogenomics, facilitating a deeper understanding of the genetic underpinnings of drug responses and ADRs. Unlike old sequencing techniques, which could only examine a few genes at a time, NGS can sequence many genes simultaneously and generate a substantial amount of genetic data in a short period. It is crucial for this capability to identify genetic changes that can impact both the way a drug is metabolized and its effects on the body. With the growth of pharmacogenetic testing, NGS is now a crucial method for personalizing medicine, matching drugs to a person's genetic information, and thereby significantly reducing the likelihood of harmful side effects. The use of NGS in healthcare could benefit patients by providing them with more effective treatments and reducing potential negative side effects. NGS has a significant impact on both drug development and clinical practices, particularly in oncology, where selecting chemotherapy is crucial. Pharmacogenomics enables clinicians to select the most effective drugs and doses for cancer treatment, thereby reducing the risk of side effects and enhancing the efficacy of the treatment. For instance, knowing certain variations in the TPMT gene helps decide on the proper use of thiopurine drugs for leukemia and autoimmune conditions. If NGS is used, healthcare providers can give patients with low TPMT activity a different dose to avoid possible severe side effects. These proactive measures exemplify how NGS technologies can mitigate ADRs through informed decision-making that leverages individual genetic information, as evidenced in pharmacogenetic studies emphasizing the importance of genotype-phenotype correlations in clinical outcomes (Tamm et al., 2017). In addition, the progress made by NGS in pharmacogenomics also presents new challenges that need to be addressed. Interpreting all the genetic data can be challenging, mainly because it is not always clear what the identified variants mean for patients. Additionally, utilizing NGS results in routine clinical practice is challenging due to the need for robust bioinformatics systems and the requirement for doctors to learn how to interpret and comprehend genetic information. In spite of these challenges, NGS is a vital element in today's pharmacotherapy because it can increase patient safety and the effectiveness of drugs. More studies and improved guidelines for NGS in pharmacogenomics are necessary to maximize its benefits. Ultimately, as the field evolves, the ongoing collaboration between geneticists, pharmacologists, and clinicians will enhance our ability to predict ADRs and empower personalized medicine initiatives (Baskin et al., 2017) (Figure 11.15).

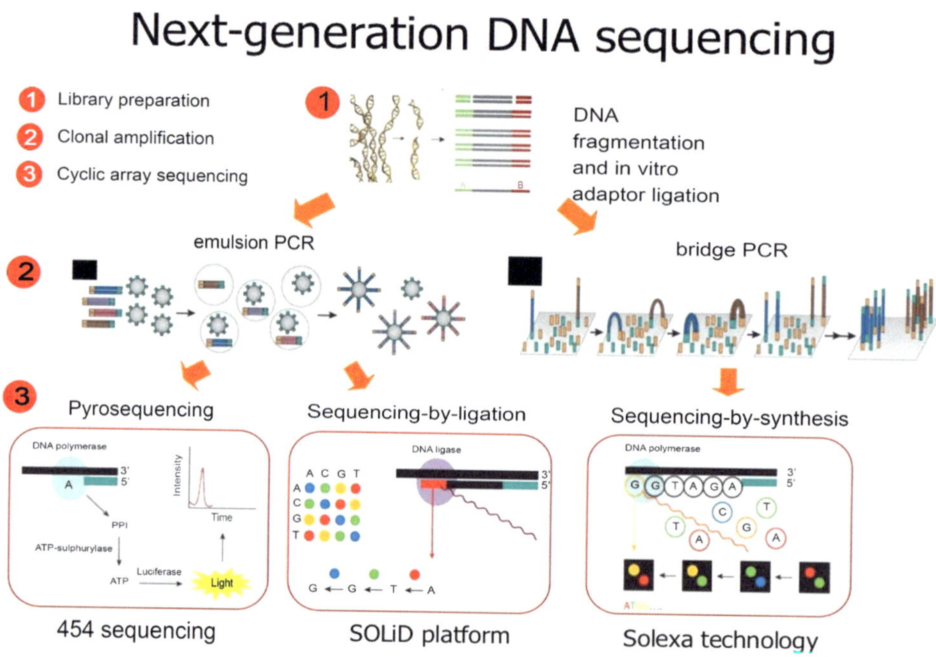

Figure 11.15. Next-generation sequencing techniques.

Source: https://cdn.technologynetworks.com/tn/images/body/ngsseo31615391054366.png.

11.4.2. Bioinformatics Tools for Data Analysis

Within the field of pharmacogenomics, bioinformatics software plays a key role in analyzing dense genetic information to make drug therapies safer and more effective. Software programs scan vast databases to identify useful genetic data, guiding individualized medicine applications. For instance, genomic analysis algorithms enable the detection of single-nucleotide polymorphisms (SNPs) that affect drug metabolism and response. The integration of bioinformatics in clinical use facilitates the evaluation of how genetic difference affects ADRs more subtly, so HCPs can tailor treatment based on individual genetic profiles. Not only does the possibility of drug-related adverse effects decrease, but so does the potential for increased therapeutic efficacy. Hence, the use of bioinformatics tools becomes a part of existing pharmacogenomics research. With the growing need for proper pharmacovigilance, computerized systems with bioinformatics capabilities have transformed the detection and regulation of ADRs tremendously.

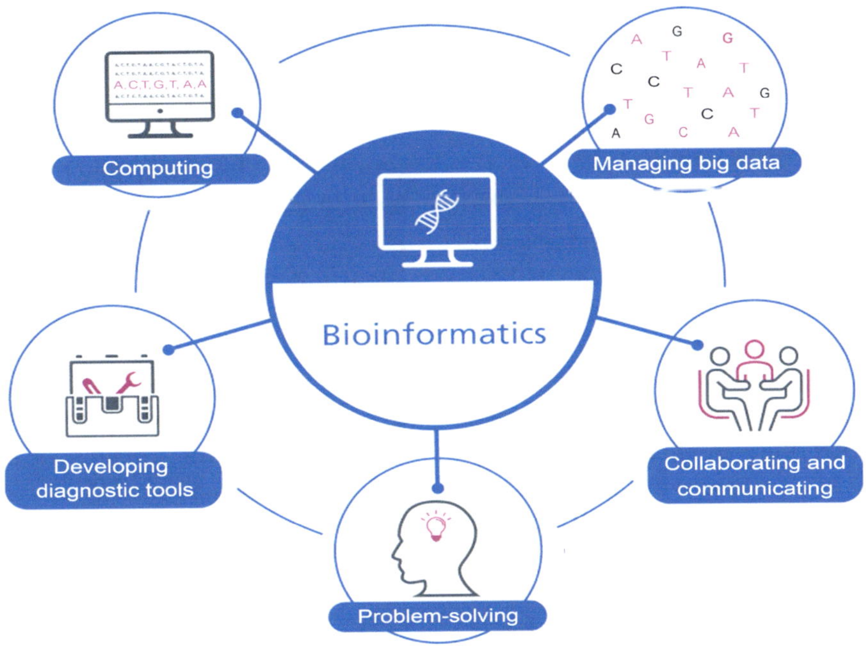

Figure 11.16. Bioinformatics tools for data analysis.

Source: https://www.genomicseducation.hee.nhs.uk/wp-content/uploads/2021/04/Bioinformatics-graphic-01-983x640.png.

Current studies highlight that such systems can dramatically increase ADR reporting rates, as evident in a 335% increase in reporting via electronic health records (EHRs) compared to manual procedures (Milić et al., 2025). Additionally, ML models such as Random Forest and XGBoost demonstrated significant performance measures, with 89% sensitivity and 92% specificity in detecting dangerous drug interactions in diabetic patients, respectively. The ability of these tools to provide real-time analytics not only makes the monitoring process faster but also engages healthcare personnel in ADR management, thereby fostering a culture of safety and efficient medication use among diverse patient populations. Moreover, the potential role of computational tools in pharmacogenomics transcends merely the identification of genetic variants to encompass economic analysis in terms of drug efficacy and safety. Existing clinical trials speak to the merit of pre-emptive screening for pharmacogenomics, which aims to curb ADRs among pediatric patients with cancer by taking advantage of actionable genetic variants (Conyers et al., 2024). The prospective approach analyzes the incidence rate of ADRs as well as tests the cost-effectiveness of tailored interventions relative to standard treatment. By integrating bioinformatics tool information properly into clinical decision-making processes, HCPs can not only forecast patient responses but also conserve healthcare resources spent in managing ADRs. In all, the use of bioinformatics tools in pharmacogenomics represents a significant leap towards safer therapeutic regimens that align with the principles of personalized medicine (Figure 11.16).

11.4.3. Clinical Applications of Pharmacogenomic Tests

Due to pharmacogenomic testing, healthcare providers now have a better way to manage drug treatments. Thanks to these tests, doctors can use personalized medicine to determine the most effective treatment for each patient. For instance, individuals who exhibit specific genetic traits can be prescribed medications that are more likely to be effective while minimizing the risk of ADRs. The deployment of Clinical Decision Support (CDS) systems, such as the Epic Genomics module at institutions like the University of Florida, illustrates how EHRs can effectively incorporate pharmacogenomic data into routine clinical workflows. This approach not only educates clinicians about the implications of genetic variations on drug responses but also enhances patient safety and treatment efficacy, supporting the overarching goal of personalized healthcare (Hall et al., 2025). Despite some people still questioning its usefulness, comprehensive sequencing is being used more frequently as pharmacogenomic testing continues to improve. Comprehensive sequencing reveals more genetic changes than targeted genotyping, including those that are rare and may affect a person's reaction to medications. Still, utilizing this extensive information in clinical settings is not easy, as it is challenging to comprehend and integrate into medical care. Today's pharmacogenomic panels differ, and the usefulness of the genetic information they contain can vary significantly. As research progresses, addressing these challenges is essential to ensure that comprehensive pharmacogenomic testing can provide actionable insights that improve patient care (Zhou et al., 2024). Still, several factors are hindering the widespread use of pharmacogenomic tests, including technical issues and economic challenges. Since it is challenging to interpret some genetic variants, especially when the genes are complex, misinterpretations may occur, leading to harm in treatment choices. Additionally, since it is not always clear how much pharmacogenomic testing costs or whether insurance will cover it, this adds further challenges for doctors to utilize it. To fully realize the promise of pharmacogenomics in reducing ADRs and enhancing patient outcomes, it is imperative to cultivate a robust framework that addresses these challenges and fosters the integration of pharmacogenomic insights into standard care practices (Zhou et al., 2024).

11.5. Regulatory and Ethical Considerations

The swift progress of pharmacogenomics invites a careful review of regulatory and ethical principles underpinning this maturing science. With personalized medicine striving to match therapeutic interventions with each patient's unique genetic makeup, the authenticity of pharmaceutical marketing becomes ever more important. The WHO and the South African Health Products Regulatory Authority (SAHPRA) have established pivotal ethical standards to strengthen the marketing of medicines. However, with the growing popularity of social media and online advertising, the burden of implementing these guidelines becomes greater. A study that experimented with drug advertising during the COVID-19 pandemic revealed that the majority of ads were not compliant with the moral standards set by WHO and SAHPRA, detailing key monitoring and regulatory gaps, particularly in the context of active ingredient disclosures, ADRs, and safety practices (Chimukuche et al., 2024). Furthermore, the ethical landscape of pharmacogenomics extends beyond practice in marketing to encompass issues of information privacy, consent, and global access to genetic testing and medications. Patients must have faith that their genetic information will be handled in utmost secrecy and utilized judiciously to guide treatment decisions. The implications of genetic discrimination, whether in healthcare or employment, must be addressed with caution to ensure that both the individual's rights and moral codes are protected. Furthermore, regulatory agencies are encouraged to adapt as rapidly as the science on genomics evolves to ensure ongoing patient safety. Through addressing these regulatory challenges, stakeholders can introduce a more ethical drug development in pharmacogenomics, ultimately enhancing drug compliance and reducing drug-related adverse effects (Jeffrey, 2024). Putting regulatory and ethical concerns at the forefront of the pharmacogenomics discussion is paramount to realizing its full potential while safeguarding public health. The intersection of multi-omics approaches, for example, those offered by protein interaction and microbiome information, requires a systematic approach to patient treatment, where efficacy and safety take on heightened priority. Clinical practice itself needs to meet these challenges and develop therapeutic strategies that are not only personalized but also equitably accessible to all patients, regardless of their socioeconomic status. Continuous surveillance of drug advertising, in coordination with interprofessional collaboration between regulatory agencies, medical professionals, and pharmaceutical companies, is crucial for developing guidelines that promote judicious advertising strategies. Through collaboration with an ethics system, the field of pharmacogenomics can contribute significantly to minimizing ADRs and maximizing therapy outcomes in diverse patient groups (Chimukuche et al., 2024; Jeffrey, 2024).

11.5.1. FDA Guidelines on Pharmacogenomic Testing

The FDA guidelines on pharmacogenomic testing represent a critical intersection between personalized medicine and the mitigation of ADRs. When genetic information is used in choosing medicine, doctors can select the best drug for each patient and prevent most ADRs. They recommend using genetic data to guide prescribing, especially for medicines that are known to be influenced by a patient's genes regarding their metabolism, efficacy, and safety. Since ADRs result in significant healthcare costs, primarily due to hospitalizations and emergency visits, these guidelines aim to ensure better patient safety and effective treatment. Specifically, pre-emptive pharmacogenetic testing can identify at-risk patients and guide drug selection, thus significantly reducing the incidence of ADRs as highlighted in recent studies (Chenchula et al., 2024). The FDA has established a system that promotes pharmacogenomic testing and also requires education of healthcare providers about its impact on patient care. This effort is based on the knowledge that traditional prescribing usually ignores how genes play a role in how drugs are processed. When pharmacogenomic testing is used in clinics, it enables doctors to utilize data to effectively manage medications and intervene before any serious side effects occur. The minimising ADRs and verifying economic legitimacy study, among others, has shown that pre-emptive pharmacogenomic testing reduces the risk of ADRs and improves patient outcomes. By aligning clinical practices with FDA guidelines, healthcare systems reinforce their commitment to improving patient safety through informed prescribing (Conyers et al., 2024). Following the FDA's guidelines for pharmacogenomic testing improves the standard of care given to patients.

Knowing that drug metabolism and response differ from person to person due to genes, HCPs can prevent events that might harm patients. Additionally, these guidelines help the economy by reducing hospitalizations and unnecessary medical expenses, which supports the long-term sustainability of healthcare. With more research in pharmacogenomics, it will be important for regulatory bodies and HCPs to keep working together to define and spread the best practices. Ultimately, the integration of pharmacogenomic testing, as endorsed by the FDA, represents a paradigm shift in clinical medicine that promises to revolutionize patient management and significantly reduce the risk of ADRs (Chenchula et al., 2024) (Figure 11.17).

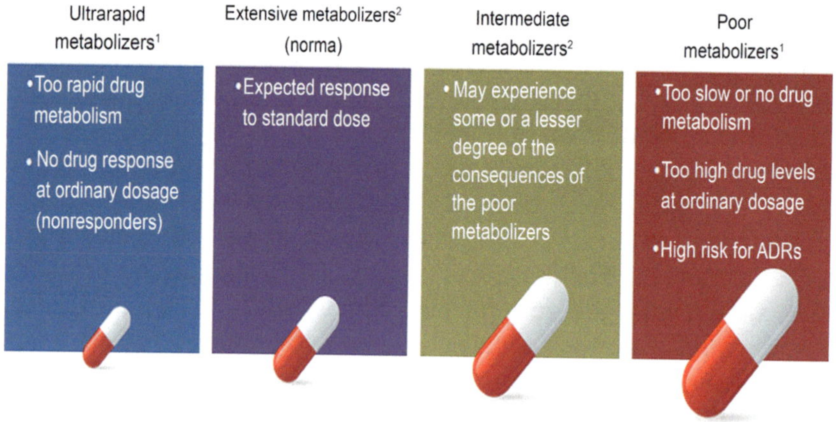

Figure 11.17. FDA guidelines on pharmacogenomic testing.

Source: https://www.tarnowcenter.com/images/stories/vitamins/001.jpg.

11.5.2. Ethical Implications of Genetic Testing

Pharmacogenomics in the clinic brings not only potential benefits to targeted therapy but also genuine ethical issues surrounding genetic screening. One central concern is patient autonomy because patients can be pressured into genetic testing to optimize drug therapies, with issues around informed consent and the quality of information made available to patients. Pharmacogenomic data could reveal drug susceptibilities to ADRs and can support decisions that could lead to beneficial or detrimental outcomes. Moreover, the interpretation of genetic data needs to be conducted with caution, especially in heterogeneous populations like the African population. Studies have identified genetic profile differences among various ethnic populations, necessitating the need for culture-specific approaches to genetic testing, as well as the application of pharmacogenomics (Thandeka et al., 2025). Therefore, there is a need to ensure that patients clearly understand the outcomes of genetic testing in order to uphold their autonomy and informed health choices. Another significant ethical implication of genetic testing in pharmacogenomics is the potential for stigmatization and discrimination. With the advent of genomic information, there is a risk that individuals can be unfairly associated with particular medical conditions or discriminated against by their employers or insurance providers. Ethical guidelines are necessary to address these concerns, which entail strict protocols for protecting sensitive genetic information from misuse. In addition, with the growing use of pharmacogenomic testing, population stratification can occur in which some sections can be privileged in the treatment strategy based on genetic susceptibility. This could enhance health disparities among marginalized populations unless pharmacogenomic benefits are equally accessible (Kayani et al., 2025). Consequently, the responsibility for ethical duty falls upon policymakers and HCPs to make sure that pharmacogenomic testing is only used to promote equity and justice and not perpetuate ingrained systemic biases. Lastly, privacy and data protection concerns in genetic testing cannot be overlooked. With more digitalization of genetic information, threats of data breach and illegal access to people's health information have significantly increased. If patients think their information may be misused or revealed, they may object to genetic testing. To provide control over the use, distribution, and storage of genetic data in healthcare systems, ethical guidelines ought to be created. Furthermore, transparency is needed for the purposes for which genetic data are being collected. This calls for collaboration between stakeholders, including ethicists, geneticists, and healthcare providers, in developing best practices that foster trust and ensure protection of individual rights (Thandeka et al., 2025). Lastly, resolution of these ethical concerns is essential to foster a responsible pharmacogenomics practice that enhances patient welfare, privacy, and equity in healthcare provision (Figure 11.18).

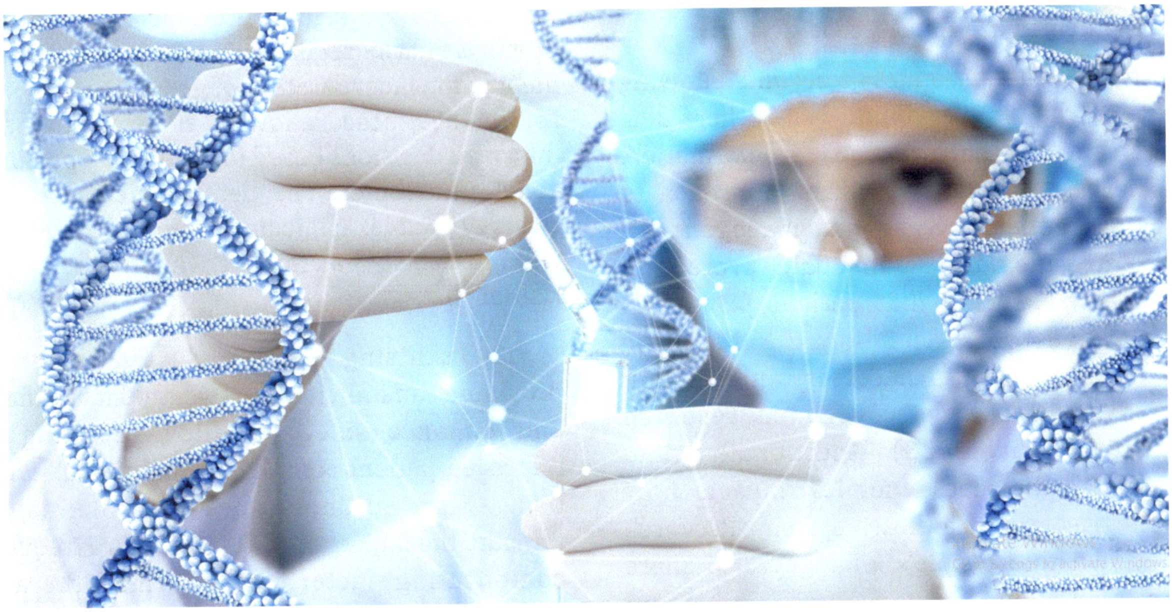

Figure 11.18. Ethical implications of genetic testing.

Source: https://mdaquest.org/wp-content/uploads/2023/11/iStock-970394890-e1700500274874.jpg.

11.5.3. Patient Privacy and Data Security Issues

The intersection of patient privacy and data security is paramount in the realm of pharmacogenomics, particularly as it relates to ADRs. Since genetics is used more in medicine, there is a growing risk that sensitive information will be misused. People are often concerned about their genetic information being used to discriminate against them or for the benefit of other people. This issue is particularly significant for British South Asians, who are excited about the potential benefits of pharmacogenomics but remain concerned about data privacy. Rather than merely seeking to advance health outcomes, researchers must prioritize establishing trust through transparent communication, which is critical for gaining community buy-in and fostering a collective commitment to data security, as suggested by findings from focus groups emphasizing the need for trust in pharmacogenomic initiatives (Caulfield et al., 2023). Furthermore, the field of pharmacogenomics is influenced by a complex system of regulations that further complicates data security.

Since each country has its guidelines for pharmacogenetic testing, patients' data is sometimes protected differently. It is challenging for regulatory organizations, such as the UK Medicines and Healthcare products Regulatory Agency and the US Food and Drug Administration (FDA), to ensure that privacy is protected when new medicines are introduced.

In this situation, ethics go beyond following the rules; they influence how researchers deal with and manage important genetic information. The necessity for a harmonized approach to evidence generation in pharmacogenetics inherently includes strong data protection standards, ensuring that patient privacy is safeguarded while enabling the scientific community access to necessary information for advancing pharmacogenomic research (Johnson et al., 2025). Additionally, data privacy in pharmacogenomics impacts how people trust the healthcare system. Research has shown that people's willingness to share their genetic information is largely influenced by their concerns about data security and the risks associated with its potential misuse. A discrete choice experiment also highlighted that the amount of evidence required to inform a patient's decision in pharmacogenetics may vary. Many participants were willing to share their data when they felt their privacy was protected, which suggests that strong privacy measures are necessary. The integration of effective data security protocols, along with ongoing community education and outreach, will be essential for fostering a culture of mutual trust, ultimately enhancing patient engagement and the successful implementation of pharmacogenomic interventions (Johnson et al., 2025).

11.6. Future Directions in Pharmacogenomics

As pharmacogenomics continues to mature, much of the emphasis is on enhancing the specificity of drug treatment by matching medicines to specific genetic profiles. By this method, not only is the therapeutic effect hoped to be improved, but also the reduction of ADRs, which remain a significant concern in clinical practice. Pharmacogenomics trends of the future include the incorporation of genetic testing into routine healthcare, allowing clinicians to make informed decisions based on a patient's personal genetic attributes. The personalized medicine strategy enables clinicians to utilize drugs that will most likely be effective while reducing the risk of ADRs.

By utilizing genetic data, healthcare providers can individualize treatment regimens and enhance safety profiles, resulting in improved patient compliance and overall well-being. Such advances have the potential to mitigate the impact of ADRs, which are frequent complicating factors of pharmacotherapy. Another potential of pharmacogenomics is the possibility of using artificial intelligence (AI) and ML to examine large data sets. Genetic variant discovery by AI technologies may facilitate improved identification of genetic variants associated with ADRs and drug effects and thereby improved optimization of individualized treatment regimens. Future research should focus on developing AI algorithms to integrate genetic, phenotypic, and environmental data to predict improved individual drug responses. In addition, ML's ability to manage complex datasets may aid in achieving a deeper understanding of the polymorphisms associated with ADRs, which could lead to new solutions. Developing such predictive models can significantly change pharmacovigilance, as AI can efficiently identify potential safety concerns and correlate them with pharmacogenomic results. These data-driven issues will be overcome by being the crucial factor in ensuring that pharmacogenomics is able to counter the threats of ADRs and enhance patient treatment. Ultimately, collective action in policy-making and research is necessary to ensure the success of pharmacogenomics in clinical settings. Pharmaceutical companies, regulatory organizations, healthcare providers, and patients must collaborate to establish standardized protocols for genetic testing and pharmacogenomic interpretation. Such coordination shall also assist in creating in-depth guidelines for the safe use of pharmacogenomic data in prescribing. HCPs must be trained to educate others about the importance of pharmacogenomics in minimizing ADRs, with the ultimate goal of improving patient care. Importantly, as the pharmacogenomics science improves, ethical issues of data privacy and consent must always be in focus to protect patient rights. Enhanced communication and interaction amongst these multidisciplinary stakeholders will pave the way towards innovative solutions that leverage the promise of pharmacogenomics while effectively addressing the problem of ADRs (Figure 11.19).

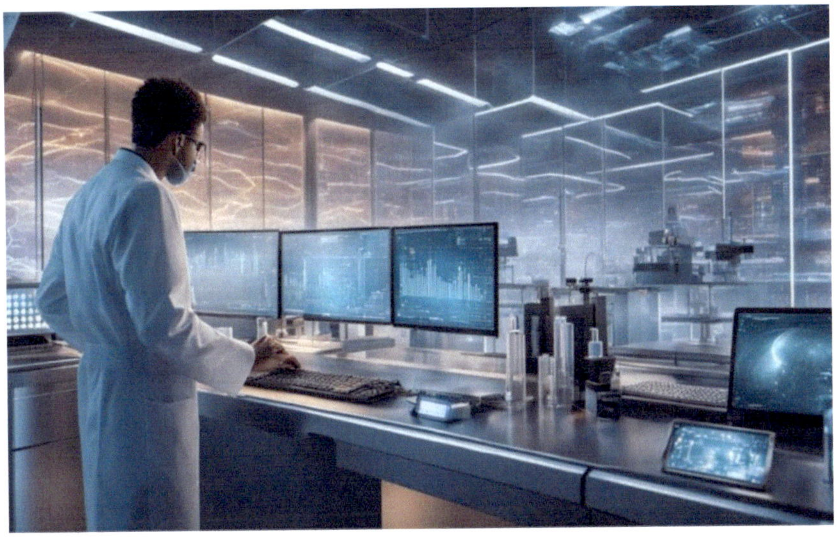

Figure 11.19. Future directions in pharmacogenomics.

Source: https://americanpharmacogenomicsassociation.com/wp-content/uploads/2024/01/Challenges-and-Future-Directions-of-Pharmacogenomics-1024x585.jpg.

11.6.1. Emerging Research Trends

Emerging research trends in pharmacogenomics are increasingly highlighting the necessity for personalized medicine tailored to individual genetic profiles, particularly in the context of ADRs. Due to genetic differences, the way drugs are metabolized is now influencing how treatment is administered. For example, recent studies rely on bibliometric analyses to identify the most important topics in drug-drug interactions and how genetic features are linked to the results of drug treatment. This is meant to strengthen the safety of drugs and also to bring together researchers worldwide to handle the challenges of ADRs in different groups. The integration of personalized medicine paradigms seeks to optimize therapeutic strategies, ultimately aiming for a substantial reduction in the incidence of ADRs through targeted approaches, thereby leading to enhanced patient safety and care overall (Li et al., 2024). Additionally, the use of pharmacogenomics helps improve the accuracy of treating hypertension in individuals with diverse genetic backgrounds. Today, it is clear that learning about genetic polymorphisms linked to drug metabolism can significantly improve how well patients stick to their treatment and how effective it is. It is known that variations in the genes responsible for antihypertensive drug responses can lead to significant differences in treatment outcomes among different ethnic groups. Noticing these distinctions helps clinicians design better treatment plans, which may help reduce the chances of ADRs. This highlights the crucial need for continued research into genetic determinants of drug responses and the establishment of normative guidelines that incorporate pharmacogenomic insights into routine clinical practice, ensuring that each patient receives optimal and safe antihypertensive therapy (Ashiq et al., 2023). Pharmacogenomics is advancing, and the primary goal is now to integrate all-omics technologies into clinical settings. With high-throughput genotyping and next-generation sequencing, it is now possible to gain a deeper understanding of how genes influence a person's response to drugs and potential adverse effects. It is now vital for researchers, healthcare providers, and patients to find ways to collaborate with the data. Moreover, direct-to-consumer genetic testing is making genetic information easier for people to access, which is increasing interest and talk about how pharmacogenomics affects daily medical care. As these technologies evolve, research must prioritize ethical considerations and patient education to ensure informed use of genetic data, ultimately fostering a healthcare environment that prioritizes personalized medication strategies focused on reducing ADR risks while enhancing therapeutic success (Li et al., 2024).

11.6.2. Potential for Reducing ADRs in Clinical Practice

Pharmacogenomics is highly likely to reduce drug adverse reactions (ADRs) in clinical use. Based on genetic information, doctors can tailor drug therapy to better predict which patients are likely to be harmed by a specific medication. Through tailoring prescriptions using pharmacogenomic testing, patients can circumvent the trial-and-error method of prescribing, as the test identifies how one's genetic makeup influences their response to medication. For instance, genetic differences for drug metabolizing genes could lead to reduced efficacy or increased toxicities of a given drug, and therefore understanding a patient's genetic profile becomes important. Initiatives such as the PharmacoGenetics for Every Nation Initiative (PGENI) demonstrate efforts towards realizing pharmacogenomic strategies globally, particularly for developing countries with limited financial resources. These interventions enhance patient security and treatment outcomes by facilitating the broader implementation of personalized medicine in various healthcare systems (Borg et al., 2012). Development of pharmacogenomics in routine clinical practice, particularly within the NHS of the UK, is a paramount achievement towards ADR minimization. With the increasing frequency of genetic screening in the healthcare system, pharmacists and doctors will be able to refer to critical genetic information that will guide medication decisions. Most clinicians currently work extensively with full utilization of genetic data not impacting drug effects. Genetic variation is estimated to account for up to 50% of inappropriate drug reactions, and this is why the application of pharmacogenomic data in practice decision-making is significant. This shift in practice will play an important role in enhancing the accuracy of drug prescription, leading to more effective and safe treatment for patients, consequently significantly reducing the frequency of ADRs in the long term (Wright et al., 2020). Besides that, awareness and education on pharmacogenomics are required to help it reach its maximum capability in reducing ADRs. The interpretation of pharmacogenomic test results and the effectiveness of application by healthcare providers can be facilitated. Training programs that incorporate the role of genetic tests in pharmacotherapy can help empower clinicians to adopt a culture of personalized medicine. As a supplement, increasing public awareness of the benefits of pharmacogenomics can help empower patients as they make informed choices about their health. By collaborating to address the genetic basis of drug response, stakeholders in the healthcare system can make treatment more integrated. This change not only enhances patient outcomes but maximizes the control of drugs as well, paving the way for a reduced burden of ADRs in the clinical setting and outlining the future of patient care towards an individualized and efficient paradigm (Borg et al., 2012).

11.6.3. Integration of Pharmacogenomics into Standard Care

Integrating pharmacogenomics into standard healthcare practices represents a transformative approach to personalized medicine, particularly concerning ADRs. Since drug response varies among individuals, pharmacogenomics enables doctors to tailor treatment plans to a patient's genetic profile. Recognizing genetic polymorphisms related to drug metabolism and effectiveness, for example, those of the CYP450 family, helps healthcare providers avoid many ADRs.

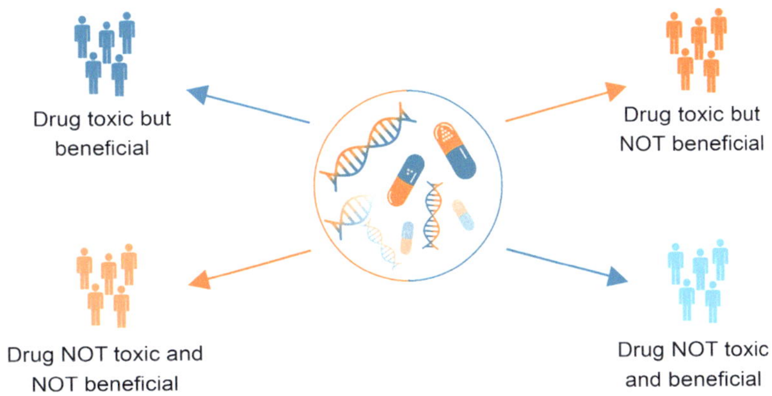

Figure 11.20. Integration of pharmacogenomics into standard care.

Source: https://media.licdn.com/dms/image/v2/D5612AQH4AUvc9G6JyQ/article-cover_image-shrink_720_1280/article-cover_image-shrink_720_1280/0/1719791003562?e=2147483647&v=beta&t=00j7yhDOgqlPProLXOskGcrX91DOqbL0jl0CrPVEeeY.

The United Kingdom's National Health Service (NHS) is initiating efforts to review the evidence for national implementation of pharmacogenomics, aiming to align genetic testing with routine clinical decision-making. However, concerns persist about the unequal availability of these tests across different demographics, which may perpetuate existing disparities in care quality and patient safety (Magavern et al., 2023). Pharmacogenomic testing should be used to improve how patients respond to drugs and avoid the risks of ADRs. In particular, certain groups have started pre-emptive testing for clopidogrel variants, as the results of poor drug response can be very significant for high-risk patients. It is evident that some loss of function alleles affect people differently, and London populations have needs that are not the same as those in more similar areas. As pharmacogenomics moves toward a nationally coordinated framework, equitable access to testing becomes paramount to ensure that diverse patient populations benefit from precise medication strategies that are informed by genetic insights (Adithan et al., 2015). Although pharmacogenomics could play a big role in lowering ADRs, there are still many obstacles that prevent its widespread use. HCPS need to get thorough education on how to use and understand genetic data in their clinical work. Additionally, the advancement of EHRs offers a unique opportunity to integrate pharmacogenomic information seamlessly into standard care pathways. This way, physicians can utilize clinical decision support systems (CDSS) to prescribe patients the right medications based on their genetic information. However, gaining buy-in from stakeholders across the healthcare continuum is necessary to overcome existing logistical and regulatory challenges, thereby ensuring that pharmacogenomic integration achieves its intended goal of improving patient safety and therapeutic efficacy (Magavern et al., 2023) (Figure 11.20).

Summary

The conclusion of this examination into pharmacogenomics and ADRs highlights the transformative potential of personalized medicine in clinical settings. As the area develops, it is becoming increasingly clear that using personalized therapy approaches is not only helpful but also necessary. Using pharmacogenomic information in healthcare can help reduce the number of ADRs by helping doctors predict each patient's reaction to drugs. This move to personalized therapy should make drugs safer and more effective, which will transform the way drugs are developed and given to patients. Pharmacogenomics is becoming increasingly important, and it remains vital to match its use with today's healthcare practices for proper application and comprehensive patient care. One of the most important aspects of utilizing pharmacogenomics is the collaboration among healthcare providers, researchers, and policymakers. Since pharmacogenomics is being adopted slowly in most clinics, it is essential to have organized frameworks that facilitate the country's widespread adoption. As shown by the 100,000 Genomes Project in the UK, there is a big chance to expand the use of pharmacogenomics in healthcare beyond small academic centers. The UK Pharmacogenetics and Stratified Medicine Network, along with similar cooperative networks, enables patients and industry experts to collaborate in creating and promoting policies that increase the adoption of pharmacogenomics and enhance treatment outcomes for many individuals. All in all, the combination of pharmacogenomics and clinical practice offers a key opportunity to lower ADRs and improve the way treatments are given. The rise in interest in this field should lead to strategies that address the issues between research and its application in routine care. Due to personalized medicine, it is now more crucial than ever to employ innovative methods in developing and testing drugs. For pharmacogenomics to benefit patient care in various groups, it is essential to address challenges in education, training, infrastructure, and policy. All in all, cooperating and being informed will help pharmacogenomics achieve its goals in improving medication management and lowering ADRs, making the future healthier.

The use of pharmacogenomics is crucial in personalizing medicine, particularly in oncology, as it enables doctors to select the most suitable drugs for each patient's unique genetic profile. Pharmacogenomics aims to enhance the effectiveness and safety of medicines, particularly for children, as standard dosing may not be effective for them. This approach becomes particularly important given the complex landscape of pediatric cancer treatment, which frequently involves multiple pharmacologic agents that can lead to a significant incidence of ADRs. A national multicenter trial, as outlined by Conyers et al. (2024), is examining the effect of pre-emptive pharmacogenomic testing on ADR incidence in children diagnosed with cancer. The main objective of this trial is to cut down on serious ADRs, so the treatment is easier for these patients and their outcomes are better. For pharmacogenomics, it is essential to understand the relationship between specific genes and how drugs interact to enhance treatment plans. For instance, the introduction of isocitrate dehydrogenase (IDH) inhibitors has opened avenues for targeted therapy in acute myeloid leukemia (AML) patients, particularly those with IDH mutations. Research highlighted by Peng et al. (2024) emphasizes the connection between these targeted therapies and the adverse effects profile associated with each drug. Analyses done by the WHO on databases help to explain the characteristics of ADRs caused by various IDH inhibitors. By examining ADRs for various medications, clinicians can prescribe treatments that are more effectively tailored to each patient's specific needs. The addition of pharmacogenomic information in healthcare settings is meant to reduce ADRs and also deal with the financial effects of using personalized medicine. Cost-effectiveness assessments, as indicated by Conyers et al. (2024), are essential in evaluating the broader impact of pharmacogenomics on healthcare systems. When healthcare providers compare the cost difference between standard care and preemptive pharmacogenomic testing, they can determine if these advanced methods are financially reasonable. They are necessary because they ensure that resources are used wisely, leading to better patient outcomes. Overall, when pharmacogenomics is used with close monitoring of ADRs, it can greatly improve treatments for oncology patients and many others.

CLOSER LOOK

PHARMACOGENOMIC TESTING MADE CLINICIANS

Pharmacogenomic testing has significantly enhanced clinicians' ability to tailor medical treatments based on a patient's genetic profile, making healthcare more precise and individualized. This form of testing examines how a person's genes affect their response to drugs, helping clinicians predict which medications will be most effective or potentially harmful. By identifying genetic variants in drug-metabolizing enzymes, such as those in the cytochrome P450 family (e.g., CYP2D6, CYP2C19), clinicians can adjust drug type or dosage to maximize efficacy and minimize adverse effects. This is particularly valuable in managing conditions like depression, cancer, cardiovascular disease, and chronic pain, where response to medications varies greatly among individuals.

For example, pharmacogenomic testing can reveal that a patient is a poor metabolizer of certain antidepressants or opioids, prompting the clinician to choose an alternative drug or reduce the dose to avoid toxicity. In oncology, testing for genes such as TPMT or DPYD can guide chemotherapy regimens, preventing life-threatening complications. This approach not only improves therapeutic outcomes but also reduces the trial-and-error process traditionally involved in prescribing, saving time and healthcare resources.

Clinicians equipped with pharmacogenomic data are better prepared to make informed, evidence-based decisions. This has led to increased integration of pharmacogenomics into electronic health records and clinical decision support systems, enabling real-time access to genetic insights during prescribing. However, widespread adoption still faces barriers such as cost, limited genetic literacy among healthcare providers, and disparities in access to testing. Despite these challenges, pharmacogenomic testing represents a major advancement in personalized medicine. By aligning treatments with genetic profiles, it empowers clinicians to provide safer, more effective care—ushering in a new era where medication decisions are guided not only by symptoms but by the patient's unique genetic makeup.

References

1. Elzagallaai, A. A., Abuzgaia, A. M., & Rieder, M. J. (2025). A comprehensive update on the human leukocyte antigen and idiosyncratic adverse drug reactions. *Expert Opinion on Drug Metabolism & Toxicology*. https://doi.org/10.1080/17425255.2025.2455388Adithan, C., & Sandhiya, S. (2015). Drug-induced diseases (DID): Need for more awareness & research. *The Indian Journal of Medical Research, 142*, 7–9. https://www.semanticscholar.org/paper/9c5fdb41c8be0c3116335d105e40f60a4ff9f28f (accessed on 9 June 2025).
2. Alanazi, A. J., Almutairi, N. H. B., Alakroosh, A. A., Alyamani, I. M., & Alotibi, F. S. N. (2019). The role of pharmacogenomics in personalized nursing care: Laboratory techniques and clinical applications. *International Journal of Health Sciences.* https://www.semanticscholar.org/paper/8584d938ac9d3d5bc3c91ee70236c3b8a8744020 (accessed on 9 June 2025).
3. Anunobi, O. (2024). Pharmacogenomics as a tool in addressing genetic variation-dependent adverse drug reactions. *Dutse Journal of Pure and Applied Sciences.* https://www.semanticscholar.org/paper/756fa202f5f82e203cb389d916e256ce6710db53 (accessed on 9 June 2025).
4. Ashiq, K., Ashiq, S., & Mustafa, N. (2023). Pharmacogenomics and the concept of personalized medicine for the management of hypertension. *Pakistan Heart Journal*. https://www.semanticscholar.org/paper/4b930ba15268196e7e1ec6f51d040207902bbe3e (accessed on 9 June 2025).
5. Baskin, Y., & Kocal, G. C. (2017). Polymorphisms in pharmacogenetics of personalized cancer therapy. https://core.ac.uk/download/322431568.pdf (accessed on 9 June 2025).
6. Bastaki, K., Velayutham, D., Irfan, A., Adnan, M., Mohammed, S., Mbarek, H., Qoronfleh, M. W., et al. (2024). Forging the path to precision medicine in Qatar: A public health perspective on pharmacogenomics initiatives. *Frontiers in Public Health, 12*. https://doi.org/10.3389/fpubh.2024.1364221.
7. Bate, A., & Stegmann, J. U. (2021). Safety of medicines and vaccines–Building next generation capability. *Trends in Pharmacological Sciences, 42*, 1051–1063. https://doi.org/10.1016/j.tips.2021.09.007.
8. Becquemont, L., & Negrini, S. (2017). HLA-associated drug hypersensitivity and the prediction of adverse drug reactions. https://core.ac.uk/download/151085525.pdf (accessed on 9 June 2025).
9. Borg, J. J., Fenech, A. G., Grech, G., Mitropoulos, K., et al. (2012). Relevance of pharmacogenomics for developing countries in Europe: Implementation in the Maltese population. https://core.ac.uk/download/46602333.pdf (accessed on 9 June 2025).
10. Bramon, E., Caulfield, M., Hill, S., McNamee, R., et al. (2020). Pharmacogenomics in the UK National Health Service: Opportunities and challenges. https://core.ac.uk/download/343121631.pdf (accessed on 9 June 2025).
11. Brunham, L. R., Chan, A., Chan, S. L., Ng, W., et al. (2019). Economic burden of adverse drug reactions and potential for pharmacogenomic testing in Singaporean adults. https://core.ac.uk/download/305124429.pdf.
12. Caulfield, M. J., Clinch, M., Durrani, F., et al. (2023). British South Asian ancestry participants' views of pharmacogenomics clinical implementation and research: A thematic analysis. https://core.ac.uk/download/590960200.pdf (accessed on 9 June 2025).

13. Chavhan, A. R., & Uplenchwar, P. M. (2024). AI-driven signal detection in pharmacovigilance: Advancements, challenges, and future directions. *International Journal of Pharmacy and Pharmaceutical Research.* https://www.semanticscholar.org/paper/bb9f0886f24576d1b2df1738bedc4fff37706690 (accessed on 9 June 2025).

14. Chenchula, S., Atal, S., & Uppugunduri, C. (2024). A review of real-world evidence on preemptive pharmacogenomic testing for preventing adverse drug reactions: A reality for future health care. *The Pharmacogenomics Journal, 24.* https://www.semanticscholar.org/paper/10a7d2d5070c6fe8a61ceba870e527270107ee2c (accessed on 9 June 2025).

15. Chimukuche, R. S., Ndlazi, J., Mtolo, L. T., Bird, K., & Seeley, J. (2024). Evaluation of drug and herbal medicinal promotions on social media during the COVID-19 pandemic in relation to World Health Organization ethical criteria and South African Health Products Regulatory Authority guidelines in South Africa: Cross-sectional content analysis. *Online Journal of Public Health Informatics, 16.* https://www.semanticscholar.org/paper/8662531dbab3693f385f04c469fc4258e50078f1 (accessed on 9 June 2025).

16. Conyers, R., Halman, A., Moore, C., Stenta, T., Felmingham, B., Collier, L., Khatri, D., et al. (2024). Minimizing adverse drug reactions and verifying economic legitimacy—Pharmacogenomics implementation in children (MARVEL-PIC): Protocol for a national randomized controlled trial of pharmacogenomics implementation. *BMJ Open, 14.* https://www.semanticscholar.org/paper/4e3923653120d13b032dac687a3322c76d119bb1 (accessed on 9 June 2025).

17. Dash, S. R., & Sahu, M. K. (2025). Investigating the role of pharmacogenomics in optimizing pediatric medication therapy: A pilot study. *Journal of Neonatal Surgery.* https://www.semanticscholar.org/paper/c58bd4605f794a6e0bd63f8be75291039dd1c0ae (accessed on 9 June 2025).

18. Evans, B. J. (2006). What will it take to reap the clinical benefits of pharmacogenomics? https://core.ac.uk/download/46955240.pdf (accessed on 9 June 2025).

19. Evans, W., Meslin, E. M., Kai, J., & Qureshi, N. (2024). Precision medicine—Are we there yet? A narrative review of precision medicine's applicability in primary care. *Journal of Personalized Medicine, 14*, 418. https://doi.org/10.3390/jpm14040418.

20. Hall, B., Eken, E., Cavallari, L. A., Duarte, J. D., Wiisanen, K. W., Cicali, E. J., & Nguyen, K. A. (2025). Implementing pharmacogenomics clinical decision support: A comprehensive tutorial on how to integrate the Epic Genomics Module. *Clinical Pharmacology and Therapeutics.* https://www.semanticscholar.org/paper/3ad28aa249da53ecbcd9b0363df51fd9a42dedd5 (accessed on 9 June 2025).

21. He, M., Shi, Y., Han, F., & Cai, Y. (2025). Prediction of adverse drug reactions based on pharmacogenomics combination features: A preliminary study. *Frontiers in Pharmacology, 16.* https://www.semanticscholar.org/paper/66c31d7018178cd393b67071c19e89003b9f804c (accessed on 9 June 2025).

22. Hulot, J. S. (2010). Pharmacogenomics and personalized medicine: Lost in translation? https://core.ac.uk/download/pdf/8394873.pdf.

23. Issa, A. M. (2020). Personalized medicine and the practice of medicine in the 21st century. *McGill Journal of Medicine, 10.* https://doi.org/10.26443/mjm.v10i1.625.

24. Johnson, D. (2025). The implementation of pharmacogenetics: Evidence and preferences. https://core.ac.uk/download/543787822.pdf (accessed on 9 June 2025).

25. Kayani, M., Sangeetha, G. K., Sarangi, S., Sarmada G, L., Sharma, S., Adedara, V. O., Abdallah, S., et al. (2025). Pharmacogenomics and its role in cardiovascular diseases: A narrative literature review. *Current Cardiology Reviews*. https://www.semanticscholar.org/paper/7ef045df1f3695c681f6e048377e27e765abbc89 (accessed on 9 June 2025).
26. Koch, V. G. (2012). Incentivizing the utilization of pharmacogenomics in drug development. https://core.ac.uk/download/56355492.pdf (accessed on 9 June 2025).
27. Leonova, E. (2024). Comprehensive evaluation of pharmacological risks: Enhancing drug safety through interdisciplinary collaboration and advanced methodologies. *Power System Technology*. https://www.semanticscholar.org/paper/49c30d47e91c62475ebd9721da57897b8b42d830 (accessed on 9 June 2025).
28. Li, L., Zhou, Y., Ye, L., & Xie, Z. (2024). Tracing the evolution: A comprehensive bibliometric analysis of drug interaction clinical studies. *The Journal of Clinical Pharmacology, 64*. https://www.semanticscholar.org/paper/bf20a28c3a5026d90fc99fbe6fe019a1814a5b67 (accessed on 9 June 2025).
29. Magavern, E. F., Marengo, G., Sivathasan, C., Mezzanzanica, M., Wright, A. J., Keen, J., Sharma, V., et al. (2025). A United Kingdom nationally representative survey of public attitudes towards pharmacogenomics. *QJM: Monthly Journal of the Association of Physicians*. https://www.semanticscholar.org/paper/393aea1593ace482699c26dce633fa44dff971af (accessed on 9 June 2025).
30. Magavern, E., & Caulfield, M. (2023). Equal access to pharmacogenomics testing: The ethical imperative for population-wide access in the UK NHS. *British Journal of Clinical Pharmacology, 89*. https://www.semanticscholar.org/paper/639abac379f3bbb6990b363db6443a1030a554e9
31. Malinga, T. V. B., Othman, H., Paximadis, M., Tiemessen, C., Ramsay, M., Hazelhurst, S., & Twesigomwe, D. (2025). Characterization of NAT, GST, and CYP2E1 genetic variation in Sub-Saharan African populations: Implications for treatment of tuberculosis and other diseases. *Clinical Pharmacology and Therapeutics, 117*, 1338–1357. https://www.semanticscholar.org/paper/814fec1c13b053edc305effba6db178a17198483 (accessed on 9 June 2025).
32. Marsh, A., Singer, D. R. J., Taylor, P. C., et al. (2010). Personalized medicine: The impact on chemistry. https://core.ac.uk/download/45676.pdf (accessed on 9 June 2025).
33. Meurer, M. (2003). *Pharmacogenomics, Genetic Tests, And Patent-Based Incentives*. https://core.ac.uk/download/322516871.pdf.
34. Milić, K., Sinanović, Š., Prodović, T., & Derdemez, I. (2025). Digital systems in pharmacovigilance: Enhancing adverse drug reaction detection in endocrine disorders. *Medicinski Glasnik Specijalne Bolnice za Bolesti Štitaste Žlezde i Bolesti Metabolizma*. https://www.semanticscholar.org/paper/54739a07a9adb2259ab6cc64a2a3e37b2061e163 (accessed on 9 June 2025).
35. Nafea, A. A., AL-Mahdawi, M., Al-Ani, M. M., & Omar, N. (2024). A review on adverse drug reaction detection techniques. *ARO–The Scientific Journal of Koya University*. https://www.semanticscholar.org/paper/96cf251a54d1563ff26179ecad5c1519c8bbadfc (accessed on 9 June 2025).
36. Ozdemir, V., & Williams-Jones, B. (2008). Pharmacogenomic promises: Reflections on semantics, genohype and global justice. https://core.ac.uk/download/151544094.pdf (accessed on 9 June 2025).

37. Peng, M., Guo, Q., Dang, Z., Zhang, B., Li, M., Wang, Z., Lu, X., et al. (2024). A real-world study of adverse drug reactions of two isocitrate dehydrogenase inhibitors based on the US FDA adverse event reporting system and VigiAccess databases. *Frontiers in Pharmacology, 15*. https://www.semanticscholar.org/paper/e9288db66f5001213021560d0378dc215447a29d (accessed on 9 June 2025).

38. Roman, Y. M. (2025). Pharmacogenomics and rare diseases: Optimizing drug development and personalized therapeutics. *Pharmacogenomics*. https://www.semanticscholar.org/paper/c71fd0dae54e6705f7178aedee454e26ee69dcb0 (accessed on 9 June 2025).

39. Sadée, W., Wang, D., Hartmann, K. E., & Toland, A. E. (2023). Pharmacogenomics: Driving personalized medicine. *Pharmacological Reviews, 75*, 789–814. https://doi.org/10.1124/pharmrev.122.000810.

40. Seguin, C. S., Fidelis, G. F. S., Dagli-Hernandez, C., Vasconcelos, P. E. N. S., Morau, M. V., Matos, Y. G., Perroud, M. W., et al. (2025). Association of ABC efflux transporter genetic variants and adverse drug reactions and survival in patients with non-small lung cancer. *Genes, 16*. https://www.semanticscholar.org/paper/3e98c744ba2790c260af659f8f317348d829a9a7 (accessed on 9 June 2025).

41. Shaman, J. A. (2024). The future of pharmacogenomics: Integrating epigenetics, nutrigenomics, and beyond. *Journal of Personalized Medicine, 14*. https://www.semanticscholar.org/paper/193cfafac39208112c15d63659c00ae3422009a7 (accessed on 9 June 2025).

42. Suke, S., Kosta, P., & Negi, H. (2015). Role of pharmacovigilance in India: An overview. *Online Journal of Public Health Informatics, 7*. https://www.semanticscholar.org/paper/9cfeb16f2a8d9dfe22b7119f71bca5fe158ee959 (accessed on 9 June 2025).

43. Tamm, R. (2017). *Ute tiopuriinmetüültransferaasi aktiivsust mõjutavate biomarkerite otsingul*. https://core.ac.uk/download/83597675.pdf (accessed on 9 June 2025).

44. Tempark, T., John, S., Rerknimitr, P., Satapornpong, P., & Sukasem, C. (2022). Drug-induced severe cutaneous adverse reactions: Insights into clinical presentation, immunopathogenesis, diagnostic methods, treatment, and pharmacogenomics. *Frontiers in Pharmacology, 13*. https://www.semanticscholar.org/paper/54c7089365ce28c81ca8eb2cba505bef15aca456 (accessed on 9 June 2025).

45. Wang, J., You, J., Huang, W., Yuan, C., Chen, J., Wang, F., Wang, W., et al. (2025). The characteristics of adverse reactions of three anti-prostate cancer drugs based on VigiAccess database and bibliometric analysis. *Frontiers in Pharmacology, 16*. https://www.semanticscholar.org/paper/95ab3e9d46d5b6b9eff1ff538c53f96f6b3de7cb (accessed on 9 June 2025).

46. Wright, D., & Youssef, E. (2020). *Pharmacogenomic Testing and Its Future in Community Pharmacy*. https://core.ac.uk/download/288394496.pdf (accessed on 9 June 2025).

47. Yow, H., Hamzah, S., Abdul Rahim, N., & Suppiah, V. (2023). Pharmacogenomics of response to statin treatment and susceptibility to statin-induced adverse drug reactions in Asians: A scoping review. *Asian Biomedicine: Research, Reviews and News, 17*, 95–114. https://www.semanticscholar.org/paper/d5e025efc333916ffc24608b9c5556797c0e9207 (accessed on 9 June 2025).

48. Zhao, Q., Chen, Y., Huang, W., Zhou, H., & Zhang, W. (2023). Drug-microbiota interactions: An emerging priority for precision medicine. *Signal Transduction and Targeted Therapy, 8*. https://doi.org/10.1038/s41392-023-01619-w.

49. Zhou, Y., & Lauschke, V. (2024). Next-generation sequencing in pharmacogenomics–Fit for clinical decision support? *Expert Review of Clinical Pharmacology, 17*, 213–223. https://www.semanticscholar.org/paper/c7a9fad6f35809d27e2eea41401c1d98c69a8d67 (accessed on 9 June 2025).

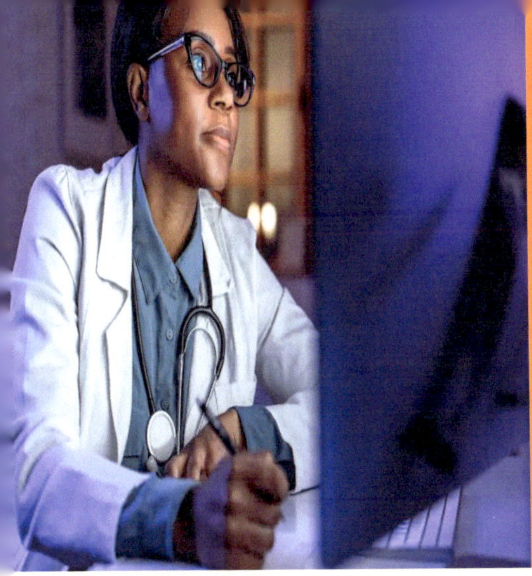

Chapter 12
POLYPHARMACY AND DRUG INTERACTIONS

Contents

Introduction

The syndrome of polypharmacy, or the concurrent use of multiple drugs by a patient, has gained increased exposure recently in the medical literature, particularly with an aging population and an outbreak of chronic illness. This is at the core of drug-drug interactions, as with every new drug added, there is an increased risk of adverse effects and unwanted results. With medical practitioners striving to optimize treatment regimens for patients with complex cases, especially those with comorbidities, the importance of pharmacologic interactions cannot be overstated. Effective management of these interactions requires clinicians to have a solid foundation in the pharmacokinetic characteristics of drugs, including their potential interactions, in order to minimize risks and optimize therapeutic outcomes. The increased focus on drug-drug interactions (DDIs) is further increased by the increased availability of novel drugs, which could make previously prescribed regimens more complicated (Gasperoni et al., 2024). In some patient groups, the confluence of polypharmacy and drug interaction occurs uniquely in such conditions as metastatic hormone-sensitive prostate cancer (mHSPC). With the introduction of next-generation Androgen Receptor Signaling Inhibitors (ARSIs), the pattern of treatment has made a sharp turn. However, the oral mode of administration of such molecules introduces levels of pharmacokinetic variables and potential DDIs. As elderly mHSPC patients also have comorbid disease, the risk of drug-induced adverse interactions is much greater. The majority of these patients can be put on not only ARSIs but also add-on therapies, further complicating drug regimens. This underscores the importance for HCPs to employ full medication reviews and remain cognizant of the ever-evolving pharmacotherapy process, especially in terms of how drugs interact with one another (Gasperoni et al., 2024). Apart from cancer therapy, other chronic diseases, e.g., HIV, illustrate the significance of polypharmacy and DDIs in prescribing practice. As antiretroviral therapy (ART) has improved, life expectancy has been significantly enhanced in patients who have HIV and comorbidities, therefore, rendering the prescribing situation a key factor to consider. Older patients with HIV infection tend to present with a multifaceted range of drug interactions during the receipt of further therapy for concomitant diseases, with the potential to cause intensified side effects and complex management scenarios. Effective clinical management in this case emphasizes the importance of understanding drug interaction mechanisms, which necessitates personalized treatment strategies to maximize patient outcomes. For clinicians, being aware of the interactions between antiretroviral drugs and other commonly used medications in older adults is essential for ensuring efficient antiretroviral stewardship and enhancing overall health management measures (Figure 12.1).

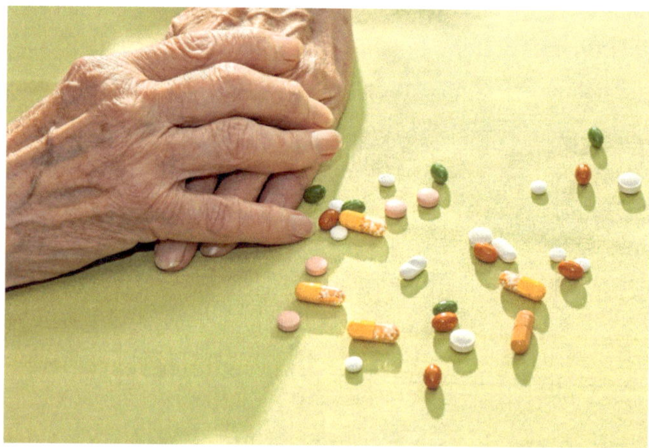

Figure 12.1. Polypharmacy and drug interactions.

Source: https://www.infectiousdiseaseadvisor.com/wp-content/uploads/sites/16/2019/11/rheumatoid_arthritis_G_187814190-1720x1146.jpg.

Definition of Polypharmacy

Polypharmacy is usually understood as a person using more than five medications at the same time. Nowadays, this situation occurs more often in elderly people who must deal with several long-term illnesses. Taking several medications at the same time can make it challenging to manage drugs, which might result in adverse effects and possible drug conflicts. In addition, having to take many medications at the same time can make life less comfortable for patients because of the mental and physical challenges involved. While trying to improve patients' drug treatments, HCPs should take into account the effects of taking multiple medications and look for better ways to manage them. Besides their numbers, polypharmacy affects the care that patients receive. It is now emphasized in public health and clinical guidelines that medication reconciliation and management should be extra careful for groups at risk of taking many medicines, such as the elderly. According to health organizations, clinicians are advised to periodically review whether the prescribed medications are still appropriate. It is especially vital to carry out this careful evaluation because several drugs taken together can create dangerous interactions. Practitioners are encouraged to take into account escalating dosages or the addition of new medications, which can exacerbate adverse effects, reinforcing the essential skill of clinical judgment (Visseren et al., 2021). For this reason, effective communication between healthcare providers and patients is essential to manage the risks associated with polypharmacy. It is vital to deal with the problem of drug interactions when looking at the effects of polypharmacy, as they tend to increase when a patient takes several medications at once. Such interactions might lower the effectiveness of treatment or even be dangerous to patients. There are drug interactions that happen due to PK, where one substance affects the other's absorption, distribution, metabolism, or excretion, and those that happen due to pharmacodynamics, where two drugs may either work against each other or together in the body. It is essential for healthcare providers to understand these interactions when dealing with patients on several medicines. Furthermore, specific studies emphasize the importance of carefully managing anticoagulants and other medications, as the potential for serious adverse events increases significantly in polypharmacy scenarios (Steffel et al., 2021). Therefore, healthcare providers should always be aware and informed to help patients receive the best care with the least possible risks from using many medications (Figure 12.2).

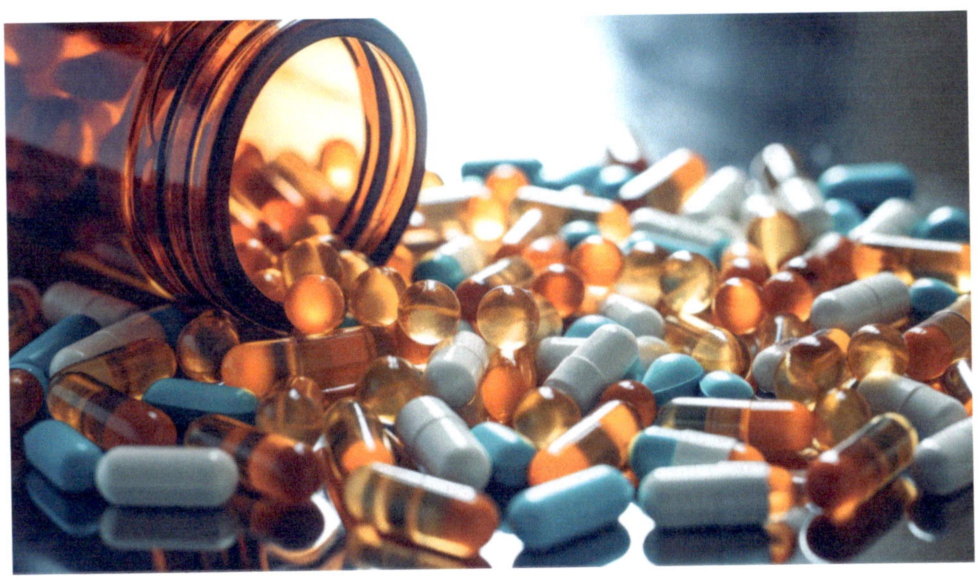

Figure 12.2. Definition of polypharmacy.

Source: https://images.prismic.io/herohealth/cfe57a96-fda0-4eda-b8f6-cb66e68ef698_AdobeStock_627493260.jpeg?auto=compress%2Cformat&fit=max&w=4630&h=2595.

Prevalence of Polypharmacy in Various Populations

The incidence of polypharmacy, or the simultaneous use of several drugs, is one of the key healthcare issues, especially in geriatric populations. With aging, individuals acquire comorbidities, which require them to receive a multitude of medications as part of their treatment regimen. A study in Tamil Nadu presents a problem, revealing that multimorbid geriatric patients often struggle to manage their polypharmacy. With targeted counseling interventions, authors reported substantial improvement in medication adherence, enhancing patients' knowledge about polypharmacy hazard and resulting in a significant reduction in potentially inappropriate medications. This supports the function of polypharmacy management in minimizing detrimental health consequences such as drug interactions, thus compromising patient quality of life and safety (Prakash et al., 2024). Apart from the elderly, polypharmacy is also becoming prevalent in young adult patients, particularly those with long-standing diseases such as diabetes. Ethnic and genetic factors contribute to the varying responses of patients to medications, which can complicate treatment regimens. Research on Indian populations has identified significant interethnic pharmacogenetic variation in predicting responses to non-insulin antidiabetic drugs (NIADs). The research revealed a high rate of alleles that are linked with drug response to adverse medication among these populations, indicating a relatively heightened risk of drug-drug interaction if the patients are being administered more than one drug concurrently. This creates a clear need for population-oriented solutions to polypharmacy that consider genetic variation in drug response and potential interactions (Bhoyar et al., 2024). The implications of polypharmacy extend beyond patient health and pose a significant threat to the healthcare system as a whole. Additional medication prescriptions can mean additional healthcare costs in the form of adverse drug reactions (ADRs), hospitalization, and prolonged treatments. Practitioners are therefore confronted with the need to balance the usefulness of polypharmacy with the potential for drug interaction and overall patient safety. Good practice, such as regular medication reviews and patient education, is critical for minimizing the hazards of polypharmacy. As evidence that shows improved outcomes through structured counseling is supported, incorporating education programs into the delivery of healthcare can regulate the complexity of polypharmacy and maximize health benefits across different populations (Prakash et al., 2024).

Importance of Studying Drug Interactions

The need to understand drug interactions is greater when people take several drugs, especially older adults who are the main users of multiple medicines. Because many older adults take many medications, they are more likely to face the risks of drug interactions. It is shown in the literature that older adults have difficulties following their medication routine. It can be more sensitive to drugs, which can cause more health issues and make treatment harder. Since these patients are more at risk, it is crucial to know the effects and actions of drugs on them. As outlined in recent studies, investment in methodologies that assess medication quality is essential, as these can inform clinical practices and reduce the prevalence of potentially harmful medications among older patients (Denig et al., 2024). Additionally, understanding drug interactions requires input from individuals working in various healthcare fields. Medical professionals should collaborate in reviewing and evaluating the effectiveness of patients' medication plans. Collaboration among doctors is important to spot drug interactions that may not become clear from usual prescribing. As highlighted in pharmacogenetics research, individualized treatment plans informed by genetic testing can mitigate risks associated with drug interactions, particularly among patients with complex health conditions (Knisely et al., 2016). Using a team approach, HCPs can solve existing drug problems and also prevent new ones from happening because of polypharmacy. Besides immediate safety, the study of drug interactions also influences overall healthcare outcomes and the associated costs. Dealing with ADRs can decrease the number of hospital admissions and healthcare costs, which is particularly important given the increasing health spending. Following evidence-based guidelines for medications is important for achieving better treatment outcomes and avoiding additional healthcare problems. Consequently, more research on drug interactions should be done and its findings should be shared promptly among HCPs. Proactively addressing polypharmacy and drug interactions ultimately serves to enhance the quality of care delivered to patients, aligning with the overarching goal of healthcare systems to provide safe and effective treatment options (Denig et al., 2024).

12.1. Causes of Polypharmacy

The subject of polypharmacy, described as the simultaneous use of several drugs by a patient, is affected by several interrelated factors. The most common cause is the increased population of elderly people, who are also subject to higher incidences of chronic diseases, thus calling for multiple forms of therapeutic interventions. With growing age, patients usually develop comorbidities like hypertension, diabetes, and cardiovascular disorders simultaneously, which all together call for a polypharmacy strategy to treat them effectively. Moreover, healthcare systems unwittingly create polypharmacy through weak models of care, whereby patients visit multiple specialists without a coordinated medication management plan. Such disorganization is likely to result in elevated rates of prescription and contribute to the risk of adverse drug interactions and events among older patients, who are already susceptible to drug-related complications. Apart from considerations of age, the sheer complexity of chronic disease management also gives rise to polypharmacy. Patients with chronic health issues tend to have multiple pharmacological interventions, so they accumulate prescriptions over time. The issue is compounded by the prescribing cascade process, whereby a physician prescribes additional drugs to treat side effects of current medications. The cycle can cause medication use to accelerate rapidly and make regimens complex, making it more difficult to comply and more susceptible to drug interactions. Notably, studies have demonstrated that medication burden among specific patient populations, such as dialysis patients, significantly correlates with frailty and nutrition status, suggesting that polypharmacy not only complicates treatment but also greatly impacts patient outcomes. As per reports, the count of medications significantly predicted hospitalization and survival, quoting the strong correlation of polypharmacy with deteriorating health (Chun et al., 2022). Finally, the prescribing style of medical professionals primarily establishes the face of polypharmacy. Excessive prescribing by clinical guidelines and pharmaceutical promotion may lead to higher utilization of medicines without due consideration of the risk of drug-drug interaction. While guidelines, such as those of the European Society of Cardiology (ESC), provide valuable information on handling specific conditions, they cannot replace the clinician's fundamental task of weighing individual patient needs and circumstances (Visseren et al., 2021). The interactive dynamic relationship between clinical judgment, patient preference, and integral reviews of medications is thus crucial in the avoidance of polypharmacy. To treat the etiology of polypharmacy, alongside the understanding of the clinical and systemic problems involved, it is imperative that communication among HCPs should be fostered to optimize patient care and minimize harm.

12.1.1. Aging Population and Chronic Diseases

More and more, the population is aging, which means older adults often deal with several chronic illnesses and, as a result, take many medications at once. As people grow older, they may develop conditions like hypertension, diabetes, and arthritis, which require the use of different drugs to treat them properly. Because there are now more complicated treatment plans, the chance of drug interactions and side effects also increases. When healthcare resources are scarce, the role of pharmacists becomes especially crucial in managing medications. Inadequate attention to the implications of polypharmacy can exacerbate health issues, underscoring the importance of thorough medication reviews and patient education in the geriatric population, as explored in studies assessing the efficacy of clinical pharmacy interventions (Khanal et al., 2019).

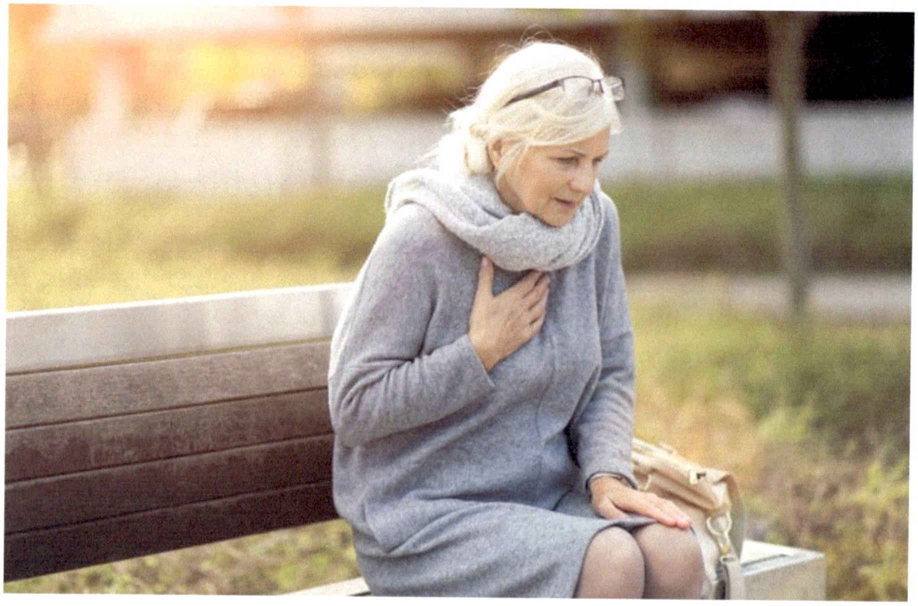

Figure 12.3. Aging population and chronic diseases.

Source: https://drprem.com/globalhealthcare/wp-content/uploads/sites/17/2015/04/Effects-of-chronic-disease-and-an-aging-population.jpg.

Additionally, using many medications at once can significantly affect an older person's quality of life and ability to do daily tasks. Research indicates that the presence of multiple medications, often exceeding five, is correlated with increased risks of falls and decreased physical mobility, as highlighted by the Timed Up-and-Go test outcomes in older adults (Chen et al., 2016). When seniors have many chronic diseases and take several medicines, they may have a hard time living on their own and staying healthy. It stresses that HCPs should recognize at-risk patients and carry out actions that can prevent the harmful effects of taking too many medications. For instance, optimizing pharmacotherapy through regular assessments can substantially enhance mobility, reduce fall risk, and improve health outcomes among the elderly (Chen et al., 2016). All in all, dealing with polypharmacy in elderly people with chronic diseases calls for a variety of strategies. Healthcare providers should pay attention to the number of drugs prescribed and the potential effects of those drugs on the health of elderly patients. When pharmacists are part of the healthcare team, medication management becomes more effective and patients experience better results. Because polypharmacy is a significant issue in geriatric care, it is necessary to keep researching and making changes to the healthcare system. By fostering awareness and implementing strategic interventions, healthcare systems can better serve the growing population of older adults, ultimately improving their health and quality of life (Khanal et al., 2019) (Figure 12.3).

12.1.2. Prescribing Practices and Healthcare Provider Behavior

In polypharmacy, provider behavior and prescribing behavior are key determinants of patient outcomes. As the prevalence of cases of polypharmacy, where more than one medicine is administered concurrently, continues to rise, attention has fallen on how providers manage medication regimens. Providers are typically confronted with challenges of safe prescribing, particularly when they have to manage the elderly, who are at risk of ADRs. Proper coordination and communication among the healthcare teams play a significant role in overcoming such challenges. By applying evidence-based prescribing, providers can reduce the risks of polypharmacy, thereby enhancing patient safety and quality of care.

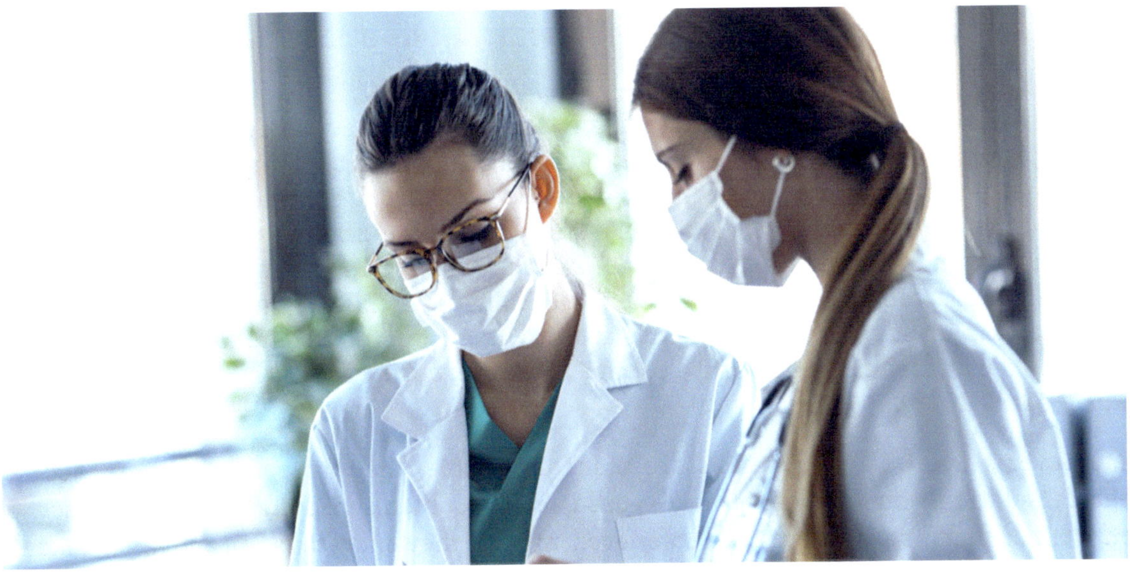

Figure 12.4. Prescribing practices and healthcare provider behavior.

Source: https://firstline.org/assets/images/blog/changing-prescribing-behavior.png.

In addition, systematic approaches to monitoring and reviewing medicines help prevent potential drug interactions and other issues, thereby highlighting the providers' contribution to managing polypharmacy (Anmolsingh et al., 2017). Despite sensitivity to the implications of polypharmacys, there are significant knowledge and application gaps between providers' knowledge and implementation of prescribing guidelines that do exist. Studies show that while most healthcare providers are sensitized to available tools, such as the BEERS criteria, there is inconsistency in the effectiveness with which the tools are translated into practice. A recent study surveyed primary care providers about the BEERS criteria and found that, although the majority recognized the importance of BEERS in older adults, gaps exist in their proficiency in its application (Black et al., 2023). This difference highlights the need for enhanced educational materials and training in polypharmacy management. By fostering a culture of continuous learning and reflection, HCPs can enhance prescribing behavior, not just being conscious of potential harms but also being competent in performing actions to manage polypharmacy and improve patient outcomes. Both healthcare provider behavior and relations between prescribing practices are also complicated by issues in healthcare delivery systems. Many providers work within fragmented systems that lack adequate support for monitoring patients with complex drug regimens. This fragmentation can lead to oversights and miscommunications that exacerbate the issues associated with polypharmacy. Without shared definitions and standards regarding polypharmacy, providers are likely to be unable to distinguish appropriate use of drugs from inappropriate combinations. This situation is one of the contributors toward possible drug interaction adverse effects, which have the potential to badly hurt patients and hike healthcare spending caused by resultant complications. Thus, healthcare systems must develop improved definitions and implement uniform protocols for polypharmacy treatment to help practitioners in their efforts to maximize prescribing behavior and improve patient outcomes (Anmolsingh et al., 2017; Black et al., 2023) (Figure 12.4).

12.1.3. Patient Factors, Including Self-Medication, and Over-the-Counter Drugs

The complex relationship between patient factors and polypharmacy underscores the significance of self-medication and the use of over-the-counter (OTC) drugs in contemporary healthcare. Many patients choose to treat their symptoms or conditions on their own rather than seeking help from a doctor. Even though it can ease your pain quickly, there are many issues about how safe and effective it is. When older adults with several health problems start their medication, it can cause more drug-related problems. In many cases, these individuals may not fully disclose their use of OTC medications or supplements to healthcare providers, thereby complicating the medication reconciliation process and potentially leading to dangerous overlaps in therapeutic regimens (Aljadhey et al., 2018).

Moreover, since OTC medications are more accessible, they have helped more people get healthcare solutions, but they have also caused more problems related to polypharmacy. Some patients think that OTC products are safe, even though they may cause problems if taken with prescription drugs. OTC analgesics and herbal supplements may have important interactions that most people are unaware of. If this misunderstanding exists, it can cause ineffective monitoring of medications and more cases of preventable adverse reactions. In studies highlighting medication errors, inappropriate prescribing often stems from an incomplete understanding of a patient's comprehensive medication list, which includes both prescription and self-medicated products (Doherty et al., 2017). Using self-medication and OTC drugs is now more important when considering patient-centered care. When patients participate in managing their medications, they gain a deeper understanding of what they want to achieve and why it is essential to adhere to their treatment plan. If healthcare providers encourage patients to speak about self-medication, it allows them to deal with polypharmacy concerns and help patients decide what is best for their health. If we consider what motivates patients, such as a desire to be in control and achieve results immediately, we can enhance their adherence to medications and mitigate the risks associated with taking multiple drugs simultaneously. Thus, prioritizing shared decision-making not only aligns therapeutic approaches with patient expectations but also reduces the burden of adverse drug events in vulnerable populations (Doherty et al., 2017) (Figure 12.5).

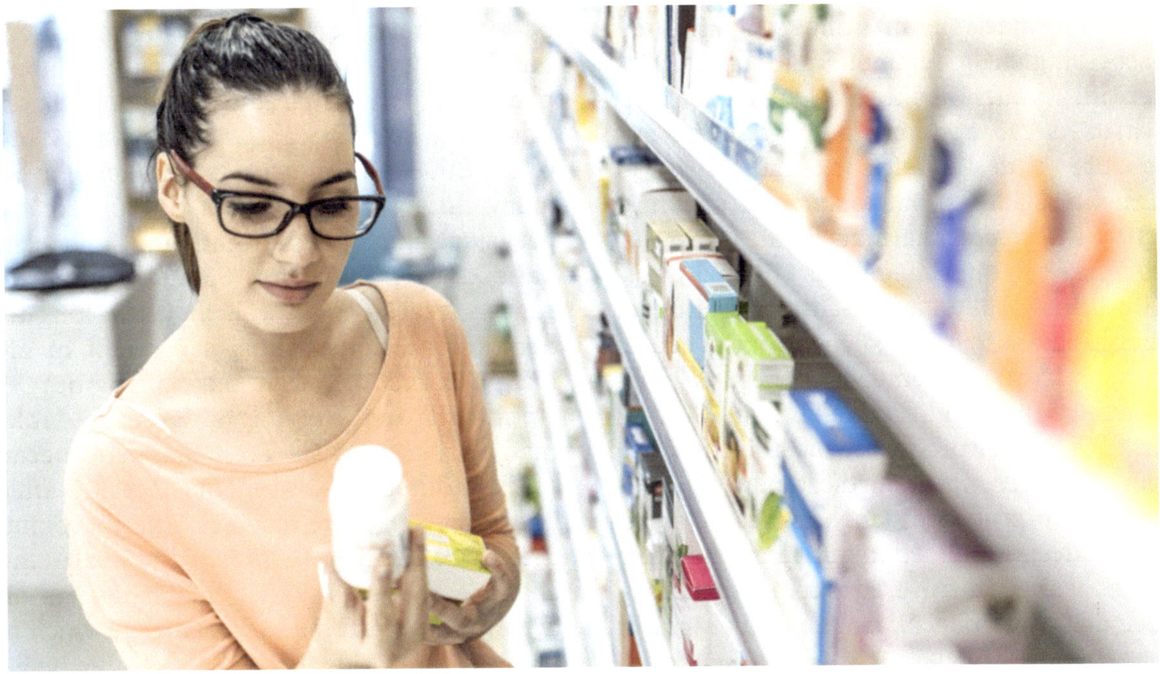

Figure 12.5. Patient factors, including self-medication and over-the-counter drugs.

Source: https://images.ctfassets.net/4f3rgqwzdznj/3Qzxk78gKhSbGKE3Cz4Vl0/2469f0a23329dcf 6368def4d1dbd670a/reading_otc_labels_pharmacy_aisle-983235484.jpg.

12.2. Types of Drug Interactions

Drug interaction is a complicated process, particularly in those studies on polypharmacy, in which a combination of drugs taken simultaneously causes significant clinical problems. Drug interactions can be categorized into several types: pharmacodynamic and pharmacokinetic drug interactions. Pharmacodynamic drug interactions refer to one drug's effect being facilitated or hindered by another drug, potentially leading to unexpected therapeutic effects or heightened toxicity. For example, the concurrent use of anticoagulants and antiplatelet drugs raises the risk of bleeding, highlighting the importance of monitoring in polypharmacy cases. Clinicians need to be aware of these interactions, especially since older patients often have multiple comorbidities that necessitate complex regimens. The awareness of drug actions that intersect at the therapeutic level can inform safer prescribing and better patient outcomes in populations with increasing healthcare needs (Khanal et al., 2019). Pharmacokinetic interactions are alterations in drug absorption, distribution, metabolism, and excretion, with potential consequences of either increased toxicity or therapeutic failure. For instance, certain drugs may induce or inhibit hepatic enzymes involved in drug metabolism, thereby altering the plasma concentrations of concomitantly administered drugs. Polypharmacy patients, especially elderly patients, generally bear a greater risk due to physiological changes with age, where drug clearance may be significantly impaired. Under such conditions, the role of a clinical pharmacist is of utmost significance. By assessing drug regimens and identifying potential pharmacokinetic interactions, pharmacists can optimize medication therapy to ensure both the efficacy and safety of treatment regimens, particularly in oncology practice, where polypharmacy is the norm due to complex treatment regimens (Khanal et al., 2019). Additionally, the co-administration of traditional drugs with herbal medicinal products (HMPs) and food supplements has become more evident as a cause of drug interactions. Studies indicate that older people are most likely to use concomitant prescription medication with HMPs, and therefore, prudence must be observed about possible adverse interactions. St. Johns Wort, for instance, has been discovered to comprehensively induce drug metabolism, leading to the loss of efficacy of most standard treatments. Moreover, the prevalence of such concomitant use appears to be high, with approximately one-third of older adults consuming both prescription drugs and HMPs, of which a sizable portion is susceptible to adverse interactions. Due to the growing popularity and ready availability of HMPs, healthcare providers must periodically inquire about these products to effectively manage drug interactions and safeguard the well-being of older patients being treated by them.

12.2.1. Pharmacokinetic Interactions

Pharmacokinetic interactions are very important in explaining the problems that can occur when elderly and chronically ill patients take several medications at the same time. When the body takes in, shares, processes, and eliminates drugs, this process can be influenced by many factors that can lead to dangerous drug interactions. Changes in liver function caused by hepatic cirrhosis may cause the body to react more strongly to drugs. Changes in the liver's blood supply and metabolic functions can result in more side effects and higher toxicity, mainly when several medications are taken at the same time for complicated health problems. The interplay between polypharmacy and PK underscores the necessity for clinicians to closely monitor patients to prevent harmful interactions that may arise from such therapeutic regimens (Widyati et al., 2009). Since cancer treatment involves many different approaches, polypharmacy is prevalent among cancer patients. Many cancer patients over the age of 65 have to deal with cancer treatment as well as other long-term health conditions, which can result in more drug interactions that may affect both the treatment and the patient's safety. Taking many drugs at once often happens because of chemotherapy, treatments for side effects, and drugs for other diseases. Pharmacokinetic interactions may further complicate these challenges because other medicines can alter the process of chemotherapy drugs, which may result in more side effects or less effectiveness. Therefore, the role of clinical pharmacists becomes essential in this context, as they can assess and adjust drug regimens to mitigate the risks associated with polypharmacy and ensure optimal therapeutic outcomes (Khanal et al., 2019). Additionally, addressing pharmacokinetic interactions requires a strategy that involves educating patients and collaborating with various healthcare teams. Health professionals should collaborate to design plans that consider the possibility of drug interactions based on a patient's unique way of processing drugs. Reviewing medications regularly, changing the dosage as needed, and counseling patients help a lot in avoiding adverse drug events. Using a standardized method to study how drugs interact when given together will support better medical decisions, ensure higher patient safety, and lead to improved care. As the prevalence of polypharmacy continues to rise, particularly among aging populations, an emphasis on understanding and managing pharmacokinetic interactions is imperative for effective healthcare delivery and better patient outcomes (Widyati et al., 2009; Khanal et al., 2019).

12.2.2. Pharmacodynamic Interactions

Pharmacodynamic interaction is a condition in which two or more drugs influence each other's activity but not the process of absorption, distribution, metabolism, and excretion. The interaction can result in synergistic or antagonistic effects and can be the cause of therapeutic failure or toxicity. The complexities involved in the administration of multiple drugs in elderly patients who typically have polypharmacy complicate such interactions even further. Since older people often use many drugs for chronic diseases such as diabetes and hypertension, the risk of pharmacodynamic interactions is quite high. For healthcare providers, this interaction is important because it has a direct influence on patient safety and the effectiveness of treatment. Thus, encouraging an understanding of pharmacodynamic concepts will help clinicians optimize drug efficacy regimens to maximize the therapeutic effect of each drug, without causing potential adverse effects that may lead to re-hospitalization or further complications (AlJassas et al., 2024). Second, evaluating pharmacodynamic interactions is important in the context of elderly groups, who often present with polypharmacy. Model Answer. Factors such as age-related changes in physiological processes, including receptor sensitivity and homeostatic mechanisms, can significantly influence drug responsiveness. Trends in medication among older adults have been studied to reveal high rates of particular drug categories, e.g., antihypertensives and antidiabetics, which could interact with one another and complicate treatment (Keche et al., 2024). For example, the synergistic effect of beta-blockers and calcium channel blockers increases the risk of hypotension, whereas the combined use of anticoagulants can increase the risk of bleeding. In order to guarantee safer prescribing, practitioners should take precautions against these potential interactions by reviewing medications and educating patients. With the potential problems caused by pharmacodynamic interactions, the application of systematic drug analysis of prescriptions is a vital weapon against risk reduction from polypharmacy. Continuous monitoring of patients' medication allows for the identification of potentially harmful combinations and more rational prescribing. The examination can identify drug usage trends that can lead to harmful interactions, particularly among elderly populations at higher risk. For instance, a significant percentage of elderly individuals taking herbal supplements along with other medications makes it more challenging to interact drugs because these drugs also have pharmacodynamic actions. The integration of comprehensive prescription analysis into practice can be done by clinicians to facilitate patient safety, improve control over chronic diseases, and reduce the frequency of negative outcomes as a result of polypharmacy (Keche et al., 2024).

12.2.3. Drug-Food Interactions

The phenomenon of drug-food interactions (DFIs) represents a critical aspect of polypharmacy that can significantly alter therapeutic outcomes for patients. These interactions occur when the effects of drugs are altered by certain foods or components of a diet. As an illustration, vitamin K-rich foods can work against anticoagulants, such as warfarin, and this may result in serious complications for patients with coagulation disorders. In addition, drinking grapefruit juice can stop enzymes from doing their job, which results in higher levels of certain drugs in the blood and often makes them more dangerous. Because people's diets and medications can be complex, healthcare providers should be vigilant in identifying and addressing DFIs to ensure effective treatment and patient safety. This is why it is essential to use proactive medication management strategies to address these risks. Polypharmacy increases the risks of DFIs for people who are older or have chronic diseases, since they are usually given several medications at the same time. Being elderly often makes people more prone to DFIs, mainly because their digestive and metabolic systems change with age. Such changes add more challenges to the relationship between what we eat and our medications. Also, chronic health issues may call for using medications as well as changing your diet, which can lead to more chances for interactions. Understanding how food affects the way drugs are absorbed and metabolized can have a direct impact on a patient's treatment. Therefore, plans for patients should be created by involving nutritionists, pharmacists, and healthcare providers. When doctors and dietitians team up, patients can learn more about the connection between their diet and medications, leading to better adherence to advice and successful results. It is also important to note that pharmacists play a vital role on healthcare teams, mainly by providing education and counseling. When pharmacists carefully review medications and discuss patients' diets, they can identify any potential interactions between food and drugs. More people using OTC supplements and herbal remedies makes the problem more complicated, since patients may not see the risk of these products interacting with their prescribed medicines. Teaching people about these interactions and how to avoid them can significantly enhance patient safety and health outcomes. With the help of pharmacists, handling DFIs is one way to reduce the chances of adverse events from drug interactions and ensure that patients get the best results from their treatment (Figure 12.6).

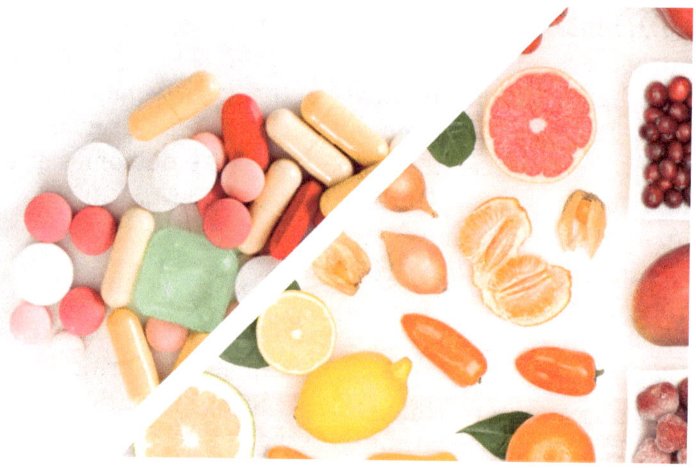

Figure 12.6. Drug-food interactions.

Source: https://burtsrx.com/wp-content/uploads/2020/10/Food-Vs-Medications.png.

12.3. Consequences of Polypharmacy

The impact of polypharmacy extends far beyond mere medication management, with significant implications for patient safety and quality of care. As patients, particularly the elderly, typically require taking numerous drugs to manage several comorbidities, the regimen complexity increases the risk of ADRs. These responses are more than just an annoyance; they may result in serious health consequences and numerous hospital stays, which are especially concerning for older people whose health may already be compromised. Indeed, polypharmacy does complicate treatment itself for cancer, where medication may be required in multiples for therapy as well as prevention of side effects, and this suggests an apparent overlap between polypharmacy and the significant burden of healthcare it creates. Careful examination of these interactions is necessary to optimize patient outcomes in the era of a more heterogeneous pharmacological environment (Khanal et al., 2019). In addition, the elderly population is specially vulnerable to the adverse effects of polypharmacy as the process of aging alters PK and pharmacodynamics, thus increasing susceptibility to ADRs. Such adverse effects have uncharacteristic presentations, which tend to complicate their detection and early intervention further. New technologies, such as the GerontoNet ADR Risk Score, attempt to define older patients at higher risk of ADRs, thereby presenting an algorithm for implementing preventive strategies. Targeting the highest-risk patients, healthcare providers can better manage polypharmacys impact and potentially reduce the incidence of ADRs that are commonly responsible for distasteful clinical consequences. In addition, enhancing clinical geriatric pharmacology education can provide healthcare providers with the knowledge necessary to address these problems effectively and improve care for this vulnerable population (Onder et al., 2012). In addition, the integration of clinical pharmacists into multidisciplinary health care teams can be an essential component in preventing the consequences of polypharmacy. In the majority of resource-limited settings, the absence of clinical pharmacists in addressing complex drug regimens can further exacerbate the issues surrounding polypharmacy. A multidisciplinary approach, combined with clinical pharmacy consultation, can facilitate the detection and resolution of potential drug interactions through a formal process for medication review and adjustment. This model of partnership not only addresses urgent problems concerning ADRs but generates a safer prescribing culture, especially in cancer treatment environments where drug combination is standard practice. Therefore, promoting the services of pharmacists in patient care can lead to enhanced patient safety and quality therapeutic outcomes, demonstrating the necessity for the multidisciplinary management of polypharmacy challenges responsibly (Khanal et al., 2019).

12.3.1. Increased Risk of Adverse Drug Reactions

The phenomenon of polypharmacy, particularly among the elderly population, significantly contributes to an increased risk of ADRs, which pose a considerable threat to patient safety. As people grow older, they commonly have several chronic diseases that call for taking many different medicines. This complexity not only raises the likelihood of drug-drug interactions (DDIs) but also the potential for mismanagement and errors in drug administration. Elderly patients are particularly vulnerable due to age-related physiological changes, including altered drug metabolism and excretion, which can exacerbate the sedative effects of medications, leading to profound complications such as gastrointestinal bleeding and cognitive impairment (Khan et al., 2025). Therefore, understanding the consequences of polypharmacy is crucial for healthcare professionals who want to lower the risk of adverse drug reactions and deliver effective therapies. Using careful monitoring and specific strategies helps reduce the chances of ADRs in people taking many drugs. Recent studies highlight the correlations between high-risk DDIs and adverse clinical events among elderly patients, demonstrating that up to 37% of hospitalizations can be traced back to problematic polypharmacy (Khan et al., 2025). Strategies such as comprehensive medication reviews and the implementation of CDSS can enhance medication safety by identifying potentially harmful interactions before they manifest into serious health issues. In addition, using Beers Criteria and STOPP/START Criteria as established rules has become a helpful method for clinicians to manage medication therapy. Applying these strategies, healthcare teams can collaborate to ensure the appropriate use of medicines and enhance the treatment outcomes for vulnerable individuals. Additionally, education helps overcome the problems of polypharmacy and improves patient outcomes. Many HCPs, including geriatricians and pharmacists, report limited access to contemporary DDI screening tools and insufficient training in geriatric pharmacology, which are critical barriers to effective polypharmacy management (Khan et al., 2025). While managing medications, interdisciplinary teams should make a point to increase awareness of possible drug interactions and when it is necessary to reduce or stop taking certain drugs. Improving pharmacovigilance in healthcare systems can be achieved by providing clinicians with additional training and promoting policy changes that address these issues. In the end, solid measures that improve providers' knowledge and simplify the use of drugs are important for lowering the risks of ADRs in polypharmacy (Figure 12.7).

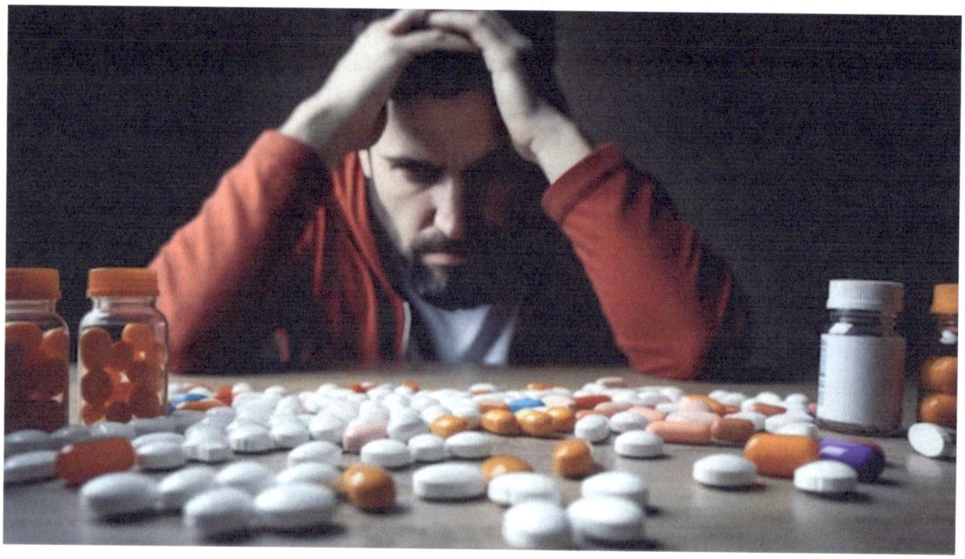

Figure 12.7. Increased risk of adverse drug reactions.

Source: https://safetherapeutics.com/wp-content/uploads/2023/12/Managing-Medication-Risks-Tackling-Adverse-Drug-Reactions-in-Psychiatric-Hospitals-Safe-Therapeutics.jpg.

12.3.2. Impact on Medication Adherence

Older patients who take many medications at once often find it hard to follow the drug plan, which can seriously harm their health. With time, seniors might receive several medications in one visit since they have many chronic illnesses, which makes their drug treatment more complicated. Research has shown that about 80% of elderly patients have drug-related issues (DRPs), with drug interactions and dose calculation being the most common issue found among them. Due to this complexity, patients often struggle to follow the prescribed dosage and goals. Therefore, when patients fail to adhere to their treatment, it typically leads to unfavorable health outcomes. The increased burden of using several medications facilitates the vicious cycle of non-adherence, elevating morbidity risks as well as influencing the overall well-being of the patients, highlighting the need for strategic interventions (Bertorio et al., 2025). Therefore, it is necessary to understand the factors that cause people not to take their medication as planned to deal with the condition. The mental changes that usually happen because of polypharmacy can make it difficult for patients to follow directions for their medicines. Also, the stress of taking many prescriptions can make it hard for patients to follow their treatment plans, sometimes resulting in them skipping their medicine or dropping their routine. If people do not follow medical advice, they often have to be hospitalized, experience more health problems, and their mental and physical health decline. To control polypharmacy, it is important to educate patients on drug use and improve the way doctors and patients communicate. Educating and empowering patients, as well as optimizing medication regimens, can potentially mitigate the adverse effects of polypharmacy and improve outcomes (Siddique, 2024). For older patients with polypharmacy, healthcare systems should use different ways to help them take their medicines properly. This includes medication reconciliation, or routine review of a patient's medication regime to remove unnecessary prescriptions and avoidable drug interactions. Additionally, removing unnecessary medications from patients would make it easier for them, which in turn helps improve their adherence. Regular check-ups with healthcare professionals help patients understand how to take their medications and why following the regimen is important. Additionally, creating patient care plans tailored to the needs of elderly individuals encourages them to follow the plan. Supported by the evidence of reduced side effects and improved quality of life, successful interventions will be of great benefit to this risk population (Bertorio et al., 2025; Siddique, 2024). If the healthcare system emphasizes patient education, monitoring, and patient activation, it will be able to address polypharmacy and ensure that older patients take their medications as prescribed, leading to improved health outcomes (Figure 12.8).

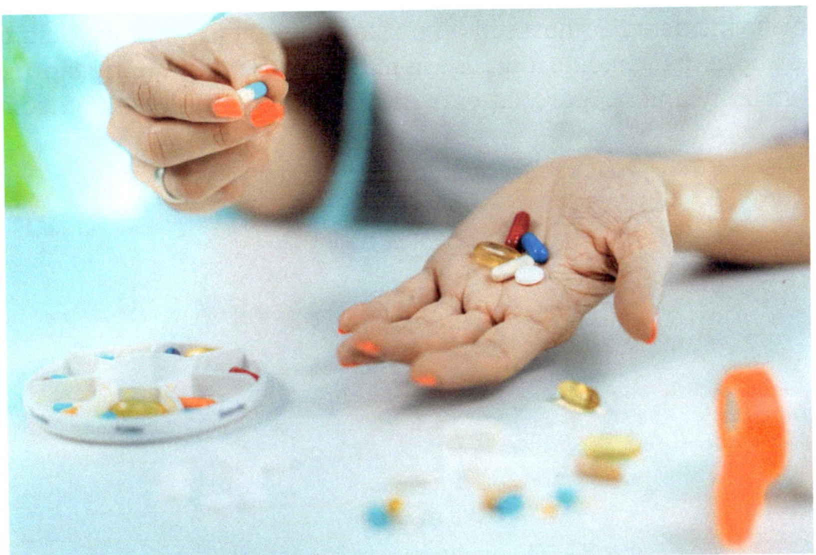

Figure 12.8. Impact on medication adherence.

Source: https://www.revenuexl.com/hubfs/Medication_Adherence.jpg.

12.3.3. Economic Burden on Healthcare Systems

Healthcare systems face significant and diverse economic challenges due to polypharmacy. Since chronic diseases have become more common among older people, the number of patients treated with several medicines has gone up a lot. As a result, concerns have arisen about the safety and effectiveness of medications, and healthcare costs continue to rise. Treating adverse drug events is more expensive for hospitals and health providers, as these events occur more often in people who take several medications together. According to studies, these ADEs may cause people to spend more time in the hospital, receive additional medical care, and put more pressure on the healthcare system. Managing difficulties caused by polypharmacy can be expensive for both patients and the healthcare system as a whole, so it is necessary to respond in a planned manner to reduce these costs and improve care. Additionally, polypharmacy has economic effects that extend beyond healthcare expenses. As an illustration, individuals dealing with ADRs may notice a decline in their quality of life, which can lead to reduced productivity and increased absenteeism from work. As a result, the economy may suffer, as caregivers may have to miss work to care for the affected individuals, thereby adding more stress to the economy. In some cases, when drugs interact, patients may not get the best results, and this can cause extra spending on ineffective treatments. All these factors together indicate that we need to implement integrated medication management strategies as soon as possible. Tackling polypharmacy is important for improving patient outcomes and for helping to lower healthcare costs. New ways to deal with polypharmacy can significantly reduce the financial burden on healthcare systems. Implementing interdisciplinary medication reviews, enhancing clinician education, and utilizing technological innovations such as CDSS can improve prescribing practices and reduce the incidence of adverse drug events. For instance, making sure patients take fewer medicines and helping them stop using some drugs can prevent the dangers linked to polypharmacy. Using the buy-and-bill model for certain treatments could encourage patients to adhere to their treatment regimen, potentially leading to improved outcomes and a lower incidence of hospital admissions. As the healthcare field evolves, it will be essential to focus on optimizing medication use in patients who take multiple drugs to maintain the system's financial stability and support patients in achieving better health outcomes (Figure 12.9).

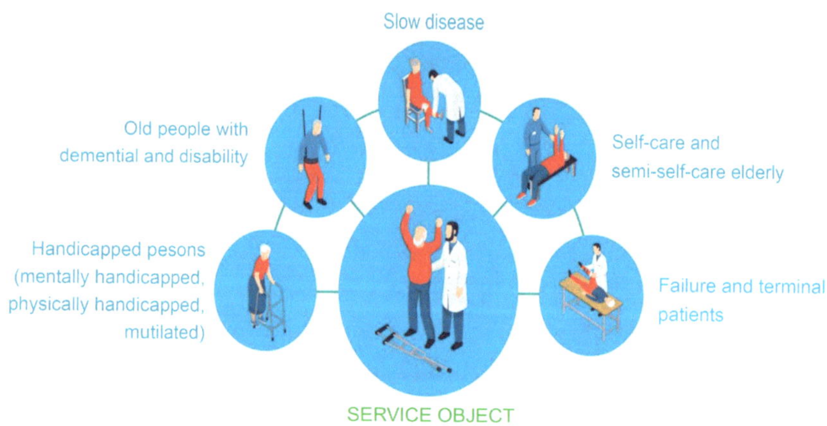

Figure 12.9. Economic burden on healthcare systems.

Source: https://pub.mdpi-res.com/sustainability/sustainability-14-16505/article_deploy/html/images/sustainability-14-16505-g001.png?1670581160.

12.4. Identifying Drug Interactions

Drugs interactions are crucial in the case of polypharmacy, particularly in high-risk groups such as comorbid patients. Because patients will take a combination of drugs for various diseases, drug-

drug interactions (DDIs) will be more probable. Research indicates that individuals with complex treatment regimens, such as cancer and HIV-infected patients (PWHC), have higher risk factors for DDIs. In a study from May 2020 to May 2024, 410 distinct interactions were identified in a 140-PWHC cohort, highlighting the burden of polypharmacy and the need for close monitoring in such high-risk populations (Cattaneo et al., 2025). This emphasizes the need for accurate identification and management techniques to reduce harmful clinical effects while maximizing therapeutic potency. It is crucial to understand the mechanisms of drug interactions to establish good clinical practice (GCP). Drug-drug interactions can alter the pharmacokinetic and pharmacodynamic profiles of the interacting drugs, resulting in unpredictable therapeutic failure or toxicity. Identification of such interactions involves not only knowledge of which drugs are involved but also the nature of the interaction between them in terms of being synergistic, antagonistic, or asymmetrically active. Recent studies have postulated that asymmetric drug interactions are particularly challenging, in that a drug may influence the effectiveness of another with no influence in opposition, complicating treatment regimens (Deng et al., 2024). It is only possible to detect such complexities through sophisticated analytical techniques that contribute to integrating various kinds of data and highlighting potential DDIs, thus enabling healthcare providers to make informed prescribing choices. There is a need to include a multidisciplinary approach for the successful identification and management of drug interactions in patients undergoing polypharmacy. Multidisciplinary teams of pharmacists, doctors, and other healthcare providers can facilitate the process of monitoring drug regimens and potential interactions. By employing various approaches such as therapeutic drug monitoring (TDM), patient education, and optimization of medication schedules, teams can prevent the risks of DDIs. Also, evidence from studies indicates that prevention of polypharmacy improves patient safety and outcomes (Cattaneo et al., 2025). The development of new prediction models, including multimodal data analysis and variational graph autoencoders, may also alter the screening and treatment of such drug interactions and shift it towards individualized patient treatment and increased therapeutic effectiveness (Deng et al., 2024).

12.4.1. Role of Healthcare Professionals in Monitoring

Today's complicated medication plans for older adults cause serious challenges for HCPs, especially in dealing with polypharmacy and its risks. Healthcare providers must be vigilant in monitoring patients to mitigate the ADRs that can arise from multiple medications. Since older adults are frequently given several drugs for different conditions, the risk of drug interactions goes up a lot. Due to these interactions, patients may require hospitalization and experience additional health issues. Comprehensive training and education in clinical geriatric pharmacology can enhance HCPs ability to recognize atypical presentations of ADRs and implement effective monitoring strategies that prioritize patient safety, ensuring that older patients receive optimal care tailored to their specific needs and conditions (Onder et al., 2012). Pharmacists are very important in healthcare monitoring, especially in oncology and geriatrics because people there often take many medications. Thanks to their knowledge, they can spot possible adverse effects that could arise from taking chemotherapy with drugs for ADRs or other conditions. Conducting this type of monitoring helps prevent negative health consequences and ensures the more effective use of medications. In places where resources are limited, clinical pharmacists should be given more responsibilities to assist elderly cancer patients who are at risk of taking many drugs at once. Integrating pharmacists into multidisciplinary teams can facilitate better communication and collaboration, ensuring that all HCPs work cohesively to improve patient outcomes (Khanal et al., 2019). To monitor patients well,

HCPs must rely on comprehensive tools, including the GerontoNet ADR Risk Score that was recently introduced. They help in finding older people who are more likely to suffer from adverse events as a result of taking multiple medications. As a result of using these screening tools, healthcare teams can pay closer attention to patients who may require extra care. It is essential to encourage healthcare providers to communicate with one another regularly. As a result of this teamwork, medical staff can adjust the patient's medication plan as needed, incorporating new assessments and information shared by the patient. Ultimately, by embracing the collective expertise of various HCPs, including physicians, pharmacists, and other specialists, the quality of care and patient safety in the context of polypharmacy can be significantly improved (Onder et al., 2012) (Figure 12.10).

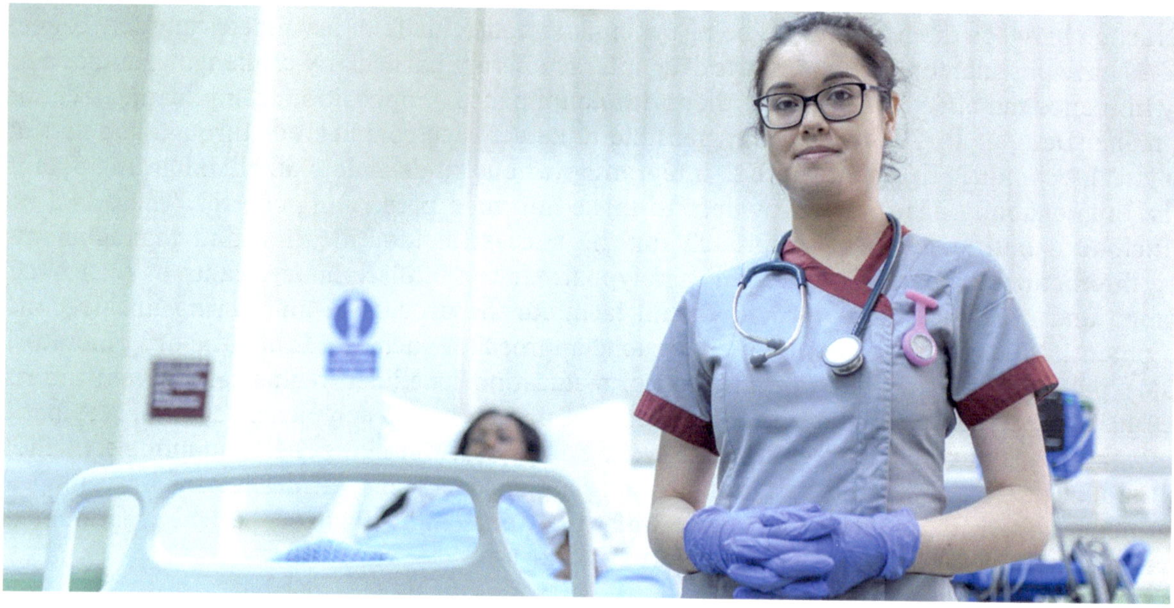

Figure 12.10. Role of healthcare professionals in monitoring.

Source: https://healthplan.co.uk/wp-content/uploads/2023/01/explaining-the-role-of-healthcare-professionals.jpg.

12.4.2. Use of Technology and Databases for Interaction Checks

With the help of advanced technology and expert databases, assessing drug interactions has become much easier, mainly in the case of polypharmacy. Because more elderly people are using multiple drugs for their long-term health problems, it is very important to ensure efficient interaction checks. The KALIS system demonstrates that using computers for decision-making can help reduce errors and adverse outcomes associated with drug use by studying each patient's profile. It provides both the guidelines for prescribing and molecular facts, which help clarify possible interactions. With interoperability with existing EHRs, KALIS facilitates effortless communication among HCPs, thereby guaranteeing a team-based approach to the management of polypharmacy (Friedrichs et al., 2019). Such technology is crucial for ensuring that patients with complex medical conditions can safely and effectively administer their medications. Apart from established systems like KALIS, the use of natural language processing (NLP) technologies is a force-of-change phenomenon in clinical situations. Using electronic medical records in secondary data analysis can significantly improve clinical care, mainly in terms of medication safety. With the help of terminology servers, hospitals can utilize ontology and NLP pipelines to detect drug interactions in incomplete or challenging medical documents, such as discharge letters. Using a knowledge-based method has proven to be very precise and accurate in finding drug-disease interactions. For instance, the detection of proton-pump inhibitors in osteoporosis achieved a 100% accuracy rate, signifying the highest utilization of such technologies in medical practice (Demuth et al., 2019). It enables clinicians to screen patients at a low cost and make informed decisions with full confidence on the best course of action. When technology and databases are used in healthcare, the risk of polypharmacy goes down, and clinical results improve. Since digital resources are being used more often in healthcare, it is necessary to keep improving them to deal with drug interactions. Clinicians utilize data analytics, information retrieval systems, and computer-based decision-support tools to conduct a more comprehensive risk assessment before prescribing. Moreover, these advancements enable the monitoring of any effects of new drugs and treatment programs as soon as they are introduced. Ultimately, utilizing these innovative methods is a means to ensure patient safety and proper care, particularly as the number of medications patients take increases, thereby enabling healthcare to meet the diverse needs of various groups (Figure 12.11).

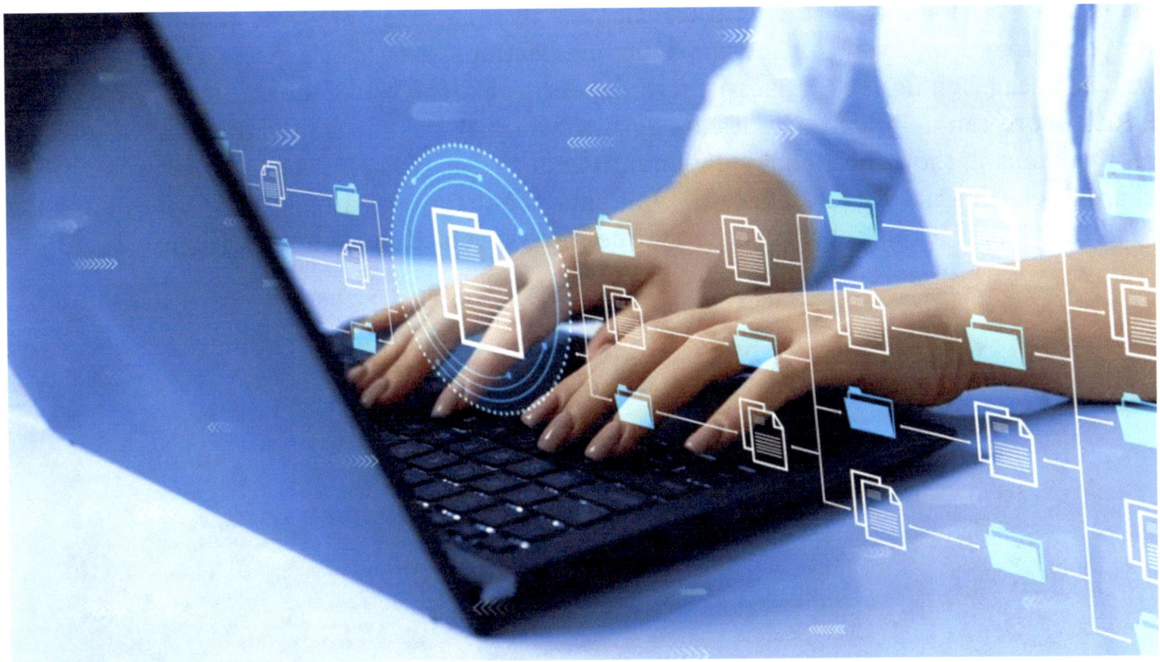

Figure 12.11. Use of technology and databases for interaction checks.

Source: https://imageio.forbes.com/specials-images/imageserve/63d7f6950f3157d4c14c5504/0x0.jpg?format=jpg&width=1200.

12.4.3. Patient Education and Self-Reporting

Proper education of patients helps reduce the risks associated with using multiple medications and potential interactions. Educating patients about their medications empowers them to understand the importance of adherence, recognize potential side effects, and identify signs of ADRs. As medications become more complex for seniors, informed patients are better equipped to manage their health outcomes. Research indicates a significant prevalence of medication errors, with prescribing errors reported to range from 2% to 94% in various studies (Aljadhey et al., 2018). As a result, when patients are well-informed, they can participate in their treatment, ask important questions, and understand their prescriptions, which may improve their adherence to the treatment plan. Patients' reports about their medications are very useful in managing polypharmacy. If patients truthfully tell their healthcare provider about the drugs and supplements they take, doctors can evaluate possible drug interactions and make the necessary changes to treatment. It is especially important for older people, since their bodies may process drugs differently and they can have unique diseases. By implementing systematic methods for self-reporting, such as medication diaries or digital health applications, providers can enhance medication reconciliation processes and ensure that prescribers are fully informed about a patient's medication landscape (Onder et al., 2012). Hence, when patients and healthcare providers communicate openly, it becomes easier to take timely actions that reduce drug-related problems. Additionally, encouraging patients to learn about and report their symptoms helps establish a cooperative relationship between them and their healthcare providers.

It is essential for this partnership to exist, as polypharmacy presents numerous challenges. When patients are involved in choosing their medications, they can express their concerns and views, which can significantly impact prescribing decisions. The use of tools such as the GerontoNet ADR Risk Score can help identify patients at risk who may benefit from additional interventions, thereby enhancing the educational component (Onder et al., 2012). If healthcare providers focus on shared decision-making and educating patients about their treatment, they can help patients manage the challenges of polypharmacy and be more involved in their care (Figure 12.12).

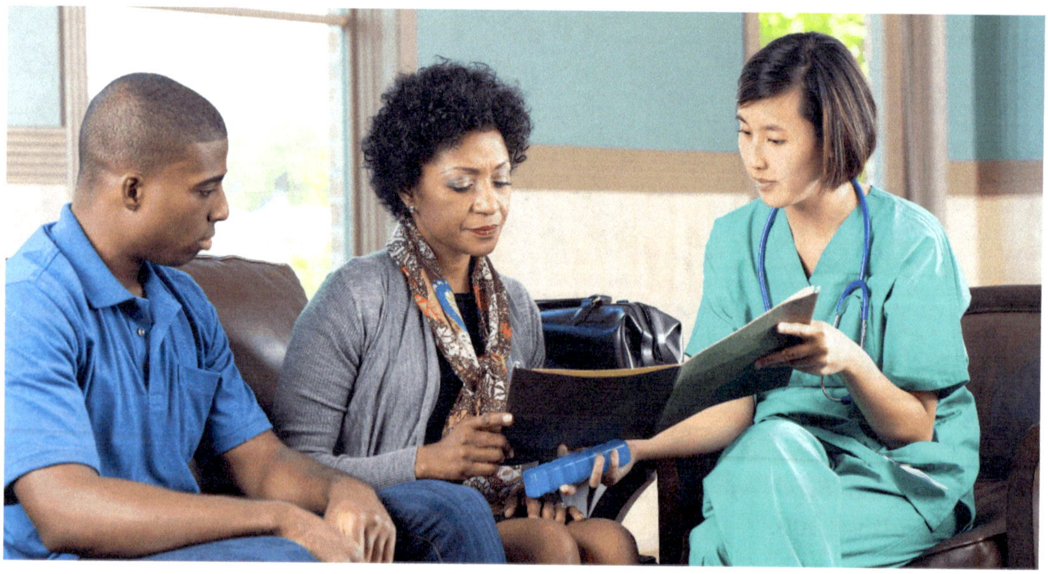

Figure 12.12. Patient education and self-reporting.

Source: https://thenerdynurse.com/wp-content/uploads/2021/08/Why-Patient-Education-is-Important-FB.png.

12.5. Strategies to Manage Polypharmacy

Polypharmacy is best handled by focusing on both the safety of patients and the effectiveness of the drugs used. It is very important to conduct thorough medication reviews as part of a strategy, as this helps identify any extra or repeated prescriptions. With this analysis, HCPs can check if every medication is suitable for a patient's condition and the outcomes they are looking for. Since pharmacists are well-informed about drug interactions and their side effects, they play a significant role in this area. If pharmacists look at medication regimens as a whole, they can suggest ways to reduce the chance of DDIs.

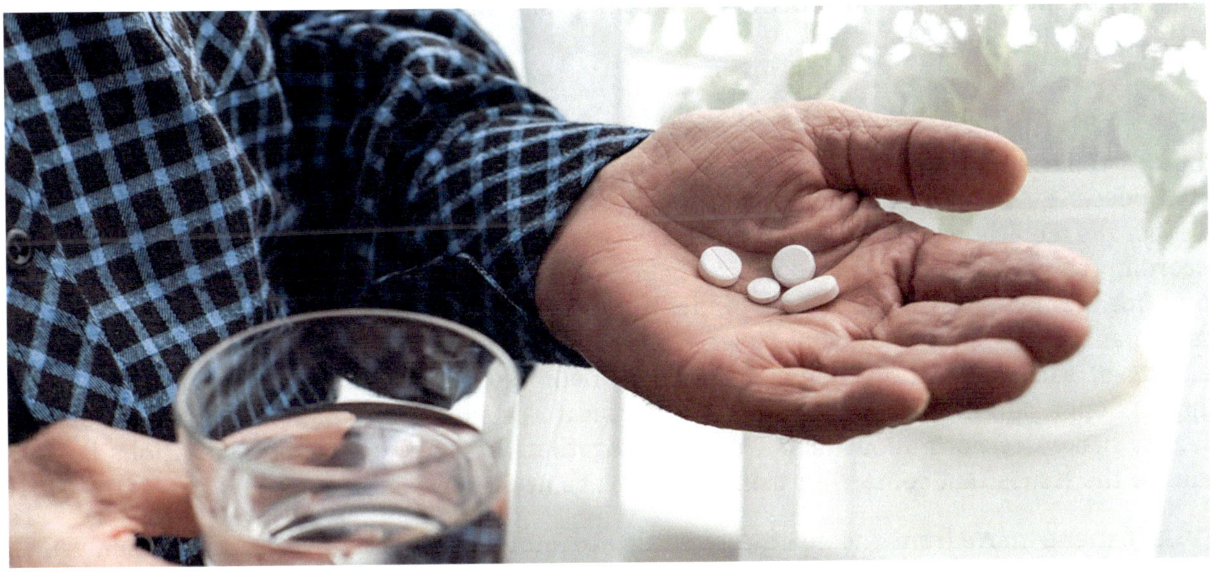

Figure 12.13. Strategies to manage polypharmacy.

Source: https://kauveryhospital.com/blog/wp-content/uploads/2023/06/Polypharmacy-in-the-Elderly-1200x545_c.jpg.

Additionally, when EHRs are linked to CDSS, it enables real-time warnings about potential DDIs, facilitating clinicians' ability to make informed decisions. Thus, these systematic reviews enhance patient care and encourage collaboration between HCPs to maximize the medication therapies (AlJassas et al., 2024). It is most important to educate and communicate with patients to manage polypharmacy. Providing patients with clear instructions about their medications, including their uses, potential side effects, and risks associated with mixing them with other drugs, is crucial for both adherence and informed decision-making. Participating in the discussion allows patients to mention any worries about their treatment and suggests OTC drugs or supplements that could interact with the prescription drugs.

This approach to patient care helps patients adhere to their medication regimen and makes them understand the importance of taking them. In addition, regular meetings among physicians, pharmacists, and other healthcare professionals are necessary to monitor the effects of medication. Such collaboration helps adjust treatments ahead of time, react to DDIs when they develop and eventually improve patient health and compliance (Shekho et al., 2024). The use of personalized medicine is very promising for managing the use of multiple drugs and avoiding problems caused by their interaction. Pharmacogenomics enables pharmacists and other healthcare professionals to tailor medications to an individual's genetic profile, thereby maximizing therapeutic benefits while minimizing the risk of adverse drug interactions. Using this approach, the safety of drugs can be improved, and it becomes easier to understand why a patient responds to a certain medicine in a particular way. Additionally, with digital health technology, patients can utilize mobile applications on their phones to more effectively track their medication, receive reminders, and report any potential interactions. As advanced strategies and technologies continue to evolve, the health system can enhance its potential to overcome the challenges of polypharmacy, ensuring patients achieve maximum therapeutic benefit without compromising safety (AlJassas et al., 2024; Shekho et al., 2024) (Figure 12.13).

12.5.1. Regular Medication Reviews

Since polypharmacy is more common these days, it is necessary to review medications regularly to avoid possible risks from drug interactions and errors. These reviews provide a means to assess whether the medications prescribed for elderly patients with various illnesses are suitable for them. According to research, differences in prescribing errors, including those that are inappropriate, point out the need for careful review of medications. An emphasis on comprehensive medication assessments can identify potential adverse drug events (ADEs) and ensure that the therapeutic benefits of each medication outweigh its risks. Being so careful helps keep patients safe and supports open and informed talks between healthcare providers and patients, which encourages them to make decisions about their treatment together. Regularly checking medications helps to manage the issues that come with using many drugs at once.

As patients move from one healthcare setting to another, the possibility of medication-related problems goes up a lot. In some cases, patients may get different medication instructions because their doctors do not communicate well with each other. Reviewing medications regularly helps find cases of drug-drug interactions that may result in harmful ADEs. Ensuring that only necessary medicines are administered and their doses are adjusted for each patient can help alleviate the issue of polypharmacy. Adopting this strategy minimizes the chances of negative interactions and improves patients' lives by helping them avoid the problems caused by using too much or the wrong medication. Additionally, regular reviews of medications can significantly impact healthcare systems and the economy. Since about 7% of ADRs are caused by drug interactions, the resulting costs are very significant.

Reviewing medications can simplify a patient's drug regimen, which may lower costs associated with emergency room visits and readmissions. Additionally, utilizing research-based strategies during medication reviews aligns with clinical goals to care for patients effectively and control the costs associated with polypharmacy. The increasing number of people who agree that these procedures are important in managing chronic illnesses makes it clear that regular reviews of medications are necessary. Many studies have highlighted that addressing these factors can enhance patient safety and improve the efficiency of healthcare systems, ultimately benefiting all parties involved (Figure 12.14).

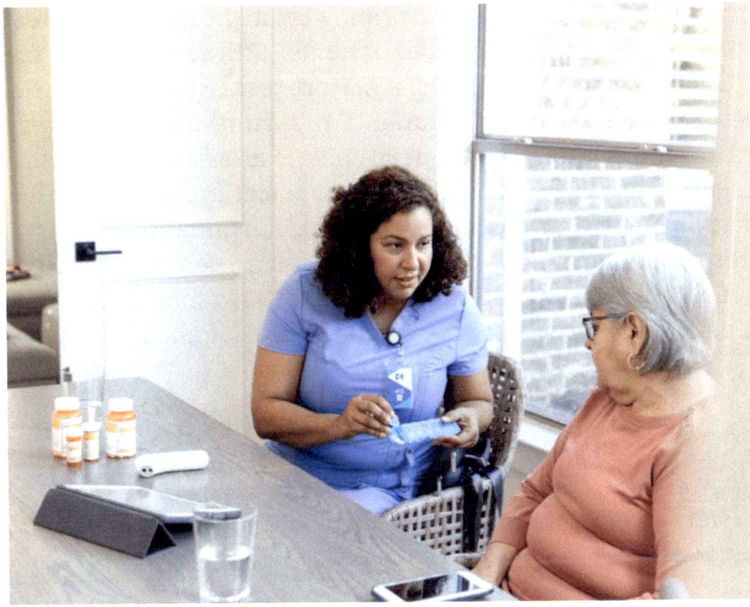

Figure 12.14. Regular medication reviews.

Source: https://allseniors.org/wp-content/uploads/2024/06/Medication-Reviews.png.

12.5.2. Deprescribing Practices

Deprescribing is increasingly gaining ground as an unavoidable response to the complexities of polypharmacy, particularly in geriatric patients. Polypharmacy has classically referred to the concurrent prescription of five or more drugs. However, it poses high risks of drug-interaction problems and side effects, particularly in elderly patients with multiple chronic comorbidities. Effective deprescribing is not merely a careful examination of a patient's medication list, but also sensitivity towards the patient's attitudes and beliefs regarding their medicines. Research indicated that 96.3% of older patients strongly believed in the necessity of their medicines, and a significant percentage (33.9%) were also bothered by potential side effects. These dynamics highlight the complex interplay between patient trust in health professionals and receptiveness to considering deprescribing strategies, underscoring the need for practitioners to engage in open communication in a patient-focused manner to foster an open setting for medication review (Boland et al., 2017). Furthermore, systematic deprescribing pathways have been found to enhance clinician confidence in addressing polypharmacy. Many healthcare providers report feeling inadequately equipped to make informed decisions regarding what medications to reduce or discontinue. A scholarly project set up to bridge this gap utilized evidence-based guidelines to develop a polypharmacy protocol intervention that significantly improved clinician confidence in identifying potentially inappropriate medications. Clinicians reported increased competence in conducting deprescribing, aligned with the latest professional recommendations. This not only reduces the polypharmacy burden but also enables safety and effectiveness in patient care. The findings suggest that with adequate equipment and education, practitioners can feel more secure in discussing drug management options with patients, making a collaborative approach to deprescribing possible, centered on patient welfare (Steiner et al., 2020). In addition to clinician-centered programs, patients' beliefs also play a significant role in successful deprescribing strategies. Scientific research identifies that an effective doctor-patient relationship affects patients' attitudes toward medicines on a broad scale, facilitating or discouraging the deprescribing process. Health professionals must establish trust and open communication to facilitate patients reporting their concerns and preferences for medications. As patients make their health decisions, it is essential to understand and address their misconceptions and fears about discontinuing medication. Clinicians hence, need to pursue a holistic strategy that not only addresses the clinical determinants of drug interactions but also focuses on the psychosocial determinants involved. Fostering patient participation in the decision-making process is crucial in overcoming deprescribing resistance and promoting overall health outcomes for individuals living with polypharmacy (Boland et al., 2017) (Figure 12.15).

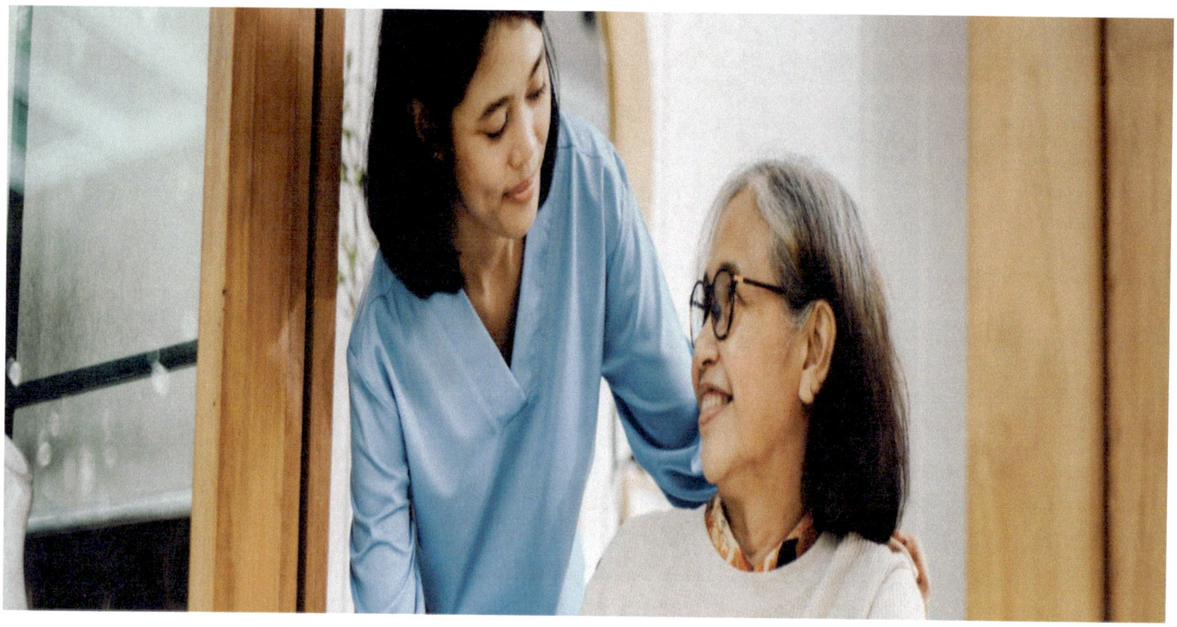

Figure 12.15. Deprescribing practices.

Source: https://gpex.com.au/wp-content/uploads/2024/05/Palliative-Care-Blog.png.

12.5.3. Collaborative Care Models

Because many elderly people take several drugs, it has become necessary to use collaborative care models in different health settings. They encourage medical teams to combine their expertise and knowledge to ensure proper use of medicines. These models encourage team members to communicate effectively and provide detailed reviews of patients' medications, especially when they are taking multiple medications. These methods cut down on mistakes with drugs and also try to prevent the risks that come from using several drugs together. When these models incorporate effective communication strategies, healthcare workers are more likely to be familiar with each patient's medication plan and can prevent serious drug-related effects that may impact the patient's health. Particularly, working together in teams has helped community pharmacists achieve better results in managing medications. Pharmacists are involved in checking patients' medications and spotting any possible drug interactions. A triage system used in regular meetings enables more attention to be given to patients who require thorough medication reviews. It simplifies the identification of medication-related problems and helps apply suitable interventions tailored to each patient's needs. Several studies have shown that when working together, pharmacists can significantly improve the management of polypharmacy, particularly in older adults. When pharmacists join healthcare teams, it becomes possible to enhance the safety and effectiveness of medications. In addition, using technology in collaborative care can make it easier to handle polypharmacy and avoid drug interactions. Utilizing electronic medical record (EMR) systems facilitates the seamless exchange of patient information among healthcare providers, allowing for real-time updates to medication lists and alerts for clinically significant drug interactions. As mentioned in quality improvement efforts, holding educational sessions for all involved can help individuals become more responsible for taking their medications. Regularly checking how patients are taking their medications makes it possible to make adjustments based on new findings and what patients report, which helps prevent adverse drug reactions. When different HCPs work together and use technology well, collaborative care models can help patients avoid problems linked to taking many medications and interacting drugs, which leads to improved health (Figure 12.16).

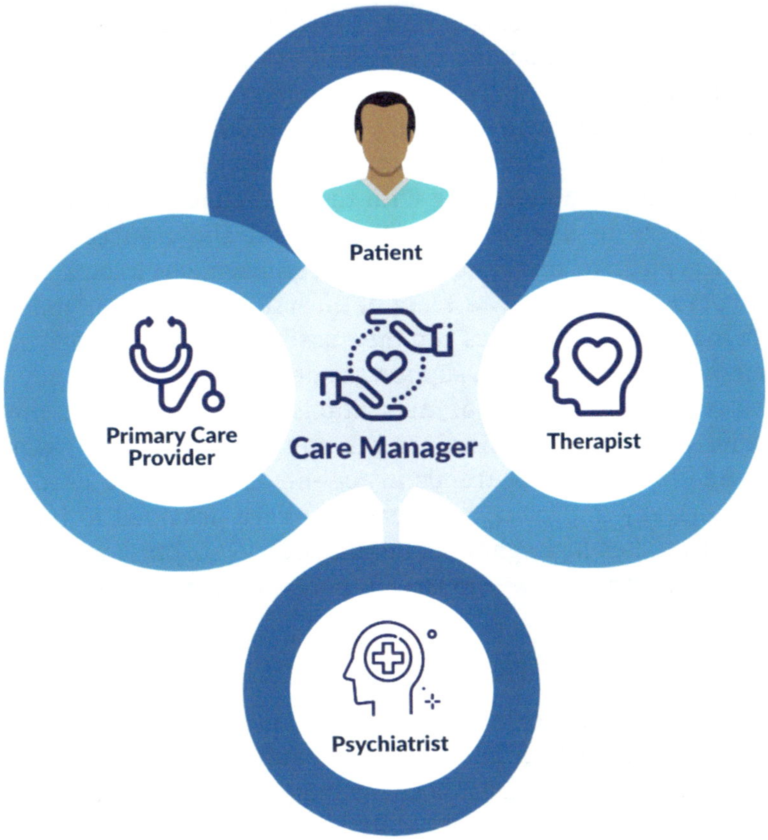

Figure 12.16. Collaborative care models.

Source: https://therapymantra.co/wp-content/uploads/2022/02/What-Is-Collaborative-Care-Model.png.

12.6. Case Studies and Real-World Examples

Because more elderly people are taking several medicines at the same time, it becomes difficult to handle drug interactions, which is clear from many case studies. A classic example is atrial fibrillation patients, most commonly treated with non-vitamin K antagonist anticoagulants (NOACs) to avert stroke. These important clinical trials were conducted in a strict manner, so patients with other health issues and those taking multiple medications were typically excluded. They also point out that findings from trials may not be applicable to real patients. Often, clinicians encounter cases that are similar to those discussed in advisory board meetings, where experts discussed managing patients who were underrepresented in the trials. This deficiency in robust supporting evidence requires physicians to base their actions on their clinical acumen and refer to available literature in order to navigate complex treatment landscapes effectively (Acar et al., 2020). Another educational case study focuses on the use of healthcare technology, specifically wearable devices that continuously monitor vital signs. The use of this technology greatly helps in managing chronic diseases, particularly for patients who are taking multiple medications simultaneously. With these devices, people can constantly monitor their heart rate and blood pressure, which may reveal potential problems that occur when using multiple medications together. When patients provide information from smart devices to doctors, physicians can make more informed decisions about medication doses. Monitoring patients in real time promotes their involvement in care and ensures they take their drugs as prescribed, which can help avoid possible drug interactions. This interface between technology and healthcare is a promising direction that can potentially render patients safer and enhance their results when dealing with the challenges of polypharmacy (Hosseinpour et al., 2019). It is necessary to look at case studies that show successful drug management in complicated patient groups to understand how polypharmacy affects them. For instance, a retrospective review could highlight how a team of diverse professionals managed the care of an older population with multiple health issues and their associated medications. Using comprehensive reviews of medications and clinical decision support, healthcare workers can advise against potential drug interactions and reduce the number of medications prescribed to patients. Such approaches lead to better outcomes for patients and reduce the number of hospital readmissions caused by adverse drug effects. Additionally, these trends in real-life cases can be used to create guidelines for drug management, thereby improving the quality of care provided to individuals at risk. The examination of such case studies highlights the importance of adapting clinical strategies to fit the special needs of vulnerable populations exposed to polypharmacy (Acar et al., 2020).

12.6.1. Case Study of a Geriatric Patient

More and more, as people age, they experience the challenges of polypharmacy, especially those in geriatrics who have many chronic conditions that require using different medicines. The case study of an elderly patient points out that it is challenging for them to manage their medicines, as they often take many drugs for several health conditions, and the side effects of these drugs. As a result, this patient could receive several drugs for hypertension, diabetes, and arthritis, which raises the chance of adverse effects and makes it harder to follow all the prescribed treatments. Additionally, since their medical conditions are interrelated, a minor change in one area can impact the safety or effectiveness of their medications in other areas, which is why it is crucial to regularly review their medications to minimize risks. Having many medications at once in elderly patients is not only a problem to organize; it can seriously affect their health, especially in oncology. Cancer, along with the treatments it necessitates, typically adds further challenges to the situation. In this patient's case, taking medications for cancer can interact with the other drugs they are taking. As highlighted by Khanal et al. (2019), the impact of polypharmacy in elderly cancer patients may not always be adequately addressed in clinical practice due to a lack of systematic evaluation and intervention strategies. This points out that healthcare providers should create better guidelines for identifying and handling polypharmacy, mainly for cancer patients, so that the benefits of treatment do not get overshadowed by the risks of taking many drugs. Treatments for polypharmacy should be standardized for all patients and also tailored to meet the individual needs of each patient in geriatric oncology. In line with recommendations from Aparicio et al. (2016), the process of deprescribing—defined as the strategic reduction of medications when potential harm outweighs the benefit—could provide a viable framework for managing complex medication regimens. When collaborating with clinical pharmacists, our case study patient's healthcare team can carefully review medications and identify patients who may benefit from deprescribing, taking into account the patient's overall health and treatment goals. If such teams are formed, the results may improve, risks from polypharmacy could drop, and patients' lives could be made better as they deal with cancer and chronic diseases (Figure 12.17).

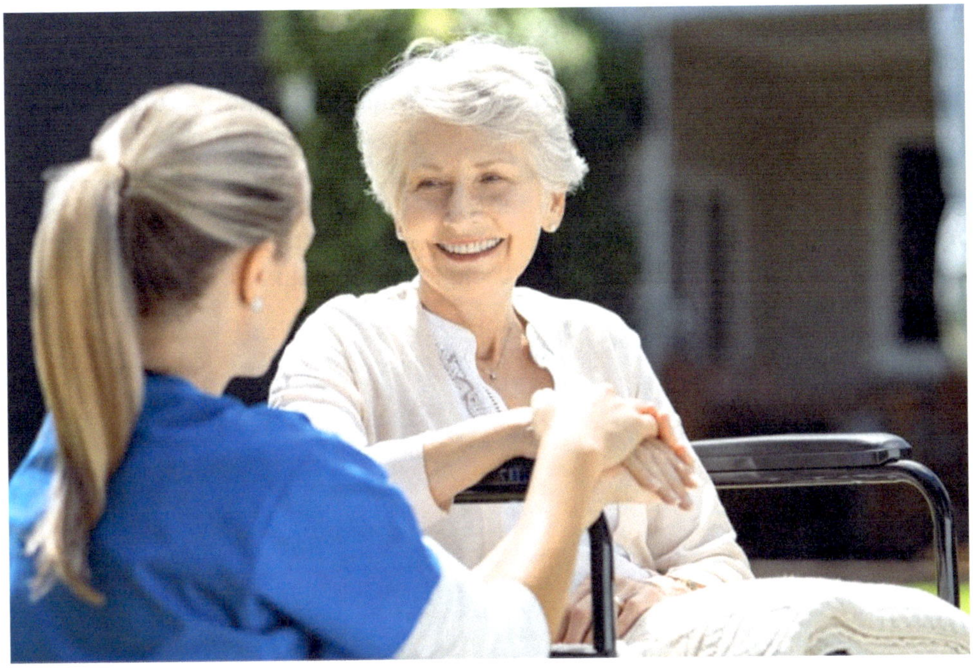

Figure 12.17. Case study of a geriatric patient.

Source: https://unicityhealthcare.com/wp-content/uploads/2020/02/Nurse-Performs-Geriatric-Care-Assessment.jpg.

12.6.2. Impact of Polypharmacy in Patients with Multiple Comorbidities

Polypharmacy, the use of numerous drugs at the same time, is a complicated phenomenon, particularly in patients with multiple comorbidities. The patient population tends to require drugs for various chronic illnesses, leading to an increased risk of drug-related morbidity. Older patients, especially those on cancer treatment, are the embodiment of this challenge; they tend to receive polypharmacy due to the need for chemotherapy drugs, management of ADRs, and management of other comorbid diseases. The medication complexity of drugs in this group may result in adverse health outcomes, including a high percentage of drug interactions and side effects, which call for effective medication management strategies in clinical settings (Khanal et al., 2019). Inability to address these conditions may disrupt patients' care and create adverse health outcomes. This overlap of aging, pharmacotherapeutic complexity, and chronic disease is best seen in HIV-infected subjects, where polypharmacy is increasingly being observed. With increasing age, health profiles of patients often include a multitude of comorbidities, which necessitate the administration of a multiplicity of drugs. A seminal study has demonstrated that regimens of antiretroviral treatment become complex because of the need to contend with these concomitant disorders and thereby increase the risk for ADRs and drug interactions. The Medication Regimen Complexity Index has been a valuable tool for assessing drug regimen complexity among this high-risk population. These are issues that necessitate healthcare providers to enhance their approach to managing medications, incorporating deprescribing and the appraisal of potentially inappropriate medications to ensure optimal patient outcomes (Mart et al., 2018). Polypharmacy among comorbid patients needs an interdisciplinary approach, and interprofessional cooperation among HCPs, such as clinical pharmacists. Clinical pharmacists play a crucial role in evaluating the appropriateness of medication and mitigating polypharmacy risks. Their expertise assists in identifying possibly inappropriate medications and preventing drug interactions from leading to unwanted effects, and thus enhances the health of the patient, especially in resource-limited environments. Additionally, integrating clinical pharmacists into general and oncology care teams can significantly enhance the overall drug management process, thereby minimizing the negative impacts of polypharmacy. With increased progress in the healthcare system, similar collaborations will be necessary to deliver quality care to patients with complex medical backgrounds (Khanal et al., 2019) (Figure 12.18).

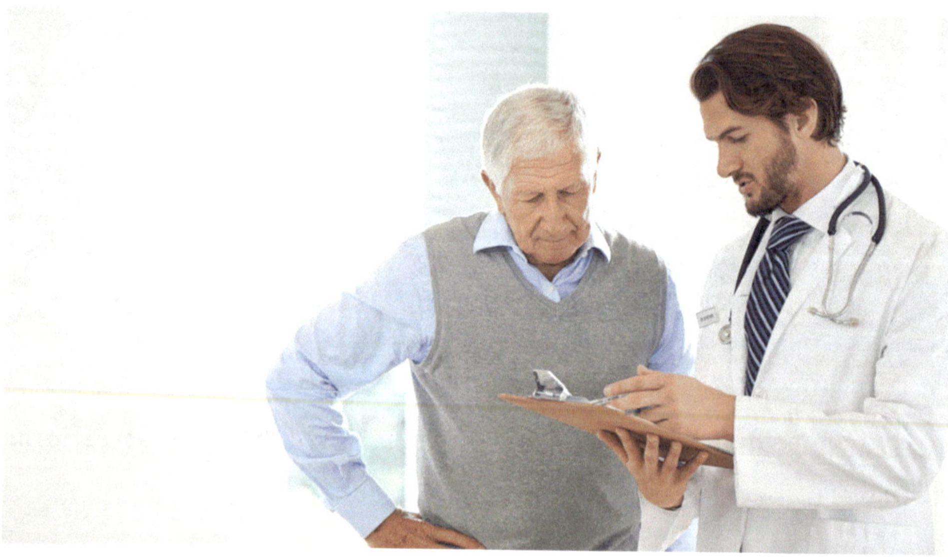

Figure 12.18. Impact of polypharmacy in patients with multiple comorbidities.

Source: https://www.physiciansweekly.com/wp-content/uploads/2017/06/doctor-patient-physician-old-elderly-geriatrics.png.

12.6.3. Successful Interventions in Reducing Polypharmacy

To address the issue of polypharmacy, it is crucial to educate patients, organize their medications, and engage caregivers. It appears that patient-centered educational programs play a significant role in improving both the safety and adherence to medicines in older adults. In a project focused on home-based elderly patients, applying a planned education program decreased the number of polypharmacy cases and improved patients' outcomes. As a result of these interventions, patients gain important information about their drugs, risks, and the need to follow the doctor's recommendations, which leads to a decrease in harmful drug interactions and medication errors. Furthermore, when caregivers are involved in these educational initiatives, patient quality of life improves, fostering a collaborative approach to medication management that is critical in addressing polypharmacy challenges among older adults (Oluoha et al., 2023).

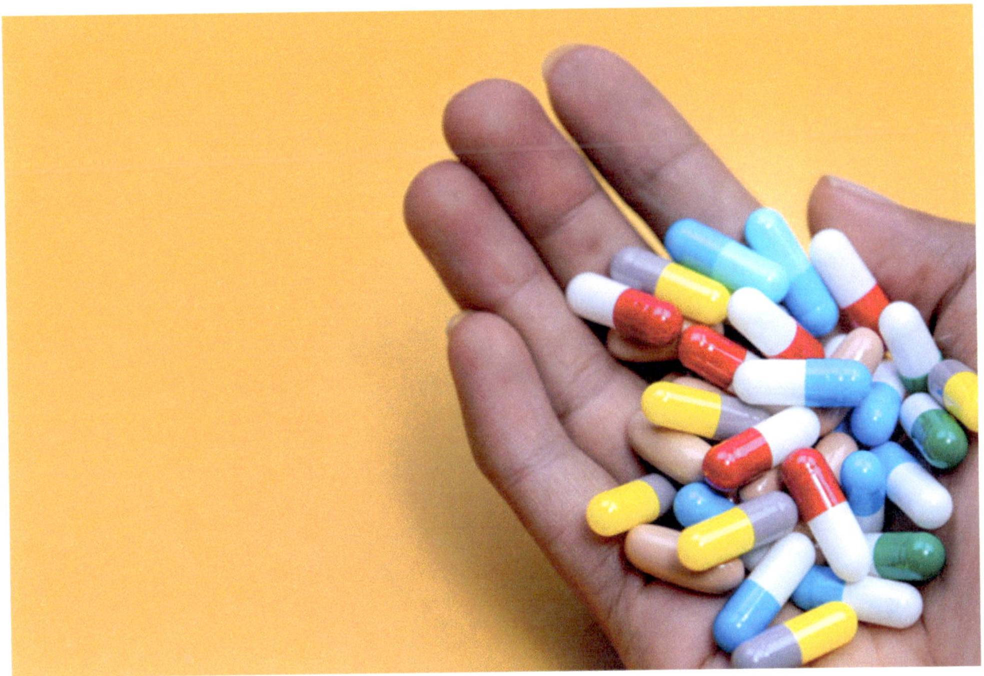

Figure 12.19. Successful interventions in reducing polypharmacy.

Source: https://www.quasrapp.com/wp-content/uploads/2022/09/polypharmacy-featured.jpg.

It is also effective to review the medications a person is taking, especially when they are older. Because polypharmacy is linked to negative health results, it is important to have set ways of assessing and managing medications. Experts in the field now emphasize the need for standardized definitions and methods to assess polypharmacy, particularly in geriatric oncology. Taking away unnecessary or risky drugs from patients is very important for managing polypharmacy. Still, because there are so many ways to define and measure these interventions, it is not easy to use them consistently. Standardization of these processes not only facilitates better assessment of polypharmacy but also enhances the effectiveness of deprescribing strategies, ultimately improving patient safety and health outcomes (Aparicio et al., 2016). It is essential to employ a multidisciplinary approach when managing polypharmacy, which involves collaboration among pharmacists, physicians, and nursing staff. When doctors and pharmacists collaborate, they can review all aspects of a patient's health, including both medical and non-medical considerations. With the help of experts from various healthcare fields, teams can determine if a patient is at risk of polypharmacy and design plans tailored to their needs. As a result, these collaborations can lead to making smarter decisions about medicines, which helps patients achieve better outcomes and reduces the potential risks associated with taking multiple drugs at once. Future research should continue to explore the efficacy of multidisciplinary interventions in geriatric care, specifically examining how these collaborative models can be implemented effectively to mitigate the adverse effects of polypharmacy further (Aparicio et al., 2016; Oluoha et al., 2023) (Figure 12.19).

Summary

All in all, polypharmacy has more effects than just the number of medicines a person is given; it also involves how those drugs interact with each other. Based on research done in prescription clinics, it is evident that managing polypharmacy depends on clear communication among healthcare providers. It is especially concerning that most patients do not understand their treatments and how they work, since this can create safety issues when prescriptions are made. The integration of sound doctor-patient relationships is essential for ensuring that patients are informed advocates for their health, thereby minimizing the risks associated with drug interactions (Abela et al., 2014). Furthermore, since the elderly population is increasing, more patients will be taking multiple medications, which makes it more challenging to manage them in primary care. The need for systematic screening tools to identify potentially inappropriate prescribing (PIP) is paramount in this context. The creation of GheOP3S greatly helps pharmacists in identifying and managing risks associated with polypharmacy for older people. By adopting such tools in community pharmacy practice, healthcare providers can significantly enhance their capacity to address the intricacies of drug interactions, fostering improved patient safety and health management overall (Boussery et al., 2015). The primary challenge here is to employ a team effort that involves regular training, clear communication, and more effective guidelines for prescribing medications. To address these challenges, both patients and healthcare providers should be open and transparent in discussing how medications are managed. Researchers should keep investigating new approaches like medication reviews and better teamwork among different HCPs to handle the issues of polypharmacy. When patients are educated and special screening tools are used, the healthcare community can help reduce the adverse effects of polypharmacy and improve both patients' health and daily living.

Polypharmacy, becoming more common among older people, is a significant concern in today's healthcare system. Using several medications at the same time is known as polypharmacy, and this dramatically increases the risk of problems with drugs and their side effects. It is often difficult for patients to stick to their treatment plans because of the many medications they are given. Older people often have several health conditions that call for several medicines, which makes harmful drug interactions more likely. According to recent analyses, the demographic of patients aged 65–74 years is particularly vulnerable, with female patients in this age bracket being at a heightened risk of ADRs due to metabolic differences and varying pharmacokinetic profiles (Alexander et al., 2022). For this reason, dealing with the effects of polypharmacy is necessary to improve patient outcomes and guarantee proper use of drugs. In addition, the complexity of drug interactions in people taking multiple drugs is very significant. Some interactions occur when medicines interact through their effects (pharmacodynamic), while others influence how the drugs are absorbed, distributed throughout the body, metabolized by the liver, and excreted (pharmacokinetic). Notably, patients on non-vitamin K antagonist oral anticoagulants (NOACs) present a critical group, as their efficacy can significantly influence the management of conditions such as atrial fibrillation. Researchers have identified specific scenarios in which concomitant medications, such as certain antihypertensives or NSAIDs, alter the pharmacological efficacy of anticoagulants, thereby increasing the risk of thromboembolic events or bleeding (Steffel et al., 2021). Knowing how these drugs interact helps healthcare providers take steps to lower the risks of polypharmacy and protect patients. It is important in polypharmacy discussions to have regular check-ups of medications and teach patients about the possible risks of taking many drugs at once. It is essential for physicians, pharmacists, and nursing staff to cooperate to ensure safe drug prescribing and to observe the effects of various drugs used together. Patient education programs can help people learn more about their drugs, stick to their treatment, and notice any adverse effects sooner. Because guidelines and pathways are changing to handle polypharmacy, all involved need to know about the latest evidence on drug interactions and how to manage them. Ultimately, through a concerted effort to minimize unnecessary medications and improve medication reconciliation processes, the adverse outcomes associated with polypharmacy can be significantly reduced, resulting in an overall enhancement of quality of care for patients (Steffel et al., 2021; Alexander et al., 2022).

CLOSER LOOK

BESIDES IMMEDIATE SAFETY

Besides immediate safety, which focuses on preventing acute harm or adverse reactions during medical treatment, broader considerations play a crucial role in ensuring long-term patient well-being and treatment success. While immediate safety aims to avoid short-term complications such as allergic reactions, incorrect dosages, or surgical errors, long-term safety encompasses potential delayed effects, cumulative toxicity, and the overall impact of treatment on a patient's quality of life. This perspective is particularly important in chronic disease management, oncology, and pharmacotherapy, where interventions may have lasting physiological, psychological, or metabolic consequences.

For instance, chemotherapy may effectively reduce tumor burden but also lead to long-term issues such as cardiotoxicity, infertility, or secondary malignancies. Similarly, long-term use of corticosteroids or certain psychiatric medications can result in metabolic disturbances, osteoporosis, or dependency. Thus, clinicians must balance short-term therapeutic goals with potential future risks, making informed choices about treatment duration, dosage, and monitoring strategies. Besides physical safety, psychological and social effects—like emotional distress, reduced functional capacity, or stigma—also need to be considered to support holistic care.

Regulatory bodies, research institutions, and healthcare systems are increasingly emphasizing post-market surveillance, real-world evidence collection, and patient-reported outcomes to better understand the long-term safety profile of treatments. In addition, technologies such as pharmacogenomics, electronic health records, and AI-driven analytics aid in predicting long-term risks and personalizing care plans accordingly. Ultimately, ensuring safety in healthcare means more than preventing immediate harm; it involves a proactive, continuous assessment of how interventions affect patients over time. By considering long-term impacts alongside immediate outcomes, healthcare providers can deliver care that is not only safe in the moment but also sustainable and supportive of patients' future health and quality of life.

References

1. Preca, Justine & Abela, Jurgen. (2014). Evaluating a prescription clinic at a primary health centre. *Malta Medical Journal, 26.* Agbabiaka, T. B., Spencer, N. H., Khanom, S., & Goodman, C. (2018). Prevalence of drug-herb and drug-supplement interactions in older adults: A cross-sectional survey. https://core.ac.uk/download/287581097.pdf (accessed on 9 June 2025).
2. Alhozim, B. M. A., Almutairi, E. T., Albutyan, Z. Y., Alzahrani, N. A., Alonizy, M. M., Albutyan, L. Y., Refaei, I. A. A., et al. (2024). The impact of polypharmacy on drug efficacy and safety in geriatric populations. *Egyptian Journal of Chemistry*. https://www.semanticscholar.org/paper/681e3bc211cfa3b37028eb1901012c369d7ac14f (accessed on 9 June 2025).
3. AlJassas, S. M., Alzaidi, N. A., Algharqan, S. M., Aljawad, S. H., Alsofyani, B. M., & Hadadi, F. A. (2024). Evaluating the impact of drug-drug interactions in polypharmacy strategies for safe medication management. *Journal of Healthcare Sciences.* https://www.semanticscholar.org/paper/6ae6fe4db7636a1bc33058f907aaf6adc75781b8 (accessed on 9 June 2025).
4. Assiri, G. A., Shebl, N. A., Mahmoud, M. A., Aloudah, N., Grant, E., Aljadhey, H., & Sheikh, A. (2018). What is the epidemiology of medication errors, error-related adverse events and risk factors for errors in adults managed in community care contexts? A systematic review of the international literature. https://core.ac.uk/download/287581034.pdf (accessed on 9 June 2025).
5. Barry, B., Cabral, K. P., Sullenberger, L., McAlister, J. L., Sandroni, T., & Patel, D. S. (2024). Clinical considerations for healthcare provider-administered lipid-lowering medications. *American Journal of Cardiovascular Drugs, 24*, 729–741. https://www.semanticscholar.org/paper/30c0e8e960fa852b10b4a0b14b0614f023ec622c (accessed on 9 June 2025).
6. Bertorio, M. J., & Agustina, A. (2025). Analisis drug related problem terhadap penggunaan obat pada pasien geriatri di Puskesmas Kapanewon Kasihan Bantul. *SEHATI: Jurnal Kesehatan.* https://www.semanticscholar.org/paper/2f5bcd2ef80044b287559d354de0d151dce3205a (accessed on 9 June 2025).
7. Bhoyar, R. C., Divakar, M. K., Gibson, G., et al. (2024). Landscape of pharmacogenetic variants associated with non-insulin antidiabetic drugs in the Indian population. https://core.ac.uk/download/619413084.pdf (accessed on 9 June 2025).
8. Black, A., Keel, P., & Pippin, J. (2023). Primary care provider knowledge and utilization of the BEERS criteria for the prevention and management of polypharmacy in the elderly. https://core.ac.uk/download/618305451.pdf (accessed on 9 June 2025).
9. Boland, F., Clyne, B., Cooper, J. A., et al. (2017). Beliefs about prescribed medication among older patients with polypharmacy: A mixed methods study in primary care. https://core.ac.uk/download/78901181.pdf (accessed on 9 June 2025).
10. Boussery, K., Mehuys, E., Petrovic, M., et al. (2015). Older patients' prescriptions screening in the community pharmacy: Development of the Ghent Older People's Prescriptions Community Pharmacy Screening (GheOP^{3}S) tool. https://core.ac.uk/download/55843875.pdf (accessed on 9 June 2025).
11. Cattaneo, D., Ridolfo, A., Dalu, D., Pruneri, C., Giacomelli, A., Cossu, M., Ruggieri, L., et al. (2025). Management of polypharmacy and potential drug-drug interactions in people with HIV and cancer: Insights from a 4-year multidisciplinary clinic experience. *Expert*

Opinion on Drug Metabolism & Toxicology. https://www.semanticscholar.org/paper/b3cda243e61ccd7c6aea8366c03a27c803896b06 (accessed on 9 June 2025).

12. Chan, G. C., Ng, J. K. C., Chow, K. M., Cheng, P. M. S., Law, M. C., Leung, C. B., Li, P. K. T., et al. (2022). Polypharmacy predicts onset and transition of frailty, malnutrition, and adverse outcomes in peritoneal dialysis patients. *The Journal of Nutrition, Health & Aging, 26*, 1054–1060. https://doi.org/10.1007/s12603-022-1859-8.
13. Chen, C., Sestini, L., & Wilde, R. (2016). Influences of body composition, multimorbidity and polypharmacy on physical mobility of older adults. https://digitalscholarship.unlv.edu/cgi/viewcontent.cgi?article=4547&context=thesesdissertations (accessed on 9 June 2025).
14. Cisneros, R., Kim, E. J., Mehta, C., et al. (2023). Medication management program among elderly at a residential facility. https://core.ac.uk/download/586155197.pdf (accessed on 9 June 2025).
15. Demuth, I., Diekmann, D., König, M., et al. (2019). Knowledge-based best of breed approach for automated detection of clinical events based on German free text digital hospital discharge letters. https://core.ac.uk/download/288114301.pdf (accessed on 9 June 2025).
16. Deng, Z., Xu, J., Feng, Y., Dong, L., & Zhang, Y. (2024). MAVGAE: A multimodal framework for predicting asymmetric drug–drug interactions based on variational graph autoencoder. *Computer Methods in Biomechanics and Biomedical Engineering.* https://www.semanticscholar.org/paper/9ff441e5c4d0302c5837a87c00b548ad8ebe084e (accessed on 9 June 2025).
17. Denig, P., & Schmidt-Mende, K. (2024). Drug utilization in older people. https://core.ac.uk/download/653280091.pdf (accessed on 9 June 2025).
18. Doherty, C. L., Gurwitz, J. H., Hirsch, G. A., et al. (2017). Optimization of drug prescription and medication management in older adults with cardiovascular disease. https://core.ac.uk/download/158967722.pdf (accessed on 9 June 2025).
19. Farrell, B., Raman-Wilms, L., Sadowski, C. A., Mallery, L., Turner, J. P., Gagnon, C., Cole, M., et al. (2023). A proposed curricular framework for an interprofessional approach to deprescribing. *Medical Science Educator, 33*, 551–567. https://doi.org/10.1007/s40670-022-01704-9.
20. Friedrichs, M., & Shoshi, A. (2019). History and future of KALIS: Towards computer-assisted decision making in prescriptive medicine. https://core.ac.uk/download/211862559.pdf (accessed on 9 June 2025).
21. Gasperoni, L., Giunta, E., Montanari, D., Masini, C., & de Giorgi, U. (2024). New-generation androgen receptor signaling inhibitors (ARSIs) in metastatic hormone-sensitive prostate cancer (mHSPC): Pharmacokinetics, drug-drug interactions (DDIs), and clinical impact. *Expert Opinion on Drug Metabolism & Toxicology, 20*, 491–502. https://www.semanticscholar.org/paper/5ae551f18e12b591bc0f834f7e48efee45e15657 (accessed on 9 June 2025).
22. Hosseinpour, F., Ilic, A. S., Jakobik, A., Jarynowski, A., Krzyszton, M., Marks, M., Moldovan, D., et al. (2019). Medical data processing and analysis for remote health and activities monitoring. https://core.ac.uk/download/224993779.pdf (accessed on 9 June 2025).
23. Keche, Y., Gaikwad, N. R., Wasnik, P., Nagpure, K. B., Siddiqui, M. S., Joshi, A., Dhaneria, S., et al. (2024). Analysis of drugs prescribed to elderly patients in a tertiary health care center in Raipur, Central India: An observational study. *Cureus, 16.* https://www.semanticscholar.org/paper/d59f4d12d82b269e91ead41eb4b00d5c67e60467 (accessed on 9 June 2025).

24. Khan, E., Ijaz, A., Jan, F., Rashid, S., & Mercado, G. M. (2025). Investigating specific drug–drug interactions and their clinical implications in polypharmacy, particularly in elderly patients. *Journal of Medical & Health Sciences Review*. https://www.semanticscholar.org/paper/dd62153842c39c65f32b46d753442d68f8c62567 (accessed on 9 June 2025).

25. Khanal, S., Shrestha, S., & Shrestha, S. (2019). Polypharmacy in elderly cancer patients: Challenges and the way clinical pharmacists can contribute in resource-limited settings. https://core.ac.uk/download/287605655.pdf (accessed on 9 June 2025).

26. Knisely, M. R. (2016). Understanding exposure to pharmacogenetically actionable opioids in primary care. https://core.ac.uk/download/84830723.pdf (accessed on 9 June 2025).

27. Kumar, N., Balraj, T. A., Kempegowda, S. N., & Prashant, A. (2024). Multidrug-resistant sepsis: A critical healthcare challenge. *Antibiotics, 13*, 46. https://doi.org/10.3390/antibiotics13010046.

28. Linfield, R. Y., Nguyen, N. N., Laprade, O. H., Holodniy, M., & Chary, A. (2024). An update on drug–drug interactions in older adults living with human immunodeficiency virus (HIV). *Expert Review of Clinical Pharmacology, 17*, 589–614. https://www.semanticscholar.org/paper/87c1225a9f9eedacf0632ff389aa6b679e6af3c4 (accessed on 9 June 2025).

29. Lorensia, A., Hubeis, A., Widyati, W., & Bagijo, H. (2009). Drug interaction study in hospitalized hepatic cirrhosis patient in Dr. Ramelan Navy Hospital. https://core.ac.uk/download/11980627.pdf (accessed on 9 June 2025).

30. Lyon, A. R., López-Fernández, T., Couch, L. S., Asteggiano, R., Aznar, M. C., Bergler-Klein, J., Boriani, G., et al. (2022). 2022 ESC Guidelines on cardio-oncology developed in collaboration with the European Hematology Association (EHA), the European Society for Therapeutic Radiology and Oncology (ESTRO), and the International Cardio-Oncology Society (IC-OS). *European Heart Journal, 43*, 4229–4361. https://doi.org/10.1093/eurheartj/ehac244.

31. Morillo-Verdugo, R., Blanco Ramos, J. R., Abdel-Kader Martín, L., & Álvarez de Sotomayor, M. (2018). El reto del envejecimiento y la complejidad farmacoterapéutica en el paciente VIH+. https://core.ac.uk/download/322845396.pdf (accessed on 9 June 2025).

32. Oluoha, E. (2023). Reducing polypharmacy amongst home-based older adults using patient-centered education. https://core.ac.uk/download/571288538.pdf (accessed on 9 June 2025).

33. Onder, G., Petrovic, M., & van der Cammen, T. (2012). Adverse drug reactions in older people: Detection and prevention. https://core.ac.uk/download/55848564.pdf (accessed on 9 June 2025).

34. Peter, T., Hemavathi, G., Kanishka, P. H., Haritha, C. S., Harshini, S. K., Janani, K., & Wani, J. A. (2025). A comprehensive clinical review on geriatric polypharmacy. *International Journal of Pharmaceutical Sciences Review and Research*. https://www.semanticscholar.org/paper/d2a293f6ebc8a8182cf0e7f593a6d2fa0bce5e99 (accessed on 9 June 2025).

35. Prakash, K., Arun, M., Sarath, A., & Simon, A. (2024). Assessing the benefits of targeted counselling in multimorbid elderly patients for polypharmacy management: A comparative analysis of pre and post intervention data. https://core.ac.uk/download/640070225.pdf (accessed on 9 June 2025).

36. Sanajou, S., & Baydar, T. (2025). Common drug-drug and drug-food interactions in antineoplastic agents: A short update review. *Hacettepe University Journal of the Faculty of Pharmacy*. https://www.semanticscholar.org/paper/db153810ea8238df486c0a8c349c239ab2be851d (accessed on 9 June 2025).

37. Sharma, M., Loh, K. P., Nightingale, G., Mohile, S. G., & Holmes, H. M. (2016). Polypharmacy and potentially inappropriate medication use in geriatric oncology. https://core.ac.uk/download/155271770.pdf (accessed on 9 June 2025).

38. Shekho, D., Mishra, R., Kamal, R., Khurana, D., Chauhan, A., & Awasthi, A. (2024). Polypharmacy in psychiatry: An in-depth examination of drug–drug interactions and treatment challenges. *Current Pharmaceutical Design*. https://www.semanticscholar.org/paper/32db7ae4fe76d88ffb2d0f2e9f928a4030a552d2 (accessed on 9 June 2025).

39. Siddique, M. I. (2024). Impact of polypharmacy on elderly patients: A comparative study of outcomes and risk management. *Asian Journal of Pharmaceutics*. https://www.semanticscholar.org/paper/2ca70fb5e522787ec311f7b55f693a1bd856b6ea (accessed on 9 June 2025).

40. Steffel, J., Collins, R., Antz, M., Cornu, P., Desteghe, L., Hæusler, K. G., Oldgren, J., et al. (2021). 2021 European Heart Rhythm Association practical guide on the use of non-vitamin K antagonist oral anticoagulants in patients with atrial fibrillation. *EP Europace, 23*, 1612–1676. https://doi.org/10.1093/europace/euab065.

41. Steiner, C. M. (2020). An evidence-based intervention to enhance provider awareness and confidence in addressing polypharmacy. https://core.ac.uk/download/288850281.pdf (accessed on 9 June 2025).

42. Toivo, T. (2020). *Avohoidon lääkitysturvallisuus: Tehostettu lääkehoidon koordinaatio ja riskien hallinta apteekin ja kotihoidon yhteistyönä* [Medication safety in outpatient care: Enhanced coordination and risk management in collaboration between pharmacy and home care]. https://core.ac.uk/download/328856161.pdf (accessed on 9 June 2025).

43. Türk, U. Ö., Acar, R. D., Akgün, T., Emren, V., Kanat, S., Karacağlar, E., Kepez, A., Kul, Ş., Özel, E., Şimşek, E., Yakar Tülüce, S., Tülüce, K., & Camm, A. J. (2020). Current clinician perspective on non-vitamin K antagonist oral anticoagulant use in challenging clinical cases. https://core.ac.uk/download/322366773.pdf (accessed on 9 June 2025).

44. Valenza, P. L., McGinley, T. C., Feldman, J., Patel, P., Cornejo, K., Liang, N., Anmolsingh, R., & McNaughton, N. (2017). Dangers of polypharmacy. https://core.ac.uk/download/322431183.pdf (accessed on 9 June 2025).

45. Visseren, F. L. J., Mach, F., Smulders, Y. M., Carballo, D., Koskinas, K. C., Bäck, M., Bénétos, A., et al. (2021). 2021 ESC guidelines on cardiovascular disease prevention in clinical practice. *European Heart Journal, 42*, 3227–3337. https://doi.org/10.1093/eurheartj/ehab484.

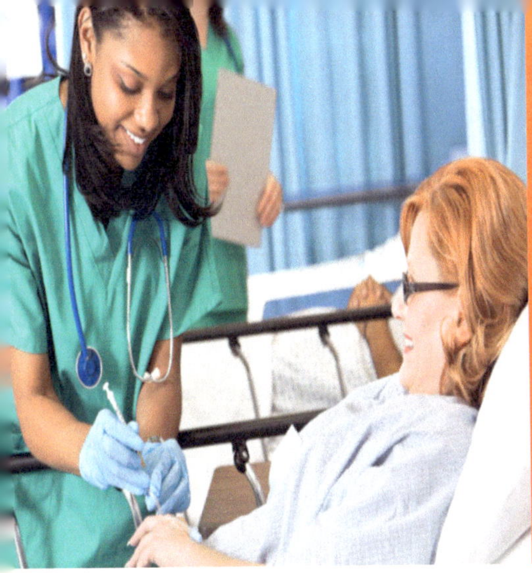

Chapter 13

DETECTION AND MONITORING OF ADRS

Contents

Introduction

The introduction to the detection and surveillance of adverse drug reactions (ADRs) highlights the paramount importance of prudence in the field of pharmacotherapy. Because more prescription drugs are being used and new treatments are being introduced, the problem of ADRs is very serious for healthcare systems everywhere. Each year, serious ADRs cause many hospitalizations, which shows why it is important to have effective systems for monitoring potential harm to patients. People need to be aware of these adverse reactions to make the most of therapy while minimizing risks. Therefore, it is crucial to develop methods for detecting ADRs, as this will inform the future of pharmacovigilance and patient safety. Due to technological advancements, ADR can now be detected using computerized and data-driven approaches, rather than traditional methods. Tools powered by ML and NLP can help a lot in finding and keeping track of important publications related to ADRs. The current research on the LiSA pipeline explains that it uses several deep learning models to search through scientific literature accurately. Because these systems assist reviewers in identifying important results, they are causing a shift in how pharmacovigilance is conducted. This is particularly crucial given the immense amount of medical literature that continues to grow, necessitating such technological intervention in order to achieve comprehensive safety surveillance (Martenot et al., 2022). Also, using ADR analysis and visualization tools makes it easier to understand the safety limits of drugs. Better ways of displaying data help researchers and HCPs find drug safety patterns and signals more easily. It is essential for quick action and informed choices, which benefit the patient. With the continued development of the field, the adoption and optimization of these techniques will be at the forefront of creating safe systems for ADR detection and surveillance to ensure the safety of therapeutic interventions remains a focus in the practice of medicine (Alexander et al., 2022) (Figure 13.1).

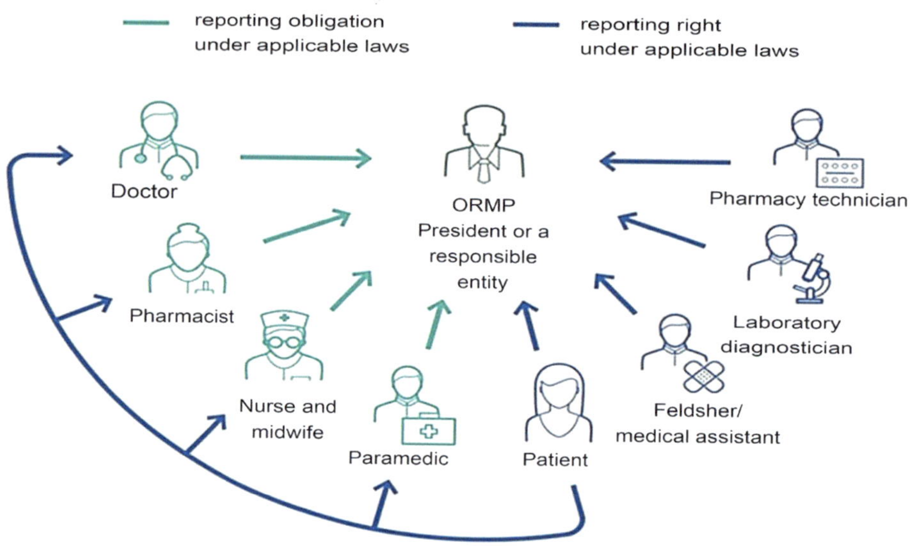

Figure 13.1. Detection and monitoring of adverse drug reactions (ADRs).

Source: https://www.nik.gov.pl/plik/id,23174.jpg.

Definition of Adverse Drug Reactions (ADRs)

The term adverse drug reactions (ADRs) refers to unintended and harmful effects that occur as a result of medication use. ADRs can take many forms, ranging from minor side effects to severe, life-threatening conditions that require medical attention. Such reactions make treatment more difficult and typically result in higher healthcare expenses and longer hospital stays. It is very important to identify and understand ADRs for the field of pharmacovigilance. It was mainly in the 1960s, after the thalidomide tragedy, that this approach started to form, pointing out the importance of organized safety monitoring. Continued advancements in scientific research and the integration of comprehensive data sources strive to refine our understanding of ADRs and enhance detection methodologies, ensuring that patient safety remains a priority in pharmaceutical care (Bate et al., 2021). ADRs are important because they can vary significantly depending on the type, severity, and the time of appearance in different individuals and groups. While some ADRs can be easily predicted using what we know about drugs, others are extremely rare and hard to expect. The fact that reactions may appear after the treatment has finished means that monitoring needs to continue during the drug's entire life. Being so careful is especially important for people with chronic diseases, since they usually take more than one medicine at the same time. Due to these challenges, pharmacovigilance has evolved, leading to efforts to enhance the systems used to capture ADR data in real-time across various healthcare settings. These advancements aim to provide a more comprehensive understanding of drug safety and support timely interventions when necessary (Kapoor et al., 2017). Additionally, new technology and data analysis tools can significantly enhance the process of monitoring and reporting on ADRs. Due to EHRs and social media, we can now gain a more comprehensive understanding of how patients perceive their medications. Using all this information, healthcare providers can identify safety concerns earlier and address them more effectively. Still, there are difficulties in making sure the data collected from various sources is of high quality and complete. More participation from patients and reporting by them could make the pharmacovigilance system even stronger. Therefore, an integrated approach that combines traditional methods with innovative technological solutions is vital to the future effectiveness of ADR detection and monitoring efforts (Bate et al., 2021) (Figure 13.2).

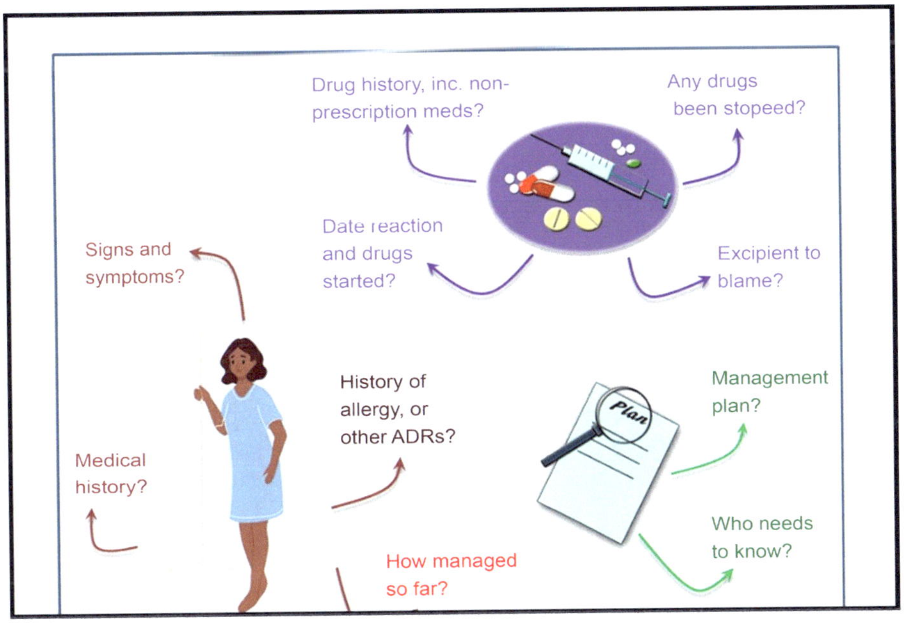

Figure 13.2. Definition of adverse drug reactions (ADRs).

Source: https://lh3.googleusercontent.com/blogger_img_proxy/AEn0k_sodiSz2IfhGeUF4B6mkY9H5vnKVmFvhr21aXb455tDSW6NemcM_3QjKVRa1oMq00bId_ChUZW876jF8iA2Qdu3GTGC4mPSV8iPwff0gCKfDRH-S28vBAoB6LrQzJxgZi9IgKB90iDXbyAvMqZHxpKZhkyMkaMLaYocz3k0b1dFu18eOlEm=w1200-h630-p-k-no-nu.

Importance of Detecting and Monitoring ADRs

Detection and monitoring of ADRs are critical in ensuring patient safety and the provision of quality care. Since ADRs can occur right away, doctors may find it challenging to help the patient and the risks to them may increase. Clinicians can discover and address any side effects by regularly monitoring the patient, which helps prevent much harm to the patient. Thus, if healthcare workers in a clinical setting are more aware of ADRs, they can report and document them quickly, which makes the environment safer for all. Not only does such forward thinking benefit an individual patient's well-being, but it also enhances drug safety at a population level, ultimately influencing regulatory proceedings and clinical guidelines informing future therapeutic practice. Paying attention to ADRs allows you to notice both drug interactions and how patients react to certain drugs, which is necessary for proper treatment. Clinicians rely on ADR monitoring data to give patients better care. It has been observed that a thorough review of ADRs reveals that some patients and drugs are connected to drug-related health issues more often. The findings of Anu et al. (2023) show that the most common ADR cases observed are caused by certain classes of drugs, which emphasizes the role of effective pharmacovigilance systems within hospitals. When HCPs look at real-time cases, they can notice patterns and improve their ways of treating patients. Additionally, the results from monitoring can aid in the approval of drugs and issuing warnings to both clinicians and patients about potential risks once the product is on the market. Using the cycle helps patients enjoy more advantages from treatment and lessen possible side effects. Healthcare workers should be motivated to use ADR awareness, since it helps secure the safety of patients now and in the future. ADRs play a crucial role in healthcare, so healthcare workers should learn about them to address and resolve pharmacological problems. The results presented by Atilla et al. (2025) demonstrate how education in the correct technique for injections and site rotation to prevent local reactions plays a crucial role, highlighting how progressive education can help mitigate undesired consequences. Allowing people to report ADRs easily encourages teamwork among HCPs who can exchange their ideas and knowledge. Because ADR monitoring and reporting are ongoing, doctors and scientists can more easily identify risks, develop more effective treatments, and provide patients with better care.

13.1. Types of Adverse Drug Reactions

Understanding the various types of ADRs is crucial in the context of pharmacovigilance and ensuring patient safety. ADRs are mainly divided into two groups called Type A and Type B reactions. The reactions seen in Type A are easy to predict based on the drug's effects.

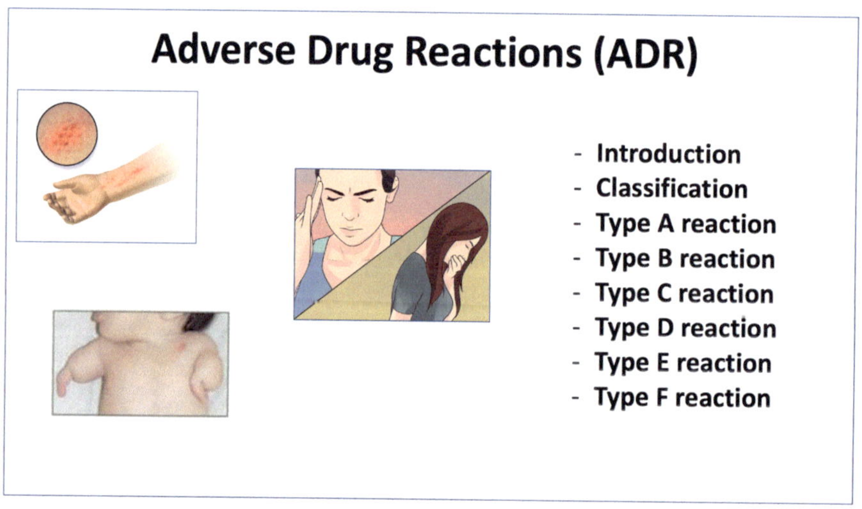

Figure 13.3. Types of adverse drug reactions.

Source: https://biopharmanotes.com/wp-content/uploads/2022/01/featured-image-of-ADR.png.

Beta-blockers may cause hypotension in certain individuals because this is a common side effect of their action. On the other hand, Type B reactions are not always expected and are not affected by the amount of drug given, for example, anaphylaxis that might happen after using anticonvulsants. This grouping is important for identifying and tracking ADRs, as it helps doctors determine which drugs may be risky for certain patients, thereby facilitating the overall management of ADRs. To identify and manage ADRs, it is essential to employ various approaches and robust monitoring methods. Pharmacovigilance helps to find and assess any issues related to drugs, which is important for controlling the risks of both Type A and Type B reactions. Post-marketing surveillance is one of the methods used to monitor the safety of approved drugs. Such techniques as cohort studies, prescription event monitoring, and voluntary reporting systems, for example, the UK's Yellow Card System, play a significant role in collecting information that helps understand the frequency and nature of ADRs. This proactive approach not only improves drug safety but fosters a culture of transparency and trust in medical treatment (Suraj et al., 2023). To deal with ADRs, HCPs have to be able to notice and respond to them quickly. Training and education about ADRs and their causes are important for finding and monitoring them. For example, being aware of the way a drug acts and is absorbed can help clinicians predict Type A reactions, and knowing about genetic backgrounds can show why some people react with Type B reactions. Having clear ways for people to report possible ADRs adds to the monitoring system and allows for quick actions to protect patients. Ultimately, a comprehensive understanding of ADR types alongside rigorous monitoring practices is vital to enhancing pharmacovigilance and ensuring patient safety in medical settings (Suraj et al., 2023) (Figure 13.3).

13.1.1. Type A (Augmented) Reactions

Type A (Augmented) reactions are a significant category of ADRs characterized by their pre-ducibility and dose dependence. Adverse reactions of Type A usually happen because the drug's actions that help the patient can also cause unwanted side effects. If a person is given an anticoagulant and is given too much, it can lead to a higher chance of bleeding.

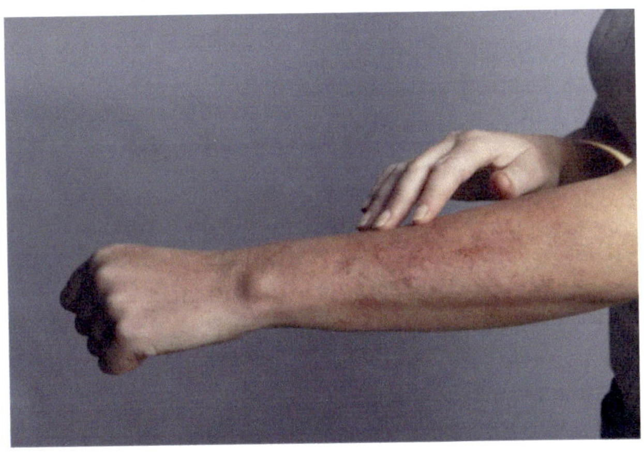

Figure 13.4. Type A (augmented) reactions.

Source: https://www.verywellhealth.com/what-is-an-adverse-reaction-3959900.

Type A reactions are necessary to understand because they typically describe how a drug works, helping health professionals choose the right dosage and decide whether to switch. Additionally, knowing what to expect from Type A reactions makes it easier to identify and monitor them, ensuring patient safety and improving the effectiveness of the treatment. These reactions occurring so frequently demonstrate the importance of having effective systems in place to monitor and report them. Healthcare groups and workers are important in this because they use reliable systems to report ADRs. A retrospective study also depicted that a high proportion of the ADRs reported were by drugs commonly used, such as antibiotics, which are highly reported to cause side effects (Monesh et al., 2020). A thorough study of the reports' data allows healthcare systems to spot trends related to drugs with higher risks. It adds to the scientific knowledge on drug safety and also prompts doctors to rethink their drug prescribing, for the benefit of both parties. Also, being able to identify Type A reactions is important for both educating and empowering patients. If patients are informed about the possible side effects of their medications, they can monitor for any adverse effects and promptly notify their doctor. As you can see, patients participating in monitoring can help introduce additional safety measures. For instance, studies have shown that heightened alertness of potential ADRs supports a culture of safety and leads patients to question their care from HCPs (Aditi et al., 2024). When practitioners educate patients and maintain open communication, it becomes easier to recognize Type A responses and address them effectively, which in turn improves the overall results of therapy and the quality of care (Figure 13.4).

13.1.2. Type B (Bizarre) Reactions

The phenomenon of Type B (Bizarre) reactions in the context of ADRs necessitates a nuanced understanding of how certain individuals exhibit unpredictable and often severe responses to medications. While Type A reactions are related to how much of the drug is given and are easy to predict, Type B reactions are unique to each person and cannot be explained by the drug's profile. Being unpredictable, these diseases are challenging to detect and monitor, as standard methods may not reveal the associated risks. Since these reactions are complex, healthcare providers need to use several methods, such as closely monitoring and documenting the patient's condition. With increased awareness of such reactions, professionals can enhance their clinical judgment, which is pivotal in reducing instances of unplanned hospitalizations due to ADRs (Zazzara et al., 2021). It is important to notice that Type B reactions may lead to rare but serious results such as SJS and TEN. Such skin problems are of great concern because they must be treated promptly to avoid serious complications or even death. In recent years, studies have expanded the understanding of these conditions by not only identifying specific drug triggers but also elucidating the role of infectious agents, such as Mycoplasma pneumoniae, in exacerbating these skin reactions (Ramien et al., 2020). The connection between medicines and infections highlights the importance of a system that can account for multiple factors, including a person's genes and environmental influences. If there is no thorough monitoring, health professionals may not be able to prevent these severe forms of Type B reactions, which highlights the need for more research and education. In addition, the results of Type B reactions can influence the entire healthcare system by increasing expenses and use of resources. Lengthy hospitalization and intensive care for Type B reactions can cause healthcare systems to face significant challenges. In older groups, the risk of ADRs can be higher because of having several drugs at the same time and other health issues that can make it harder to spot ADRs. The need for targeted interventions aimed at preventing these bizarre reactions cannot be understated, especially as the healthcare community strives for improved patient safety (Zazzara et al., 2021). If healthcare systems employ clinical vigilance, educate patients, and have robust reporting mechanisms, they can better manage the risks associated with Type B reactions. All in all, being proactive helps to safeguard patients and also makes it easier to handle adverse drug events in healthcare.

13.1.3. Type C (Chronic) Reactions

Type C (Chronic) Reactions are alarming in the field of pharmacology, as they occur slowly and may persist for an extended period. While some adverse reactions to drugs occur right away, Type C reactions are seen only after a person uses the drug for a very long time. Because of the health problems that can last, managing patients with Type C reactions is more difficult and puts extra strain on the healthcare system. Because of the efforts to monitor severe ADRs, healthcare providers need to understand the factors and results of Type C reactions to prevent lasting problems from drug therapies. Determining the predisposing factors that affect patients' reactions, such as age, drug allergy history, and chronic diseases, is crucial in developing prevention and intervention strategies that ensure patient safety and improve treatment outcomes (Sittiphan et al., 2025). Getting Type C reactions right and monitoring them closely remains the primary factor in helping patients improve. Sometimes, reactions to hormone therapy for non-metastatic breast cancer are long-lasting, proving that the use of medications for an extended period can be difficult. Many unpleasant symptoms, for example, joint pain and depression, can happen to patients, which may result in them not sticking to their treatment plan. It appears that using proactive systems, such as mobile health apps, can help patients follow their treatment better by responding quickly to ADRs. These interventions are able to enhance communication between patients and healthcare providers, thereby contributing to enhanced management of chronic reaction and concomitant health-related quality of life (HRQoL) (Gernier et al., 2023). So, using advanced technology is at the heart of the latest efforts to manage and treat Type C reactions well. In addition, studying Type C reaction data can help direct future studies and inform the development of targeted therapies. As an illustration, national registries of major ADR cases give helpful information about the occurrence of prolonged reactions, which is useful for spotting people at risk and hazardous drugs. Researchers can utilize advanced statistics to identify connections that inform the development of more effective clinical practice guidelines and dosage plans. With these models, the quality of patient care increases and the main purpose of pharmacovigilance is to stress the importance of regular monitoring. Type C reaction monitoring is thus not just a precautionary clinical action but an anticipatory one that opens the door to greater patient safety and therapy effectiveness (Sittiphan et al., 2025).

13.2. Methods of Detection

The detection of ADRs is essential for safeguarding patient safety and enhancing the therapeutic efficacy of pharmacological interventions. Several ways have been set up to check for ADRs, such as spontaneous reporting, EHRs, and observational studies. The most common approach is for HCPs to report ADRs freely, which forms a collection of data that can be checked for patterns and any possible signals. Still, the fact that this method can be biased and underreport means that it needs to be supported by other methods of study. By integrating EHRs, which provide comprehensive patient data, healthcare providers can leverage advanced analytical tools to identify correlations between drug administration and adverse events, thereby improving the accuracy of ADR detection (Vaismoradi et al., 2021). Other than spontaneous reporting and EHRs, prospective cohort studies and clinical trials use organized approaches to find ADRs. They include strict monitoring methods for different patient groups, which help in studying the effects of the drugs. In the context of cutaneous ADRs, for instance, a retrospective analysis revealed significant insights regarding the timing and classification of skin reactions associated with specific drug classes (Modi et al., 2019). It is very important to use validated tools to classify ADRs by causality, severity, and preventability to understand them better in the studied groups. They help identify ADRs and also give important information to regulators to improve how safe drugs are. Ultimately, employing various approaches in ADR detection facilitates a more comprehensive approach to handling pharmacovigilance. HCPs, researchers, and regulatory bodies must collaborate to enhance existing methods for detecting errors and promoting patient safety. It is important to teach healthcare providers about ADRs and the ways to report them to manage risks. Additionally, utilizing standard processes and technology-based systems for ADR monitoring facilitates the prompt identification of safety signals. As demonstrated in the studies examining medicines management, such innovative approaches could significantly reduce the burden of adverse drug effects and ensure patient well-being (Vaismoradi et al., 2021).

13.2.1. Spontaneous Reporting Systems (SRS)

The role of spontaneous reporting systems (SRS) in surveillance and detection of ADRs is pivotal in pharmacovigilance. People working in healthcare are mainly responsible for reporting any ADRs they observe during their work. Thanks to SRS, it is possible to find information about data in everyday situations, such as among many patients and in various therapy settings, which could help spot unusual or unknown side effects. However, these systems raise issues. Reporting bias and under-reporting reduce the effectiveness of SRS due to the possibility of a considerable underestimation of ADRs. Inadequate active involvement of the healthcare community hinders the accurate identification of a drug's actual safety profile, and therefore, there must be increased awareness and engagement among professionals in the reporting process, as discussed in the literature (Alomar et al., 2020). New techniques have emerged to strengthen SRS, primarily by utilizing technology and analyzing data. The increase in digital tools in healthcare has enabled healthcare workers to report their findings more easily and conveniently. The use of algorithms by platforms could help them identify safety issues from reports before such issues usually are noticed. Moreover, the development of AI-based information systems, as seen in Russian pharmacovigilance, suggests the promise of using predetermined data formats such as the international ICH E2B standard to aid in a more systematic way of producing reports and considering safety information (Журавлева et al., 2019). Such changes are necessary to address the issues of spontaneous reporting and to monitor the safety of drugs on the market. To guarantee the future of SRS, HCPs must keep receiving training and education. Doctors and other HCPs usually do not know about procedures and the value of ADR reporting, which makes the problem of under-reporting worse. Giving special training on the importance of pharmacovigilance and the right way to report ADRs can encourage safety in healthcare institutions. Additionally, approaches that encourage patients to participate in safety can enhance the standard reporting process. As SRS keeps changing due to the challenges they create, health professionals will be encouraged to act accordingly. These endeavors will ultimately enhance drug safety surveillance and improve the understanding of drug therapies in relation to patient outcomes, thereby creating a stronger pharmacovigilance system overall (Alomar et al., 2020).

13.2.2. Electronic Health Records and Data Mining

The integration of EHRs has transformed the landscape of healthcare, particularly in the detection and monitoring of ADRs. EHRs enable healthcare providers to collect, store, and access patient information digitally, allowing them to view complete medical records. Now, using data in healthcare opens the door for data mining to spot patterns in massive datasets about ADRs. If these technologies are used effectively, they can help keep patients safe by identifying and mitigating risks associated with certain medications. Moreover, as noted, tools that employ artificial intelligence (AI) and ML can elevate the fidelity of ADR detection beyond what is achievable through traditional methods, ultimately enhancing clinical decision-making and patient outcomes (Shuroug et al., 2023). In addition to EHRs, the utilization of Big Data Analytics (BDA) plays a crucial role in advancing ADR monitoring. Healthcare providers can gain a comprehensive understanding of how patients respond to medications by utilizing both structured and unstructured data. Using data from sensors, medical backgrounds, and notes from doctors helps provide a better understanding of ADRs. It has been found that when medical facilities use data integration and analytics, they can notice trends and similarities that might point to possible ADRs in risky groups. Therefore, leveraging BDA within the framework of EHRs is not merely a supplementary practice but a transformative approach that enhances clinical surveillance and informs better healthcare delivery (Batko et al., 2022). When EHRs and data mining technologies are combined, it becomes possible to implement proactive pharmacovigilance strategies that can benefit public health. Healthcare systems can regularly find and document ADRs as they happen, instead of waiting until later to collect the information. By analyzing data as it comes in, we can quickly notice any safety issues with medications and take action to prevent many people from being affected. With the advancement of AI, it can spot more anomalies than people, making it easier to find issues related to drugs. Establishing these dynamic systems helps ensure that both patients and providers benefit from enhanced medication safety, which is vital for effective and responsible healthcare delivery (Shuroug et al., 2023) (Figure 13.5).

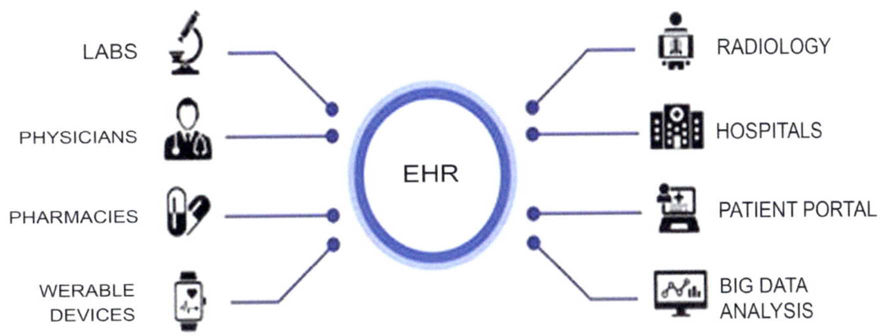

Figure 13.5. Electronic health records and data mining.

Source: https://relevant.software/wp-content/uploads/2023/08/h90m5rtToHeo5UsWfBAHAqXjCMoehW_cdRva-xSuXRiVpwzFHB_iUsiG3tzWqeHkKFKijmoME_hXnKDYjqDA36rVsJUIlL9Ehe-Qaim2E83CyuRSoP8IKsyf_KmbvgI8bmgejkbV5z63SvSjN3E4WlA.

13.2.3. Clinical Trials and Post-Marketing Surveillance

The process of drug development is intricate, with clinical trials that supply invaluable information regarding safety and effectiveness as well as post-marketing surveillance that keeps on observing even after a drug's approval. In clinical trials, the drug undergoes several tests to determine its benefits, the optimal dose, and any potential adverse reactions. The process helps researchers spot any possible risks of the drug before it is given to the public. Still, clinical trials usually happen in a controlled setting that may not show all the ADRs that can affect different groups when the drug is used widely. Therefore, the transition from clinical trials to post-marketing surveillance introduces a critical focus on continuous detection and monitoring of ADRs, a process critical to long-term drug safety reporting by pharmacovigilance systems (Wagh et al., 2024). It is essential to use post-marketing surveillance to keep an eye on and evaluate drugs after they are approved. This stage is particularly important since it involves more people and better overall health, which is often not included in clinical trials. Reviewing the ADR reports enables healthcare authorities to identify similarities, assess the severity of the events, and determine if the drug was involved. Over the last decade, advancements in digital tools and global cooperation have enhanced the reliability of pharmacovigilance. This is demonstrated by the rapid COVID-19 vaccine rollout, which clearly highlights the importance of effective post-marketing surveillance to monitor the safety and efficacy of vaccines in various populations. Therefore, while clinical trials initially form the foundation for drug approval, it is through post-marketing surveillance that safety concerns are identified early and addressed, ultimately benefiting patients (Tembe-Fokunang et al., 2022). It is important to connect clinical trials and post-marketing surveillance for the practical assessment of new ADRs to protect the public. After drugs are approved and used in various groups, more cases of drug interactions and reactions in people are being noticed. Therefore, a strategy for monitoring drugs that can quickly react to new information and safety concerns is required. Also, agencies in charge of drug safety should interact closely with health care professionals, drug companies, and patients to help with thorough reporting and sharing of information about ADRs. Lastly, the combination of clinical trials and strict post-marketing surveillance is imperative for continuous monitoring of therapeutic drugs so their benefits might outweigh the risks, establishing public confidence in drug efficacy and safety, particularly in the new era of health care (Wagh et al., 2024).

13.3. Role of Healthcare Professionals

Healthcare professionals (HCPs) play a critical role in the detection and monitoring of ADRs, serving as frontline guardians in ensuring patient safety. Their role is vital in pharmacovigilance, especially after rules were put in place that allow patients and caregivers to report ADRs. It is clear from EudraVigilance data that from 2011 to 2013, the number of reports from patients and caregivers went up, suggesting that more people are now aware of drug safety. Even so, HCPs are the primary source of ADR reports needed to understand the safety of each medication. This professional input is vital for understanding the complexities of ADRs, as it possesses the training and expertise required to evaluate the clinical implications of these reactions, thereby contributing to the overall integrity of the pharmacovigilance system (Sienkiewicz et al., 2021). The specialized knowledge of HCPs is integral when it comes to recognizing and managing immune-related adverse effects (irAEs) associated with treatments such as immune checkpoint inhibitors (ICPI). It is the duty of these experts to regularly check patients for the appearance of irAEs, as early detection can alter the course of treatment. Several oncology groups recommend closely monitoring mild irAEs to ensure they do not become severe. It is usually necessary to start prompt actions, such as stopping treatment and using immunosuppressants, when these side effects appear. Through their expertise, HCPs can ensure that patients are well supported throughout their treatment, thereby maximizing the therapeutic benefits of ICPI while minimizing associated risks (Morgado et al., 2020). Additionally, as HCPs assume new roles in detecting and monitoring ADRs, it highlights the need for teamwork among various professionals. In several healthcare environments, handling ADRs requires cooperation among pharmacists, nurses, and physicians. Working in a team provides more expertise and makes it easier to monitor tasks with shared duties and diverse opinions. Good teamwork helps the staff notice possible ADRs early and prepare suitable care plans for each patient. As healthcare systems evolve to incorporate technology and data analytics, the role of professionals will further expand, ensuring that the detection and management of ADRs adapt to new challenges and innovations, ultimately leading to enhanced patient outcomes in pharmacotherapy (Sienkiewicz et al., 2021) (Figure 13.6).

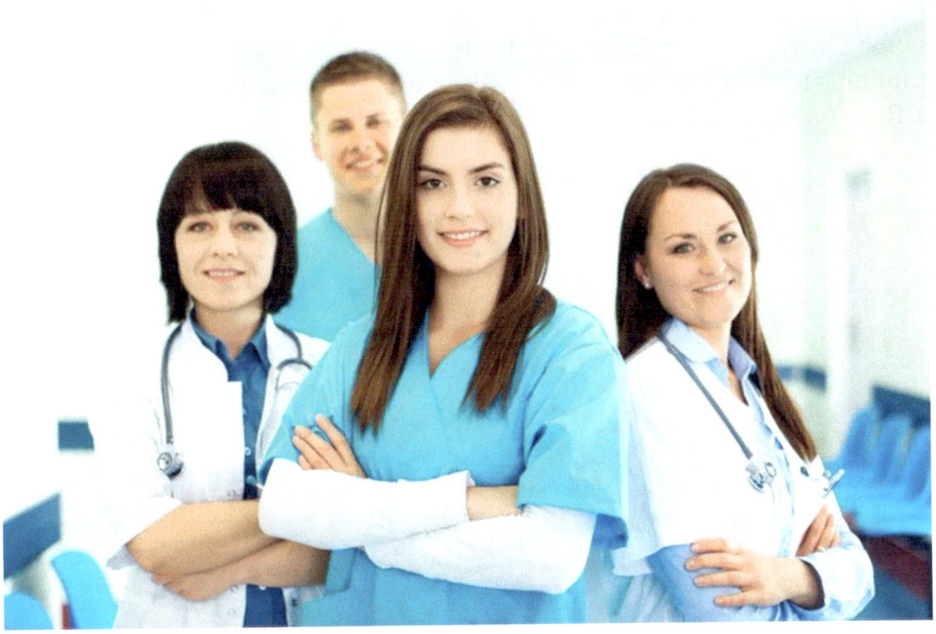

Figure 13.6. Role of healthcare professionals.

Source: https://medipharm.com.au/wp-content/uploads/2024/02/successful-medical-team.jpg.

13.3.1. Physicians and Pharmacists in ADR Reporting

Involvement of both pharmacists and doctors in the reporting of ADR is required in establishing an effective pharmacovigilance system. Most of the time, doctors are the first to notice and report ADRs, which greatly helps in keeping drugs safe. According to recent studies, 39.66% of ADR reports submitted to the South African Health Products Regulatory Authority (SAHPRA) were from doctors, indicating their primary role in identifying potential safety issues with medicines. Additionally, detailed information from doctors is useful in ADR reports, helping regulatory authorities identify any changes or patterns in drug safety. But even as they bring their input, report incompleteness remains a serious gap, and this suggests the requirement for better training modules that equip doctors with better pharmacovigilance data and report capabilities (Steyn, 2023). So far, pharmacists have not been responsible for many ADR reports, as they accounted for only 4.45% of all reports sent to SAHPRA. Since they have the necessary experience and knowledge, they are best suited to handle drug therapy and check for any drug interactions or side effects. Physicians were also happy to delegate specific tasks to pharmacists in conversations on Pakistan's TB care, demonstrating a recognition of the role pharmacists play in treating patients (Atif et al., 2022). Higher involvement of pharmacists in ADR reporting would enhance the overall pharmacovigilance system and assist doctors with certain tasks. Teaching pharmacists about their duties in monitoring and reporting ADRs would allow them to help more in patient safety programs. Physicians and pharmacists need to work together in reporting ADRs to improve care for patients and increase public health. Multidisciplinary reporting is beneficial in both positions, as it fosters honest communication and holds everyone accountable for drug-related side effects. For instance, patients are currently taking an active role in reporting, and a significant share of ADR reports are consumer inputs, thus reflecting the trend of patient involvement in healthcare (Steyn, 2023). If pharmacists and HCPs join forces, they can improve the number and quality of ADR reports, which helps collect more data and care for patients better. Emphasizing that health professionals should continually learn from and communicate with one another, it will be essential for them to prioritize safety culture and active ADR monitoring and reporting (Figure 13.7).

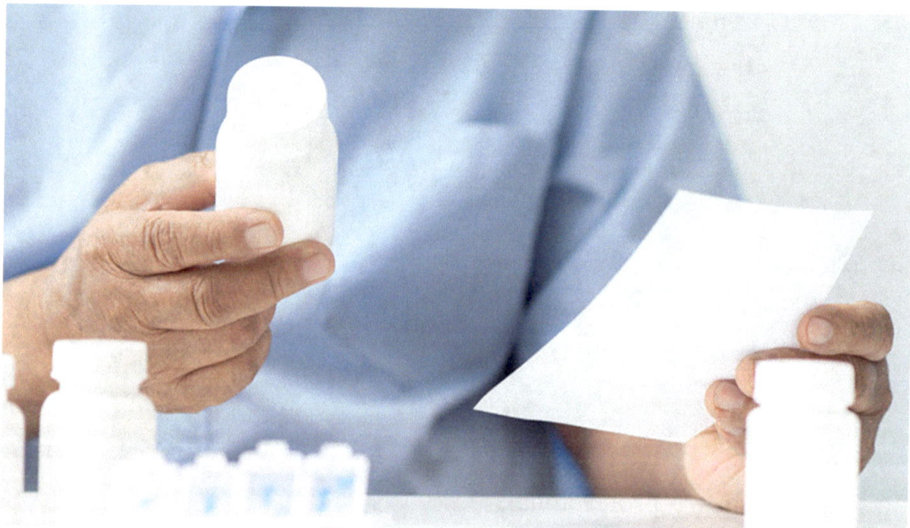

Figure 13.7. Physicians and pharmacists in ADR reporting.

Source: https://duckduckgo.com/?q=Physicians+and+Pharmacists +in+Adverse Drug+Reaction+Reporting& t=h_&iar=images&iaf=size%3ALarge&iai=https%3A%2F%2Fassets.unilab.com.ph%2Fuploads%2FU nilab%2FArticles%2FHealth_tips%2FA.%2520Thumb_WhentoReportAdverseDrugReaction.png.

13.3.2. Nurses' Responsibilities in Monitoring ADRs

The role of nurses in monitoring ADRs is critical to patient safety and overall healthcare efficacy. Nurses, as the first people to give medication to patients, are important in noticing any possible

ADRs. It is not enough for them to give medications; they must also carefully watch patients after giving them medicine for any unusual signs. Being careful in this way can help prevent major problems that may arise from unnoticed ADRs. Nurses also ensure that patients are aware of the importance of reporting any side effects to the doctor. Sharing information and keeping records of ADRs lets healthcare teams act promptly and update treatment plans, helping to ensure the best care for patients and lower the risks caused by medicines. Nurses are especially important in ADR management because the medication regimens in healthcare are getting more complex. Because more and more elderly and chronically ill people are taking several medications, there is a greater possibility of errors and interactions. Nurses are expected to assess the patient's entire medical history, along with the drugs that have been prescribed, to identify any possible drug interactions. Their critical assessments contribute to enhanced medication safety, aligning with findings that indicate approximately 1 in 10 hospitalizations in OECD countries may result from medication-related events, underscoring the need for diligent monitoring and proactive nursing interventions (Bienassis et al., 2022).

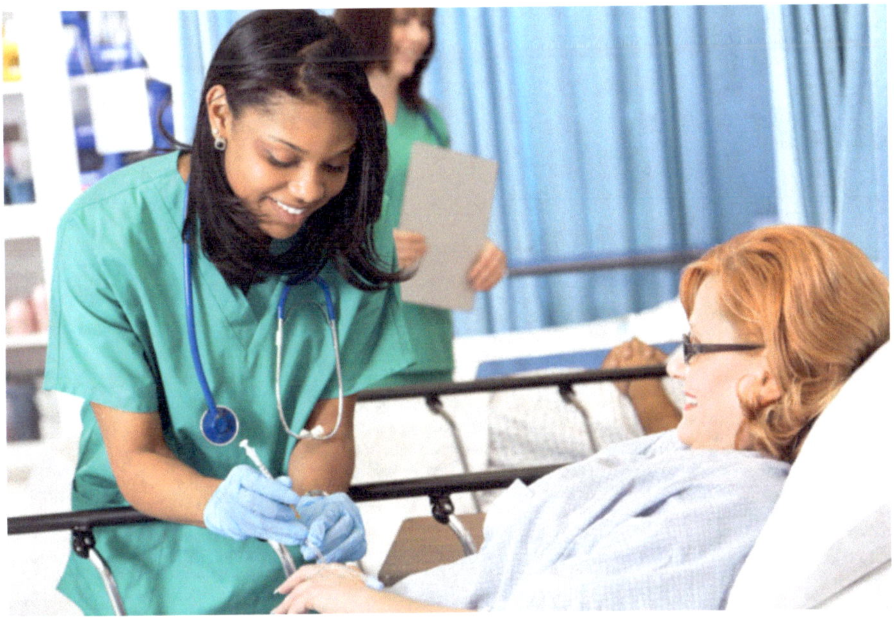

Figure 13.8. Nurses' responsibilities in monitoring ADRs.

Source: https://duckduckgo.com/?q=Nurses%27+responsibilities+in+monitoring+Adverse+Drug+Reaction&t=h_&iar=images&iai=https%3A%2F%2Fworklifelaw.org%2Fwp-content%2Fuploads%2F2017%2F03%2FNurse-administering-medication-to-patient-through-an-IV-000020786741_Large-1080x720.jpg.

So, it is important to use nursing assessments in daily work to spot patients who might have ADRs and give them timely help. Another important part of a nurse's role is to collaborate with other HCPs when monitoring ADRs. Nurses typically assist patients, pharmacists, and physicians in communicating about drug safety and any potential issues that may arise. Their findings may guide doctors when they need to adjust a patient's treatment or medication due to adverse reactions. Because the healthcare field is constantly changing, nurses must know a lot about how drugs work and what side effects they may cause to better watch for ADRs. If nurses are encouraged to discuss medication safety, it will help to solve the problems caused by ADRs as health systems advance. This collaborative approach not only enhances patient outcomes but also reflects a commitment to refining clinical practices and reducing medication-related harms (Atif et al., 2022) (Figure 13.8).

13.3.3. Importance of Interdisciplinary Collaboration

The detection and monitoring of ADRs necessitate a robust interdisciplinary approach, as the complexities involved in pharmacovigilance extend beyond the purview of any single discipline. When HCPs, researchers, and policymakers join forces, the different aspects of ADRs can be properly managed. By combining the knowledge of doctors, the skills of IT experts, and the understanding of pharmacologists, a more effective and accurate method for identifying ADRs is developed. Additionally, collaborating with various experts facilitates the exchange of numerous ideas, which may lead to innovative approaches for monitoring drug safety.

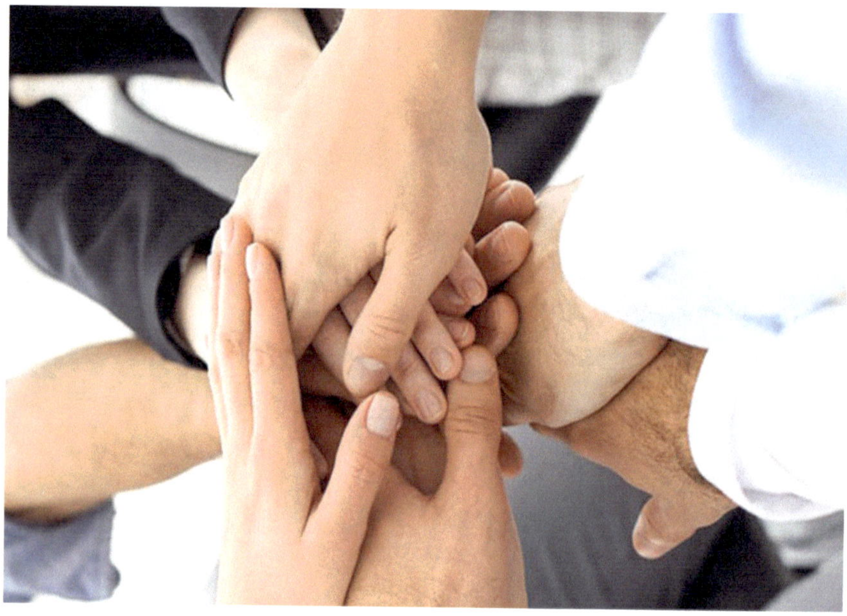

Figure 13.9. Importance of interdisciplinary collaboration.

Source: https://www.timeshighereducation.com/sites/default/files/2._interdisciplinary_collaboration_makes_a_difference_in_science.jpg.

The combination of efforts in such partnerships makes it easier to identify ADRs and leads to the creation of strategies that are informed by the details of patient care and drug development. Advancements in technology, particularly in AI and nanotechnology, exemplify the critical role of interdisciplinary collaboration in improving ADR detection. According to recent research, AI can analyze a large amount of data and identify patterns that people might not notice, which enhances the way drugs are monitored. By incorporating expertise from computer science, healthcare, and bioethics, healthcare systems can more effectively leverage AI technologies, thereby minimizing the human error that often complicates ADR evaluation (Shuroug et al., 2023). Furthermore, the application of nanotechnology in targeted drug delivery and monitoring highlights the need for collaboration among material scientists, chemists, and clinical practitioners, as these professionals work together to develop innovative techniques that can revolutionize ADR detection and provide greater precision in treatment options (Chehelgerdi et al., 2023). When these specialties merge, it becomes easier to make important improvements in patient care. The active involvement of regulatory bodies is necessary to maximize the benefits of interdisciplinary work in ADR detection and monitoring. They are crucial in establishing standards and guidelines to support teamwork in healthcare. Regulatory agencies can help different areas, such as pharmacovigilance, public health, and data science, work together, which improves the results of ADR management. Working together in this way enhances patient care and lays the groundwork for future studies and innovative ideas in drug safety. When different fields collaborate, they can build better monitoring systems that help HCPs deal with the issues related to ADRs, which keeps patients safe and healthy (Figure 13.9).

13.4. Patient Involvement in ADR Monitoring

Patient involvement in the surveillance of ADRs is now an important aspect of ensuring drugs are safe and effective within healthcare systems. Active involvement of patients enables improved coverage of the therapeutic environment, allowing for the detection of ADRs that would not have been identified through clinical trials. Patients, who are the earliest to report unusual side effects, can provide real-world experience to support ADR monitoring systems. Patient-reported outcomes also have the power to substantially influence regulatory decision-making because authorities are increasingly appreciative of the value of experience data in assessing drug risk. By promoting an open style of ADR reporting, patients are trusted by HCPs to report their experience freely, thereby contributing to better overall ADR detection and management in practice. Engaging patients in ADR monitoring not only empowers the individuals but also promotes a culture of safety and shared responsibility towards healthcare. Systems that facilitate real-time communication between patients and health care professionals are essential in capturing ADRs more effectively. For instance, electronic media and mobile applications used for reporting ADRs represent convenient and timely mechanisms for patients to convey their experiences. Using these technologies, patients can be actively involved in the management of their health while providing clinicians with vital information to tailor treatment protocols best. Additionally, this collaborative activity will help fill the vast gaps in data commonly observed with routine ADR reporting systems, particularly among vulnerable populations who may not otherwise have access to formal healthcare channels. This type of active participation is crucial in improving patient outcomes and reducing the risks associated with drug treatments. Additionally, patient preferences in ADR monitoring are part of the broader trend toward individualized or personalized medicine, where therapy is tailored to the patient. Patient-led healthcare is becoming a model for healthcare, where prescribing becomes more inclusive, informed by information on how individual patients react to medicines. Practice stimulated by patient feedback encourages manufacturers to prioritize safety in drug development and post-marketing drug surveillance. It may also guide health policies to enhance stricter surveillance systems, ultimately leading to improved public health. Effective coordination among patients, doctors, and researchers provides a synergistic platform for ADR monitoring, enabling the identification of potential complications at an earlier stage and enhancing the level of care. By recognizing patients as stakeholders in ADR identification and management, the health care system can become more responsive and accountable, and hence better protect public health.

13.4.1. Educating Patients About ADRs

The education of patients about ADRs plays a crucial role in the detection and monitoring of these events, as well as ensuring patient safety within the healthcare system. A patient who knows about possible side effects can report them, which significantly helps in pharmacovigilance. According to the study of existing information on legal aspects of medicines management, healthcare providers should be well-trained to support these initiatives. It emphasizes the importance of collaboration between patients and professionals in identifying and addressing any side effects. By empowering patients with knowledge about their medications, including potential side effects and the importance of reporting unusual symptoms, healthcare providers can foster a proactive approach to medication safety, ultimately leading to improved health outcomes and safer medication practices in clinical settings (Vaismoradi et al., 2021).

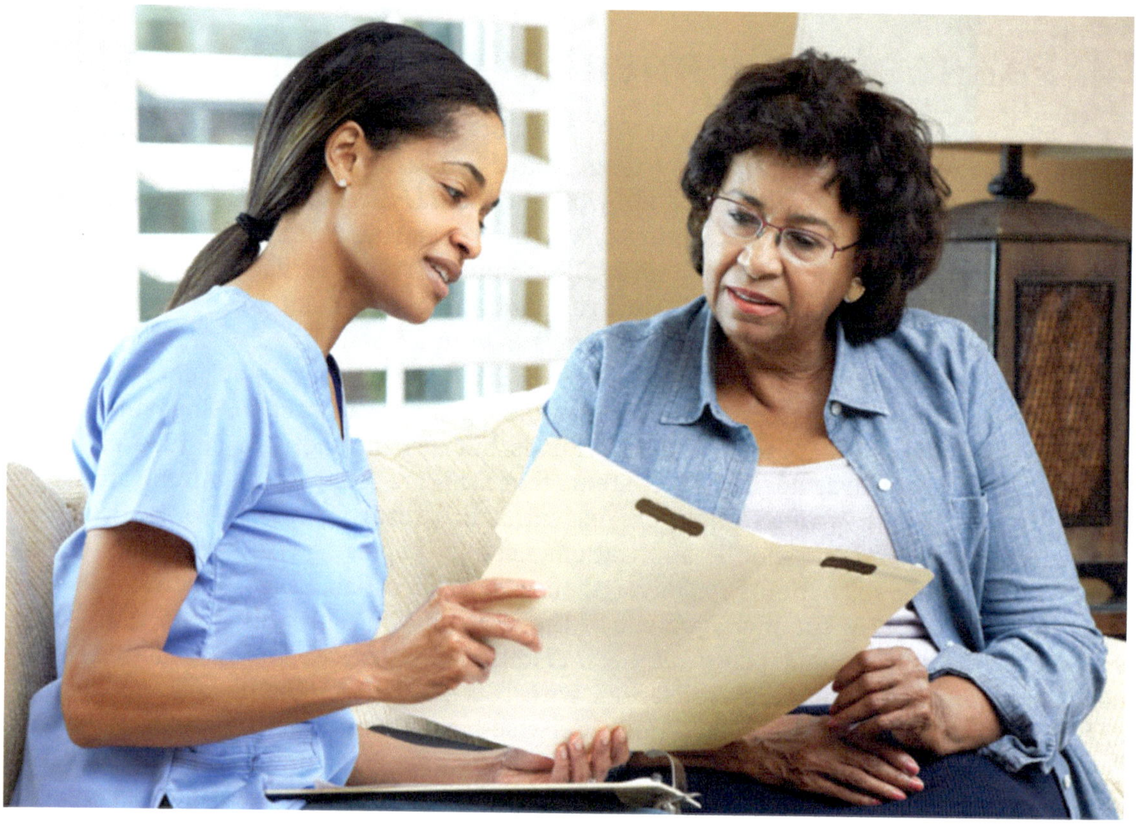

Figure 13.10. Educating patients about ADRs.

Source: https://www.ons.org/sites/default/files/2018-03/1000_iStock-177863138_1.jpg.

In addition, patient education should focus on sharing details and also teach people how to notice and report ADRs. Workshops or digital tools can improve a patient's knowledge of their drugs and their risks, which is necessary because polypharmacy can be very complex for seniors. Research indicates that effective patient engagement in healthcare decision-making correlates with a higher likelihood of reporting ADRs, thus improving monitoring systems (Livingston et al., 2020). It should be standard practice to inform patients about the signs of ADRs and instruct them on how to report them. As a result, there is improved communication between patients and healthcare providers, allowing ADRs to be handled efficiently and promptly. In addition, teaching patients about ADRs should include promoting openness and honesty among healthcare staff. It is essential for patients to feel recognized and supported when using medications, as this facilitates ADR monitoring. Prompting HCPs to discuss the risks of ADRs helps patients become aware and trust the doctors. Legal considerations in medicines management underscore the importance of incorporating patients' rights and perspectives into clinical practices (Vaismoradi et al., 2021). Because patient-centered care is now recognized as crucial, ensuring patients are involved in managing their medications is very important. Working together can result in improved safety procedures, thereby lowering the risks associated with ADRs and enhancing patients' overall health (Figure 13.10).

13.4.2. Encouraging Self-Reporting of ADRs

Encouragement of patient self-reporting of ADRs is key in optimising the detection and surveillance of such events. By actively involving patients in the reporting of ADRs, there is additional information gained by the health system regarding the impact of medication. This active involvement results in a patient-oriented culture where patients are motivated to report their experience. Additionally, through the use of multiple channels, such as direct reporting systems and educational programs, patients' understanding of what an ADR is can be facilitated. Such efforts can go a long way toward boosting the quality and quantity of data collected, thereby leading to improved patient safety practices and more informed therapeutic decisions. As hinted in research, significant adverse events have been noted among patients on various regimens for drug-resistant TB, and it is plausible that a robust self-reporting system may illuminate similar trends across different patient groups (Cox et al., 2012). The role of technology cannot be downplayed in the quest to trigger self-reporting of ADRs. With the use of smartphones and social media, there are websites that facilitate simple communication between patients and doctors. For example, mobile applications that allow patients to record symptoms and send them in real-time easily can simplify reporting. Social media presents yet another platform for the gathering of information relating to health, and thus timely analysis of drug usage patterns and associated adverse reactions among focused groups such as pregnant women (Chandrashekar et al., 1989). Through the utilization of such technological ability, the healthcare systems are capable of strengthening their ADR monitoring systems, thus enabling more effective responses to drug safety issues. Moreover, the platforms can be utilized to foster community discussions that continue to inform patients about the importance of reporting ADRs and sharing their drug experiences. Creating a self-reporting-friendly environment also entails eliminating barriers that prevent patients from reporting. In the majority of situations, a lack of awareness and misinformation about ADRs restricts patients from reporting their experiences. To mitigate these challenges, healthcare practitioners need to place a strong focus on education campaigns that demystify ADRs and clarify reporting processes. These kinds of efforts could be aimed at targeted segments, depending on specific problems, and making information more useful and usable. Health professionals could also help by proactively soliciting patient feedback during consultations, making reporting part of a standard step rather than an afterthought. Lastly, the development of an organizational culture that values patient complaints can enhance the efficiency of ADR monitoring activities, leading to optimal patient safety and improved therapeutic outcomes in various medical contexts.

13.4.3. Utilizing Patient-Reported Outcomes in Monitoring

The integration of patient-reported outcomes (PROs) into the monitoring of ADRs offers a transformative approach that prioritizes patient experiences. When patients are involved in reporting their symptoms and side effects, healthcare providers gain a better insight into how ADRs change their daily activities and quality of life. It can be used to notice patterns of adverse events that are not always found in regular observational studies. Therefore, PROs enable clinicians to quickly learn about changes in patients' symptoms and adjust their medication plans accordingly. As more patients require the use of multiple medications, using PROs is crucial to ensure safety and optimal treatment outcomes.

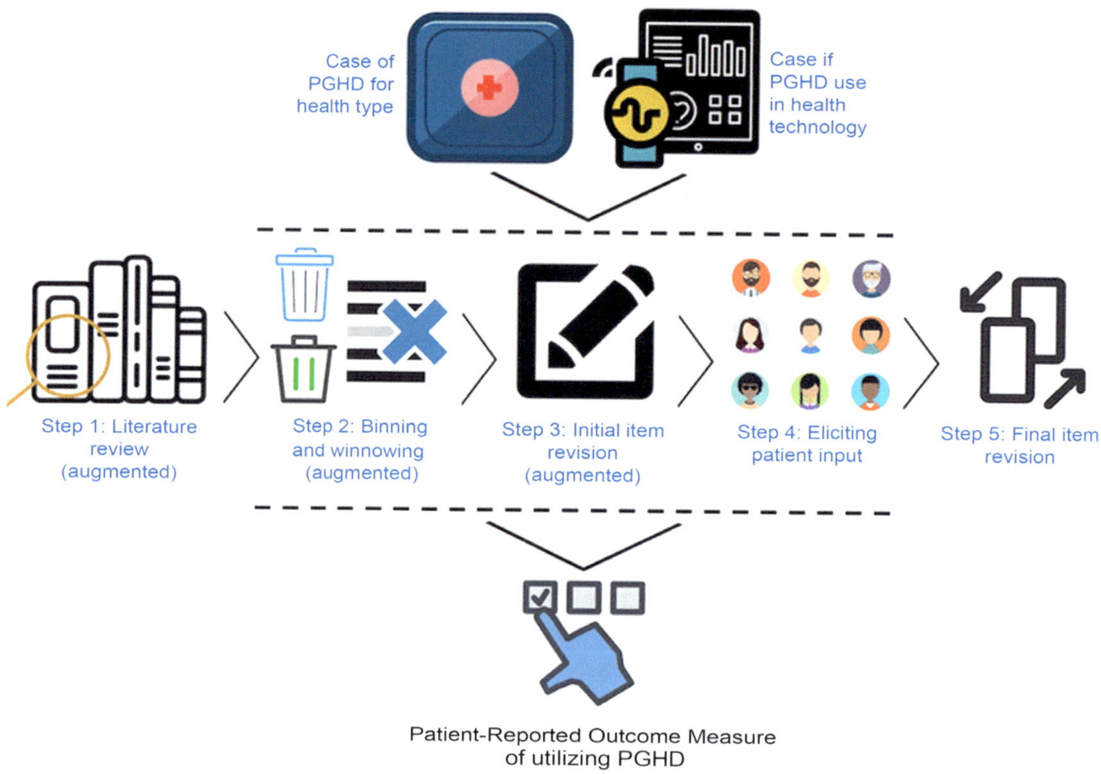

Figure 13.11. Utilizing patient-reported outcomes in monitoring.

Source: https://www.researchgate.net/profile/Gerardo-Luis-Dimaguila/publication/338808163/figure/fig1/AS:924345383784448@1597392521075/The-steps-of-the-patient-reported-outcome-measure-of-utilizing-person-generated-health.ppm.

Furthermore, using PROs in monitoring helps identify certain serious adverse events, particularly in cases where patients are infected with multiple diseases. For instance, patients receiving treatment for multidrug-resistant tuberculosis (MDR-TB) often face a myriad of potential adverse events due to polypharmacy. However, there is not much information available about what these patients go through, especially those who have HIV too. By analyzing patient-reported data, healthcare systems can gain a better understanding of the frequency and severity of adverse events in vulnerable populations (Cox et al., 2012). Using standard PRO measures in these settings could provide valuable information, inform clinical decisions, and aid in selecting treatments that minimize the risk of adverse outcomes while effectively managing both conditions. Moreover, having PROs involved in healthcare encourages patients to be more active in their care and share their experiences. Consequently, patients and their healthcare providers can communicate more effectively, which fosters teamwork and can significantly impact the treatment process. With evidence suggesting that significant percentages of drug-related problems are preventable, focusing on patient reports can enhance vigilance in clinical monitoring (Yassin et al., 2018). For example, regularly using patient-reported outcomes can help detect issues such as non-adherence to medication or experiencing adverse side effects sooner than usual. Being proactive in this way helps identify ADRs as well as enhance patient care, leading to improved health outcomes and satisfaction (Figure 13.11).

13.5. Regulatory Framework

The regulatory framework surrounding the detection and monitoring of ADRs plays a pivotal role in ensuring patient safety and the efficacy of pharmaceuticals. Regulatory bodies such as the FDA in the United States and the European Medicines Agency (EMA) in Europe establish guidelines and processes that govern the clinical testing and post-marketing surveillance of drugs. They require drug companies to report any problems that arise during clinical trials, as well as any incidents that occur after the drug is released into the market. If these rules were not followed, more ADRs could go unnoticed, which would be very dangerous for public health. As a result, a strong set of regulations supports the detection of ADRs and encourages trust between healthcare providers and patients, so safety is always a primary concern in medicine. Moreover, the evolution of AI holds the potential to enhance the regulatory framework for detecting and monitoring ADRs. As mentioned by Shuroug et al. (2023), AI technologies are increasingly integrated into clinical practice, where they can analyze vast datasets to identify patterns that may escape traditional monitoring systems. As a result, HCPs have an easier time entering information about ADRs when reporting. When AI is used in regulation, it helps identify risks with greater detail, leading to proactive action rather than reactive responses only after an incident. Still, this new method introduces legal and ethical concerns about data privacy and bias in algorithms that regulators should address to ensure AI does not compromise patient safety. All in all, the effectiveness of the system in detecting and monitoring ADRs depends on constant improvement and updates, particularly in light of emerging technologies. Regulatory bodies must remain vigilant in updating guidelines to incorporate emerging tools such as AI while addressing the associated challenges, as highlighted by Zeppenfeld et al. (2022). If regulatory bodies, healthcare workers, and technology experts join forces, the healthcare system may improve its ability to find and address ADRs in a timely way. A solid and well-designed set of regulations that includes innovative technologies can help keep the public healthy, ensure safe use of medications, and improve healthcare for patients.

13.5.1. Role of the FDA in ADR Monitoring

The activities of the FDA in tracking ADR are key in ensuring medication safety. The FDA governs post-marketing surveillance of drugs by pharmaceutical products through programs like the Adverse Event Reporting System (FAERS). The FDA uses data collected from both healthcare professionals and consumers to see if there are any risks with medications after they are approved. It is essential to regularly review these reports to identify trends and any unusual side effects that may not have been detected in clinical studies. Thanks to this information, the FDA can adjust drug labeling or issue safety notices to promote better healthcare for everyone and more informed decisions by patients and healthcare professionals. Last but not least, the FDA's regulation plays a key part in the entire pharmacovigilance system in America. A significant part of the FDA's role in ADR monitoring involves interacting with pharmaceutical companies, healthcare professionals, and regulatory agencies. The FDA advises manufacturers to report any adverse events related to their products, which is important for checking their safety. Also, the FDA works with international organizations and educational bodies to find and inspect ADRs all around the world. Initiatives such as Risk Evaluation and Mitigation Strategies (REMS) are among the measures through which the FDA collaborates with drug manufacturers to ensure that medications are prescribed and used safely, particularly when risks are identified. By cooperating, the monitoring of ADRs improves, and the drug industry becomes both safer and more transparent. Additionally, the FDA utilizes state-of-the-art methods to enhance the process of identifying ADRs and tracking them. With the help of big data and ML, the agency can improve its ability to find new safety signals as soon as possible. Since the methods for monitoring drugs have evolved following the COVID-19 pandemic, the FDA must adapt to new challenges and emerging types of medications. During the current battle against COVID-19, it is obvious that rapid tracking of ADRs involving vaccines and treatments developed for SARS-CoV-2 shows the need for strong government oversight. Due to the rapid progress in medicine, the FDA's strong focus on ADR monitoring ensures that patients are kept safe and treated with effective medications (Figure 13.12).

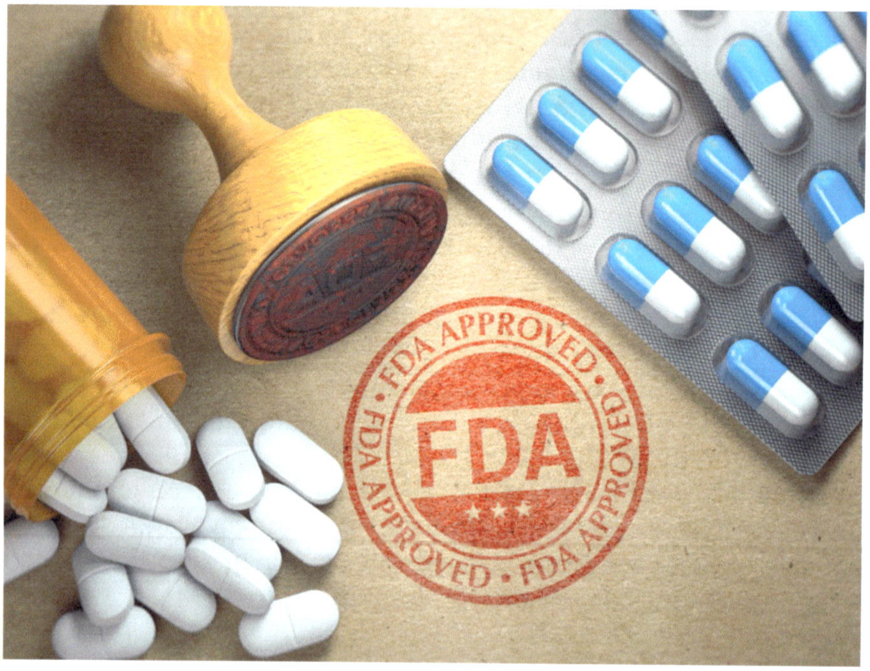

Figure 13.12. Role of the FDA in ADR monitoring.

Source: https://www.sofpromed.com/wp-content/uploads/2024/01/The-FDA-drug-approval-process.png.

13.5.2. International Guidelines and Organizations

International guidelines and organizations play a central role in identifying and tracking ADRs worldwide. A robust infrastructure for pharmacovigilance is offered by the WHO, and this is directed at systematic monitoring to improve patient safety. The WHO enables countries, particularly those with limited resources, to establish effective pharmacovigilance systems by developing guidelines that harmonize practices worldwide. Implementation of these guidelines facilitates the overcoming of such obstacles as underreporting and lack of awareness about ADRs among HCPs, which remain widespread in the majority of regions. In addition, WHO's cooperation with the country's health authorities accelerates the capacity-building activities aimed at increasing local pharmacovigilance systems to international best practice standards and thus increasing overall therapeutic intervention safety. In the Developing World, adherence to international standards of pharmacovigilance facilitates progress in monitoring drug safety in diverse healthcare settings. A critical analysis of Tanzanias pharmacovigilance system shows the success and areas of implementation, emphasizing international cooperation as a success factor. The Tanzania Food and Drugs Authority (TFDA) is primarily responsible for pharmacovigilance and regulatory affairs; however, studies reveal key problems, including inadequate training, a lack of easily accessible reporting forms, and insufficient dissemination of guidelines to healthcare providers. Despite the TFDAs' efforts, the relatively low rate of reporting of ADRs suggests the urgent need for enhanced international support and well-structured frameworks to promote local reporting systems and address training deficiencies. This alignment with international standards has the potential to provide a platform on which the healthcare provider is both capable and willing to contribute to ADR monitoring actively. Technological interventions are fast becoming the requisite tools aligned with international pharmacovigilance that will enhance the detection and monitoring of ADRs. Mobile health applications are transforming the way adverse effects are communicated in the developing world by allowing prompt communication between healthcare practitioners and regulatory authorities. Such innovations not only simplify the reporting process but also bring critical safety information closer to the patient. Technology integration into the pharmacovigilance system allows global agencies to make resources and training available to HCPs, thereby developing solutions as presented in reports like TFDA and NACP. Additionally, fostering a culture of safety that counters the stigma surrounding the reportability of ADRs is crucial. By synergistic effort in terms of guidance, education, and incorporation of technology, the global health community can achieve positive changes in the existing systems for reporting and managing ADRs effectively.

13.5.3. Impact of Regulations on Drug Safety

The landscape of drug safety is profoundly shaped by regulations designed to safeguard public health, especially concerning the detection and monitoring of ADRs. It is important to carry out comprehensive pharmacovigilance activities because regulations require it for identifying new ADRs, mainly in the first 10 years after a new drug is approved. Even though these steps are considered sufficient for new medicines, generics and older drugs can still pose risks because their safety may have changed. Problems may occur when the integration of manufacturing and pharmacovigilance quality systems is not done well during the product's lifecycle. By failing to monitor these established products diligently, regulatory frameworks may inadvertently leave room for serious adverse reactions arising from manufacturing defects or quality control lapses, highlighting a critical area for improvement in drug safety management, as noted by Sardella et al. (2021). In addition, regulators should not only oversee the approval process but also monitor drug safety after it is approved for market. Although many believe that long-standing medications are safe, new risks can emerge, primarily due to changes in their production and distribution methods. Therefore, regulations should ensure that pharmacovigilance is carried out thoroughly and can respond to changing situations. If people do not use drug safety reporting for older medicines, it may be difficult to identify any potential dangerous situations. Health professionals' supervision, as described in guidelines such as those from the ESC and EAS, is crucial in addressing these issues. These guidelines encourage clinicians to maintain a high standard of vigilance and consider updated safety information, reinforcing the vital importance of ongoing education and awareness in drug safety practices, as per François Mach et al. (2019). Overall, the connection between drug safety and regulatory frameworks is constantly evolving and requires regular review and improvement. Proper regulations encourage the collection of extensive data about ADRs, which helps us learn more about the medications over time. To deal with this, we should focus on strong approval steps and keep an eye on drugs throughout their use. It is essential for regulations to encourage collaboration among manufacturers, pharmacovigilance experts, and healthcare providers to address new safety issues promptly as they arise. Emphasizing proactive actions, regulatory bodies can enhance the quality of public health safety, ensuring that all types of drugs are thoroughly examined and monitored in the evolving world of drug safety, as discussed in the field (Figure 13.13).

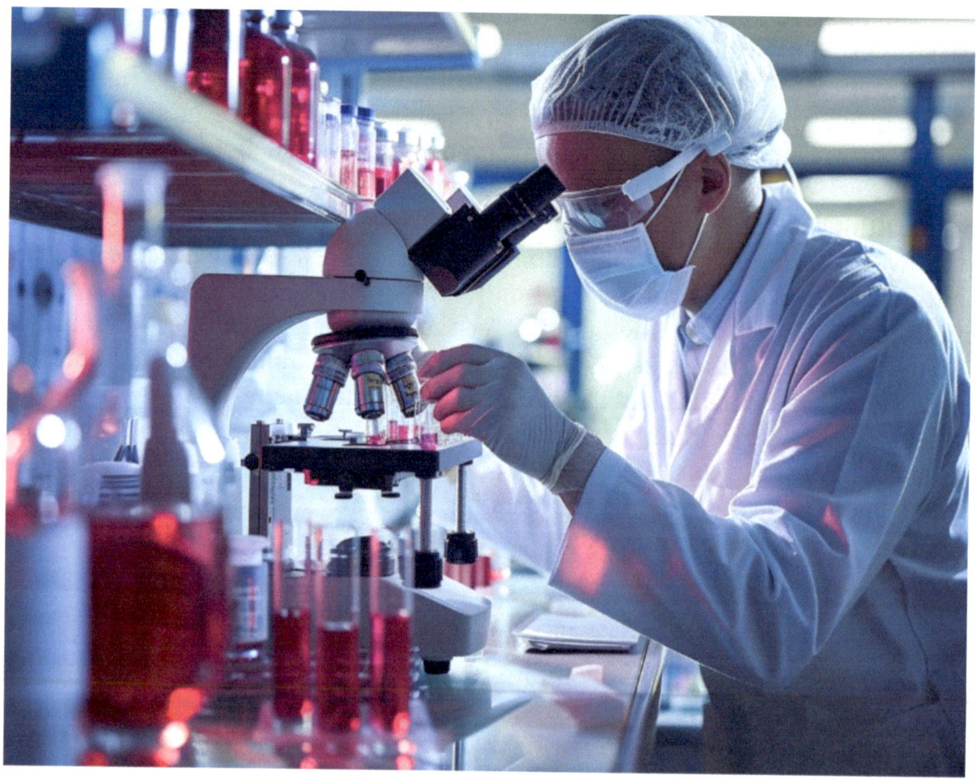

Figure 13.13. Impact of regulations on drug safety.

Source: https://www.cryptopolitan.com/wp-content/uploads/2024/05/philipcryptopolitan_Drug_safety_and_regulatory_83e679d8-1b77-4e7b-955d-8b4013e5ccf7.jpg.

13.6. Challenges in ADR Detection and Monitoring

Detection and monitoring of ADRs are confronted with a series of challenges that can hinder effective pharmacovigilance. Underreporting by patients and healthcare providers is one of the greatest hindrances. The majority of clinicians may not be aware of the requirement for reporting or perceive adverse effects as usual or not significant enough to report. Consequently, this leaves absolutely enormous gaps in data that limit the possibility of detecting patterns or signals for ADRs. Moreover, since it is founded upon SRS, the image of a drug's safety profile remains incomplete. These challenges require a cultural shift within healthcare settings to emphasize the importance of ADR reporting as part of patient safety in general, ultimately creating a more engaged model for drug safety surveillance. Another challenge is the quality and access to data used in ADR detection. Traditional pharmacovigilance systems usually depend on structured data sources that are either non-representative or inconsistent from the overall patient population. For instance, spontaneous reports are very heterogeneous in terms of completeness and detail, which makes it difficult for detailed analysis and signal detection. This issue is further exacerbated by the integration requirement of real-world data (RWD) from different sources, e.g., EHRs, patient registries, and social media, which provide valuable information on ADRs. Their integration requires standardization and validation for the promise of reliability for use in pharmacovigilance. Enhancing data quality collection and reporting will be essential for effective ADR detection and monitoring, thereby improving the overall pharmaceutical safety system. Despite enhanced pharmacovigilance methods, ethical and regulatory issues for ADR monitoring present serious challenges. The integration of technological advances, such as AI and ML, into systems presents a huge potential for higher detection rates and efficacy. However, AI must be used cautiously, as issues regarding data privacy, algorithm bias, and the ethical utilization of patient data are of overriding significance. The development of proper regulatory paradigms is necessary to safeguard patient information while also harnessing the full potential of emerging technologies. As emphasized in the literature, such ethical issues necessitate a sensitively balanced set of advantages for increased ADR monitoring, considering the risk to privacy and the equity of access to healthcare (Komi et al., 2025; Kumar et al., 2025). Future innovations must prioritize solving such complexities to build a robust and adaptable pharmacovigilance system in meeting the dynamic nature of drug safety.

13.6.1. Underreporting of ADRs

The underreporting of ADRs poses significant challenges to the detection and monitoring of medication safety. Although patients may experience various side effects, healthcare providers often overlook these, resulting in insufficient data to analyze them. Since medication-related events can result in avoidable hospitalizations, it is very important to improve the way such incidents are reported. Research indicates that as many as 1 in 10 hospitalizations in OECD countries can be attributed to medication-related events, demonstrating the extensive human and economic ramifications of this issue (Bienassis et al., 2022). If there is no reliable way to record ADRs, HCPs may not identify any patterns and will be unable to prevent risks properly. The main reason for underreporting ADRs is that healthcare systems are biased, with some providers uncertain about the importance of reporting them. A lot of HCPs are not sure if an ADR is related to a drug, so they are less likely to report these cases. Additionally, there are insufficient incentives for practitioners to participate in reporting ADRs, which diminishes their interest in this important task. The problem is exacerbated by the fact that patients' experiences can vary, and side effects are often subjectively judged, which makes the reporting process more challenging. Consequently, the substantial clinical and economic consequences of underreported ADRs contribute to unnecessary health care expenditures and compromise patient safety, as highlighted by the projection that avoidable admissions due to medication-related events cost over USD 54 billion in OECD countries (Bienassis et al., 2022). Furthermore, the analysis of large databases such as the FDA's Adverse Event Reporting System (FAERS) reveals critical insights into the underreporting dilemma. Continuous examination of ADRs can uncover potential safety signals, particularly for specific drug classes, as seen in the investigation of Janus kinase inhibitors (JAK inhibitors) and their associated thromboembolic events. This supports the need for solid frameworks to help detect and address ADRs. As the healthcare industry evolves, it is crucial to enhance methods for collecting and analyzing ADR data to safeguard patients and enhance their outcomes. To make reporting more common and ensure drugs are safe, all involved should provide education, make reporting easy, and put clear rules in place that help healthcare providers report ADRs correctly (Figure 13.14).

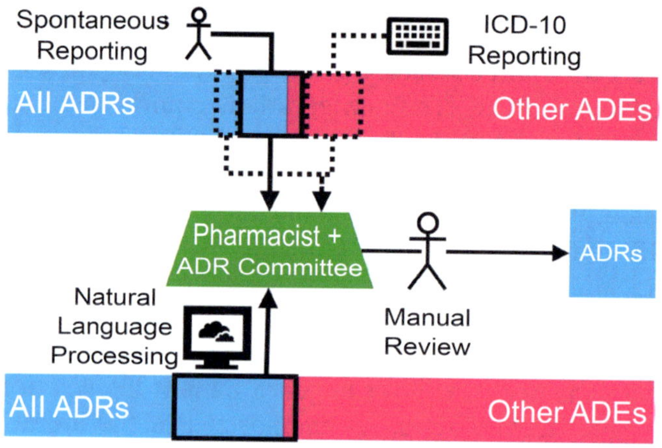

Figure 13.14. Underreporting of adverse drug reactions (ADRs).

Source: https://www.medrxiv.org/content/medrxiv/early/2021/12/13/2021.12.11.21267504/F1.large.jpg.

13.6.2. Variability in Reporting Practices

The disparity in reporting processes significantly impacts the observation and monitoring of ADRs. Different countries and institutions have different reporting protocols and guidelines, which may lead to gaps in the data as well as disparities. Some have limited resources or capacity for training to enable extensive reporting, and therefore, they possess small data sets that are not representative of the whole scope of ADR events. For instance, variations in regulatory requirements and the implementation of pharmacovigilance systems can create challenges in collecting ADR data reliably. The variation renders the process of assessing drug efficacy and safety challenging, as recognized by the significance of standard procedures in the analysis of the microbiological pharmaceutical quality by Sharaf (2018). It is only by adopting a simultaneous approach to data collection that the global medical community can contribute to a collective understanding of ADRs, ultimately leading to enhanced patient safety. In addition, the effectiveness of spontaneous ADR reporting schemes is invariably compromised by the lack of detailed information in the reports themselves.

The majority of submissions to databases, such as VigiBase®, may not contain relevant context of the patient population, drug dosage, and concomitant illness. This exclusion affects not just the detection of patterns of adverse event reports but also suppresses the detection of potential quality issues regarding drugs. As was the case with efforts by the Uppsala Monitoring Center to improve algorithms for identifying substandard drugs in their databases, complete and accurate data are essential. Poor reporting undermines the attempts to adequately evaluate the safety and therapeutic efficacy of drugs, as discussed by Juhlin et al. (2015). A more systematic approach to enhancing the quality of ADR reporting can significantly support pharmacovigilance activities worldwide. Finally, the participation of national centers in ADR reporting is a crucial factor in addressing practice diversity. The analysis of ADR clusters by national centers can lead to the verification and falsification of suspected cases of substandard drugs, ultimately enhancing knowledge about ADR causality. Participation of reporting centers in the evaluation process, as seen from the study by Uppsala Monitoring Center, provides a collaborative setting where information could be integrated and utilized to a greater extent. Through facilitation of a more active system by communication between primary reporters and national centers, the pharmacovigilance arena can shift towards a more efficient and reliable model. Improved communication channels and reporting structures will enable enhanced monitoring and ADR detection rates in broad populations, integrating frequently divided and changeable in nature data (Figure 13.15).

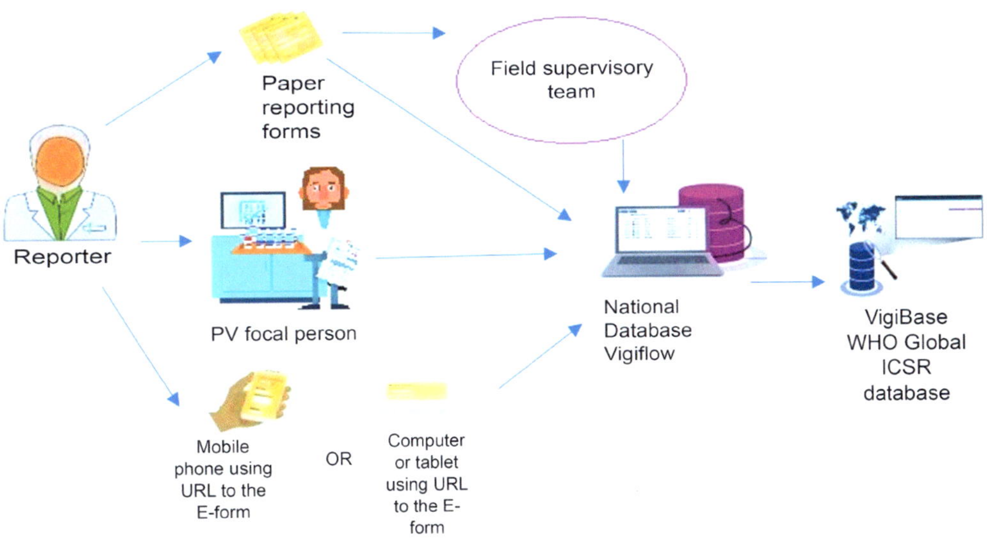

Figure 13.15. Variability in reporting practices.

Source: https://www.mdpi.com/ijerph/ijerph-19-03264/article_deploy/html/images/ijerph-19-03264-g001.png.

13.6.3. Limitations of Current Detection Methods

Despite significant advancements in pharmacovigilance, current detection methods for ADRs exhibit notable limitations that hinder efficacy in drug safety monitoring. Since the data is not well-organized, it is challenging to gather complete information about ADRs. Most of these methods rely on individuals submitting reports when they notice something, which can lead to missing information or biased accounts. Besides, the current frameworks usually use the same kind of data, which does not represent the wide range of patients who have ADRs. This inadequacy is particularly concerning as specific demographic groups, such as women and children, have historically been underrepresented in clinical trials, resulting in overlooked ADRs that could inform clinical practice and regulatory decisions (Pretis et al., 2022). Because data is still largely stored in traditional databases and reported manually, there are significant issues with data quality and the ability to identify signals. Current methodologies struggle with the inconsistent and incomplete data inherent in individual case safety reports (ICSRs). Moreover, not using advanced technologies such as ML and automation properly means that data analytics cannot fully help with detecting signals. If we rely solely on numbers and not on quality, it can be challenging to identify crucial safety signals, which may delay the necessary actions. As articulated in recent literature, there is an urgent need to improve the quality and accessibility of data used in pharmacovigilance to elevate the overall effectiveness of ADR detection efforts (Bate et al., 2021). The amount and complexity of safety data are increasing, making it challenging for many existing systems to handle them. It is evident that pharmacovigilance has not changed quickly enough to include data from EHRs and what patients report. Such problems make it harder to identify ADRs right after someone takes the drug. In addition, since adverse events are often not categorized in sufficient detail, it is challenging to determine the exact causes of them. To effectively advance the detection of ADRs, innovative approaches that leverage digital technologies, encourage patient engagement, and create more inclusive data collection frameworks must be prioritized within pharmacovigilance initiatives (Pretis et al., 2022).

Summary

The need for effective detection and monitoring of ADRs is paramount in ensuring patient safety and optimizing therapeutic outcomes. Several studies, including a detailed analysis in a tertiary care hospital, have proven that females and persons between 18 and 65 are more likely to suffer from ADRs. Since skin and connective tissue reactions are most common, there is a need to continually monitor and improve the way pharmacovigilance is conducted. This underscores the necessity for healthcare systems to implement robust monitoring frameworks that capture and analyze ADR data efficiently, thereby mitigating the risks associated with medication therapies (Kumar et al., 2023). Moreover, reviewing and documenting ADRs helps medical professionals determine the best treatment options. The high number of ADRs associated with amoxicillin-clavulanic acid suggests that doctors should use personalized approaches for their patients. Looking at the reasons and severity of ADRs helps to understand how each patient responds to their treatment. Additionally, the implications of antibiotic monitoring, as highlighted in observations about Salmonella infections and skin reactions, illustrate that multidisciplinary approaches can enhance patient care and promote safer prescribing practices (Min et al., 2021). All in all, the main goal of detecting and monitoring ADRs is to encourage safety in healthcare settings. Using detailed data analysis is crucial for reducing the discrepancy between when ADR occurs and when it is reported. Because pharmacotherapy is constantly changing, HCPS must be alert to ADRs by learning more and using better reporting methods. Ultimately, these efforts contribute to improved health outcomes and reinforce the commitment to patient-centered care in pharmacovigilance (Min et al., 2021; Kumar et al., 2023). The detection and monitoring of ADRs is a multifaceted process that requires an understanding of various methodologies and the epidemiological principles that underlie them. In this field, it is crucial to have robust detection systems to ensure patient safety and optimal treatment outcomes. There is much focus in current literature on the connection between wrongful use of medicines and the harm it can result in. If there is a standard Heinrich ratio for these types of mistakes, it would make it much easier for healthcare workers to identify and measure harm, allowing them to focus their efforts more effectively. Consequently, an accurate measurement of ADRs derived from errors that did not result in harm could enable healthcare providers to extrapolate potential improvements in patient safety following intervention (Barber et al., 2006). Also, pharmacoepidemiology has become an important part of tracking and finding out about ADRs. It emphasizes the importance of having integrated methods to share data, which facilitate extensive studies. However, some recent comments suggest that current data protection laws may hinder pharmacoepidemiological research by restricting the sharing of data. The present system of laws does not always encourage the sharing of important information for patient safety. To enhance the capabilities of detection and monitoring processes, there is a pressing need for a reorientation of data protection strategies towards facilitating rather than restricting essential health research (Sethi et al., 2014). Along with new laws, teamwork among HCPs is very essential for developing and improving ADR detection and monitoring. Working with different parties helps spread good practices and maintain a consistent approach to reporting. Additionally, the formation of task forces for drug safety can help enhance the methods used to monitor drugs. Since ADR detection involves multiple aspects, healthcare institutions must utilize modern technology and refine their communication methods. They are needed to identify ADRs and ensure the environment is safe for patients, leading to better medical outcomes. The discussion about this topic shows that strategic cooperation is needed to create an ADR monitoring system that can handle new challenges in medicine.

CLOSER LOOK

NON-METASTATIC BREAST CANCER

Non-metastatic breast cancer refers to breast cancer that has not spread beyond the breast tissue or nearby lymph nodes. This early-stage diagnosis is critical, as it offers a higher chance of successful treatment and long-term survival compared to metastatic disease. Non-metastatic breast cancer is typically categorized into stages I, II, or III, depending on tumor size, lymph node involvement, and other biological features such as hormone receptor status and HER2 expression. These factors guide the treatment plan, which may include surgery, radiation therapy, chemotherapy, hormone therapy, targeted therapy, or a combination of these approaches.

Surgical options for non-metastatic breast cancer include lumpectomy (breast-conserving surgery) or mastectomy, often followed by radiation to eliminate residual cancer cells. Systemic therapies like chemotherapy or hormone therapy are determined based on tumor characteristics and are used to reduce the risk of recurrence. In hormone receptor-positive cancers, medications such as tamoxifen or aromatase inhibitors can be used to block hormone-driven tumor growth. HER2-positive cancers may benefit from targeted agents like trastuzumab, which specifically inhibit the HER2 protein.

The prognosis for non-metastatic breast cancer is generally favorable, especially when diagnosed and treated early. However, patients may still face challenges such as treatment side effects, fear of recurrence, and the emotional toll of cancer. Regular follow-ups, imaging, and lifestyle interventions are essential for monitoring recovery and maintaining health. Advances in genomic testing and personalized medicine are also improving the ability to predict outcomes and tailor treatments more precisely. Overall, managing non-metastatic breast cancer involves not only eradicating the disease but also supporting the patient's physical and emotional well-being throughout the treatment journey and beyond, offering hope for long-term survival and quality of life.

References

1. Alomar, M. J., Tawfiq, A. M., Hassan, N., & Palaian, S. (2020). Post marketing surveillance of suspected adverse drug reactions through spontaneous reporting: Current status, challenges and the future. *Therapeutic Advances in Drug Safety, 11*. https://doi.org/10.1177/2042098620938595.
2. Alowais, S. A., Alghamdi, S. S., Alsuhebany, N., Alqahtani, T., Alshaya, A., Almohareb, S. N., Aldairem, A., et al. (2023). Revolutionizing healthcare: The role of artificial intelligence in clinical practice. *BMC Medical Education, 23*. https://doi.org/10.1186/s12909-023-04698-z.
3. Anu, R., Murgesh, V., Vishwanath, M., & R. K. (2023). A retrospective study of adverse drug reactions reported in a tertiary care hospital. *National Journal of Physiology, Pharmacy and Pharmacology.* https://www.semanticscholar.org/paper/a35613f6c12d5dd044c805423262f440e501fef9 (accessed on 9 June 2025).
4. Atif, M., Munir, K., Malik, I., Al-Worafi, Y. M., Mushtaq, I., & Ahmad, N. (2022). Perceptions of healthcare professionals and patients on the role of the pharmacist in TB management in Pakistan: A qualitative study. *Frontiers in Pharmacology, 13*. https://doi.org/10.3389/fphar.2022.965806.
5. Baraka, V., Fakih, B., Francis, F., Filbert, K., Kabanywanyi, A., et al. (2013). Strengthening pharmacovigilance system to capture safety data from HIV clients on ART in Tanzania: Identification of gaps in safety reporting system. https://core.ac.uk/download/pdf/19726103.pdf (accessed on 9 June 2025).
6. Barber, N., Franklin, B. D., Gallivan, S., Taxis, K., et al. (2006). Can the Heinrich ratio be used to predict harm from medication errors? https://core.ac.uk/download/1747122.pdf (accessed on 9 June 2025).
7. Bate, A., & Stegmann, J. U. (2021). Safety of medicines and vaccines–building next generation capability. *Trends in Pharmacological Sciences, 42,* 1051–1063. https://doi.org/10.1016/j.tips.2021.09.007.
8. Batko, K., & Ślęzak, A. (2022). The use of big data analytics in healthcare. *Journal of Big Data, 9*. https://doi.org/10.1186/s40537-021-00553-4.
9. Büyükgebiz, A., & Demir, A. (2025). Severe lipoatrophy in a growth hormone deficient toddler girl treated with a non-pegylated long-acting growth hormone. *Children, 12*. https://www.semanticscholar.org/paper/ea6b7495c3e16580b98615a68dd97df9c5bdbf30 (accessed on 9 June 2025).
10. Chandrashekar, P., Bharadwaj, P., Magge, A., Sarker, A., Gonzalez, G., et al. (1989). Social media mining for identification and exploration of health-related information from pregnant women. https://core.ac.uk/download/pdf/86423814.pdf (accessed on 9 June 2025).
11. Chehelgerdi, M., Chehelgerdi, M., Allela, O. Q. B., Pecho, R. D. C., Narayanan, J., Rao, D. P., Thamaraikani, T., et al. (2023). Progressing nanotechnology to improve targeted cancer treatment: Overcoming hurdles in its clinical implementation. *Molecular Cancer, 22*. https://doi.org/10.1186/s12943-023-01865-0.
12. Cox, H. S., Da Silva, E., Isaakidis, P., Khan, F., et al. (2012). Adverse events among HIV/MDR-TB co-infected patients receiving antiretroviral and second line anti-TB treatment in Mumbai, India. https://core.ac.uk/download/pdf/9418392.pdf (accessed on 9 June 2025).

13. De Bienassis, K., Esmail, L., Lopert, R., & Klazinga, N. (2022). The economics of medication safety. *OECD Health Working Papers*. https://doi.org/10.1787/9a933261-en.
14. De Pretis, F., van Gils, M., & Forsberg, M. (2022). A smart hospital-driven approach to precision pharmacovigilance. *Trends in Pharmacological Sciences, 43*, 473–481. https://doi.org/10.1016/j.tips.2022.03.009.
15. Deng, M., Li, J., Ding, N., & Wang, Z. (2021). A case analysis of a patient with salmonella infection and allergy to antibiotics. *Volume (39)*, 1–4. https://www.semanticscholar.org/paper/d12cb0247f8afb0f9a4017c278663c1f43712958 (accessed on 9 June 2025).
16. Gernier, F., Grellard, J., Dupont, C., Castel, H., Fernette, M., Lahaye, F., Charles, R. M., et al. (2023). Impact of web application support versus standard management on adherence with adjuvant hormone therapy in patients treated for breast cancer: The WEBAPPAC study. *BMC Cancer, 23*. https://www.semanticscholar.org/paper/7c39e09a370a80630bc749c06d2a5df0f6494512 (accessed on 9 June 2025).
17. Gordon, D. E., Jang, G. M., Bouhaddou, M., Xu, J., Obernier, K., White, K. M., O'Meara, M. J., et al. (2020). A SARS-CoV-2 protein interaction map reveals targets for drug repurposing. *Nature, 583*, 459–468. https://doi.org/10.1038/s41586-020-2286-9.
18. Hu, B., Guo, H., Zhou, P., & Shi, Z. L. (2020). Characteristics of SARS-CoV-2 and COVID-19. *Nature Reviews Microbiology, 19*, 141–154. https://doi.org/10.1038/s41579-020-00459-7.
19. Jha, P. (2022). Pharmacovigilance in developing countries: Drivers and barriers. https://core.ac.uk/download/560380635.pdf (accessed on 9 June 2025).
20. Juhlin, K., Karimi, G., Andér, M., Camilli, S., Dheda, M., Tan, S. H., Isahak, R., et al. (2015). Using VigiBase to identify substandard medicines: Detection capacity and key prerequisites. *Drug Safety, 38*, 373–382. https://www.semanticscholar.org/paper/f145ba6a57ca8fea2469598a41e91f734a7f2e56 (accessed on 9 June 2025).
21. Kamble, S. U., Bais, S. K., & Hugar, S. R. (2023). Review on adverse drug reactions. *International Journal of Advanced Research in Science, Communication and Technology*. https://www.semanticscholar.org/paper/b240d14c7b821b1dc1a42959265dff9ebf7cfba7 (accessed on 9 June 2025).
22. Kapoor, K. K., Tamilmani, K., Rana, N. P., Patil, P. P., Dwivedi, Y. K., & Nerur, S. (2017). Advances in social media research: Past, present and future. *Information Systems Frontiers, 20*, 531–558. https://doi.org/10.1007/s10796-017-9810-y.
23. Komi, L. S., Mustapha, A. Y., Forkuo, A. Y., & Osamika, D. (2025). Reviewing pharmacovigilance strategies using real-world data for drug safety monitoring and management. *International Journal of Scientific Research in Computer Science, Engineering and Information Technology*. https://www.semanticscholar.org/paper/0c163012ac2ec6d920f693be5c1d319b4ecddad2 (accessed on 9 June 2025).
24. Kumar, D. S., Shobha, P., & Sunitha, M. (2023). A retrospective analysis of adverse drug reactions reported to an adverse drug monitoring center of Pharmacovigilance Programmed of India in a tertiary care hospital. *International Journal of Scientific Research*. https://www.semanticscholar.org/paper/9f151560cb44649344baf5b867ddb9bc520b8d76 (accessed on 9 June 2025).
25. Likhitkar, M. K., Shakur, A., Roy, S., Mohan, L., Kumar, M., & Likhitkar, L. (2020). Analysis of

reporting of adverse drug reactions in a tertiary care hospital: One year survey. *International Journal of Scientific Research, 5*, 25–30. https://www.semanticscholar.org/paper/43bbed1d34ccac83f52949c6879bf5dc5ff5782d (accessed on 9 June 2025).

26. Livingston, G., Huntley, J., Sommerlad, A., Ames, D., Ballard, C., Banerjee, S., Brayne, C., et al. (2020). Dementia prevention, intervention, and care: 2020 report of the Lancet Commission. *The Lancet, 396*, 413–446. https://doi.org/10.1016/s0140-6736(20)30367-6.

27. Lyon, A. R., López-Fernández, T., Couch, L. S., Asteggiano, R., Aznar, M. C., Bergler-Klein, J., Boriani, G., et al. (2022). 2022 ESC guidelines on cardio-oncology developed in collaboration with the European Hematology Association (EHA), the European Society for Therapeutic Radiology and Oncology (ESTRO) and the International Cardio-Oncology Society (IC-OS). *European Heart Journal, 43,* 4229–4361. https://doi.org/10.1093/eurheartj/ehac244.

28. Mach, F., Baigent, C., Catapano, A. L., Koskinas, K. C., Casula, M., Badimón, L., Chapman, M. J., et al. (2019). 2019 ESC/EAS guidelines for the management of dyslipidemias: Lipid modification to reduce cardiovascular risk. *European Heart Journal, 41*, 111–188. https://doi.org/10.1093/eurheartj/ehz455.

29. Martenot, V., Masdeu, V., Cupe, J., Gehin, F., Blanchon, M., Dauriat, J., van der Horst, A. J., et al. (2022). LiSA: An assisted literature search pipeline for detecting serious adverse drug events with deep learning. *BMC Medical Informatics and Decision Making, 22*. https://doi.org/10.1186/s12911-022-02085-0.

30. Modi, A., Desai, M., Shah, S., & Shah, B. (2019). Analysis of cutaneous adverse drug reactions reported at the regional ADR monitoring center. *Indian Journal of Dermatology, 64,* 250. https://doi.org/10.4103/ijd.ijd_682_16.

31. Morgado, M., Plácido, A. I., Morgado, S., & Roque, F. (2020). Management of the adverse effects of immune checkpoint inhibitors. *Vaccines, 8*, 575. https://doi.org/10.3390/vaccines8040575.

32. Murray, C. J. L., Ikuta, K. S., Sharara, F., Swetschinski, L. R., Robles Aguilar, G., Gray, A. P., Han, C., et al. (2022). Global burden of bacterial antimicrobial resistance in 2019: A systematic analysis. *The Lancet, 399,* 629–655. https://doi.org/10.1016/s0140-6736(21)02724-0.

33. Patil, A. B., Rajashekhar, N., & Sushma, A. (2024). Cutaneous adverse drug reactions: Clinical pattern and causative agents in a tertiary care center in Central Karnataka. *International Journal of Scientific Research.* https://www.semanticscholar.org/paper/17e106e06b6f8cc6049d5435dc3d80a7bf895dd5 (accessed on 9 June 2025).

34. Ramien, M., & Goldman, J. (2020). Pediatric SJS-TEN: Where are we now? *F1000Research, 9*, 982. https://doi.org/10.12688/f1000research.20419.1.

35. Sardella, M., Belcher, G., Lungu, C., Ignoni, T., Camisa, M., Stenver, D. I., Porcelli, P., et al. (2021). Monitoring the manufacturing and quality of medicines: A fundamental task of pharmacovigilance. *Therapeutic Advances in Drug Safety, 12*. https://doi.org/10.1177/20420986211038436.

36. Senthil Kumar, R. K., & Velusamy, S. (2025). Harnessing artificial intelligence for enhanced pharmacovigilance: A comprehensive review. *Indian Journal of Pharmacy Practice.* https://www.semanticscholar.org/paper/9614f1ca45a263a1ba1ee160fdd3230eb89f5916 (accessed on 9 June 2025).

37. Sethi, N. (2014). The promotion of data sharing in pharmacoepidemiology. https://core.ac.uk/download/28977826.pdf (accessed on 9 June 2025).

38. Setyawan, J., Azimi, N., Strand, V., Yarur, A., & Fridman, M. (2021). Reporting of thromboembolic events with JAK inhibitors: Analysis of the FAERS database 2010–2019. *Drug Safety, 44*, 889–897. https://doi.org/10.1007/s40264-021-01082-y.

39. Sharaf, S. (2018). Detection and identification of Clostridium perfringens in some locally oral pharmaceutical samples. *International Journal of Pharmaceutical Sciences and Research, 57*, 89–103. https://www.semanticscholar.org/paper/47f215ffc94c8fa24e58deb2fea2b74906897b3a (accessed on 9 June 2025).

40. Sharma, A., Kumar, A., Akanksha, A., Kumar, A., Shukla, A., & Rajawat, D. S. (2023). Adverse drug reaction (ADR) and pharmacovigilance: A current prospectives. *International Journal of Pharmaceutical Sciences and Medicine.* https://www.semanticscholar.org/paper/47754a0d831f72ba5c14d55c6ff3a46ef27194a3 (accessed on 9 June 2025).

41. Sienkiewicz, K., Burzyńska, M., Rydlewska-Liszkowska, I., Sienkiewicz, J., & Gaszyńska, E. (2021). The importance of direct patient reporting of adverse drug reactions in the safety monitoring process. *International Journal of Environmental Research and Public Health, 19*, 413. https://doi.org/10.3390/ijerph19010413.

42. Sittiphan, S., Lim, A., Khurram, H., Dureh, N., & Dittakan, K. (2025). Epidemiology of reported serious adverse drug reactions due to anti-infectives using nationwide database of Thailand. *PLOS One, 20.* https://www.semanticscholar.org/paper/39dc8c352b6861393174ef74923d2657f9ff2cb7 (accessed on 9 June 2025).

43. Steyn, H. (2023). Profile of adverse drug reaction reports in South Africa: An analysis of VigiBase® for the year 2017. *South African Medical Journal.* https://doi.org/10.7196/samj.2023.v113i5.16522.

44. Tembe-Fokunang, E., Nyuki, B. A., Fokam, J., Fonmboh, D. J., Kaba, K. N., Fokunang, L. B., Mbopi-Kéou, F., et al. (2022). An overview of pharmacovigilance and adverse drug reaction monitoring of drugs and vaccines during the COVID-19 pandemic. *Journal of Advances in Medical and Pharmaceutical Sciences.* https://www.semanticscholar.org/paper/019b923f231f157e43ce83b6328d826ead4ff435 (accessed on 9 June 2025).

45. Vaismoradi, M., Jordan, S., Logan, P., Amaniyan, S., & Glarcher, M. (2021). A systematic review of the legal considerations surrounding medicines management. *Medicina, 57*, 65. https://doi.org/10.3390/medicina57010065.

46. Wagh, S. C., & Kadbhane, S. (2024). A review on pharmacovigilance. *International Journal of Advanced Research in Science, Communication and Technology*. https://www.semanticscholar.org/paper/16fe0ed08770beb3cf32367c044ea3e3d56076e1 (accessed on 9 June 2025).

47. Yassin, A., Abushaiqa, I., Ackroyd-Stolarz, S., Al Anany, D., Al Anazi, A., Al Hamid, A., Al Khaja, K., et al. (2018). Systematic review of the safety of medication uses in inpatient, outpatient and primary care settings in the Gulf Cooperation Council countries. https://core.ac.uk/download/287581298.pdf (accessed on 9 June 2025).

48. Zazzara, M. B., Palmer, K., Vetrano, D. L., Carfì, A., & Onder, G. (2021). Adverse drug reactions in older adults: A narrative review of the literature. *European Geriatric Medicine, 12*, 463–473. https://doi.org/10.1007/s41999-021-00481-9.

49. Zeppenfeld, K., Tfelt-Hansen, J., Riva, M., Winkel, B. G., Behr, E. R., Blom, N. A., Charron, P., et al. (2022). 2022 ESC guidelines for the management of patients with ventricular arrhythmias

and the prevention of sudden cardiac death. *European Heart Journal, 43*, 3997–4126. https://doi.org/10.1093/eurheartj/ehac262.

50. Журавлева, М. В., Романов, Б. К., Gorodetskaya, G. I., Муслимова, О. В., Крысанова, В. С., & Demchenkova, E. Yu. (2019). Topical issues of drug safety, possibilities of improving of pharmacovigilance. *Safety and Risk of Pharmacotherapy, 7*, 109–119. https://doi.org/10.30895/2312-7821-2019-7-3-109-119.

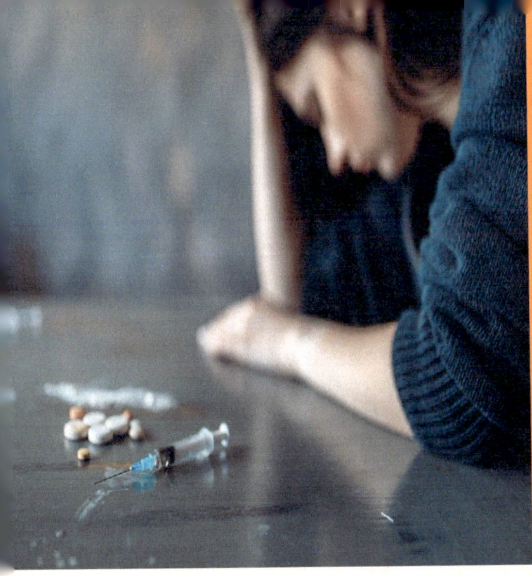

Chapter 14

PREVENTION AND RISK MINIMIZATION IN DRUG USE

Contents

Introduction

Since drug use can be complicated, it leads to many health issues that must be addressed with new and practical approaches. As with the opioid epidemic in America, millions of individuals have substance use disorders (SUDs), leading not only to severe health conditions but also socio-economic consequences cascading through communities. The main goal of treating both is systemic drug abuse and the acute illness of addicts is to prevent and reduce risks. The essay discusses different ways to reduce risks from drug use, pointing out that treatment should be flexible because substance use changes over time. As noted in recent reviews, without specific intervention, populations exposed to the risk of illicit drug use remain highly exposed to the harms of illicit drug use, which have only been exacerbated by social disadvantage, such as the COVID-19 pandemic (Alexander et al., 2020). For prevention, treatment, and harm reduction to work effectively, healthcare workers, policymakers, and communities need to be integrated into a unified system. Most discussions about drug use focus on evidence-based methods that help cut down on substance use disorder and also lower the risks to health. To support recovery, stakeholders conduct educational and outreach activities within the community. Additionally, introducing technology, especially during public health crises, enables the provision of care and support in new ways. It is essential to make these advancements because traditional face-to-face services have been interrupted, and this shows that healthcare needs to adjust. Best practice implementation in accordance with public health agencies' policies assures that risk management is tailored and effective, thereby enhancing healthier results among risk populations (François et al., 2019). In addition, preventing drug use goes beyond just not using drugs; it helps strengthen both people and the community. An approach that includes teaching, medical support, and community assistance helps stakeholders become more resilient to factors that lead to addiction. It is essential to recognize that challenges such as poverty and discrimination in society can impede the recovery process. It is argued in this essay that a health-based model should be expanded to give priority to those suffering from substance abuse, only possible through ongoing advocacy and policy adjustments based on empathy and facts. Concentrating on the systemic aspects of drug consumption enhances connections within the community and leads to a fairer, healthier society (Figure 14.1).

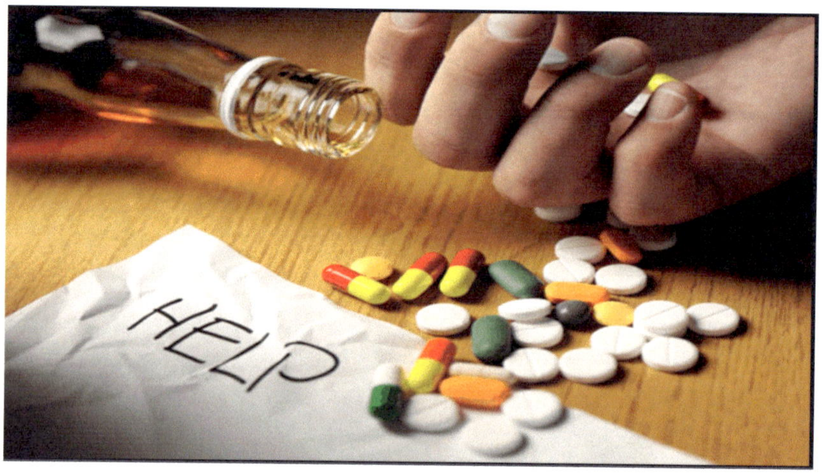

Figure 14.1. Prevention and risk minimization in drug use.

Source: https://connexionsterapiesintegrades.com/wp-content/uploads/2021/04/DROGAS.fw_.png.

Definition of Drug Use and Its Prevalence

The term drug use refers to various actions that involve taking substances meant for either therapy or for enjoyment. Taking drugs for medical reasons is usually controlled by healthcare providers, but using drugs for fun is not regulated and can cause many health problems for the public. At times, it becomes difficult to tell these apart, especially when someone takes prescription drugs without being prescribed them. According to Visseren et al. (2021), the implications of drug use extend beyond personal health, influencing social and familial dynamics while contributing to widespread public concern regarding substance dependence and abuse. It is essential to have clear definitions of drug use so that we can create effective ways to limit the harm caused by illicit drugs and encourage better behavior. Over the past few decades, drug use has become much more common due to changes in society and the increased availability of drugs. Many statistical reports show that a large part of the population uses drugs at some stage in their lives, for reasons such as fitting in or dealing with mental stress. The rates of education can vary significantly, depending on factors such as a person's age, financial situation, and place of residence. Notably, studies highlight a rise in the use of opioids, stimulants, and synthetic drugs, reflecting ongoing challenges to public health systems (Rebecca et al., 2020). Being aware of these trends is crucial, as they inform policy decisions and aid in creating programs to prevent substance abuse. Prevention and reduction of drug-related risks should rely on knowing the definitions and how common these problems are. Many prevention programs are successful because they adapt their plans to meet the needs of various communities, taking into account factors that impact drug use. Initiatives in the community, educational actions, and changes in policies are key to dealing with all aspects of drug use. If early intervention and support are included in the approach, stakeholders can try to lessen the problems linked to substance use. Additionally, ongoing research is fundamental in adapting prevention strategies to shifting trends, ensuring that programs remain relevant and effective (Rebecca et al., 2020; Visseren et al., 2021) (Figure 14.2).

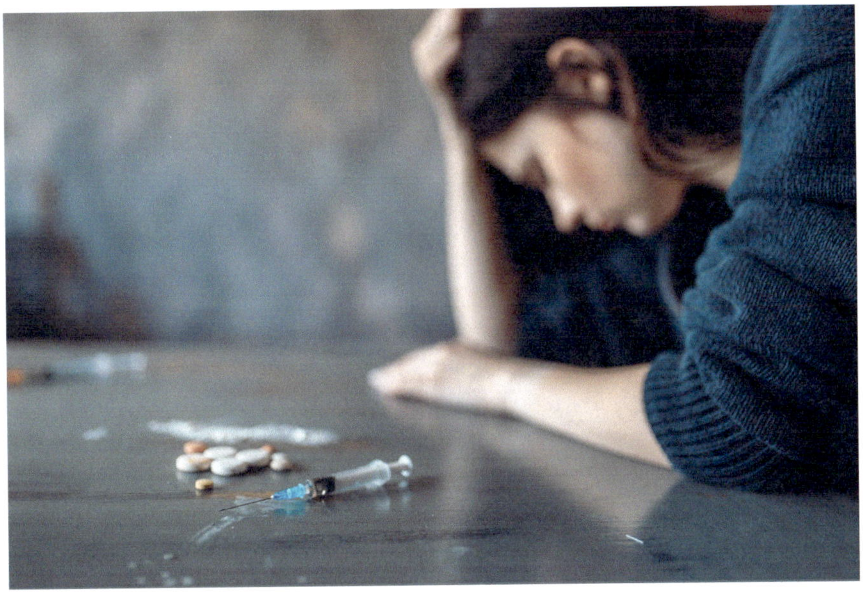

Figure 14.2. Definition of drug use and its prevalence.

Source: https://www.ilivewell.co.za/wp-content/uploads/2020/05/drug-addiction-header.jpg.

Importance of Prevention and Risk Minimization

Preventing and reducing the risk of drug use are essential, mainly to avoid harmful results and improve public health. Prevention programs are essential in shielding people from the dangers of using drugs, especially those who have previous health problems. For example, programs that regularly inform people about the dangers of certain drugs can help lower both the initiation of drug use and its abuse. When there is information on safe practices from both healthcare workers and schools, drug-related adverse reactions happen much less often. The use of prevention-based strategies in high-risk cases proves that they play a helpful role in ensuring drug safety for everyone. It is important to use risk reduction procedures when dealing with the difficulties in drug treatment. These procedures encompass a range of measures designed to reduce the frequency and severity of ADRs. With the help of effective pharmacovigilance, healthcare workers can monitor drug safety and take prompt action if adverse reactions occur. Additionally, by leveraging devices like electronic health records (EHRs) to monitor and document patients' histories, clinicians are able to anticipate drug interactions and contraindications, thus improving patient care. The knowledge collected from ongoing monitoring can assist doctors in making changes to a patient's treatment plan. With these measures, both patients and the overall image of drug safety are protected, leading to risk-aware policy changes and informed prescriptions. It is also necessary to integrate education and awareness activities with actions to prevent and reduce risks when it comes to drug use. When health professionals educate patients and their families about their medication and its proper use, it becomes safer for everyone. Learning about the best methods for spotting and handling ADRs improves healthcare professionals' (HCPs) management of drug-related problems. Recent events have demonstrated the importance of utilizing teams of diverse experts to address the challenges of drug therapy. Education with emphasis, alongside vigilant monitoring and integrated intervention practices, is essential to achieve best outcomes in prevention and risk minimization concerning drug use (Choudhary et al., 2023; Cacciapuoti et al., 2025) (Figure 14.3).

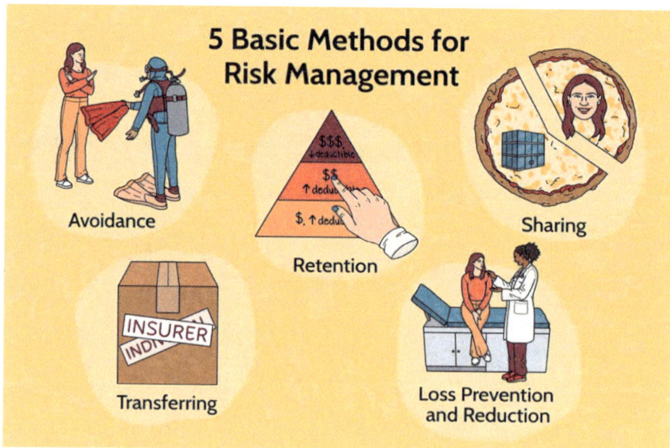

Figure 14.3. Importance of prevention and risk minimization.

Source: https://projectriskcoach.com/wp-content/uploads/2022/12/identify-risks.jpg.

14.1. Understanding Drug Use

A good understanding of drug use requires looking at all the factors that play a role, such as biological, psychological, and social reasons. An individual's genes and genetic changes can make them more likely to become dependent or addicted. Furthermore, mental health conditions like disorders might make a person more likely to use drugs, which complicates matters. The influence of friends, cultural traditions, and a person's financial situation should not be ignored when looking at drug use. After analyzing these factors, you can create better ways to prevent drug use, which consider both the individual's risks and the overall environment in which drugs are used. Moreover, the implications of adverse drug events (ADEs) highlight the importance of understanding drug interactions and their multifactorial impacts, especially in vulnerable populations such as the elderly. As people age, their bodies may respond differently to medications, so they are more likely to have ADEs such as falls or need hospital care, which significantly reduce their quality of life. The drug burden index (DBI) emerges as a crucial measure that aids HCPs in evaluating the cumulative risk associated with polypharmacy. With DBI in electronic medical records, doctors can prevent many dangerous outcomes and offer better care to their patients. This proactive approach not only underscores the necessity for informed and engaged healthcare delivery but also promotes the prevention of complications that arise from inappropriate medication use, addressing both clinical effectiveness and the overarching quality of care as highlighted in discussions surrounding medication management (Rasu et al., 2025). When attempting to lower the number of new infections, it is critical to acknowledge that drug use contributes to HIV transmission. Behavioral interventions, coupled with biomedical strategies, such as pre-exposure prophylaxis (PrEP) and post-exposure prophylaxis (PEP), can significantly mitigate the risk of HIV transmission among high-risk populations. The fact that many people do not routinely use condoms, despite their continued importance, necessitates the development of new preventative strategies for each group. By using different approaches, we can respond in many ways to drug risks and also address the causes of substance use and its connection to high-risk behaviors. By developing a comprehensive understanding of how drug use contributes to health risks, public health initiatives can more effectively target interventions to reduce new infections and enhance the overall wellbeing of at-risk populations (Chin, 2024) (Figure 14.4).

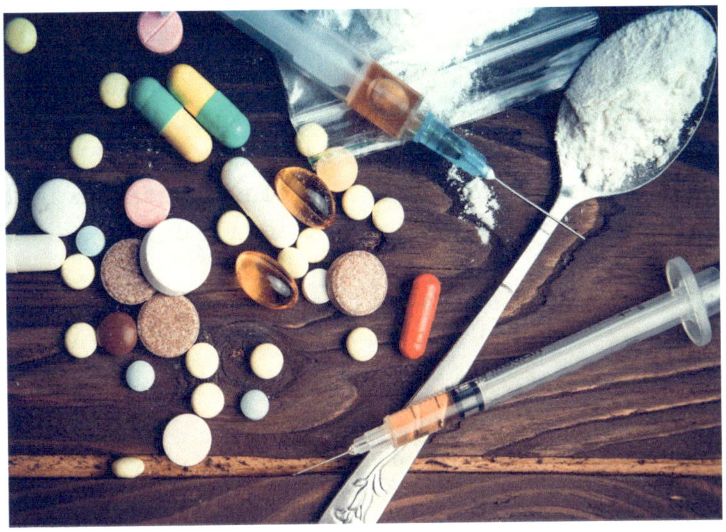

Figure 14.4. Understanding drug use.

Source: https://cdn.britannica.com/05/213705-050-4331A79A/drug-concept-drug-abuse-addition-heroin-injection-doping-opium-epidemic.jpg.

14.1.1. Types of Drugs Commonly Used

The use of drugs in the current era transcends across various classes, which have their own characteristics and implications. Some of the most common types are stimulants, depressants, hallucinogens, opioids, and cannabinoids. Stimulants such as cocaine and methamphetamine boost alertness and energy levels but have high addiction rates and cardiovascular-related problems. Depressants like alcohol and benzodiazepines reduce brain activity, which leads to drug dependency and impairment of cognitive functions. Significantly, hallucinogens like LSD and psilocybin create perceptual states of change but can produce psychological discomfort in the mentally ill. With society confronting the implications of drug use, knowing these classes is imperative to effect preventive measures and lessen connected risks. Substance use disorders not only differ by drug class but also parallel various underlying reasons that determine consumption. For instance, opioids—prescription medications and heroin—have risen in popularity, resulting in a horrifying rise in overdose deaths.

They relieve physical pain temporarily but initiate grave health crises when used for anything other than medical purposes. Cannabinoids, particularly marijuana-derived, have become more popular for both recreational and medicinal purposes. While widely viewed as safer choices, the legal framework and risk of dependency must be closely examined, particularly within the context of public health initiatives. In seeing the degree of flexibility in drug forms and their social impact, prevention increasingly becomes an issue of pressing concern that encompasses education, harm reduction, and effective regulation. Furthermore, the changing drug use landscape calls for an analysis of the effects that drugs have on specific demographics. These susceptible groups, such as adolescents and those with underlying mental health conditions, are also more likely to be at risk for drug use in a number of ways. For instance, the combination of substance and mental health disorders has been well documented because some drugs tend to worsen these conditions and perpetuate a cycle of addiction. This richness is underscored in your guidelines on the management of bipolar disorder, which highlight how drug use can break medical treatment, as described by Lakshmi et al. (2018). Here, these observations underscore the necessity of an overt, subtle strategy towards education and prevention that not only takes into consideration drug types but also the demographic and therapeutic context of their consumption. Lastly, developing sensitivity and support within communities can also do much to stem drug usage and harm (Figure 14.5).

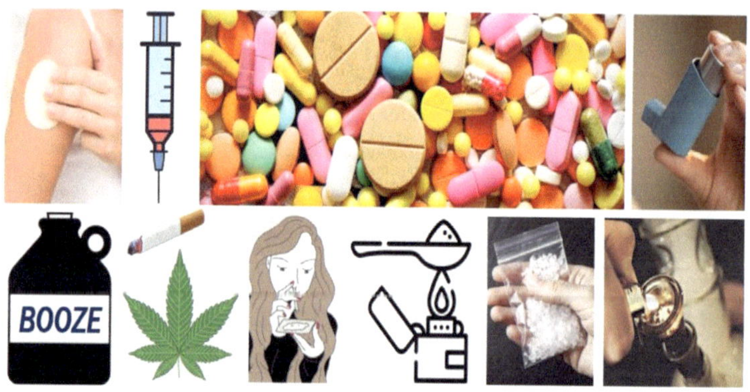

Figure 14.5. Types of drugs commonly used.

Source: https://marketbusinessnews.com/wp-content/uploads/2020/10/Drug-types-of-drugs-image-for-article-4984989484.jpg.

14.1.2. Reasons Individuals Engage in Drug Use

A person's choice to use drugs is affected by many different personal, social, and environmental factors. Many individuals use drugs to help them handle stressful events or mental health problems. For a lot of people, using substances helps them forget about their problems for a short time. The fact that mental health disorders are common makes the problem worse, since individuals with anxiety or depression may try drugs to ease their symptoms, not realizing that drugs will not help. For this reason, it is important to understand the psychology of drug use to create effective strategies that address both the drugs and the reasons behind people's addiction. Also, the influence of social factors is important in the beginning of drug use, especially among teenagers and young adults. Many people are influenced by their peers to use drugs, since substance use is often seen as an important part of growing up or fitting in with a group. When drug use is accepted or even celebrated in certain groups, individuals might think that using drugs can make them part of the crowd. This situation highlights the importance of building communities that foster healthy living and provide people with alternative options for addressing problems. If everyone values resilience and wellness, drugs will be less attractive as a way to join groups. Lastly, how easy it is to obtain drugs can significantly affect a person's chances of using them. Where drugs are easy to find, people may not see the dangers and might be more likely to try them and get addicted. In addition, when people are poor or do not have access to education, they may turn to drugs to try to leave their difficult situations. Understanding these factors is crucial when developing prevention programs to reduce drug use. Working on both the supply of drugs and the social and economic problems of at-risk groups helps to reduce risks and promote safer living and healthier drug habits (Figure 14.6).

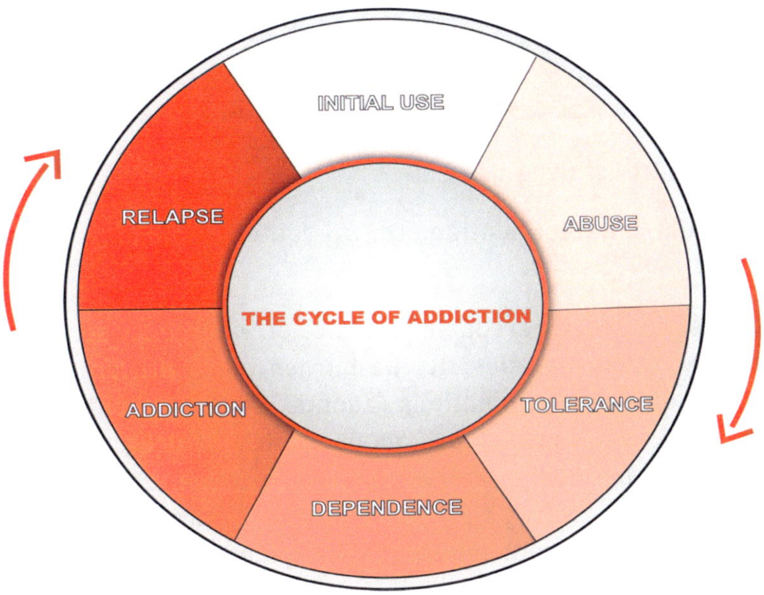

Figure 14.6. Reasons individuals engage in drug use.

Source: https://assets.website-files.com/5b342487cecf50c44231496a/602d955e6818e44bfc82ff88_QUMl5dnNKdfviOCb1YWRqoGofg2K0vemZXN2JZO8fQ4BCdsG1G9a9EEIZPK44jSDW9OJuHBNVsFYq3mPDIG86jU2zsFmGVOAaBuUp-WGiGPtwWElB690kN-neNubsHx0d25tb_N.png.

14.1.3. Societal Impacts of Drug Use

Drug abuse has many social consequences that touch the user, the user's family, and the community as a whole. The most important issue is that the healthcare system is often forced to use its resources to treat diseases and disorders related to drugs. Many patients who are victims of acute substance abuse are brought to the hospital emergency room, which results in more extended hospital stays and more expenses. Studies suggest that we need to employ intervention strategies to address these common health problems, and government agencies have recommended some of these strategies to enhance public health efforts.

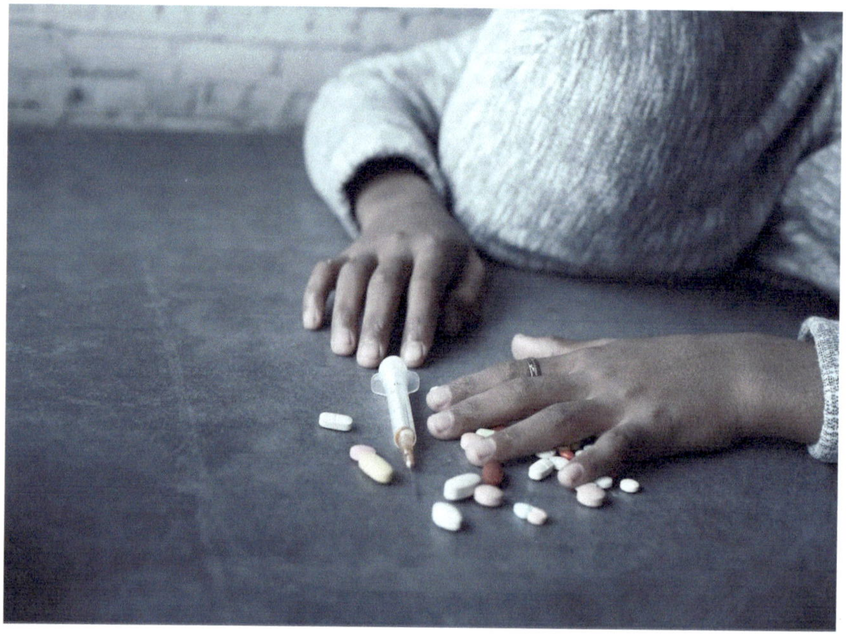

Figure 14.7. Societal impacts of drug use.

Source: https://i0.wp.com/kiitanfoundation.org/wp-content/uploads/2023/07/drug-addiction-menace.jpg?fit=1500%2C1000&ssl=1.

These include strategies aimed at reducing reliance on emergency services through preventive education and outreach, which can alleviate the burden on healthcare institutions and lead to healthier outcomes for vulnerable populations (Zaoutis, 2009). It helps avoid immediate health issues and also encourages everyone to care about the use of drugs. Drug addiction also has a significant effect on society by making it feel less secure. When drug use spreads in a country, crime rates increase, especially in drug trafficking, robbery, and violent acts, as addicts try to get money for their drugs. Such crimes contribute to creating inequality and fostering suspicion among community members, ultimately weakening unity within the community. In addition, regular drug use can result in families splitting up since addiction can cause abuse or neglect between family members. For this reason, social services are trying to deal with both the abuse and the additional problems that come with it. Through preventive community programs centered on rehabilitation, societies can mitigate these effects and build a more kinder society for drug addicts (Sisson et al., 2005). Apart from the health and safety issues, using drugs can reduce a person's ability to work and earn money in the long run. Drug abuse causes more financial problems than treatment and prevention, since it leads to reduced productivity at work, more people being unemployed, and extra costs for social and legal services. If drug use is widespread, the workforce may miss more days, do less work, and quit more often, which negatively affects the economy and its stability. It is difficult for employers to get dependable staff, and companies in drug-affected areas make less money. Therefore, it is necessary to have economic strategies that focus on prevention, provide jobs, and offer educational opportunities. By investing in such programs, communities can construct healthier and more resilient societies, ultimately addressing the root causes and broader implications associated with drug use (Sisson et al., 2005; Zaoutis, 2009) (Figure 14.7).

14.2. The Role of Education in Prevention

Learning in schools is crucial for preventing substance abuse, especially related to drugs, since it helps people make wise choices. Programs that teach about addiction, the dangers of drugs, and their effects on society can significantly decrease the number of addictions. It helps people realize the truth and also trains them to recognize the many pressures and influences related to drug use. Research indicates that effective educational strategies can lead to decreased experimentation with drugs and an overall healthier community perspective on substance use, as evidenced in recent studies highlighting the success of school-led initiatives where young people engage in discussions about drugs in a safe and informative environment (Visseren et al., 2021).

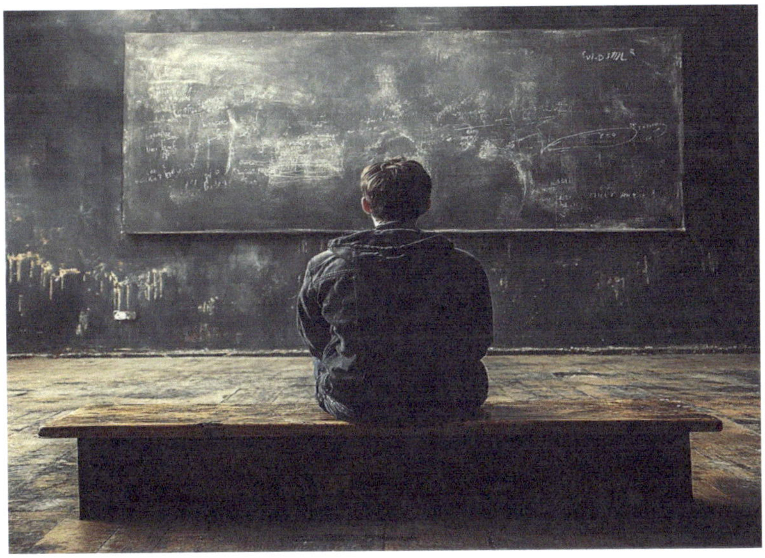

Figure 14.8. The role of education in prevention.

Source: https://www.mothersagainstaddiction.org/wp-content/uploads/2024/09/The-role-of-education-in-addiction-prevention.png.webp.

Additionally, education can be provided in schools, as well as at community workshops and through specialized programs for individuals at risk. These projects are most important in areas where drug-related issues are common and people have less access to helpful information and resources. If parents, educators, and community leaders join forces in programs, it can help young people become stronger and more resilient. Besides, the use of technology in education, for example, through the internet and social networks, makes it easier to reach a larger audience. By creating a culture that prioritizes education as a preventive tool, communities can cultivate environments that discourage drug use and support positive decision-making (Alexander et al., 2020). In addition, education helps prevent problems by teaching important skills that people need to handle peer pressure and emotional issues. Learning coping skills, how to manage stress, and how to solve conflicts can give individuals the ability to avoid drugs. Taking this approach to education means it is a key part of reducing risks when it comes to drug use. It is also necessary to regularly check and update educational programs so that they remain valuable and practical in different times. By fostering a proactive stance toward education, societies can build a foundation for healthier choices and ultimately reduce the burden of drug-related harms (Alexander et al., 2020; Visseren et al., 2021) (Figure 14.8).

14.2.1. School-Based Drug Education Programs

It is important to teach about drugs in schools because youth, who are very susceptible to evil influences, are at risk of substance abuse. The purpose of these programs is to make sure young people know how to avoid drugs and stay healthy. Such programs work well at preventing drug experimentation and addiction because they promote healthy alternatives. When a thorough curriculum is used that includes facts on drugs and social and psychological information, the result is a balanced approach to education. Moreover, having teachers who are trained helps students get proper and encouraging guidance, so the effects of these programs in preventing drug abuse and changing behavior become stronger. Moreover, it is clear that involving different stakeholders in planning and implementing drug education in schools is crucial.

It has been proven that effective intervention designs depend on the collaboration of health professionals, teachers, and ex-drug abusers. Identify an example or a case of how observations learned through focus group interviews confirmed that Ex-Drug Users (EDUs) and Health Professionals (HPs) shared common problems, which challenged drug prevention programs and emphasized the necessity of mutual support. Programs must address the factors inside schools and the factors outside schools that influence drug use. Involvement of parents and communities at the local level can enhance these efforts by developing a system that supports children facing various challenges. Such efforts are necessary to lower drug use in youth and make our communities safer. In addition to increasing awareness of drug use's harmful effects, school drug education programs can promote healthy behaviors and reinforce protective factors against drug abuse. Because they learn how to make choices, handle conflicts, and manage stress, students in these programs can handle adolescent issues with self-assurance. By incorporating health education into the school curriculum, the prevention and well-being message can be effectively supported. Such programs help narrow the gap between different economic groups by teaching all students how to make good decisions about their health and well-being. Ultimately, establishing active school health education programs not only protects the future of adolescents but also contributes to the overall health of society as a whole (Raymond et al., 2021; Tahlil et al., 2021) (Figure 14.9).

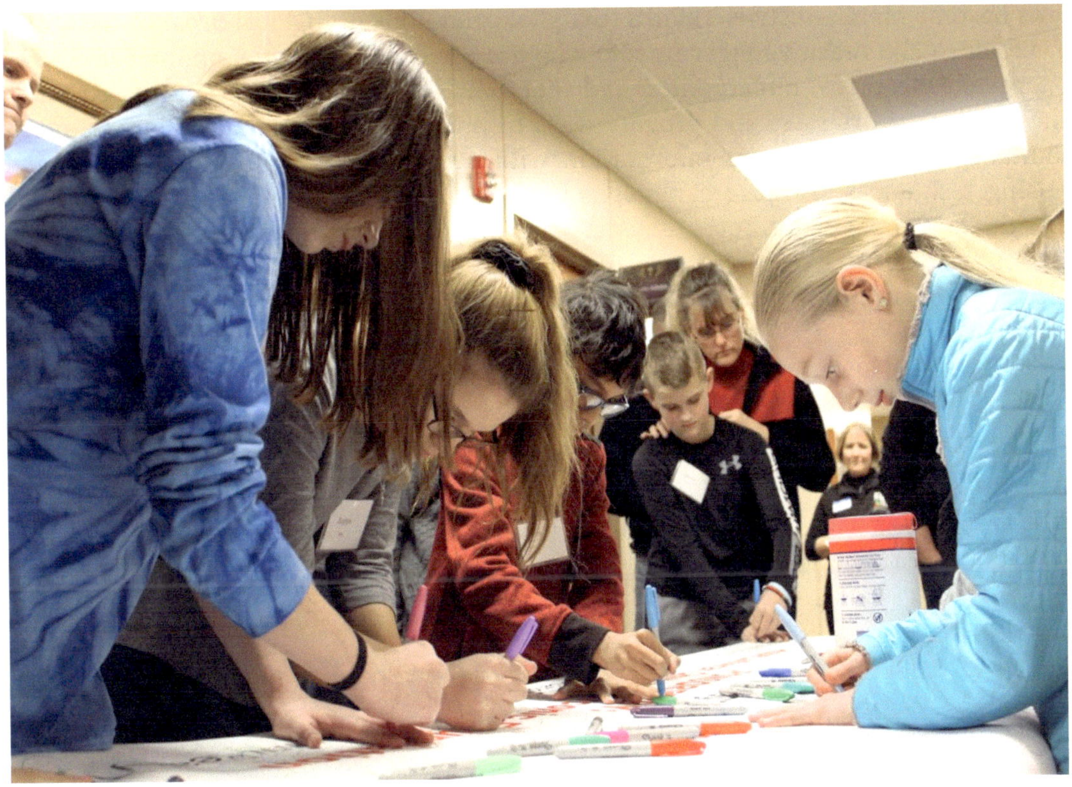

Figure 14.9. School-based drug education programs.

Source: https://www.abc-counseling.com/wp-content/uploads/2024/06/The-Role-of-Education-in-Substance-Abuse-Prevention.jpg.

14.2.2. Community Outreach and Awareness Campaigns

Community awareness programs are essential for preventing and lowering the risk of drug use. The specific circumstances and challenges of these communities allow campaigns to design messages that appeal to local people. By introducing programs that inform individuals about the risks of substance misuse and the resources available to them, people are encouraged to make informed choices. Moreover, when people are involved in their community, they feel more comfortable talking about drug issues, and this reduces the stigma, allowing them to reach the services they need. When these community activities are combined, they help people learn more and become stronger against drug use by choosing healthier lifestyles and being responsible. Besides educating people, it is essential for outreach campaigns to collaborate with local organizations, schools, and healthcare providers. They enable a united stance on drug challenges and gather valuable feedback from the public. Some collaborative activities are workshops, interactive seminars, and health fairs, which help people of all ages participate in talks about drug prevention and awareness. By leveraging what the community already has, campaigns can reach a wider audience and ensure their messages are shared by reputable sources. In addition, an inclusive method enables community members to discuss their experiences, which helps everyone understand the local drug issues better and choose the best ways to address them. These actions represent a crucial step toward sustainable methods of preventing diseases. Besides, using social media to connect with people can help awareness campaigns become more effective. Thanks to digital communication, local organizations can attract a larger audience and reach younger people who are often influenced by online content. With the help of targeted messages, infographics, and interactive media, these campaigns educate people about the dangers of drug use and provide ways to prevent it. Additionally, digital strategies can help maintain support and share information with people, encouraging them to adopt healthy habits. Using technology in these campaigns enables them to reach a wider audience and stay current with the latest digital developments. This way of working serves as a base for helping communities become informed and able to address substance abuse, by stressing the need for prevention and lowering the risks of drug use (Figure 14.10).

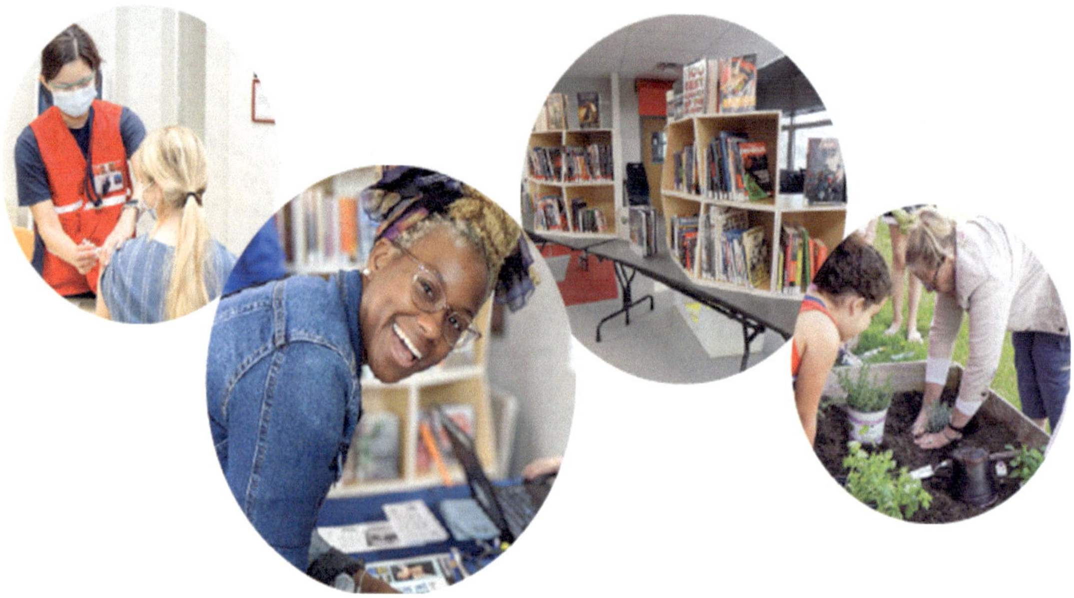

Figure 14.10. Community outreach and awareness campaigns.

Source: https://www.fairfaxcounty.gov/library/sites/library/files/Assets/images/branch-out/fall21/fall21_cc_outreach-banner.jpg.

14.2.3. The Effectiveness of Educational Interventions

To deal with the challenges of preventing and reducing drug use among teens, effective education strategies are critical. Schools that focus on the dangers of drug use can significantly change students' views and actions regarding drug abuse. It was found in the conclusion of the qualitative study that both ex-drug users and health workers are in favor of drug prevention programs in schools. Apart from telling young people about the risks of drug use, such interventions help them discuss rehabilitation and the support they can receive. The engagement of multiple stakeholders—parents, educators, and health services—also amplifies the impact of these learning efforts, underscoring the importance of prioritizing coordinated community efforts to sustain momentum in reducing teen drug use (Tahlil et al., 2021). Besides the usual ways of teaching, public health promotion models are more effective when addressing drug use. The Opioids and Police Safety Study shows how police training can be combined with education to improve the way opioid overdoses are dealt with. In order to treat drug addicts instead of detaining them, the researchers intend to train police personnel on workplace safety and public health issues. This dual focus not only minimizes the immediate health risks associated with drug use but also fosters healthier relationships between law enforcement officials and drug users, providing an environment conducive to successful intervention (Simmons et al., 2021). So, including instructional materials that appeal to professionals from various fields makes drug prevention more effective. It is important to note that the success of EIs to stop drug use also depends on regularly checking and updating the approaches using new information and research. Both school programs and initiatives such as the OPS indicate that it is important to keep an eye on the results and make changes as needed based on what participants say and new issues that arise. Studies that mix different research methods over time give a clear picture of how attitudes, knowledge, and behavior change in participants. The results gathered not only teach the best ways to act but also support using proven methods to address the risks linked to drug use. Therefore, evidence-based interventions underscore the effectiveness and sustainability of education interventions aimed at preventing drug addiction in at-risk populations, ultimately paving the way for healthier communities (Simmons et al., 2021; Tahlil et al., 2021) (Figure 14.11).

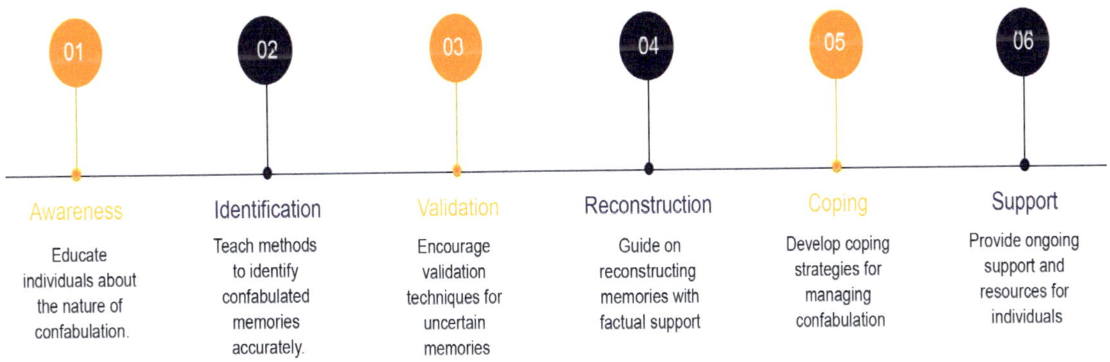

Figure 14.11. The effectiveness of educational interventions.

Source: https://www.slideteam.net/media/catalog/product/cache/1280x720/e/d/educational_interventions_for_confabulation_ppt_guidelines_acp_slide01.jpg.

14.3. Policy and Legislation

It is essential to create and carry out effective policies and laws to reduce the risks of drug use. They established a method for managing drug-related health issues, ensuring that actions are based on science and ethics. These policies are effective because they can be changed as new scientific findings and health trends appear. For instance, professional organizations, such as the European Society of Cardiology, have emphasized the need for health professionals to consider guidelines that reflect updated clinical knowledge while exercising their judgment (Visseren et al., 2021). By incorporating contemporary research and best practices, regulations can be developed to enhance public health and meet the specific needs of individual communities. Also, public health laws should consider the different social and economic factors that lead to drug use and health risks. This is especially necessary in helping developing countries, since not having enough healthcare facilities and enough medicine can make the issue worse. As highlighted in various studies, inappropriate practices surrounding antimicrobial use can lead to resistance, emphasizing the importance of targeted interventions within local contexts (James et al., 2017). By understanding the differences among regions, it becomes possible to create policies that address drug problems and also help communities become aware of their health and how to protect it. In the end, different stakeholders need to cooperate to make sure drug-related policies are carried out and enforced. For policies to be comprehensive, healthcare workers, lawmakers, community groups, and people dealing with drug use should be involved. If policies are developed with the input of many people, they are more likely to be accepted by the public and followed. Such action can also help address issues such as stigma that prevent successful intervention. Policymakers must ensure that legislation is not only evidence-based but also considers the socioeconomic dynamics that influence drug use (Visseren et al., 2021). When stakeholders from various sectors come together, sound policies can be developed to address risks and prevent substance misuse, ultimately benefiting the community's health.

14.3.1. Overview of Drug-Related Laws and Regulations

It is necessary to understand the rules and regulations about drugs to manage drug abuse and prevention. The Controlled Substances Act of the United States ranks drugs according to their abuse, medical benefits, and level of risk, which determines the laws around their use. The system influences the mode of prescription writing by HCPs and the law enforcers' approach to addressing drug use crimes.

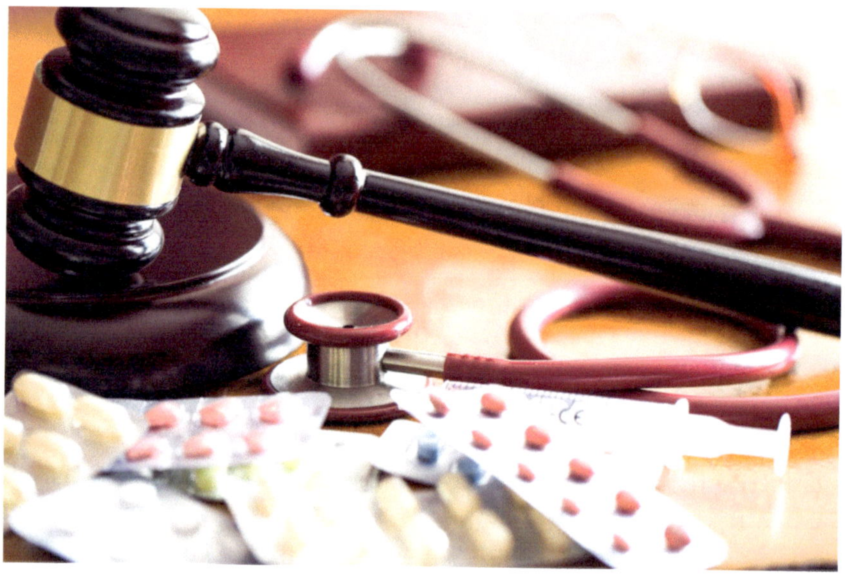

Figure 14.12. Overview of drug-related laws and regulations.

Source: https://cdn.glasspress.io/health-street.net/blog/federal-vs-state-drug-laws-image-featured.jpg.

The opioid crisis has caused people to try to change these regulations, which has resulted in thinking about making it easier to get buprenorphine and methadone. With a focus on public health rather than punishment, these modifications seek to combat the dangers of drug abuse and implement a more compassionate method of treating addiction. (Alexander et al., 2020). Due to the COVID-19 pandemic, drug-related issues have become easier to notice, and laws should be updated when emergencies occur. In particular, the Substance Abuse and Mental Health Services Administration (SAMHSA) has released new guidelines that support the transfer of patients to take-home methadone maintenance regimens, recognizing the necessity of reducing in-person encounters during the pandemic. These policy changes mean that people are accepting new drug laws, which provide treatment to patients and lower the risks from addiction and overdose. Where regulations are obstacles to effective treatment and care, regulatory agencies ought to work in conjunction with policymakers in a manner that will see resources and support reach those with substance use disorders to build patient-centered care amidst a crisis (Alexander et al., 2020). Telehealth has also led to a significant shift in how drug policies are implemented. Thanks to temporary waivers, HCPs can now prescribe controlled substances using telemedicine, which has made it simpler for people with addiction to receive the necessary help. They also reveal that more people now recognize that underprivileged individuals should not be prevented from accessing healthcare. Since the rules are constantly changing, both patients and providers should be looked after when using drugs that are not approved by standard methods. Suppose drug legislation aims to make access and safety a priority. In that case, it will result in policies that help many people avoid risks and improve treatment for substance use disorders in different groups (Figure 14.12).

14.3.2. Impact of Policy on Drug Use Rates

Different areas are affected by drug use because of the various rules and regulations regarding drugs and their treatment. The COVID-19 pandemic made policymakers realize that current rules for opioid treatment programs had to be changed right away. During the pandemic, allowing patients to take methadone at home was important since it helped them keep to their treatment plans. As a result of these changes, people could access treatment more easily, and the efforts to solve the opioid crisis were maintained when the risk of relapse was higher. Furthermore, the incorporation of telehealth services facilitated continued care for individuals with substance use disorders, further illustrating how policy adaptations can meaningfully influence treatment engagement and outcomes, thereby reshaping drug use patterns across populations affected by addiction (Alexander et al., 2020). Certain treatment approaches, including methadone maintenance treatment (MMT), have been shown to dramatically reduce drug-related risk behaviors in high-risk populations, including injection drug users (IDUs). When more people get access to MMT, there is likely to be a decrease in drug use and HIV transmission. The review of the evidence revealed that MMT has contributed to less injecting drug use and sharing of syringes, which are significant causes of HIV. This connection emphasizes the importance of treatment accessibility and adherence, as enhanced support systems can lead to improved health outcomes (Karki et al., 2018). Overall, policymakers ought to realize that MMT can solve addiction problems and also prevent the adverse effects of drug use. Additionally, incorporating information from various treatment methods can facilitate the development of effective policies. As a result of the opioid crisis, people are now thinking about harm reduction methods such as exchanging needles and providing naloxone, which can save someone from an opioid overdose. The purpose of these strategies is to reduce the risks of drug use by promoting health care rather than punishing people. It has been discovered that regions with effective harm reduction strategies deal with fewer drug-related issues and deaths. By creating supportive environments that prioritize treatment over criminalization, evidence suggests that policy can effectively alter the landscape of drug use within populations, fostering healthier communities and reducing the overall impact of substance use (Alexander et al., 2020). Therefore, coming up with strategies in public health can significantly help to reduce substance use disorders and prevent them in the future (Figure 14.13).

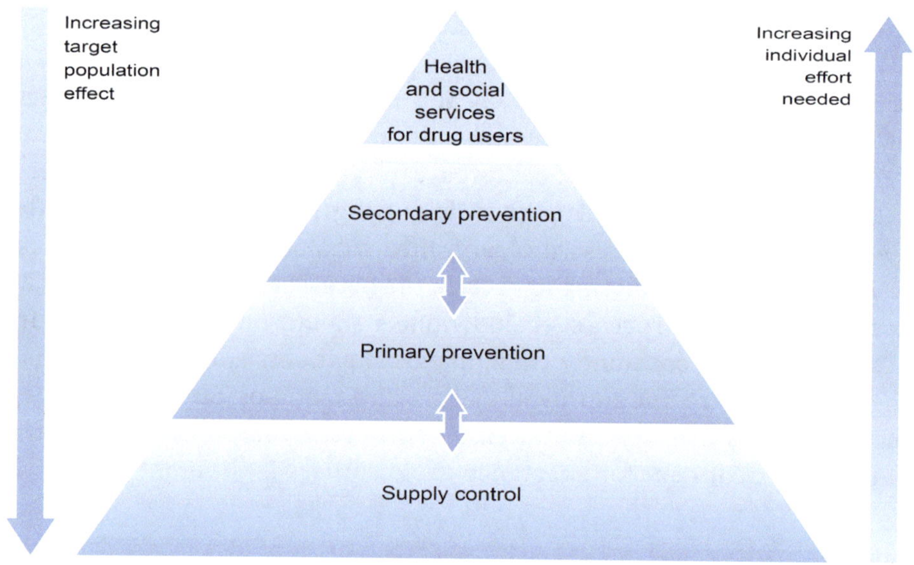

Figure 14.13. Impact of policy on drug use rates.

Source: https://els-jbs-prod-cdn.jbs.elsevierhealth.com/cms/attachment/4e36587a-c88a-479b-bebb-6321bb9c50d6/gr1_lrg.jpg.

14.3.3. The Role of Harm Reduction Policies

Harm reduction approaches are critical in the area of preventing drug use and its risks, as they provide valuable solutions to prevent the adverse effects of substance use. Harm reduction methods realize that drug use is not simple and instead focus on offering education and support to solve the issue. The primary focus of harm reduction programs is to ensure users' safety by encouraging them to discuss their actions and make informed decisions. A good example is needle-exchange programs, which help prevent infectious diseases and also provide users with access to other health services, leading us to focus on all aspects of harm reduction in public health. Because of the controversy, applying such a strategy helps people use drugs with more understanding and gives them ways to recover. Also, the introduction of harm reduction policies encourages drug consumers to adopt protective habits. It has been found that individuals use different techniques to manage their drug intake so that they can stay safe and reduce the risks. They may involve checking the quality of drugs, giving correct doses, and treating adverse effects, which lets users handle drug use more safely. It is helpful for policymakers and health workers to isolate these strategies because it gives them details to create programs that address the needs of each group. These targeted approaches can make preventive interventions more potent and a solid boost for the overall goals of harm reduction programs, as illustrated in studies on snorted cocaine users (Pinz et al., 2024). Besides, harm reduction needs to be seen as both a collection of strategies and a new approach to handling substance use disorders. Instead of focusing solely on making something illegal, harm reduction programs align with both public health and human rights. Because of this philosophy, different prevention and treatment programs can be developed to meet the needs of people in various communities. Additionally, when harm reduction interventions are effective, they involve collaboration among health experts, various community groups, and users, which helps everyone work together to achieve better outcomes. As emphasized in the latest reviews, this model promotes education and awareness about substance use, and in turn, is an integral aspect of mental healthcare for affected individuals (İkbal, 2024). The use of this approach makes harm reduction practices a main support for fighting the public health problems caused by drugs.

14.4. Risk Factors for Drug Use

It is essential to know the risk factors for drug use to prevent and reduce risks for adolescents. Several factors, including family life and the influence of friends, play a significant role in making someone vulnerable to substance use. In such cases, adolescents can learn to accept drug use as normal because of their surroundings. Besides, friends and other people in the same age group can push us, making it feel normal to try drugs. These types of social situations play a key role in whether someone uses drugs, which means special attention should be given to them. Public health campaigns that help families and encourage good relationships with peers can make youth more resistant to drug use and try to break the cycle of these dangerous social habits. Also, the characteristics of each person have a significant impact on their possibility of using drugs. Many times, anxiety and depression are linked to substance use because people may use drugs to help themselves feel better. Besides, people who are impulsive and like excitement are more likely to experiment with drugs. In addition, when co-occurring disorders are present, the treatment process becomes more complicated since both mental health and substance use must be treated at the same time. An increasing number of acute drug overdose and poisoning cases, particularly involving opioids, show that personal characteristics should be taken into consideration while addressing these problems. As a result, primary prevention should provide mental health care and education to those most likely to use drugs, so they learn better ways to manage problems and decide on using drugs wisely. Besides, factors in society, such as income and the ability to attend school, have a significant impact on drug use patterns among people. When people have a low socioeconomic status, they are more likely to be exposed to violence and instability, which may lead them to use drugs as a way to cope. In addition, when people do not have proper access to knowledge and support, they may continue to abuse drugs. According to recent research, places with a lot of unemployment and poverty tend to have more opioid-use disorders, demonstrating a clear link that must be noticed. Prevention can be achieved by ensuring that everyone has access to education and employment opportunities, as well as by utilizing harm reduction methods specifically designed for disadvantaged communities. As a result, if resources are used to tackle these systemic factors, the risk of drug use can be greatly lowered among many populations.

14.4.1. Individual Risk Factors (e.g., Genetics, Mental Health)

The interaction between individual risk factors, particularly psychiatric and genetic, is central to the understanding of drug use and prevention. Genetic risk factors may have a significant influence on a person's susceptibility to substance abuse disorders, and therefore, some groups may be especially vulnerable as a result of their genotype. Genetic variation has been shown to affect how the body metabolizes drugs, altering the subjective effects felt and possibly increasing the risk of abuse. The studies have also established that family patterns, as indicated by family histories of drug use, can be a context where similar patterns emerge in offspring. Therefore interventions aimed at them need to target these genetic influences in prevention. Mental illness is one of the important individual risk factors for drug use, with depression, anxiety, and post-traumatic stress disorder being disorders that push individuals towards drugs as self-medication. Drugs serve as a temporary solution to psychological suffering for most, but it is a process of escalation that exacerbates mental illness in the longer term. Effective prevention programs must incorporate mental health care since the resolution of underlying psychological issues is imperative in avoiding substance abuse. Through the delivery of mental health care in drug prevention interventions, health professionals are better placed to pursue a more holistic approach that promotes general well-being and discourages drug use as a coping mechanism. The development of comprehensive prevention strategies requires an understanding of these differentiated risk factors so that drug use may be addressed to maximum impact. Focusing on genetic and psychiatric concerns, policymakers and clinicians can develop interventions with maximum impact that target at-risk populations in addition to providing educational and supportive directives. Interventions that educate one about the role of genetic susceptibility and mental illness in drug use patterns can empower them in terms of making informed decisions. Furthermore, clinicians need to be informed about the interaction of these risk factors and be able to adjust their practices accordingly. This approach fosters a more comprehensive understanding of prevention and drug risk reduction, ultimately leading to improved health outcomes for individuals and communities overall (Figure 14.14).

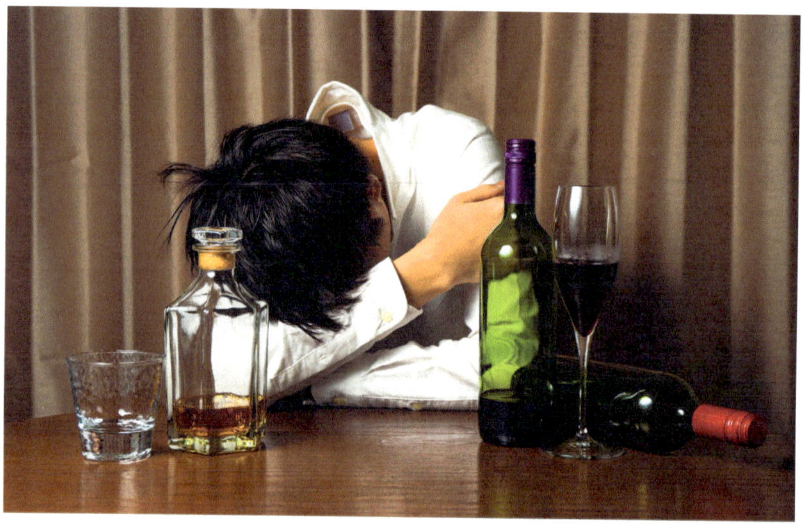

Figure 14.14. Individual risk factors (e.g., genetics, mental health).

Source: https://www.recoveryinmotion.com/wp-content/uploads/2019/02/risk-factors-for-addiction.jpeg.

14.4.2. Environmental Risk Factors (e.g., Family, Peers)

The way a family functions can significantly affect someone's risk of using drugs, depending on whether the family is supportive or not. Open discussion, trust, and mutual help in a family often act as a barrier to drug abuse. On the other hand, families that are full of conflict, neglect, or have a past of substance abuse can put individuals in more danger. When parents use drugs to cope with stress, children might think this is a proper way to handle difficulties. In addition, how much parents watch over and take part in their children's lives can have a significant impact on their drug use habits. Effective parenting strategies that emphasize monitoring, engagement, and clear expectations help in minimizing exposure to drug-using peers, thus playing a pivotal role in prevention efforts aimed at reducing drug use among youth (N/A, 2023). Another significant environmental component that increases the chance of drug use, particularly in adolescence, is peer influence. When people become teenagers, their friends have a bigger impact on their attitude and behavior about using drugs. When it is normal for peers to experiment with drugs, some people may try them in hopes of fitting in. It is shown by research that young people who spend time with others who abuse drugs are more likely to do the same. Because of peer pressure, some may give up their own judgment and start using drugs to fit in with their friends. Therefore, fostering peer networks that prioritize positive behaviors and healthy choices becomes crucial in drug prevention strategies, aiming to create social environments resistant to the allure of drug use (Paul et al., 2017). Programs and schools in the community help address the risks associated with family and peer groups. Schools may include drug prevention classes that teach students how to make informed decisions, develop resilience, and feel more empowered in their communities. In addition, giving students the chance to participate in clubs, sports, and various group activities helps them avoid spending time with drug users. Workshops and counseling services that support families can help mitigate the risks associated with family problems. By addressing the multifaceted dimensions of environmental risk factors, targeted prevention efforts can cultivate resilience among youth, equipping them with the skills needed to navigate peer pressure and familial challenges effectively (N/A, 2023) (Figure 14.15).

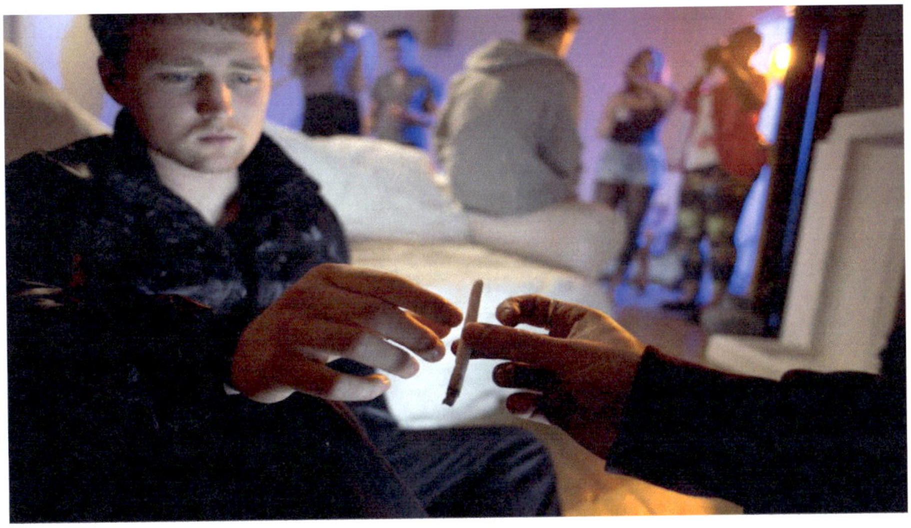

Figure 14.15. Environmental risk factors (e.g., family, peers).

Source: https://cdn-prod.medicalnewstoday.com/content/images/articles/323/323467/peer-pressure-drugs.jpg.

14.4.3. Socioeconomic Factors Influencing Drug Use

Socioeconomic status plays an important role in influencing drug abuse patterns in various groups, both at the individual and at the community levels. In the majority of cases, individuals of lower socioeconomic status are more susceptible to drug abuse since they are exposed to less education, fewer employment opportunities, and access to health care services. These limitations will create a scenario where drug usage is utilized as a coping mechanism for stressors such as economic instability, social deprivation, or inadequate support systems. Inability to secure a consistent job or decent income may lead individuals to find solace through substance use and thereby perpetuate an addiction and socioeconomic inequality. Poor communities are confronted in a way that requires multidimensional interventions to restrict access to drugs and provide alternatives that promote vocational and educational opportunities to combat the root causes of drug use and facilitate recovery instead (Visseren et al., 2021). Furthermore, in certain socioeconomic circumstances, drug use cannot be explained without taking into account social networks and community dynamics. Peer and family patterns seem to encourage young individuals to engage in drug-trying behavior in settings where drug use is common. Normalization of drug use by such a group of peers can reduce perceived risk and result in the experimentation of substances as a normative practice. This socialization is particularly evident in economically downtrodden communities where there are minimal positive role models and where involvement in illegal activities becomes a survival tactic. Prevention initiatives need to address these dynamics within the community by fostering healthy relationships and mentoring programs that discourage teenagers from getting involved in drugs. Consequently, education-focused initiatives fostered in the community, highlighting social responsibility and emotional strength, can be instrumental in preventing drug use (Alexander et al., 2020). Systemic determinants of drug use, including the provision of public policy and access to health care, also have a significant influence on drug use patterns across various socioeconomic groups. Policies that lack proper health care coverage can foster drug-related problems among low-income populations. Denial of access to substance use treatment and mental health services perpetuates cycles of addiction, leaving individuals untreated and increasingly entrenched in dependence. Furthermore, harsh drug policies are likely to disproportionately weigh upon marginalized groups, continuing to enmesh drug criminalization with socioeconomic concerns. Prevention efforts are necessary to ensure that policy changes fully address criminal justice concerns, prioritizing treatment over criminalization and promoting equal access to healthcare resources for all socioeconomic strata. By creating a favorable policy environment that expands opportunity for prevention, treatment, and recovery services, we can combat system disparities that fuel drug use and promote healthier communities (Visseren et al., 2021).

14.5. Strategies for Prevention

Developing and using effective ways to prevent drug use is very important when dealing with adolescents. In this context, education is crucial, mainly in secondary schools, because young people there are more at risk of substance abuse. Programs, such as those described by Skager (2013), emphasize the importance of providing honest, reality-based information through interactive and engaging methods. By paying attention to what teenagers go through and forming a supportive community for them, these initiatives help students make informed decisions about what is best for them. Besides, using restorative practices in schools for discipline encourages students to take responsibility and get support from the community, rather than face harsh punishments, which helps create a better environment for personal development and resisting drugs. It is also important for healthcare, education, and community organizations to join forces in the strategies for preventing drug use. As a result, preventive steps are well-integrated and become part of people's daily routines. For example, health systems can make sure that people in the community learn about the dangers of drug use by organizing regular outreach activities. In the same way, schools can collaborate with nearby health agencies to organize workshops that explain the physical and mental effects of substance abuse. When these efforts are combined, people gain a good understanding of drugs, and stigma is reduced, which helps to encourage discussions and stop youth from trying drugs. It is also necessary to focus on the main risk factors connected to drug use as part of preventative strategies. Mental health problems, a person's economic situation, and family life are important factors that increase the risk of substance abuse. For instance, in surgical settings where the management of acute pain is concerned, as mentioned by Baratta et al. (2016), recognizing the risk of opioid dependence is crucial. If we focus on mental health screenings, family support, or financial assistance, it can significantly lower the number of people using drugs. If we focus on these core issues, prevention strategies turn into systems that help people and encourage them to live healthily (Figure 14.16).

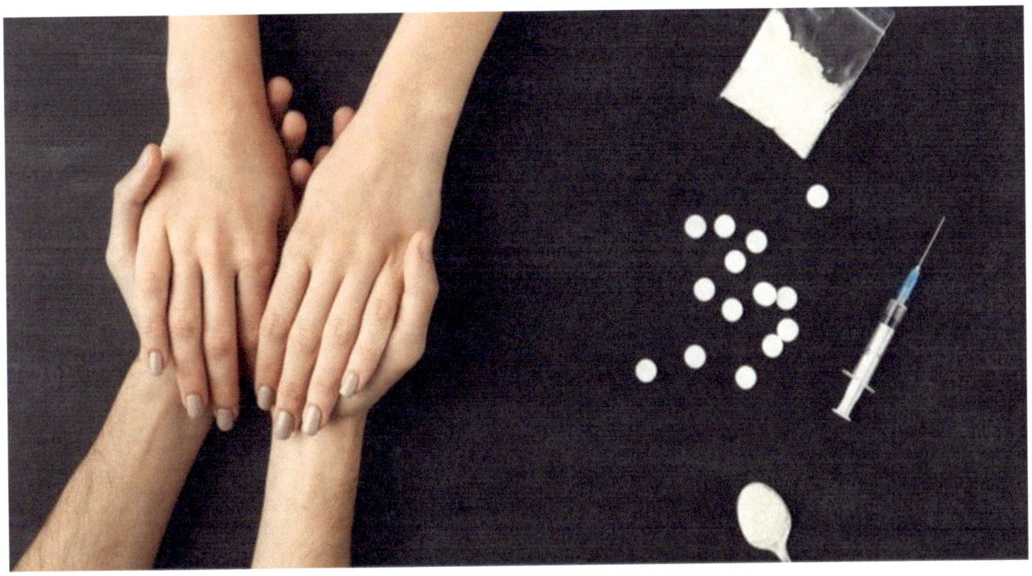

Figure 14.16. Strategies for prevention.

Source: https://www.thewilloughatnaples.com/wp-content/uploads/Shutterstock_1061638367.jpg.

14.5.1. Early Intervention Programs

Implementation of early intervention programs is crucial in drug prevention and risk reduction. Early intervention programs are intended to identify and act on alcohol or drug use disorders early, when they are not yet magnified into significant issues. The central idea behind early intervention is to provide timely intervention that lowers the potential for drug harm. These programs also typically include education components that increase awareness of the risk factors involved in substance use, enabling individuals to make informed choices. Moreover, early intervention programs often rely on community resources, fostering coordination to support social support systems that are essential for individuals at risk. Through their early focus on substance use behavior, these programs not only improve preventive health behaviors but can trigger significant declines in healthcare spending for the treatment of severe drug disorders. Responsiveness and adaptability to meet the wide range of population needs are among the most important elements of effective early intervention programs. Specialized intervention design is the evidence suggesting that it dramatically increases success by taking into account individual and community contexts. For instance, youth programs may have school-based components that are amplified by peer influence, while adult-oriented programs utilize workplace programs or community health screens. Through their responsiveness to the unique contexts from which members arrive, these programs are more effective in terms of engagement and retention. Further, early intervention strategies constantly evolve due to ongoing research on drug use patterns and demographic shifts.

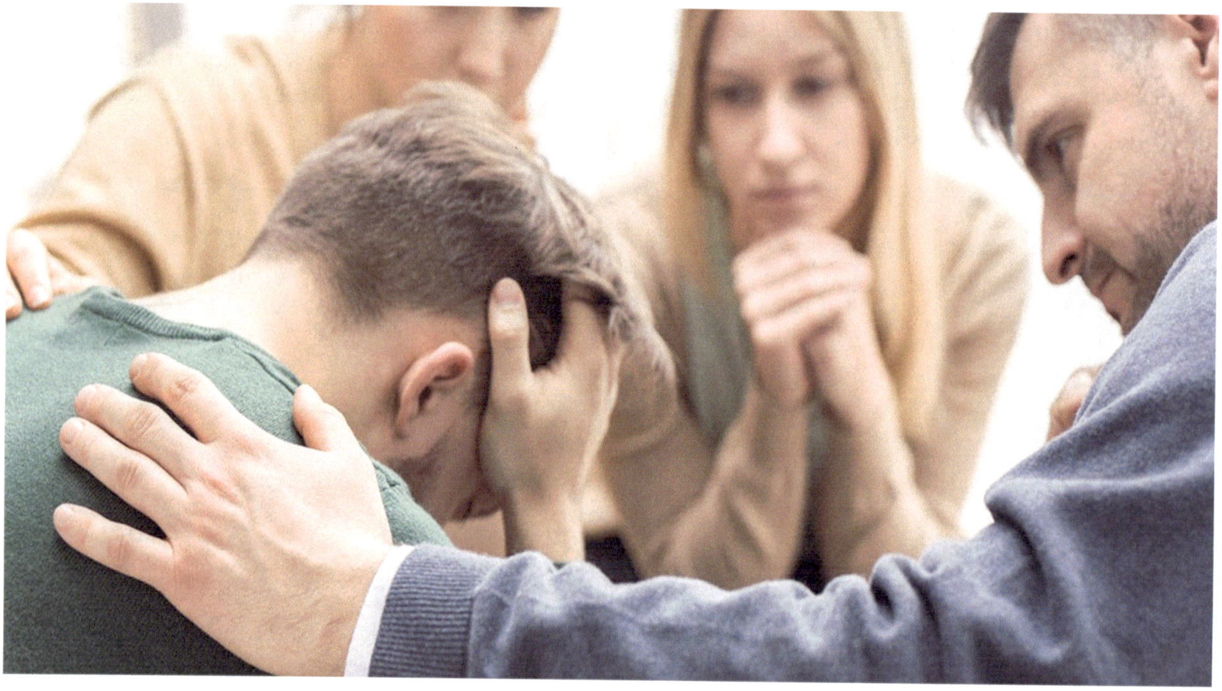

Figure 14.17. Early intervention programs.

Source: https://1.bp.blogspot.com/-qygds60PS7Q/YPpvzSPNyYI/AAAAAAAAACQ/FBy4CDs5a905sLy_s7mblkOeEpBscasuwCLcBGAsYHQ/w1200-h630-p-k-no-nu/intervention-strategies-for-drug-addiction-1200x600.jpg.

A key factor in such flexibility is the process of data gathering and evaluation, enabling instant assessment of the program's effectiveness. Such a dynamic feature increases the scope for ongoing improvement within the context of preventing substance use. The functioning of HCPs in early intervention programs cannot be overemphasized. Health professionals such as physicians, nurses, and counselors are at the forefront of recognizing early signs of substance abuse and can refer early to appropriate resources. They are equipped to provide overall evaluations in consideration of the physical and psychological aspects of drug use. The interdisciplinary programs also cater to multidisciplinary practice and teamwork, which is paramount in formulating individualized care plans. This relationship does not extend to the healthcare settings; for example, agreements with schools can make spaces where adolescents feel secure talking about substance use. Finally, integration of HCPs into early intervention programs is key to ensuring identification of drug use is guaranteed, as well as guaranteeing that assistance is being provided where necessary so that individuals are actively moving through difficulties before they are settled (Figure 14.17).

14.5.2. Support Systems and Counseling Services

Having support and counseling services is very important for preventing and lowering the risk of drug use. The systems are put in place to offer individuals advice and support while dealing with substance use and recovery. If compassionate counseling is available, individuals can notice how they use substances and learn ways to deal with stress and triggers. Additionally, being part of a support group enables individuals to discuss their challenges and feel encouraged by others who are experiencing the same difficulties. This is very important since it helps people with addiction avoid feeling alone and judged by others.

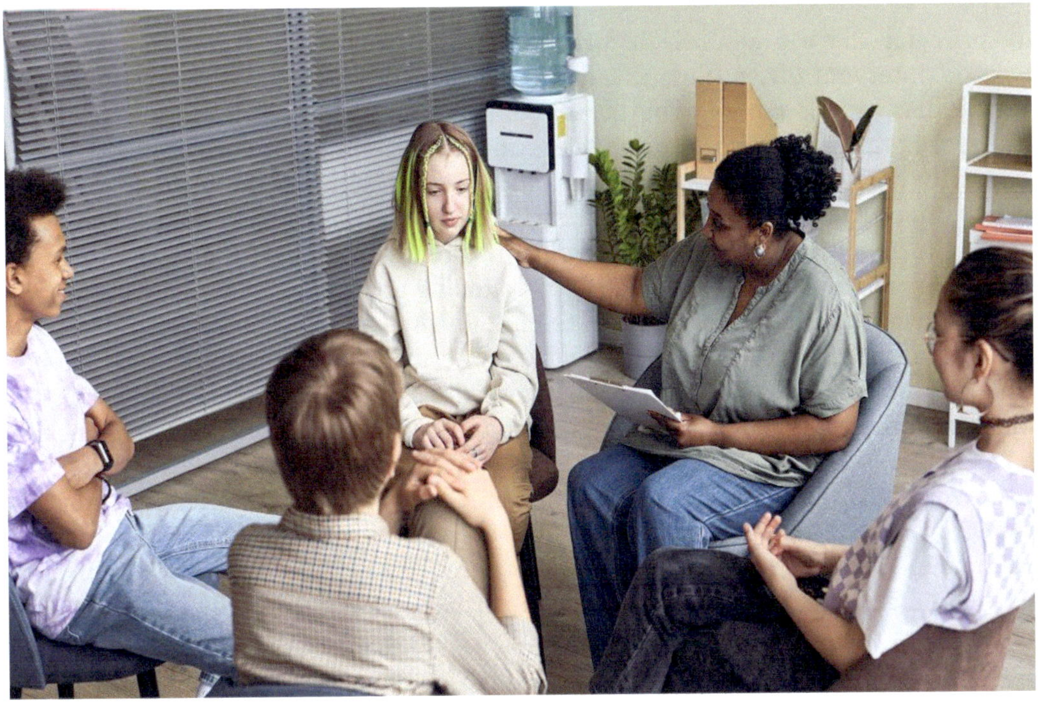

Figure 14.18. Support systems and counselling services.

Source: https://openminds.org.au/wp-content/uploads/2022/12/mental-health-support.jpeg.

Support groups are extremely helpful in encouraging people to share and in supporting early actions that lead to lasting recovery. Using evidence-based approaches is important in counseling for dealing with substance use disorders. Counselors trained in the specifics of addiction can utilize various therapeutic approaches, including cognitive-behavioral therapy (CBT) and motivational interviewing (MI), to tailor their interventions to individual needs. Taking this personalized path makes it easier for a person to see their strengths and weaknesses and motivates them to improve. When people have access to trained specialists and a planned treatment, they are more likely to handle life's problems without using drugs. Increasingly, these counseling services are utilizing technology, such as telehealth, to enable clients to receive help from anywhere and continue to receive regular care. While support and counseling matters, their results depend on how well the community provides healthcare and access to resources. For example, integrating support services with healthcare services can make it easier for people to access help. If healthcare providers, policymakers, and community organizations collaborate, it is possible to establish a system that promotes health equity and provides access to treatment for those who need it most. Moreover, studies and reports nowadays recognize the significance of comprehensive case management and emphasize that addressing social factors, such as housing and employment, is crucial for recovery. Such collaborative approaches underscore the vital role of a coordinated community response in preventing drug use and supporting individuals on their recovery journeys François et al., 2019; Alexander et al., 2020) (Figure 14.18).

14.5.3. Role of Healthcare Providers in Prevention

Healthcare providers have a key role in prevention and drug use risk reduction as enablers of evidence-based interventions within the healthcare setting. They are optimally positioned to identify individuals at risk through routine screenings and assessments, which can lead to early intervention. For instance, healthcare providers utilizing screening measures can identify substance use disorders or drug use-related complications. This proactive strategy enables providers to introduce the topic of drug use and its effects, establishing an open and trusting environment necessary for effective prevention. By being such trusted members of the community, healthcare providers not only improve patient outcomes by reducing the incidence of drug abuse but also act in aid of more macro-level policies that aim to contain the societally destructive consequences of drug-related issues. In addition to individual evaluations, medical professionals are also responsible for implementing preventive measures within healthcare systems. Through participation in quality improvement initiatives, like the screening of ICU patients at risk for delirium, clinicians can directly deal with drug use-related complications. For example, the application of a sleep-wake cycle bundle has been shown to substantially lower ICU delirium rates, reflecting an effective intervention in a high-risk environment (Bennett et al., 2015). These types of program reflect the commitment of healthcare staff to continuous improvement by adherence to best practice. Their involvement in program development ensures that prevention of drug use is not an individual intervention but a sustained process with the support of systematic assessment and adaptation, and thus meeting the multifaceted character of drug use problems in healthcare. Furthermore, education is a critical aspect of the healthcare provider's role in drug abuse prevention. Providers are not only direct service providers but also educators and advocates for their patients. By equipping themselves with current knowledge regarding the treatment and prevention of substance abuse, medical professionals are able to educate patients on the risks of drug abuse properly, the importance of adhering to prescribed medication, and alternatives to treating pain or nervousness without the aid of addictive drugs. Through this dual function as treatment and education, patients become empowered to make well-informed decisions concerning their health and wellness. The call for additional training and support for healthcare staff in this area highlights their responsibility to develop a culturally sensitive and skilled patient population, ultimately contributing to the broader goal of drug harm reduction (Devine et al., 2020).

14.6. Harm Reduction Approaches

Using harm reduction methods has become a key part of how public health tries to reduce the risks linked to drugs. Harm reduction is different from traditional abstinence-only models because it tries to minimize any harm from drug use, rather than aiming to stop it completely. It admits that drug use is affected by many social, economic, environmental, and psychological elements. Harm reduction provides individuals with helpful advice, so they can decide how to use drugs more safely. Programs that emphasize the provision of clean syringes, supervised consumption spaces, and education on drug purity exemplify the principles of harm reduction, which promote safer practices without stigmatizing users or denying their autonomy (Pinz et al., 2024). Harm reduction strategies are effective, as seen by the actions of cocaine users. An examination of experienced cocaine snorters showed that they have a range of ways to protect themselves from the risks of using cocaine. Part of these strategies was to check the quality of substances, manage the amount used, and use tactics to reduce the risks of using several drugs together. If people take these precautions, they can significantly lower their chances of facing risks, legal issues, or health problems. This study demonstrates the innate potential of drug users to manage their experiences in a responsible manner, indicating that providing information and tools to drug users improves their capacity to reduce risks and safeguard their health. (Pinz et al., 2024). In addition, promoting harm reduction is in line with public health goals that see substance use disorders as a problem that should be handled in many ways. If harm reduction is added to current treatment and prevention plans, HCPs can give a complete answer to drug use problems. This way of working helps people overcome the effects of substance use and also motivates them to live healthier lives and, if needed, look into abstinence. The main factor in the success of harm reduction is how well it supports users, respects their choices, and encourages partnership between healthcare providers and those dealing with substance use. As such, harm reduction represents a crucial paradigm shift towards a more compassionate and pragmatic response to drug-related challenges within society (İkbal, 2024).

14.6.1. Definition and Principles of Harm Reduction

Harm reduction is a liberal drug policy ideology that aims to lower the negative consequences of drug consumption rather than solely aiming at the eradication of drug use. The central premise of this ideology is that individuals will consume drugs regardless of the risks involved, and therefore, harm reduction models attempt to provide realistic solutions that can lower harm. Examples include measures such as needle exchange programs, safe consumption sites, and naloxone dispensing for Opioid Overdose prevention. Harm reduction, as an opioid-oriented public health strategy, appreciates the multidimensionality of addiction and addresses determinants of the social environment that increase drug harm. Therefore, the application of harm reduction principles not only creates a more humane approach to drug use but also underscores a commitment to improved community health outcomes (Visseren et al., 2021). The harm reduction principles arise from a profound understanding of the drugs use realities in society. One of the guiding principles is to appreciate that abstinence is not the only suitable solution for those who have issues with substance use. Harm reduction offers a route of multiple levels of participation and recovery, and it emphasizes that any action towards safer use of drugs, i.e., using clean needles or accessing support services, can have significant health benefits. In addition, harm reduction efforts are centered on the autonomy and dignity of the individuals by allowing them to exercise their own will over what they do with their drug use. This approach contradicts the often punitive nature of traditional drug policy. It provides a framework that enables users to approach help and intervention more effectively, thereby reducing risks and promoting healthier communities (Rebecca et al., 2020). In addition, harm reduction facilitates extensive education and sensitization efforts that equip individuals with the knowledge they require to manage their drug consumption responsibly. This includes EIs addressing the harms caused by a particular drug, as well as how to embrace safer practices. Public health campaigns for de-stigmatizing drug consumption can encourage individuals to seek assistance without fear of censure or prosecution. Harm reduction can construct an integrative model embracing these tenets in collaboration with healthcare practitioners, community agencies, and policymakers. This community approach not only enhances individual safety but also promotes shared social responsibility in dealing with the intricate problems of drug abuse in society (Visseren et al., 2021) (Figure 14.19).

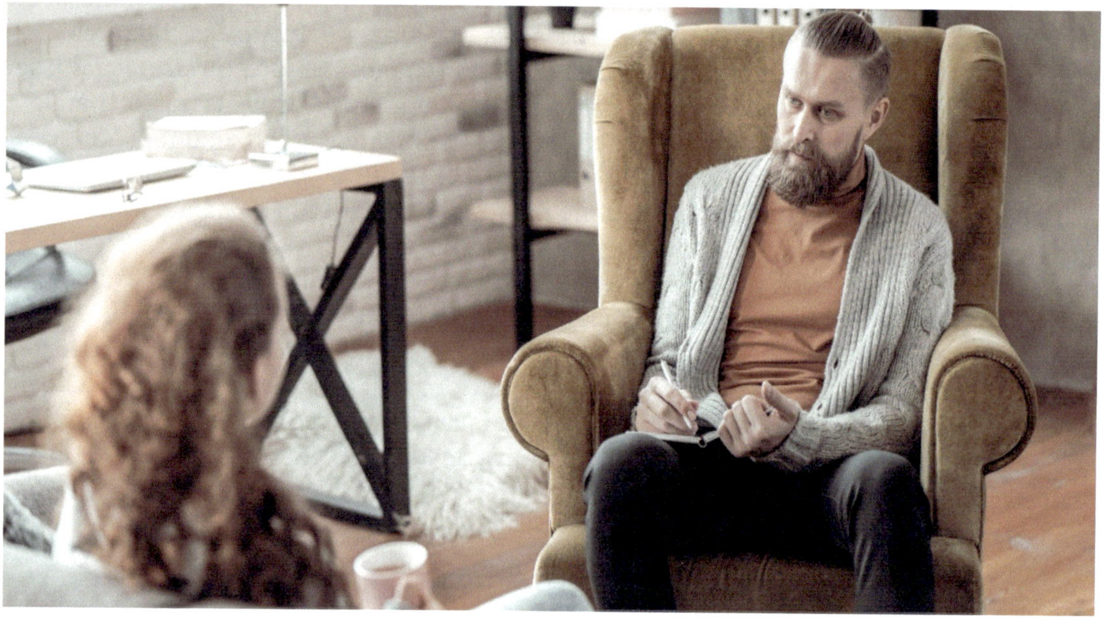

Figure 14.19. Definition and principles of harm reduction.

Source: https://www.northridgeaddiction.com/wp-content/uploads/harm-reduction-therapy.jpg.

14.6.2. Examples of Harm Reduction Strategies (e.g., Needle Exchange)

Harm reduction is a way to reduce the negative consequences of drug use for people's health, social life, and legal status. Needle exchange programs are a well-known example that gives people who take drugs access to clean needles. They support several goals: they lower the risk of HIV and hepatitis C infections, encourage safe injection habits, and help people get healthcare. By exchanging needles, these programs assist users in avoiding immediate health hazards, which in turn motivates them to seek additional assistance and ultimately leads to treatment and rehabilitation.Therefore, these programs are important for public health, as they prefer to show empathy towards people who use drugs instead of punishing them. In addition, harm reduction includes supervised consumption sites that give drug users a safe place to use under the supervision of medical staff. They aim to save lives and encourage safe drug use by giving immediate access to medical help and assistance. It has been found that supervised consumption sites lead to less drug use in public areas and fewer deaths by overdose. Moreover, these centers usually help users get involved with the larger healthcare system by connecting them to services for addiction and mental health. Therefore, supervised consumption sites tackle current dangers and also assist in long-term rehabilitation by offering healthcare and support services that fit the needs of those dealing with addiction. In recent times, technology is helping to reduce harm among people who use drugs. Due to the COVID-19 pandemic, healthcare systems have had to adapt and introduce new approaches, including digital platforms that provide access to harm reduction resources. Virtual environments are being utilized to provide education on safe drug use, offer telehealth consultations, and distribute essential supplies. Due to digital transformation, more people can benefit from harm reduction, as it enables those who may not have access to regular healthcare services. The integration of technology into harm reduction strategies emphasizes the importance of adaptability in the face of evolving public health challenges and underscores the potential for reaching a broader population through innovative models of care, as illustrated by trends in healthcare observed during the pandemic (Bansal et al., 2022; Magnolini et al., 2022) (Figure 14.20).

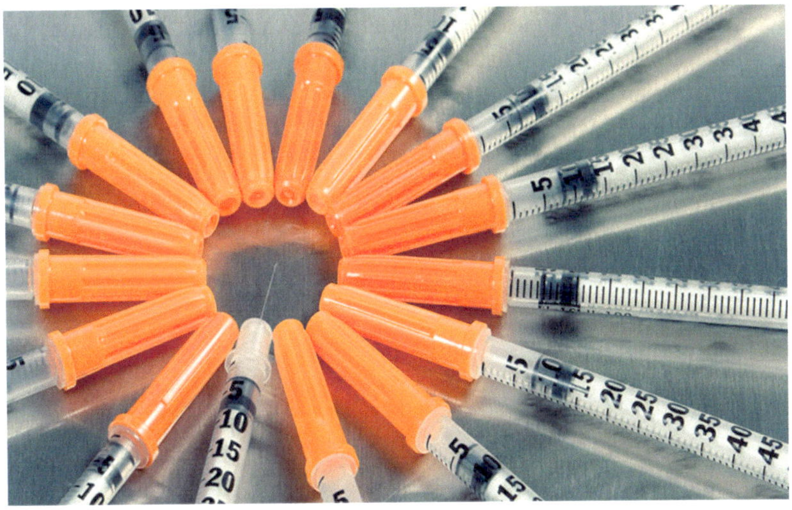

Figure 14.20. Examples of harm reduction strategies (e.g., needle exchange).

Source: https://needleexchangeredlandssunshinecoast.wordpress.com/wp-content/uploads/2022/03/hero_syringe_940x529.jpg.

14.6.3. Evaluation of Harm Reduction Effectiveness

The measurement of the effectiveness of drug use as a harm reduction is a key component of public health intervention that aims to limit the adverse outcomes of drug taking. Through the application of various methodologies, researchers can quantify the degree to which interventions such as needle exchange programs or drug consumption facilities help to reduce morbidity and mortality among drug users. For instance, when qualitative research and extensive dataset analysis are combined, a comprehensive picture of how harm reduction strategies influence user behavior and health outcomes is provided. Studies have found that individuals involved in harm reduction programs have lower rates of infectious disease and overdose episodes than users without access to such programs. This in-depth evaluation illuminates the importance of evidence-based interventions, which are vital to inform policymakers regarding the efficiency of harm reduction as a viable alternative to prohibitionist approaches to drug use. The upsurge in the trend of emerging substances, such as e-cigarettes, necessitates a critical evaluation of their position in policies of harm reduction. While such devices have become widely marketed as safer alternatives to mainstream tobacco products, their public health implications must be scrutinized. Current evidence has suggested that the introduction of e-cigarettes can perhaps contribute to quitting smoking. However, their unregulated sale and promotion mechanisms might paradoxically promote an increase in nicotine usage by non-smokers and youth. The need for proper regulation of e-cigarettes is paramount as it can avert harm in the form of increased tobacco smoking initiation among young people while enabling these products to be used as quit-smoking aids for current smokers. Failure to properly evaluate and control e-cigarettes may undermine the entire end of harm reduction, and the intricacy of truly curtailing drug-related harm (Lindblom et al., 2015). Finally, assessment of harm reduction interventions also relies on identifying at-risk populations and customizing interventions to match their specific needs. As an encompassing paradigm, it not only optimizes the effectiveness of harm reduction interventions but also enhances involvement in affected drug-using communities. This is achieved by ensuring well-developed partnerships between healthcare providers, social service agencies, and affected persons to ensure interventions are available and culturally sensitive. Additionally, mixed methods involving the use of both quantitative and qualitative data can be employed to determine access barriers and resources among these populations, thereby fueling continuous improvement in programming. Lastly, a sound assessment framework that is informed by the needs of vulnerable populations will yield more effective harm reduction policies that make for an enabling environment for those who are willing to decrease the harms of drug use (Beral et al., 2013).

Summary

Since drug use has many aspects, it is necessary to closely examine how to prevent drug problems and reduce risks for everyone's safety. A good prevention program uses different methods that take into account social, psychological, and environmental reasons for drug use. They should seek to decrease the number of people who start using drugs, as well as make sure users are safe and the effects of substance misuse are limited. Discussions that focus on educating people about the possible risks and outcomes of drug use have a substantial impact on what individuals choose to do. When communities create a safe space for sharing information, people can join forces to reduce the shame linked to drug use and ask for help whenever necessary. When everyone works together, we can lessen the adverse outcomes of drug use and encourage people to live healthier lives. It is essential to continue researching in order to continually improve prevention strategies. Studies on antibiotic resistance and anesthesia complications indicate that new medical approaches and societal changes can help mitigate the risks associated with the use of drugs and medicines. Using advanced techniques to monitor resistance to medications can help doctors and nurses refine the current guidelines for patient care. When stakeholders examine the long-term results of current practices, they can identify and implement more effective strategies. For example, understanding how microbes become resistant can help doctors administer the right amounts of drugs at the right times, which is why being responsive to drug use is important in many areas. Also, when the healthcare, education, and law enforcement sectors collaborate, it greatly helps in preventing and reducing risks. When experts from different fields cooperate, they can easily exchange information, resources, and successful methods, which leads to a more effective way to address drug problems. Community outreach enables stakeholders to focus on the needs of various groups, thereby making prevention and risk reduction programs more effective. Drawing on knowledge from multiple areas can lead to innovative solutions that help combat drug use and promote safety and responsibility. Ultimately, an encompassing and coordinated approach is essential to foster resilience within communities, ensuring that prevention and risk minimization efforts yield sustainable results in drug use management, as shown in the contexts discussed by Bezerra et al. (2024); and Circella et al. (2025).

When discussing how to prevent and reduce risks in drug use, it becomes clear that taking action ahead of time is very important. Rapid response teams are a good example of how to tackle drug-related problems. If a multidisciplinary team, similar to the CLABSI Rapid Response Team, is used, stakeholders can identify and prevent patient-specific problems before they become serious. With this strategy, the number of adverse events decreases because high-risk people are given timely interventions. The focus on predictive modeling and interdisciplinary collaboration exemplifies how systematic approaches can enhance drug safety and reduce associated risks, aligning with broader goals of public health initiatives aimed at preventing substance abuse and ensuring safe practices in treatment contexts (Lauren et al., 2024). Additionally, studying surveillance strategies reveals that prevention measures should be regularly reviewed and adjusted. Results from research, such as the CoV-Surv Study, show why it is essential to continue monitoring groups to identify any potential dangers. With the help of various tests and by engaging the community, public health officials can gather valuable information that informs their strategies and helps save money. It is possible to use this model to prevent drug use by finding out about trends and new problems linked to substance abuse. Such an approach not only aids in determining prevalence rates but also provides insights necessary for policymaking, creating a foundational framework for enhancing the overall effectiveness of drug prevention programs (Deckert et al., 2021). All of this puts together a clearer picture of how to reduce risks when using drugs. Both types of responses stress the need to be flexible and plan ahead to handle the different aspects of drug abuse. Getting healthcare workers and community leaders involved helps create an environment that is conducive to preventive actions. If stakeholders share knowledge and work together, they can handle the factors that contribute to drug misuse. Taking part in such collaborative efforts is necessary to promote prevention and lower the risk of drug-related harm. Combining these strategies provides an opportunity to make significant progress in public health, ensuring that efforts to prevent drug use are well-planned and tailored to the community's needs.

CLOSER LOOK

SOCIO-ECONOMIC CONSEQUENCES CASCADING

Health crises, such as pandemics, chronic disease outbreaks, or widespread mental health disorders, often trigger cascading socio-economic consequences that extend far beyond the immediate medical impacts. When large segments of a population are affected by illness, productivity declines, healthcare costs rise, and economic instability can follow. For individuals, especially those from low-income communities, the financial burden of medical treatment, combined with lost income due to illness or caregiving responsibilities, can push households into poverty. This creates a cycle where poor health leads to economic hardship, which in turn limits access to quality healthcare, nutritious food, and stable housing—further worsening health outcomes.

At the community and national levels, health crises strain public health infrastructure and social services, disrupt education, and reduce workforce participation. For example, the COVID-19 pandemic led to massive job losses, interrupted schooling, and deepened economic disparities, particularly in already vulnerable populations. Small businesses suffered, supply chains collapsed, and healthcare systems were overwhelmed, highlighting how interconnected health and economic stability truly are. These cascading effects often linger long after the immediate crisis has passed, leading to prolonged recovery periods.

Moreover, socio-economic consequences disproportionately impact marginalized groups, exacerbating existing inequalities. Women, minorities, and low-skilled workers often bear the brunt of job insecurity and limited access to healthcare. Policy responses must therefore address both health and socio-economic dimensions—providing universal healthcare access, social safety nets, employment protections, and community support systems. Investing in health resilience is not only a moral imperative but also an economic necessity. Recognizing and preparing for the broader socio-economic impacts of health crises enables more effective, equitable responses and strengthens societal stability in the long term. These cascading consequences remind us that public health and economic health are deeply interdependent, and one cannot thrive without the other.

References

1. Alexander, G. C., Stoller, K. B., Haffajee, R. L., & Saloner, B. (2020). An epidemic in the midst of a pandemic: Opioid use disorder and COVID-19. *Annals of Internal Medicine, 173*(1), 57, 58. https://doi.org/10.7326/m20-1141.
2. Aljefri, A., Nahhs, S. F., Kheimi, R. M., Alhamdan, A. Y., Alharbi, T. S., Alkahtani, S. S., Alajmi, S. T., et al. (2024). An overview of acute drug overdose and poisoning in emergency medicine. *Journal of Healthcare Sciences*. https://www.semanticscholar.org/paper/85858d551c8af0fef0f1253b1b66e52e25a6b08e (accessed on 9 June 2025).
3. Alowais, S. A., Alghamdi, S. S., Alsuhebany, N., Alqahtani, T., Alshaya, A., Almohareb, S. N., Aldairem, A., et al. (2023). Revolutionizing healthcare: The role of artificial intelligence in clinical practice. *BMC Medical Education, 23*. https://doi.org/10.1186/s12909-023-04698-z.
4. Alzheimer's Association. (2023). 2023 Alzheimer's disease facts and figures. *Alzheimer's & Dementia, 19*, 1598–1695. https://doi.org/10.1002/alz.13016.
5. Ayukekbong, J. A., Ntemgwa, M., & Atabe, A. N. (2017). The threat of antimicrobial resistance in developing countries: Causes and control strategies. *Antimicrobial Resistance and Infection Control, 6*. https://doi.org/10.1186/s13756-017-0208-x.
6. Bansal, G., Rajgopal, K., Chamola, V., Xiong, Z., & Niyato, D. (2022). Healthcare in metaverse: A survey on current metaverse applications in healthcare. *IEEE Access, 10*, 119914–119946. https://doi.org/10.1109/access.2022.3219845.
7. Baratta, J. L., Schwenk, E. S., Viscusi, E. R., & Wenzel, R. (2016). Managing opioid-tolerant patients in the perioperative surgical home. https://core.ac.uk/download/46975930.pdf (accessed on 9 June 2025).
8. Bennett, V. (2015). Prevention of ICU delirium through implementation of a sleep promotion bundle. https://core.ac.uk/download/72052389.pdf (accessed on 9 June 2025).
9. Beral, V., Berkel, H. J., Bullard, J., Coleman, M. P., Gulliford, M., Møller, H., & Phekoo, K. (2013). Cancer recording and mortality in the General Practice Research Database and linked cancer registries.
10. Bezerra Bezerra, R. A., Damasceno, J. E. S., Ferreira de Farias, N., & Da Nóbrega Dias, M. (2024). Sedation and laryngospasm in pediatric surgery. *Health and Society*. https://www.semanticscholar.org/paper/1ebd31155406409be554c54729abcf025d328bda (accessed on 9 June 2025).
11. Cacciapuoti, F., Crispo, S., D'Andrea, D., Materazzi, C., Chianese, S., Cotena, S., Gottilla, R., et al. (2025). Dual device intervention for stroke prevention and bradycardia: A case report. *Monaldi Archives for Chest Disease = Archivio Monaldi per le Malattie del Torace*. https://www.semanticscholar.org/paper/d19ca6da1c8ae2e43cb9bc97e7ed94deb607b2f2 (accessed on 9 June 2025).
12. Campbell, S. J., Biritwum, N. K., Woods, G., Velleman, Y., Fleming, F., & Stothard, J. R. (2017). Tailoring water, sanitation, and hygiene (WASH) targets for soil-transmitted helminthiasis and schistosomiasis control. *Trends in Parasitology, 34*, 53–63. https://doi.org/10.1016/j.pt.2017.09.004.
13. Chimezie, R. O., & Uzochukwu, M. E. (2021). Preventing behavioral-risks incidence among school

children: The role of school-based health promotion program. *Journal of Biosciences and Medicines*. https://www.semanticscholar.org/paper/dad5aef2adc0adecb08e3ee7bd6e9343b5275da9 (accessed on 9 June 2025).

14. Chin, B. S. (2024). Prevention and infection control of HIV infection and AIDS. *Journal of the Korean Medical Association*. https://www.semanticscholar.org/paper/0428dc21bebcd4a4113f7ecd9be7e94d086719c0 (accessed on 9 June 2025).

15. Choudhary, E., Jain, S., Mahto, S., & Ahuja, D. (2023). Adverse drug reactions: Identification, prevention and management. *International Journal for Multidisciplinary Research*. https://www.semanticscholar.org/paper/c835120d9f3f5f0880190b0977200d217de15b2c (accessed on 9 June 2025).

16. Circella, E., Lucatello, L., Montanucci, L., Belloli, C., & Capolongo, F. (2025). Simulation of a field condition to evaluate the risk of enrofloxacin-resistant Pasteurella multicide strain selection in food producing rabbits treated via drinking water. *Frontiers in Veterinary Science, 12*. https://www.semanticscholar.org/paper/764e05b8253cdc7cb73448a5f35dc11b973ed3c5 (accessed on 9 June 2025).

17. Deckert, A., Anders, S., De Allegri, M., Nguyen, H., Souares, A., McMahon, S., Boerner, K., et al. (2021). Effectiveness and cost-effectiveness of four different strategies for SARS-CoV-2 surveillance in the general population (CoV-Surv Study): A structured summary of a study protocol for a cluster-randomised, two-factorial controlled trial. *Trials, 22*. https://www.semanticscholar.org/paper/eae7e706fcbaf89abf59f5fed10fe0b216c5aaef (accessed on 9 June 2025).

18. Devine, T., Jordan, J., Knoderer, C., et al. (2020). The value driven pharmacist: Basics of access, cost, and quality (2nd ed.). https://core.ac.uk/download/287886562.pdf (accessed on 9 June 2025).

19. Edwards, L. M., Garcia, L., Murray, T. S., & Kandil, S. B. (2024). Adopting a proactive safety approach: Creating a CLABSI rapid response team. *Pediatric Quality & Safety, 9*. https://www.semanticscholar.org/paper/32ba16aead39572a67d776ba54865ab003c474e7 (accessed on 9 June 2025).

20. Gedik, İ. (2024). A preventive mental health service for substance use disorder: Harm reduction. *Journal of Nursing Care Research*. https://www.semanticscholar.org/paper/dd1897eb39b829c2a34b1c198ac458894e76400d (accessed on 9 June 2025).

21. Glikson, M., Nielsen, J. C., Kronborg, M. B., Michowitz, Y., Auricchio, A., Barbash, I. M., Barrabés, J. A., et al. (2021). 2021 ESC guidelines on cardiac pacing and cardiac resynchronization therapy. *European Heart Journal, 42*, 3427–3520. https://doi.org/10.1093/eurheartj/ehab364.

22. Huynh, H., Valutite, D., Schemelev, A. N., Davydenko, V. S., Ostankova, Y., Truong, T., Tran, T., et al. (2023). Prevalence of HIV-1 drug resistance among early diagnosed HIV-infected children enrolled through the national program for prevention of mother-to-child transmission in Southern and Central Highland provinces—Vietnam within 2017–2021. *HIV Infection and Immunosuppressive Disorders*. https://www.semanticscholar.org/paper/54de65773ca08a5d6ab5b7007089dd73036e07a1 (accessed on 9 June 2025).

23. Karki, P., Shrestha, R., Huedo–Medina, T. B., & Miller, M. D. (2018). The impact of methadone maintenance treatment on HIV risk behaviors among high-risk injection drug users: A systematic review. *Evidence-based Medicine & Public Health, 2*. https://doi.org/10.14800/emph.1229.

24. Lindblom, E. N. (2015). Effectively regulating e-cigarettes and their advertising—and the First Amendment. https://core.ac.uk/download/132075607.pdf (accessed on 9 June 2025).

25. Mach, F., Baigent, C., Catapano, A. L., Koskinas, K. C., Casula, M., Badimón, L., Chapman, M. J., et al. (2019). 2019 ESC/EAS guidelines for the management of dyslipidaemias: Lipid modification to reduce cardiovascular risk. *European Heart Journal, 41*, 111–188. https://doi.org/10.1093/eurheartj/ehz455.

26. Magnolini, R., Falcato, L., Cremonesi, A., Schori, D., & Bruggmann, P. (2022). Fake anabolic androgenic steroids on the black market–A systematic review and meta-analysis on qualitative and quantitative analytical results found within the literature. *BMC Public Health, 22*. https://doi.org/10.1186/s12889-022-13734-4.

27. Perkins, R. B., Guido, R. S., Castle, P. E., Chelmow, D., Einstein, M. H., García, F., Huh, W. K., et al. (2020). 2019 ASCCP risk-based management consensus guidelines for abnormal cervical cancer screening tests and cancer precursors. *Journal of Lower Genital Tract Disease, 24*, 102–131. https://doi.org/10.1097/lgt.0000000000000525.

28. Pinzón-Gómez, C., Bencomo-Cruz López, M., Gamboa Bayona, M. P., & Gantiva, C. (2024). Exploring risk prevention and harm reduction behaviours among snorted cocaine users. *Revita Internacional de Investigación en Adicciones*. https://www.semanticscholar.org/paper/2191d482b1b139d066717579bca302ecdc61537b (accessed on 9 June 2025).

29. Rasu, R., Xavier, C., & Rianon, N. (2025). Dynamic changes in medication burden leading to fall and hospital readmissions in older adults: Toward a strategy for improving risk and managing costs. *Journal of Managed Care & Specialty Pharmacy, 31*(1), 96–100. https://www.semanticscholar.org/paper/3aef5f38e14cfa7a7e2f2c832ee21e71e51d4e62 (accessed on 9 June 2025).

30. Rodrigues, C. M. C., & Plotkin, S. A. (2020). Impact of vaccines: Health, economic and social perspectives. *Frontiers in Microbiology, 11*. https://doi.org/10.3389/fmicb.2020.01526.

31. Sacco, M. A., Gualtieri, S., Santos, A., Mendes, B., & Aquila, I. (2025). Adolescent fentanyl use: Toxicological risks, epidemiological trends, and public health strategies. *Cureus, 17*. https://www.semanticscholar.org/paper/e33b6ee2f054668e20e23adcdd2226062dfd294b (accessed on 9 June 2025).

32. Sikes, R. S. (2016). 2016 guidelines of the American Society of Mammalogists for the use of wild mammals in research and education. *Journal of Mammalogy, 97*, 663–688. https://doi.org/10.1093/jmammal/gyw078.

33. Simmons, J., Elliott, L., Bennett, A. S., Beletsky, L., Rajan, S., Anders, B., & Dastparvardeh, N. (2021). Evaluation of an experimental web-based educational module on opioid-related occupational safety among police officers: Protocol for a randomized pragmatic trial to minimize barriers to overdose response. *JMIR Research Protocols, 11*. https://www.semanticscholar.org/paper/3d86a6ae15236c188ae34bff4f31720b18edaf89 (accessed on 9 June 2025).

34. Sisson, J., Wyatt, T., Guidot, D., Bagby, G., Helander, A., Tønnesen, H., & Spies, C. (2005). Bench to bedside: Mechanisms and consequences of alcohol-altered host defenses. *Alcoholism: Clinical and Experimental Research, 29*(7), 1090–1097. https://www.semanticscholar.org/paper/02cbf22a4fe7194b93ca79a24d8fbed0a00b9629 (accessed on 9 June 2025).

35. Skager, R. (2013). Beyond zero tolerance: A reality-based approach to drug education and school discipline. https://core.ac.uk/download/71363092.pdf (accessed on 9 June 2025).

36. Tahlil, T., & Aiyub, A. (2021). Ex-drug users' and health professionals' perspectives about school-based drug use prevention programs: A qualitative study. *Frontiers in Public Health, 9*. https://www.semanticscholar.org/paper/ca06333482cf9ed2b125ed967cdf5c9e1957188c (accessed on 9 June 2025).

37. Visseren, F. L. J., Mach, F., Smulders, Y. M., Carballo, D., Koskinas, K. C., Bäck, M., Bénétos, A., et al. (2021). 2021 ESC guidelines on cardiovascular disease prevention in clinical practice. *European Heart Journal, 42*, 3227–3337. https://doi.org/10.1093/eurheartj/ehab484.

38. Whelton, P. K., Carey, R. M., Aronow, W. S., Casey, D. E., Collins, K. J., Dennison Himmelfarb, C., DePalma, S. M., et al. (2017). 2017 ACC/AHA/AAPA/ABC/ACPM/AGS/APhA/ASH/ASPC/NMA/PCNA guideline for the prevention, detection, evaluation, and management of high blood pressure in adults: A report of the American College of Cardiology/American Heart Association Task Force on Clinical Practice Guidelines. *Hypertension, 71*. https://doi.org/10.1161/hyp.0000000000000065.

39. Yatham, L. N., Kennedy, S. H., Parikh, S. V., Schaffer, A., Bond, D. J., Frey, B. N., Sharma, V., et al. (2018). Canadian Network for Mood and Anxiety Treatments (CANMAT) and International Society for Bipolar Disorders (ISBD) 2018 guidelines for the management of patients with bipolar disorder. *Bipolar Disorders, 20*(2), 97–170. https://doi.org/10.1111/bdi.12609.

40. Zaoutis, T. (2009). Antibiotic resistance: Who will pay the bills? *Clinical Infectious Diseases, 49*(8), 1185–1186. https://www.semanticscholar.org/paper/049413e739e1143f47ff61da004aaadb3a7a313a (accessed on 9 June 2025).

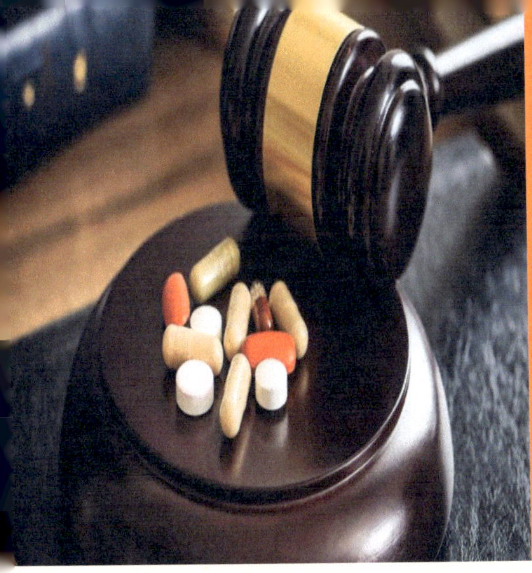

Chapter 15

REGULATORY AND ETHICAL ASPECTS OF DRUG

Contents

Introduction

The production and testing of drugs in the pharmaceutical industry are guided by numerous regulations and ethical guidelines. It is essential for drug companies to consider the public's health, new developments, and financial earnings when adhering to these regulations. Since regulatory agencies, drug firms, and the public all interact in this situation, trust becomes particularly significant because it influences the decision-making process. For instance, National Institute for Health and Care Excellence (NICE) is a real-life example of a regulatory body that must confront complexities and uncertainties when considering drug affordability and efficacy, observing that trust is significant in resolving these concerns and fostering an open atmosphere where pharmaceuticals are considered (Abraham et al., 2015). In addition, the global spread of pharmaceutical research and development, particularly in developing countries, has facilitated adherence to strict ethical and regulatory standards. As more multinational drug companies conduct drug development in Mexico, the ethics of clinical trials have become increasingly important. As a result, these traditions help develop technology and technical skills in the host countries, but also raise important concerns about the strength of their laws and the rights of those participating in trials. Significant challenges are presented as these developing nations strive to balance local traditions with international anticipated ethical standards, thus complicating the global landscape of pharmaceutical research (Santiago-Rodriguez et al., 2025). The way regulation and ethics work together impacts both the main stakeholders and the entire healthcare system and society. For drug therapies to be used properly, people must trust pharmaceuticals, which is why authorities should always explain their work and standards openly. There is also a greater need for clear rules because pharmaceutical firms can sometimes influence the way regulations are formulated. A never-ending debate on the ethical issue of drug regulation is therefore necessary, as this ensures that public interest remains paramount in the presence of balancing forces from market dynamics and scientific advancements (Abraham et al., 2015) (Figure 15.1).

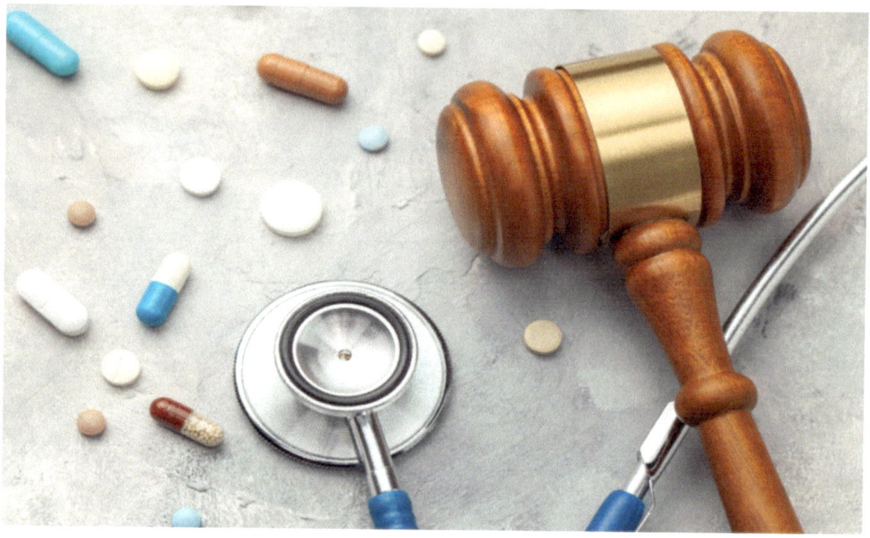

Figure 15.1. Regulatory and ethical aspects of drug.

Source: https://www.fdli.org/wp-content/uploads/2020/05/Overview-of-Drug-Law-and-Regulation-scaled.jpeg.

Definition of Drugs and Their Classifications

When used in pharmacology, drugs are defined as substances that alter the body's functions when administered, inhaled, or administered through other routes. Sorting drugs into groups is necessary for both regulations and medical care, since it helps to group them based on their structure, how they work, and whether they can be abused. For example, the categories in this classification could be narcotics, stimulants, depressants, and hallucinogens, with different features and effects for both lawmakers and medical staff. This system facilitates understanding of how drugs work and their approval and monitoring processes, highlighting the need for a robust regulatory system to protect the public. The history of drug classification reveals how rules have evolved in response to shifting attitudes and emerging scientific discoveries. Earlier, drugs were grouped depending on how they were used or made, for example, herbal or synthetic. As research advanced, it was realized that a more detailed and evidence-based way to group mental illnesses was needed. Nowadays, agencies such as the FDA in the United States use both science and ethics in their regulations. When deciding whether a drug should be available without a prescription or only with a doctor's prescription, both safety and efficacy information, as well as ethical considerations regarding access and the risk of misuse, are taken into account. Additionally, due to the growing complexity of drug classifications, it is becoming increasingly challenging for regulatory agencies to protect the public's health. The arrival of biologics and gene therapies may cause traditional systems to struggle with substances that are not easily classified. It has become clear that incorporating public views is crucial in developing regulations, primarily due to the ethical issues associated with access, equity, and the risks of new treatments. As highlighted in recent studies, criteria such as equity, efficacy, and patient-reported outcomes are fundamental in guiding healthcare decision-making and priority-setting, ensuring that regulatory mechanisms remain responsive and fair in an increasingly complex drug landscape (Baltussen et al., 2012; Meghani et al., 2014) (Figure 15.2).

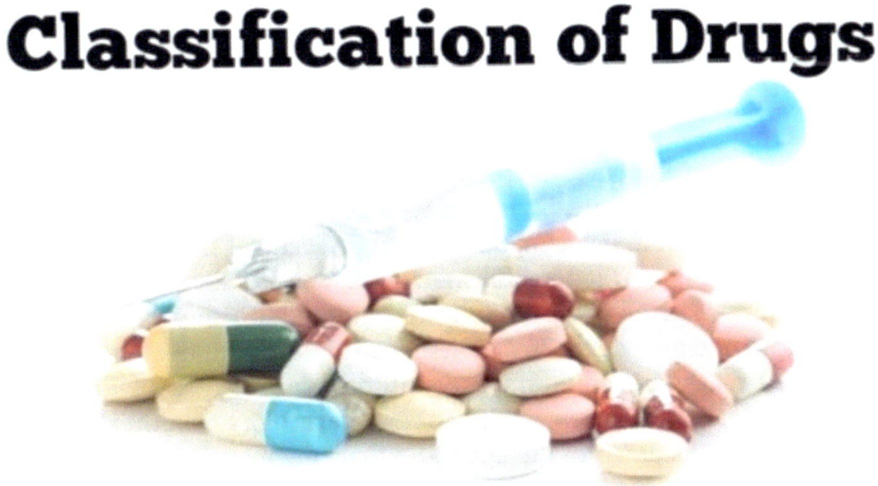

Figure 15.2. Definition of drugs and their classifications.

Source: https://www.publichealth.com.ng/wp-content/uploads/2020/10/Classification-Of-Drugs-1024x709.jpg.

Importance of Regulation in the Pharmaceutical Industry

It is essential to control the drug sector to ensure the health of the public and the effectiveness of drugs. Regulatory bodies, such as the U.S. Food and Drug Administration (FDA), are tasked with enforcing strict measures that govern the development, testing, and approval processes of drugs. To prevent risks linked to drug use, this control process is necessary because uncontrolled drugs can seriously harm your health. Such agencies ensure that drugs are thoroughly tested for safety and effectiveness before they can be sold to the public. This approach to patient care helps them and also fosters trust in medical therapy, which is crucial for maintaining ethical standards. It is also the job of regulation to keep an eye on and address any adverse effects that drugs may have after being approved. Through the system for reporting adverse events, authorities can collect information on how drugs affect people once they are released and take action if necessary. It is necessary to continue monitoring as new medical advancements and health issues arise. With the help of regulation, the costs of drug development are controlled and the public can gain access to the value of medicines. By controlling pricing and promoting healthy competition, regulatory frameworks help people get cheaper medicines and address differences in public health. It is essential to note that sociological aspects are crucial, as they reveal the broader implications of drug regulation. Regulations shape the connections among HCPs, consumers, and pharmaceutical companies and also make sure that ethical and social values are followed in drug development. As addressed in current sociological discussions, the challenges of medicalization and consumerism accentuate the value of a sociological approach to pharmaceutical regulation (Abraham et al., 2025). This discussion points out the importance of being sensitive to regulations as the world changes, so that ethics in the industry keep up with new technologies. As reiterated by scholars, the constant engagement with sociological issues in drug regulation will illustrate the required three-way interaction of science, ethics, and society as we move forward in the 21st century (Abdo-Rabbo et al., 2015).

Overview of Ethical Considerations in Drug Development

The topic of drug development ethics encompasses various aspects and addresses the needs of all stakeholders, including regulators, manufacturers, researchers, and healthcare professionals. Ensuring patients are safe and informed is a main ethical issue during the development of drugs. Doctors need to be responsible in clinical trials as well as when prescribing and promoting drugs. When it comes to treatments that manage myopia, ethics are critical since most patients are minors. Due to the guidelines and ethical rules established by agencies, doctors are required to explain the risks, benefits, and alternatives of treatments to patients and their guardians, ensuring they are well-informed before making decisions. Consequently, stakeholders must prioritize ethical considerations to foster trust and maintain accountability in drug development (Drove et al., 2019). Additionally, ethical issues often arise when determining whether the benefits of new drugs outweigh the potential risks. Trying to speed up drug development for urgent medical needs may lead to less strict clinical trials. Since ML and other new technologies are now used in drug discovery, the need to introduce new therapies to the market grows even stronger. While ML can speed up finding suitable drug candidates, it is important to pay attention to ethical issues about data quality and privacy.

With changes in the pharmaceutical sector, it is crucial to assess how researchers ensure fairness in their studies and maintain the accuracy of all data. Thus, addressing these ethical concerns is essential to promote responsible innovation in drug development (Kunduru et al., 2023). In addition, the ethical issues in drug development include ensuring that healthcare is accessible and equitable for all. Since research and development are costly, not all groups have equal access to new therapies. Ethics should ensure that all people, regardless of their financial situation, can get the effective treatments they need. Furthermore, the marketing of new drugs should adhere to ethical guidelines to prevent misleading statements that could exacerbate health inequalities. Because of this, people pay more attention to how regulatory bodies and pharmaceutical companies cooperate to ensure that all people can access new medical treatments. Thus, an ethical approach to drug development requires a holistic understanding of these issues, whereby social responsibility and transparency are interwoven into every stage of the process to ensure that the advancements made are beneficial for all (Drove et al., 2019) (Figure 15.3).

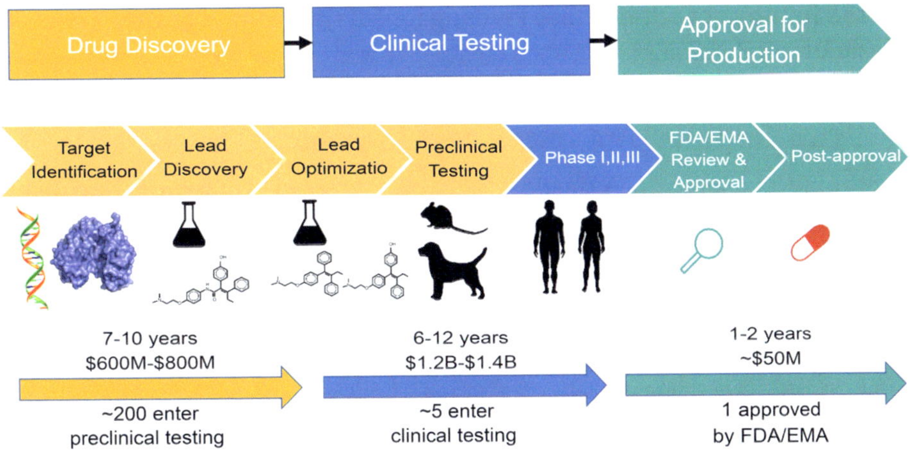

Figure 15.3. Overview of ethical considerations in drug development.

Source: https://pub.mdpi-res.com/ijms/ijms-23-13568/article_deploy/html/images/ijms-23-13568-g001.png?1667899871.

15.1. Historical Context of Drug Regulation

Drug regulation has always been influenced by the major trends that have formed public health and safety laws. At the beginning of drug consumption, not much regulation existed, so many questionable substances were sold to the public. The 1906 Pure Food and Drug Act was a significant achievement in America, as it demonstrated the government's commitment to protecting people from dangerous and misleading products. It aimed to reduce health risks by requiring labels and banning the mixing of ingredients, which helped create modern regulations. Due to new health emergencies, people have become more aware of the challenges in checking the safety and effectiveness of drugs, which has resulted in wider regulation over the years. When the pharmaceutical industry underwent changes in the mid-20th century, the rules for regulating it also became more complex. In the late 1950s, the thalidomide drug caused many birth deformities, which made it clear that drugs must be well tested before they are allowed on the market. As a result, the 1962 Kefauver-Harris Amendments to the Food, Drug, and Cosmetic Act made it significantly stricter, requiring drug companies to demonstrate that their drugs were both safe and effective before being approved. As a result of this new regulation, drugs were evaluated more thoroughly with evidence, and this helped the FDA and similar bodies to focus on both public health and encouraging new developments. From this history, it is clear that there has always been a conflict between the desire for rapid medical progress and the need for strong control. Trust plays a crucial role in bridging the connection between ethics and the regulation of drugs. According to recent research, such as that conducted by NICE, trust plays a crucial role in the relationships between drug manufacturers and regulatory authorities. It is important for these institutions to trust each other, though this trust may be fragile, especially when it comes to important decisions about expensive drugs. The historical context of drug regulation reveals an ongoing evolution of trust relationships, where regulatory agencies must balance public trust against potential prejudice resulting from industry influence. Such intricacies further suggest broader systemic issues, demonstrating how trust might function to sustain or the aims of regulatory systems in ensuring safe and effective medical interventions, as evidenced by the findings of studies that investigate (dis)trust in regulatory decisions (Abraham et al., 2015; Terzic et al., 2017).

15.1.1. Early Drug Regulations and Their Impact

The first drug regulations were introduced when people were suffering from health crises and widespread illegal activities in the pharmaceutical industry. Many harmful ingredients in patent medicines sold in the late 19th and early 20th centuries caused people to push for stricter rules. As a result of this backlash, the Pure Food and Drug Act of 1906 was enacted to prevent false labeling and protect consumers' interests. The first regulations helped create an agreement between pharmaceutical companies and the public, encouraging both parties to be responsible and honest. Even so, these laws showed that society was unsure about drug safety and effectiveness, which made it hard to determine what regulators and drug companies should do to protect the public. Although early regulations brought clear benefits, the process of implementing them revealed that the regulatory system had its own challenges and difficulties.

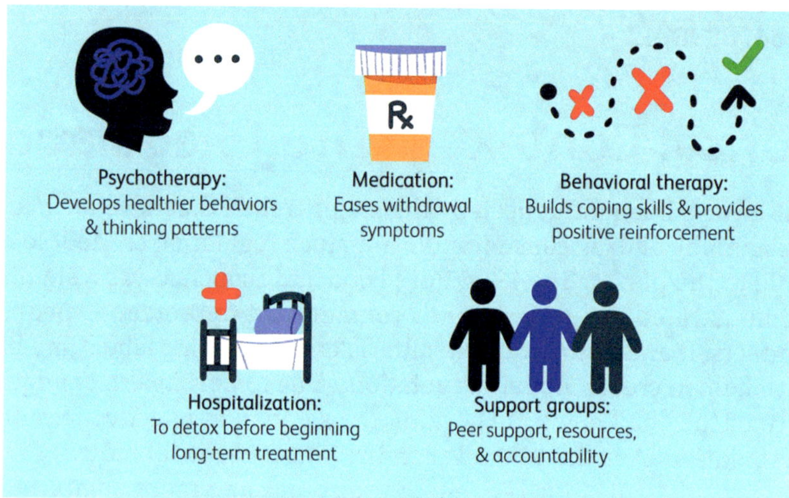

Figure 15.4. Early drug regulations and their impact.

Source: https://www.verywellhealth.com/thmb/s-1nwHWIhWGGa41GOmxVUHVaDA4=/1500x0/filters:no_upscale():max_bytes(150000):strip_icc()/the-effects-of-drug-addiction-5214343-Final-63ee57687f0a4daa90b104897ad6579e.jpg.

For example, the Pure Food and Drug Act did not address the effectiveness of drugs, and this concern was not addressed until the Food, Drug, and Cosmetic Act of 1938 was introduced. The Act was a pivotal step in the history of regulation, mandating a comprehensive review of drug safety before it could be approved for the market. Even so, it was shown that these categories could be strict or flexible, depending on the medical system and how the public in each area received them. Due to these enduring yet sometimes contentious rules, the discussion about the ethical aspects of drug development and approval persists, highlighting the importance of effective governance in protecting consumers. As drug regulations evolved, more attention was given to finding a balance between new ideas and ethical concerns, particularly in clinical trials. The process of internationalizing drug research and development is causing global pharmaceutical companies to conduct more clinical trials in developing countries, as in the case of Mexico. It raises questions about whether the rules and ethical standards in local places are robust enough, given the challenges developing countries face in enforcing global standards in clinical research. There is a contradiction in that, while rules are put in place to ensure drugs are safe and work well, they must also reflect the social and cultural backgrounds of people from different backgrounds. For this reason, the history of early drug regulations continues to influence today's discussions on how to ethically manage drug development, incorporating local traditions and cultures, and highlighting the close connection and evolution of these principles (Figure 15.4).

15.1.2. Key Legislation Shaping Drug Regulation (e.g., Pure Food and Drug Act)

Much of the regulatory framework in the American pharmaceutical industry is based on important legislation, particularly the Pure Food and Drug Act of 1906. Thanks to this law, federal authorities were given the responsibility of overseeing food and drug safety, as well as attempting to prevent the use of misleading labels and dangerous ingredients. With the Act, manufacturers were held responsible for the first time in the quality of their goods. Most notably, it was a precursor to the creation of the FDA, which would go on to establish strict safety and effectiveness standards for drugs. Over the years, amendments and new laws have been enacted to enhance the FDA's authority and ensure greater safety for individuals facing health emergencies. The Pure Food and Drug Act is the primary law that guides today's drug regulation, seeking a balance between new drug developments and consumer safety. Passing the Federal Food, Drug, and Cosmetic Act of 1938 after the Pure Food and Drug Act significantly improved the way drugs were regulated. Because of the Act, all new drugs had to be tested for safety before being allowed on the market, a measure taken after many deaths occurred in the sulfanilamide tragedy. When the Act required manufacturers to demonstrate that their drugs were safe and effective, it both improved the approval process for drugs and established the basis for today's clinical trials. Over the years, the Act has been amended to address various issues, such as the development of biopharmaceuticals, demonstrating its ability to adapt to new challenges without compromising its primary purpose of protecting people's health and safety. Moreover, the ethical issues involved in drug regulation are now more important, especially for medicines given to children and children's treatments. Laws to develop drugs for this group have been strongly opposed, mainly due to economic and ethical reasons. Since there is a great need for medicines that are safe and effective for children, drug companies are discouraged from doing research in this area by the risks and low profits involved. In addition, ethical concerns regarding informed consent further complicate the situation, underscoring the need to establish robust legal frameworks that facilitate children's ethical involvement in clinical trials. Addressing these intricate issues is essential for developing pediatric innovation as well as making the regulatory mechanism evolve in a manner that prioritizes the health and well-being of younger patients, ultimately to provide better-quality pediatric treatments (Entorf et al., 2025).

15.1.3. Evolution of Regulatory Agencies (e.g., FDA, EMA)

The evolution of regulatory agencies such as the FDA and the European Medicines Agency (EMA) reflects the dynamic interplay between scientific advancements and the need for public safety. Initially, the FDA was established to address safety issues related to food and drugs; however, as matters became more complex and new medical technologies emerged, its responsibilities expanded. Recognizing that merely approving drugs was insufficient, the FDA implemented a rigorous procedure that evaluated both the safety and effectiveness of drugs. As a result, the agency demonstrated its commitment to health protection, as well as its dedication to advancing progress in drug research. Such an approach aligns with the broader objective of ensuring therapeutic advancements do not compromise safety, aligning with the evolving mission of regulatory bodies to respond to advancements in health solutions (Terzic et al., 2017). The formation of the EMA in the early 2000s was crucial for establishing consistent rules for medicines across Europe and for streamlining the process of approving new drugs. Consolidation was necessary to make sure the rules for pharmaceuticals are the same everywhere, as development is now more global. When the EMA consolidates the regulations of EU member states, it enhances the process of conducting clinical research and approving drugs for stakeholders. This initiative ensures that patients in Europe receive new therapies sooner and addresses ethical issues related to equal access to drugs. The integration of scientific standards in the regulatory process has become essential, reflecting an evolving understanding of public health obligations intertwined with the progression of medical science (Oliveira et al., 2023). Regulatory agencies are always at the forefront of dealing with ethical matters in drug development as things progress. As personalized medicine, gene therapy, and advanced technologies emerge, regulators must continually update their rules. Both the FDA and EMA are responsible for checking safety and effectiveness as well as considering the ethical issues that arise with new treatments. It involves making sure patients agree, access to treatment is fair, and there is a good balance between new treatments and the health of the public. In addressing these complexities, regulatory agencies play a crucial role in fostering an environment where scientific advancements can be translated into safe and effective treatments while ensuring that ethical practices remain a foundational aspect of their operations (Terzic et al., 2017) (Figure 15.5).

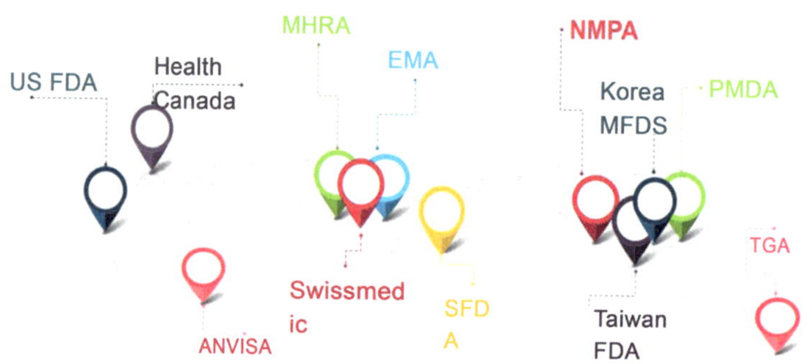

Figure 15.5. Evolution of regulatory agencies (e.g., FDA, EMA).

Source: https://globalforum.diaglobal.org/wp-content/uploads/2023/05/RWD-RWE_Regulatory-Policy-Strategy_MAP_GF.pptx-1-980x551.jpg.

15.2. Regulatory Frameworks

Having and assessing drug development regulations is the main way to ensure that pharmaceutical products are safe and effective. The entire clinical trial process relies on having robust regulations, which necessitate passing rigorous preclinical checks, obtaining ethical approval, and meeting international standards. Due to the variety in geopolitical rules, the differences in regulations could cause significant problems, especially in trials that involve many countries. For example, when various countries have different rules, the way governance is organized can impact the results of clinical research. For this reason, researchers should address these issues to ensure that their findings are scientifically accurate and that ethical standards are adhered to for the benefit of human participants. These varied regulatory environments necessitate that stakeholders continue to adapt and utilize standard procedures for clinical trials, also known as good clinical practice (GCP), to facilitate enhanced global collaboration in pharmaceutical research (Rosemann et al., 2014). Since drug innovation is now closely tied to advanced technology, the regulations surrounding it should also be strengthened. Artificial Intelligence (AI) in healthcare services and products is a prime example of this imperative, as AI modalities participate in various drug development areas, ranging from screening prospective compounds to tailoring patient treatment regimens. Still, there are major concerns about privacy, bias, and transparency associated with its integration, and these issues should be addressed by regulatory organizations. For instance, AI implementation in drug discovery poses explainability concerns in AI-driven decision-making, which is pivotal in upholding patients' and HCPs' trust. Secondly, with the advancement of AI technologies, regulatory frameworks need to institute rules that guarantee fairness while safeguarding bioethical concerns, thereby promoting responsible drug development and innovation (Kanagarajah et al., 2024). Furthermore, regulations for medical research should be able to respond to new situations and to the ethical problems that come with new technologies. Since there are many different rules in stem cell medicine, this situation can encourage new ideas while also raising ethical concerns. Researchers typically act in two ways, supporting both local and global norms, depending on their research interests and their geographical location. The fact that regulations vary between places can give rise to various economic benefits at different places, but it can also expose people to activities that are not regulated and cause harm. Thus, the creation of comprehensive and integrated regulatory regimes is necessary for safeguarding against the loss of moral control and test subject safety in pursuit of the benefits of being the first with regard to medical research (Rosemann et al., 2014).

15.2.1. Overview of the FDA's Role in Drug Approval

The FDA serves a pivotal role in the drug approval process, acting as a regulatory body that ensures the safety and efficacy of pharmaceuticals before they reach the market. It is the agency's job to review new drugs by using a framework that requires laboratory work, preclinical tests, and clinical trials in several phases. Each phase is designed to collect information on pharmacokinetics, pharmacodynamics, and potential adverse effects.

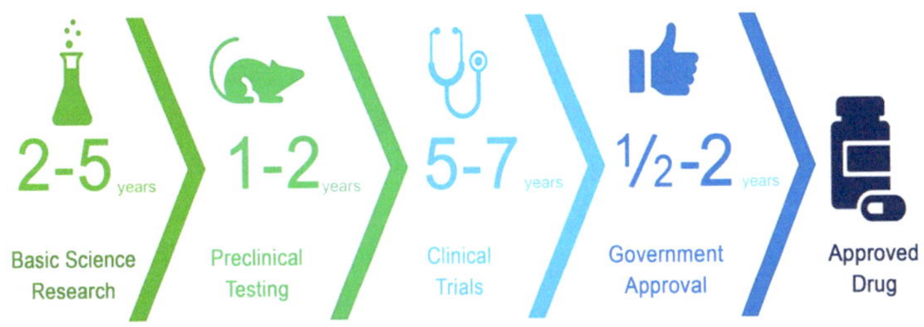

2-5 years
Basic Science Research
1-2 years
Preclinical Testing
5-7 years
Clinical Trials
½-2 years
Government Approval
Approved Drug

Figure 15.6. Overview of the FDA's role in drug approval.

Source: https://impactcare.co.in/wp-content/uploads/2024/11/Detailed-Overview-of-the-FDA-Generic-Drug-Approval-Process.webp.

Through strict rules and regulations, the FDA strives to ensure public safety and promote the development of new treatments. Nonetheless, making sure both quick access to new treatments and proper evaluation are met is still a tough issue. As new drug development becomes increasingly complex, the FDA may need to adapt its processes to incorporate bioprinting and personalized medicine, potentially enhancing patient care in the future. Over the past few years, people have been paying closer attention to the FDA, claiming that its choices are too easily affected by politics and industry connections. This doubt primarily stems from the FDA's decision to use accelerated approval and more surrogate endpoints to assess drug effectiveness. These steps can help speed up the introduction of new therapies, yet they might lower the safety and effectiveness of these drugs. Experts say that these methods put speed ahead of complete evaluation, so the drugs might not meet the expected standards. Additionally, using postmarket surveillance to assess risks introduces challenges regarding who is responsible and how trustworthy the system is perceived by the public. The key issue is to ensure the FDA maintains its objectivity when responding to the growing need for faster drug approvals in today's medical world. As the FDA explores innovative techniques to streamline the drug approval process, emerging technologies such as AI play an increasingly significant role. Virtual clinical trials and molecular modeling are emerging methods that can help regulatory agencies make more informed decisions. These ways of working help to use resources efficiently and protect volunteers from harmful things, which supports the safety of the public. Even so, using AI and computer models in this field raises serious ethical concerns about bias, transparency, and the risk of compromising safety standards. The FDA must utilize new technologies without compromising the proper approval of drugs. The agency's ability to handle these issues effectively will significantly influence the pharmaceutical industry and foster trust and reliance, ultimately shaping healthcare in the future (Figure 15.6).

15.2.2. International Regulatory Bodies and Their Functions

International regulatory bodies have the authority to establish and impose standards of drug efficacy, safety, and ethical practice within the pharmaceutical industry. Bodies such as the WHO and the International Conference on Harmonisation (ICH) serve as beacons of responsibility, maintaining regulatory harmonization among member states. By establishing models for clinical trials, drug approval, and post-marketing surveillance, such organizations ensure that pharmaceutical products are both safe for the public to use and effective in treating diseases. Such collaboration fosters global confidence in health interventions and mitigates risks associated with drug therapy, underscoring the importance of international regulatory efforts in achieving optimal health worldwide. The ethical dimensions of drug control are inherently linked with the functions carried out by international regulatory bodies. An important aspect of their function is deliberations in support of legislation that ensures fair access to medicines, as well as the protection of patient rights. The regulatory paradigms established by these institutions advance fair practices in drug pricing and accessibility, particularly in low- and middle-income countries (LMICs) where access to basic medicines is limited. Ensuring that policies on health financing are guided by objectives such as good governance and social health protection is important when addressing health inequalities. By providing legal mechanisms and regulatory guidance, international institutions can help nations develop approaches that are centered on ethical values while maintaining broader healthcare accessibility in mind, thereby furthering the overall welfare of populations across different jurisdictions. Moreover, the regulatory context is constantly evolving, requiring international organizations to adapt and address emerging challenges. With pharmaceutical developments continuing to accelerate, stringent regulatory systems that facilitate the authorization of novel treatments are a growing concern. Organizations must balance the imperative of creating new treatments with the need to ensure patient safety and efficacy. Such dynamic engagement is portrayed by matters concerning competition in health financing, as observed from the actions taken by various nations. Regulatory bodies should provide sustainable regulation while advocating against unwholesome competition that could undermine public health. Given that the regulatory environment is still in flux, the role of international organizations in forming policy and ethical frameworks remains crucial for protecting healthcare quality and access globally (Picciotto et al., 2000; Bultman et al., 2012).

15.2.3. Comparison of Regulatory Processes Across Different Countries

Drug development and approval regulations differ significantly from one country to another, typically due to variations in their political, economic, and social environments. In the United States, for example, the FDA plays a pivotal role in the rigorous assessment of pharmaceuticals. All safety and effectiveness data are carefully checked before the drug can be sold. Meanwhile, in places such as China, the rules are less stringent, which can expedite trials but may also lead to issues with safety and supervision. The difference between these regulations highlights the difficulties in getting drugs approved internationally and its impact on people's health and research. The coexistence of varied regulatory norms across borders results in a landscape where collaborative efforts in clinical research must navigate these disparities while adhering to the specific demands of each jurisdiction (Rosemann et al., 2014). Additionally, when countries collaborate in clinical trials, they often mix their standards, which can make it challenging to adhere to all the rules. For example, organizations involved in transnational research may need to comply with the different rules established by various regulatory bodies. An important study on stem cell medicine cooperation between the USA and China explains how researchers manage their work in different regulatory systems. It is clear from this research that local and international regulations can work together, showing the complicated relationship between them. Such regulatory diversity necessitates a thorough understanding of how these practices impact scientific integrity and ethical considerations, particularly in relation to patient involvement and informed consent (Rosemann et al., 2014). Since regulations differ from one country to another, it isn't easy to maintain the same ethical standards in clinical trials. Additionally, it is crucial to consider the ethical aspects of drug regulation, as clinical research is increasingly becoming a global endeavor. The Electronic Health Records for Clinical Research (EHR4CR) initiative exemplifies efforts to streamline trial management through data-driven methodologies in Europe. Although stakeholders are in favor of this platform, they highlight issues related to data privacy, security, and ethical governance that are particularly important in their respective countries. Senior healthcare officials from various European countries agree that there are benefits to improving trial conduct by better utilizing data. Nevertheless, the need to address ethical issues in every regulatory system highlights the complex relationship between new technologies and their associated rules. Therefore, it is essential to compare these regulations to facilitate international agreement and safeguard both patients and the integrity of research.

15.3. Clinical Trials and Drug Testing

Testing the effectiveness and safety of new drugs

for human use is the primary reason behind drug testing and clinical trials. Adhering to the rules set by regulators is a crucial aspect of conducting clinical trials. Rules and regulations are essential for ensuring the safety of participants, conducting trials properly, and adhering to the standards of scientific research. People who volunteer, especially those from vulnerable groups, should be informed about the potential risks and benefits of their participation. This is a main principle in ethical study protocols. When trials grow from more minor to larger phases, it is important to pay close attention to deciding who can or cannot be included, especially for groups that may gain more or less from participating, to guarantee fairness and safety. Ethical issues are not merely regulatory compliance, but also the integrity of the research process itself. Clinical trials often have a hard time dealing with complex ethical issues, particularly when the study involves treatments that may likely significantly impact participants' health and welfare, like in placental therapeutics research. Researchers, regulatory officials, and patient groups need to talk extensively about the ethical problems that come with the possibility of fetal injury and potential help for the mother. Ethical issues can change when the first people are selected for a trial and the risks are not fully known. Stakeholders must strike a balance between caring for participants and advancing research, so they should be aware of the rules and ethical standards governing clinical research. Apart from being reviewed ethically and by regulators, clinical trials depend heavily on having a solid infrastructure, especially advanced methods for testing drugs. These methods, for example, ex vivo dual human placenta perfusion experiments or in vitro experiments, are crucial in ensuring the safety of test drugs before they are administered to people. At the same time, scientists must ensure that strict scientific standards are met while also considering the ethical implications of using animal models. Choosing the right models, whether they are non-human primates or other techniques, raises ethical concerns about animal care and the potential for achieving good results. Clinical trial design, thus, driven by regulation and ethics paradigms, therefore, needs to incorporate these new approaches while promoting a culture of responsibility among scientists, all of which is essential towards the realization of actionable clinical outcomes in drug development, particularly in cases warranting careful ethical scrutiny, as in research into myopia control treatment and placental therapeutics (Drove et al., 2019; David et al., 2021) (Figure 15.7).

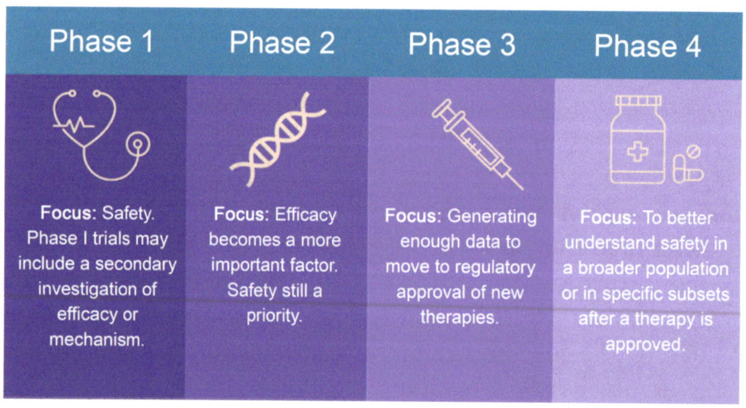

Figure 15.7. Clinical trials and drug testing.

Source: https://lustgarten.org/wp-content/uploads/2022/05/infographic-clinical-trials-1-1024x683.png.

15.3.1. Phases of Clinical Trials and Their Significance

Clinical trials play a crucial role in the development of new drugs, ensuring they are both effective and safe for the public. Clinical trials are organized into four phases that help answer specific research questions and check how well a drug performs. In the first phase, the primary objective is to assess safety, determine the drug's effects, establish an optimal dose, and evaluate its tolerability in a small group of healthy volunteers. Phase II involves testing the effectiveness of the drug in a larger group of patients, providing the first indication of its usefulness. Significantly, this structured approach not only ensures regulatory compliance but also addresses the ethical responsibility to protect trial participants while advancing scientific knowledge (N/A, 2006). The third phase of testing, known as Phase III, is often believed to be the most crucial because it involves many participants and is meant to check if the drug works as expected. At this point, the new drug is administered to individuals who may receive either a standard treatment or a placebo, allowing its effectiveness to be tested across multiple groups. When deciding on drug approval and launching them in the market, regulatory bodies such as the FDA depend mainly on data from Phase III trials. In addition, these trials adhere to the ethical principle that participants must be informed of the possible risks and benefits before they participate. The data collected during this phase significantly contributes to the broader understanding of the drug's therapeutic potential and adverse effects, thus serving as a foundation for ongoing safety monitoring post-approval (Bedding et al., 2018). In the final stage, Phase IV trials or post-marketing surveillance, the safety and effectiveness of drugs are still checked as they are used in the market. They are needed to identify unusual side effects and to assess how the drug works in actual clinical practice. With the arrival of new information, Phase IV trials may prompt changes in how the drug is labeled, how it is recommended for use, or its removal from the market if safety issues are identified. As a result, they are essential in regulations, as they are responsible for continually monitoring drug safety to protect public health. In combination, the structured progression through these phases establishes a carefully balanced approach to drug development that integrates regulatory compliance with ethical considerations, thereby fostering a more reliable and responsible healthcare system (N/A, 2006).

15.3.2. Ethical Considerations in Conducting Clinical Trials

The moral standards for the conduct of clinical trials are a top priority because they ensure participants' rights and welfare are protected throughout the research process. Using a placebo in a clinical trial is one of the key ethical issues that must be addressed. The challenge is particularly uphill in psychiatric trials, as participants' capacity to give informed consent is hampered by mental disease. Although a placebo arm can provide valuable information about a new treatment, it complicates the decision of whether to administer the treatment to those who truly need it. Thus, scientists must navigate these ethical waters with caution, balancing the scientific merit of the trial against their moral obligation of ensuring the well-being of participants, as highlighted by the requirement for strict scrutiny and training in conducting clinical trials (Bleich et al., 2009). In addition to ethical issues related to informed consent and placebos, the use of EHRs in clinical trials introduces another level of ethical consideration. The EHR4CR initiative aims to simplify patient recruitment and enhance the efficiency of clinical operations by leveraging existing healthcare data. Still, this progress in technology poses significant challenges related to privacy, security, and the management of information. Employing these websites has been both welcomed and feared by healthcare stakeholders because of the risks to patients' private information. Ethical issues arise when researchers must ensure that the data is used ethically and that safeguards are in place to protect participants' identities, while maintaining the integrity of the trial process (Dugas et al., 2015). Additionally, researchers are expected to adhere to ethical standards when conducting clinical trials. It requires researchers to follow national and international rules, for example, the Declaration of Helsinki, which stresses the importance of openness and responsibility in research. Besides obeying the rules, creating an ethical environment within research teams is crucial. This requires ensuring the well-being of participants, allowing them to discuss ethical issues, and resolving any conflicts of interest. Ethical standards are important guidelines that support the trust necessary for clinical research to be effective. The success of clinical trials depends on investigators conducting their research within an ethical framework that respects and protects the participants themselves, ultimately contributing to the credibility and generalizability of their findings (Bleich et al., 2009).

15.3.3. Informed Consent and Patient Rights in Drug Testing

It is essential to get informed consent when testing drugs in medicine. It means that patients should be allowed to decide for themselves if they want to participate in clinical trials. It is necessary to share both the possible risks and benefits of a treatment and also ensure that patients understand them. Since drug testing involves new medications, the risks are very high, so it's necessary to follow strict consent rules. Healthcare providers must adhere to numerous rules and ethics while ensuring that patients' autonomy is not compromised. When the need to speed up drug development conflicts with the duty to fully inform patients, it becomes clear how important it is to respect people's rights while still improving medicine. Additionally, the concept of informed consent is closely tied to patient rights, particularly the right to privacy and the protection of health information. When patient data is used in drug testing and later applied for purposes other than those originally agreed upon, this may create ethical concerns. There are serious moral concerns about the NHS using patient data for commercial purposes, as it is not always clear whether patients fully understand and willingly agree. Since organisations such as the NHS rely on industry to develop new ideas from patient data, it is essential to maintain patient trust by adhering to strong ethical principles. This situation exemplifies the moral conflict inherent in ensuring comprehensive patient rights while striving to advance healthcare innovations, as highlighted by Cockbain et al. (2014). Finally, discussions about informed consent should also take into account the increased involvement of participants in clinical research. Drug testing is now expected to consider ethical issues that go beyond regulations and also take into account what patients go through and their fundamental rights. As articulated by Birke et al. (2011), there is a growing recognition that the emotional and social dimensions of participants' experiences in clinical trials should inform ethical practices. It suggests that we should focus on how researchers and participants interact and influence each other regarding consent. When open communication and empathy are encouraged, regulatory bodies and research institutions can adjust their work to match new ethical standards, helping participants in drug trials become better informed and more involved.

15.4. Post-Market Surveillance

Post-market surveillance is a key mechanism for ensuring long-term safety and efficacy of pharmaceutical medicines following their approval for public use. The phase, which is known as Phase IV in drug development, involves the scientific monitoring of medicines available on the market and is crucial in uncovering potential side effects that were not identified during preclinical or clinical trials. Regulatory bodies, such as the FDA, need to harvest real-world evidence on drug utilization so that ongoing monitoring of the benefit-to-risk ratio is possible. It is not secondary data; it is a valuable public health measure of protection and can initiate rapid regulatory action whenever necessary. Therefore, robust post-market surveillance systems can prevent significant public health crises based on previously unknown drug safety issues. The ethical issues entailed in post-market surveillance are directly connected to the pharmaceutical companies' and regulatory agencies' roles. These stakeholders must prioritize transparency and ethical standards in their surveillance practices to foster trust within the healthcare system. For instance, ethical allocation of resources and sharing of safety data can be areas of conflicting argument, particularly in situations where there are limited medical resources in the case of public health emergencies. For instance, suggested by discussions of pandemic preparedness, the conflict between population health and individual rights is a conflict-inherent dilemma that can only be resolved by sensitive ethical examination and policy means. Resolution of these ethical dilemmas not only results in better patient outcomes but also underwrites public confidence in drug therapies governed by affirmatively establishing a safety commitment.

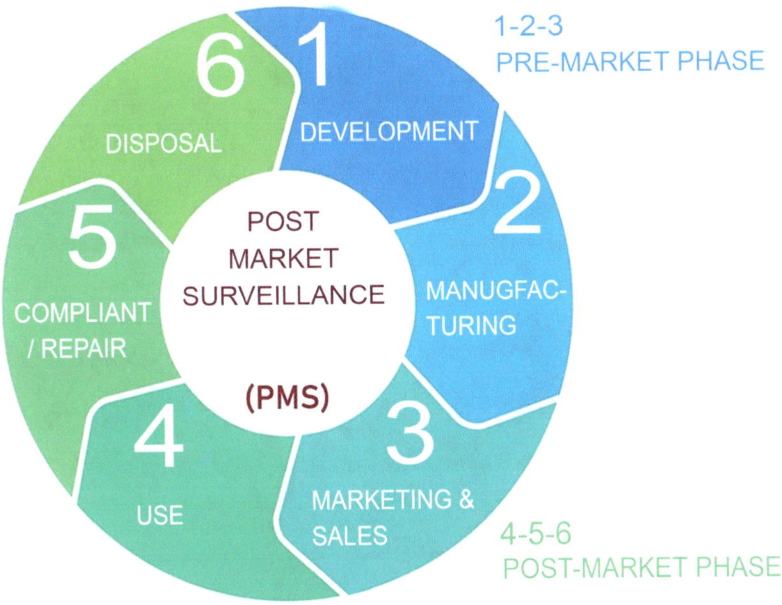

Figure 15.8. Post-market surveillance.

Source: https://www.i3cglobal.com/wp-content/uploads/2020/04/PMS-Plan.jpg.

Recent events regarding the safety of non-active implantable medical devices (NAIMDs) have underscored the need to enhance post-market evaluation processes. An ongoing comparison of drug and device surveillance procedures has revealed significant gaps, most importantly in the collection and review of adverse events concerning NAIMDs, which can hinder effective regulatory action. The integration of methodologies employed for drug safety evaluations into post-market surveillance of medical devices can facilitate an organized process that can enable regulatory agencies to react to safety concerns that may arise later on more effectively.

As unveiled by the field stakeholders, the forging of solid sources of data, like the creation of unique device identifiers (UDI), is needed to enhance monitoring of long-term patient outcomes. This kind of multi-pronged strategy emphasizes the need to transform regulatory behavior to maintain wide-ranging oversight at all stages of the product life cycle, ultimately contributing to consumer safety and confidence in medical breakthroughs (Berkman et al., 2007; Coloma et al., 2017) (Figure 15.8).

15.4.1. Importance of Monitoring Drug Safety After Approval

It is critical to keep an eye on drug safety after approval, since medical knowledge and safety issues are constantly developing. Once a drug receives approval from regulatory agencies, such as the FDA, the responsibility for ongoing safety assessment shifts partly to the manufacturers and healthcare providers. Post-marketing surveillance is crucial for identifying side effects that were not observed during the drug's testing.

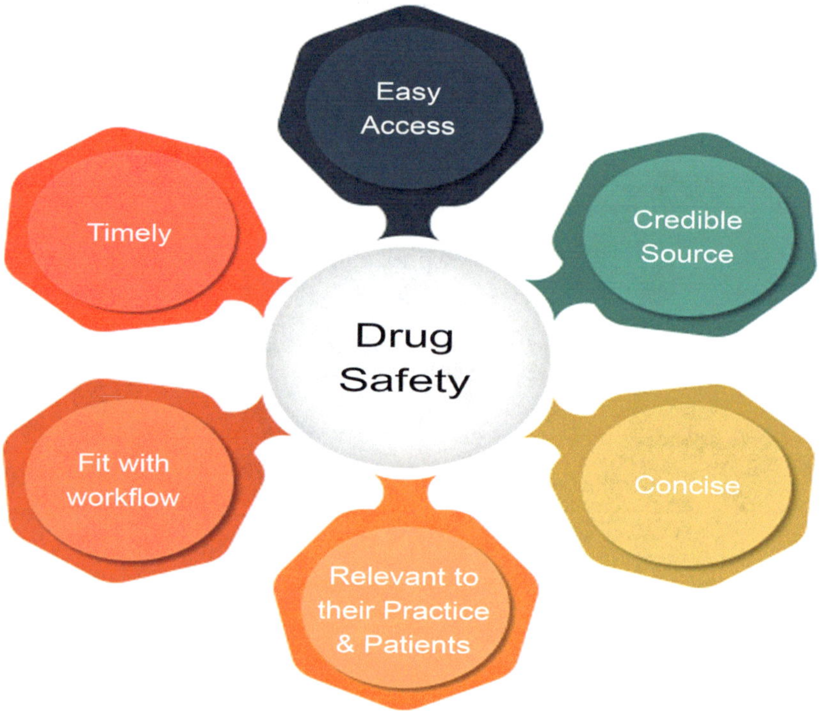

Figure 15.9. Importance of monitoring drug safety after approval.

Source: https://cdn.sketchbubble.com/pub/media/catalog/product/optimized1/9/f/9f1d6e3d7f737fa850e78a632fd393eb1df5b283a1789b8242a928f4ccbbee2f/drug-safety-mc-slide1_1.png.

Even if a medication is approved, it can still pose risks that were not initially realized, so it is essential to continue monitoring patients and the public. Moreover, reporting systems like the FDAs Adverse Event Reporting System (FAERS) facilitate the collection of data that informs regulatory actions and potential label modifications, underlining the need for a vigilant approach to drug safety beyond initial approval. Besides safety, the ethical aspects of post-approval drug monitoring are also very important. All stakeholders, such as drug makers, HCPs, and regulatory agencies, share the task of ensuring drug safety. Ethical issues are more serious when we consider minors, who can be given new treatments that have just been approved. As highlighted in the International Myopia Institutes report, ethical guidelines must govern the marketing and prescribing of medications, ensuring that clinicians understand the balance between offering innovative therapies and safeguarding patient welfare (Drove et al., 2019). Because of this ethical approach, it is essential to closely monitor how patients are informed about the benefits and risks associated with their treatment, demonstrating that an ethical duty does not end with drug approval. In addition, including post-marketing studies in the drug approval process shows a positive approach to managing drug safety. Research, such as that pertaining to new HIV prevention strategies, underscores the need for ongoing assessment and the rapid dissemination of new findings (N/A, 2006). This approach to research enhances the understanding of HCPs and patients regarding the long-term effects of drug use. Regulatory bodies can quickly address new safety information by prioritizing drug safety monitoring. Conducting safety evaluations on a regular basis is crucial for ethical medicine, as it enables prompt actions to mitigate risks associated with drugs and promotes public health (Figure 15.9).

15.4.2. Adverse Event Reporting Systems

Adverse Event Reporting Systems (AERS) are a critical component towards achieving drug efficacy and safety in the pharmaceutical regulatory environment. AERS enables medical practitioners, patients, and regulatory agencies to communicate, allowing them to report any adverse effects associated with the use of drugs.

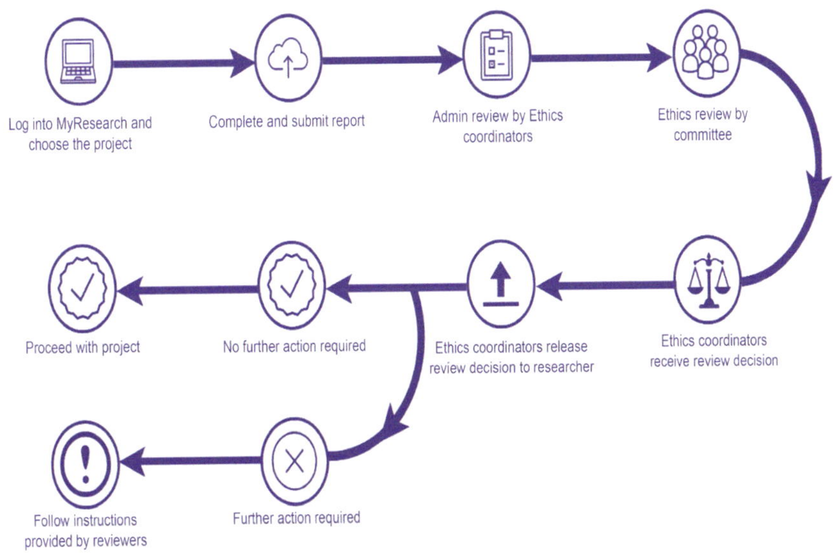

Figure 15.10. Adverse event reporting systems.

Source: https://systems-training.its.uq.edu.au/files/100110/MR-A_H-Adverse-WF.png.

The use of EHRs helped AERS perform better by gathering and reviewing data on adverse events. The findings from healthcare leaders in Europe indicate that such platforms are supported, as they are seen to increase the accuracy of reporting adverse events and address issues such as reduced workload and improved recruitment for clinical trials. Yet, the use of such systems raises pressing ethical concerns regarding patient privacy and data security that must be addressed delicately in regulatory policy (Dugas et al., 2015). The importance of AERS should not be exaggerated, mainly when it comes to consent and privacy of patients.

Since adverse event reporting involves medical information, it raises concerns about how the information is handled and used. Authorities should maintain patient information confidentiality as they collect and utilize the data necessary for public health progress. It is necessary to have clear rules for using and accessing the data. It is essential for policymakers, clinicians, and researchers to collaborate in addressing these issues and promoting scientific integrity and ethics. These initiatives not only foster confidence in the AERS but also engage the general public in a dialogue regarding ethical reporting practices and appropriate use of healthcare information (Ankley et al., 2018). Since adverse event reporting systems are continually evolving, it is essential to continually improve them for the regulatory system. The AOP (Adverse Outcome Pathway) concept has been an attractive means of developing further these systems, offering a formalized procedure to link mechanistic data with adverse effects in drug assessment. With the help of the system, complex biological interactions can be made easier to understand and utilize for regulatory purposes, which improves communication among those involved. Although AOP can be very useful, it is essential that the development and use of such frameworks focus on both scientific and ethical considerations. Engaging a wide array of stakeholders will be important in addressing these challenges and ensuring that AERS not only meet regulatory standards but also serve the greater good of public health protection (Dugas et al., 2015; Ankley et al., 2018) (Figure 15.10).

15.4.3. Role of Pharmacovigilance in Public Health

Pharmacovigilance ensures that drugs are safe and effective even after they are introduced for use in the public. This process must continue so that adverse drug reactions (ADRs) can be spotted and explained to both medical professionals and patients. Since drugs are administered by different people in various situations, pharmacovigilance provides crucial information for updating drug labels and informing regulatory decisions.

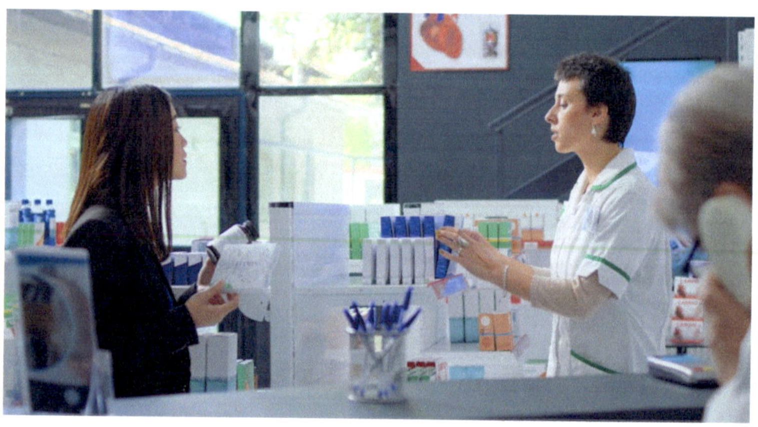

Figure 15.11. Role of pharmacovigilance in public health.

Source: https://blogs.octovion.com/wp-content/uploads/2024/03/pharmacovigilance-training-1.jpg.

Quickly noticing safety signals can greatly affect how the public sees medications, which is necessary for preserving trust in healthcare. Thus, pharmacovigilance works to keep patients safe and upholds the overall regulations intended to improve drug safety and ethical practices in the industry. Recently, the COVID-19 pandemic and other public health crises have underscored the importance of pharmacovigilance. Since mass vaccination was necessary, it became important to carefully watch how safe and effective the new vaccines were as many people were hesitant to get them. It is clear from vaccine discussions that governments must clearly explain vaccine safety to maintain people's trust and encourage many to get vaccinated. If safety issues are not addressed effectively, vaccination rates may decline, and the pandemic could persist for a longer period.

As a result, pharmacovigilance should be incorporated into public health strategies to address current health emergencies and ensure consistent drug safety. In addition, the ethical aspect of pharmacovigilance involves sharing safety data openly and ensuring the safety of individuals who are particularly at risk. When adverse effects are closely studied, pharmacovigilance enables both doctors and patients to make more informed decisions. If people are aware of drug interactions, possible side effects, and situations where medicines should not be used, they can reduce risks when taking drugs. It is the role of regulatory agencies to ensure that new drugs are safe for the public while also encouraging the development of new treatments. Participating in pharmacovigilance and acting on its findings helps create a supportive environment in the healthcare sector. In this context, pharmacovigilance encompasses all stages of drug development and use, thereby strengthening the overall framework for healthcare (Figure 15.11).

15.5. Ethical Issues in Drug Development

Developing drugs is complicated by many ethical issues that influence the process of making drugs and their advertising. Perhaps the primary ethical concern is striking a balance between patient safety and the pharmaceutical industry's pursuit of profit. Since a lot is at stake when a drug is launched, ethics issues often come up about how severe the trials are and how truthful the reports are. In the case of myopia control treatments, the moral duties of all parties involved, including manufacturers and clinicians, are clearly outlined.

These players should ensure that products administered to patients, especially children, not only work effectively but are also safe, with careful consideration given to how they inform people of the risks versus benefits of such interventions (Drove et al., 2019). It becomes more ethically complicated when healthcare professionals are required to educate patients and staff about such products. Moreover, how regulations are carried out in different countries creates a major challenge in the process of creating drugs. As a result of globalisation, the fact that regulations differ from one country to another can slow down the creation of common standards for clinical trials. The U.S.–China stem cell research collaboration is an example of how different practices carried out simultaneously can raise ethical concerns about research methods and participant protection. Researchers operating within such complex regulation regimes usually balance international normative demand with local circumstances (Rosemann et al., 2014). This situation not only challenges the scientific integrity of clinical trials but also creates serious concerns about equitable access to innovative treatments as well as researchers' moral obligations towards diverse patient populations. Money-driven interests can complicate the ethics of drug development by potentially influencing research and the regulations that govern it. There are times when making money becomes more important than caring for patients. When companies in the pharmaceutical industry focus on earning profits, it becomes possible for them to hide the risks of their drugs or claim their drugs are more effective than they are. Therefore, strong rules and regulations are necessary to ensure that ethical standards are adhered to during the development of drugs. Those involved in drug development, including healthcare workers and government officials, should prioritize ethics and patient protection over financial gain. Therefore, by promoting accountability and openness, the primary reason for these ethical issues will be eliminated, and the industry's reputation will be protected (Figure 15.12).

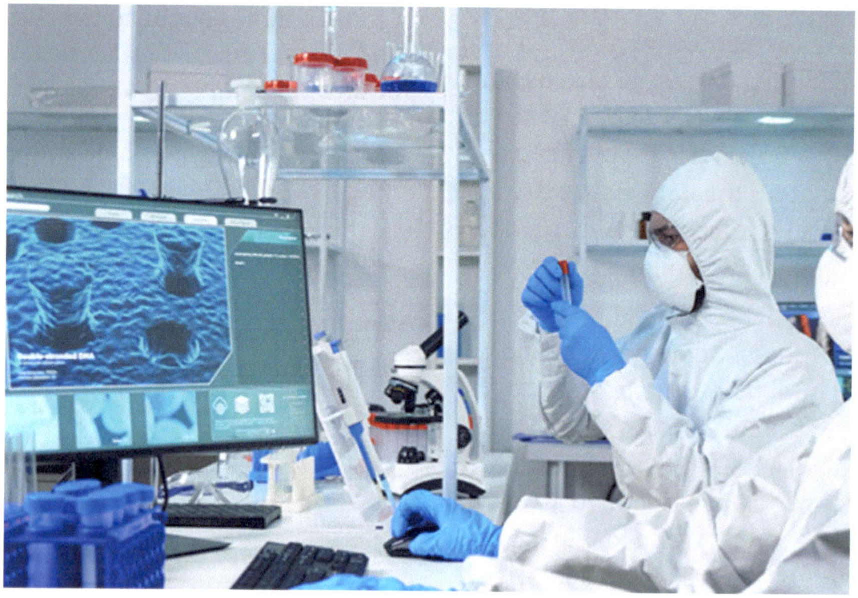

Figure 15.12. Ethical issues in drug development.

Source: https://cdn.prod.website-files.com/63217ccaf3f0f6ef21222235/66051d9642d3393158b05f73_Feb%20Blog%202.jpg.

15.5.1. Access to Medications and Equity Concerns

The connection between generating profits and caring for patients is a complex issue that impacts the ethics and laws within the pharmaceutical industry. When companies attempt to increase revenue by employing effective marketing and pricing strategies, this can lead to issues that may impact patient outcomes. This issue is most noticeable when companies prioritize profits over providing everyone with access to good healthcare. The analogy of Copernican astronomy by Sage and Hammers clearly shows why healthcare competition should be viewed differently. Misperceived competition can limit both technical advancement and social initiatives necessary for improving patient care, prompting a reevaluation of regulatory frameworks that govern the industry without compromising public health (Hammer et al., 2002). As a result, companies should ensure that their strategies incorporate ethical aspects to promote new ideas while also protecting the well-being of patients. At the same time, the field of personalized medicine stands out because it must balance its economic interests with its ethical duties. While individualized treatment plans have the potential to enhance the effectiveness of therapy, they also raise important concerns regarding fairness and access. Different entities in an industry are affected by the market and also by other important factors, such as changes in demographics and laws. Because of this, it is clear that a proper model should encompass all relevant parties, including firms, government officials, healthcare providers, and patient advocacy groups. By understanding these relationships, stakeholders can better navigate the delicate equilibrium of ensuring that profit motives do not overshadow the pivotal goal of improving patient health outcomes (Sokoli et al., 2017). Ultimately, both profit and patient welfare can be achieved if everyone involved in healthcare adheres to ethical rules and regulations. Firms in the pharmaceutical industry should be supported in focusing on research that benefits both the public and profits. These agencies ensure that pharmaceutical companies follow the rules and treat their competitors fairly. When ethics are prioritized, the industry can develop a sustainable approach that benefits both shareholders and patients. When the pharmaceutical sector pays attention to profit and welfare, it can encourage both new ideas and caring in healthcare.

15.5.2. Access to Medications and Equity Concerns

The issue of access to medication is deeply integrated into issues of equity, particularly in drug regulation and ethical practices. Inequality in access is more likely to be rooted in socioeconomic reasons that limit specific groups from seeking appropriate medications. In the majority of cases, pharmaceutical companies are more concerned with profit generation, thereby paying less attention to drug development for lower-market brackets, such as children or those with rare diseases. This lack of market incentive not only suppresses innovation but also increases inequality, keeping essential treatments out of the reach of vulnerable populations. The lack of access to medicines becomes a systemic issue, one that requires regulatory processes not just to speed up drug approval but also to ensure equitable distribution to all segments, irrespective of economic condition. Ethical considerations are paramount in determining access to medication, and with it, the challenges. The regulatory framework must consider the moral aspects of access to drugs, particularly for vulnerable populations like children who have been informally referred to as therapeutic orphans in pharmaceutical research. As detailed in recent literature, there are compelling ethical issues regarding the use of children in clinical trials who are not able to provide consent (Entorf et al., 2025). Consequently, minimal child participation in trials translates into a shortage of pediatric formulations. This raises the most profound issues of fairness and justice in medicine and highlights the need for ethically acceptable regulatory policies that balance the interests of every patient while still encouraging innovation in pediatric care. Moreover, the overlap of economic returns and ethical concerns adds to imbalances in drug availability. The economic implications of drug discovery will deter drug firms from financing therapy for small, unattractive populations such as children. This hesitance is heightened by stringent legal bans and a general atmosphere of dread surrounding ethical trials (Entorf et al., 2025). As such, novel child drugs are rare and put them at major risk of compromised health outcomes. An interdisciplinary approach must be followed, combining economic analysis with a robust ethical framework, to ensure that the welfare of poorer groups is particularly considered in the regulatory systems governing drug access. It is only through thoughtful and consultative policymaking that societies will achieve actual equity of access to necessary drugs.

15.5.3. The Role of Transparency in Pharmaceutical Practices

Being transparent in the pharmaceutical industry encourages trust among patients, healthcare workers, and those who oversee the industry. Now that there is more evidence about the ethics of clinical trials, it is essential to make the methods and results more straightforward. The shift of drug development to developing countries makes some people worry about meeting strict ethical standards. Mexico must find a way to accommodate global pharmaceutical companies and conduct local clinical trials that adhere to international rules and ethical standards. A transparent framework not only clarifies the motives behind such relocations but also holds companies accountable for their practices, thereby enhancing public confidence in the safety and efficacy of drugs (Santiago-Rodriguez et al., 2025).

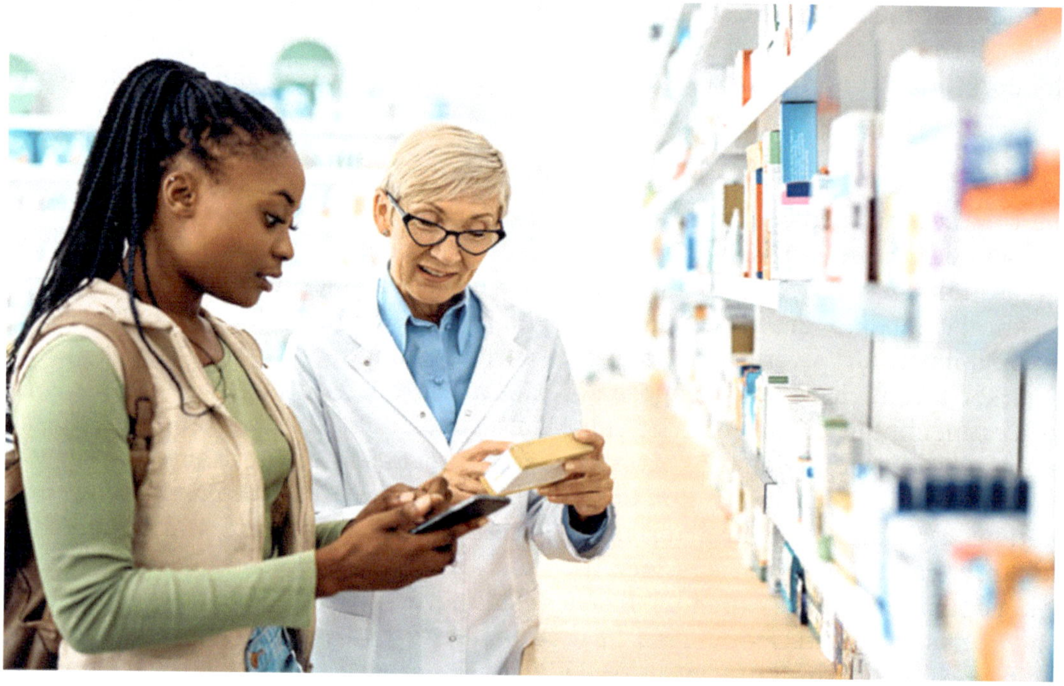

Figure 15.13. The role of transparency in pharmaceutical practices.

Source: https://www.rcainc.com/wp-content/uploads/2025/02/drug-label-768x512.jpg.

Additionally, openness is crucial when it comes to utilizing health data and earning patients' trust. The UK National Health Services' (NHS) plan to use patient data in pharmaceutical research brings up an important ethical problem. Although there is a significant opportunity to improve healthcare, the lack of strict rules regarding patient privacy and autonomy can lead people to trust healthcare institutions less. With access to massive databases, ethical questions about consent and the safety of patient information become very important for pharmaceutical companies. Without proper transparency in how this data is used and shared, patients may feel exploited rather than cared for, undermining the foundational principles of universal healthcare (Cockbain et al., 2014). It is very important to make drug pricing and marketing practices more transparent for ethical pharmaceutical operations. A lot of people and HCPs are not aware of the difficulties with drug costs, which results in distrust and misunderstanding. If pharmaceutical companies share their pricing methods and the reasons for them, they can make their work more transparent and prove to stakeholders that they act ethically. In addition, open communication about drug marketing can help reduce confusion and encourage people to decide wisely. Such transparency can lead to healthier relationships between pharmaceutical companies and their clients, ultimately fostering a more responsible and ethical industry focused on patient well-being (Cockbain et al., 2014) (Figure 15.13).

15.6. Case Studies in Drug Regulation

In the regulation of drugs, case studies give the most significant insight into the subtleties and ethical challenges facing regulatory agencies. A notable example is the controversy surrounding genetically modified (GM) food, such as the AquAdvantage salmon. The U.S. FDA asserts its evaluation procedures are always purely scientific and normative-free. However, analysis suggests that neoliberal ideologies are at the forefront of shaping the FDA's regulatory practices and thus blurring scientific assessment with broad socio-political issues.

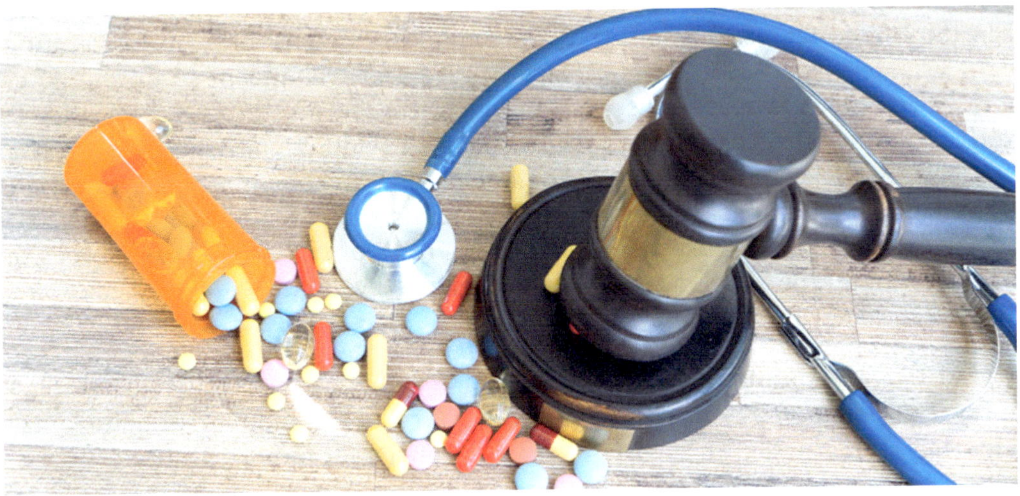

Figure 15.14. Case studies in drug regulation.

Source: https://www.darylroyer.ca/wp-content/uploads/2023/09/Understanding-The-Controlled-Drugs-And-Substances-Act-In-Canada.jpg.

The AquAdvantage salmon example illustrates how regulatory policies can be influenced by mainstream economic schools of thought and underscores the need for increased public participation in the risk assessment activities associated with GM foods, as well as their related health and safety concerns (Meghani et al., 2014). Greater complexity arises from working in the domain of evaluating expensive drugs, such as the process of NICE in England. Through ethnographic research, scholars have revealed the messy trust dynamics at work within deliberations of regulation. Trust is a crucial instrument used to navigate the uncertainties and complexities that underpin the process of evaluating cost-effectiveness, particularly in assessing new and expensive treatments. The uncertainty between trust and distrust among various stakeholders, including experts and committee members, captures broader concerns about the integrity of regulatory procedures. These tensions highlight the potential for regulatory capture, where the interests of drug manufacturers can inappropriately influence decision-making, leading to a more complex regulatory environment for drugs and therapies (Abraham et al., 2015). Drug regulation case studies not only highlight the technical aspects of evaluation but also underscore the ethical considerations involved in the decision-making process. The combination of trust, economic stakes, and public involvement also calls out the multifaceted nature of drug regulation. Agencies not only need to respond to their mandates in order to secure the safety of public health, but also need to engage actively in all questions of access, equity, and ethical implications of new treatments. As these cases involving the regulation of GM foods and cost-benefit analysis testing have demonstrated, ethical arguments in drug regulation are pervasive and necessitate a partnership model where multiple perspectives are genuinely considered. This overlap between the ethical and the regulatory is necessary to maintain public trust in public health interventions and ensure that regulatory interventions are aligned with the values of those being served (Figure 15.14).

15.6.1. Analysis of a Controversial Drug Approval (e.g., OxyContin)

The introduction of OxyContin in the 1990s was an important event in the way opioids were regulated in the United States. OxyContin was promoted as a safer method for treating ongoing pain, since it was designed with a time-release feature that was meant to lower the chances of addiction. However, the idea that drugs were harmless turned out to be wrong, since their wide use led to a national crisis caused by a lot of misuse and addiction. Regulatory bodies, such as the FDA, initially focused on clinical trials that emphasized efficacy, often neglecting the long-term implications of widespread prescribing practices and their societal impact. This narrow approach limited the regulators' ability to foresee the staggering rates of addiction and overdose that would ensue, underscoring the need for a more comprehensive evaluation of drugs like OxyContin in future regulatory frameworks (N/A, 2012).

Because of the OxyContin crisis, it is now clear that there are serious ethical issues related to the approval of opioids. When opioid prescriptions rose, the number of addictions went up, showing that the system failed to deal with the side effects of approving these drugs. The FDA primarily focused on the benefits and risks of drugs in clinical trials, rather than considering how people use them in everyday life. This approach to regulation raises doubts about the agency's duty to promote public health and consider the future effects of giving out drugs. The situation with OxyContin exemplifies a stark need for a paradigm shift, where regulatory bodies must evolve to incorporate public health implications into their approval processes (Kesselheim et al., 2018). When dealing with drugs that have a risk of addiction, like opioids, the main focus of reformed drug regulation should be public health. Some argue that the regulatory process should include factors beyond the results of clinical trials. Hence, it covers the ways doctors prescribe and patients use medication in the wider public health setting. With this model, the FDA can ensure that drugs are approved with greater responsibility and can remove them if necessary. As a result, regulations will become more accountable, and the country's efforts against the opioid crisis will improve. Incorporating these perspectives into the regulatory process could offer critical insights into the societal impacts of drug approval decisions, helping to prevent another catastrophic outcome like that seen with OxyContin (N/A, 2012) (Figure 15.15).

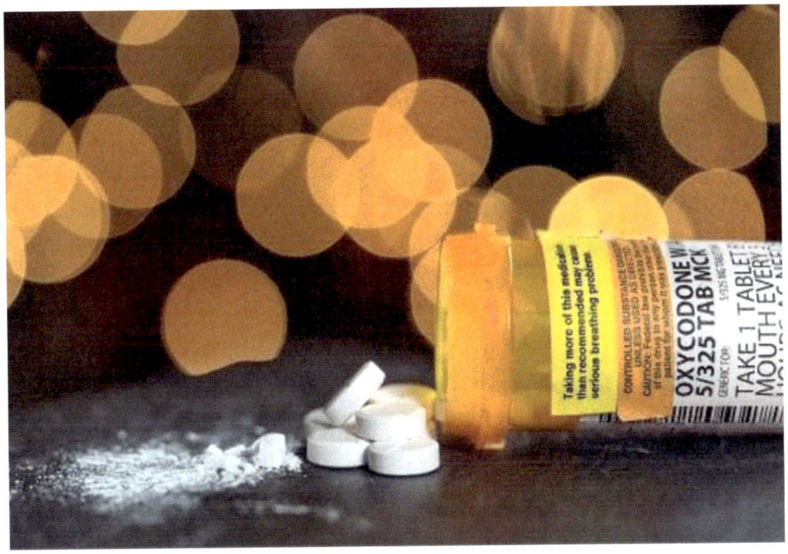

Figure 15.15. Analysis of a controversial drug approval (e.g., OxyContin).

Source: https://capobythesea.com/wp-content/uploads/2023/02/addicted-to-oxycontin.jpg.

15.6.2. Examination of a Drug Recall and Its Implications

A drug recall analysis is a complex process that reflects the intricate relationship between ethical requirements and regulatory oversight within the pharmaceutical industry. Drug recalls typically result from safety concerns, such as side effects, contamination, or incorrect labeling. The implications of such recalls extend far beyond the short-term annoyance to customers; they are a potential failure in quality assurance processes employed by drug manufacturers. A thorough review of drug recalls illustrates systemic vulnerabilities throughout the entire drug approval and oversight system. Regulatory agencies, such as the FDA, have an obligation not only to oversee market entry but also to continually review the safety and effectiveness of drugs on the market.

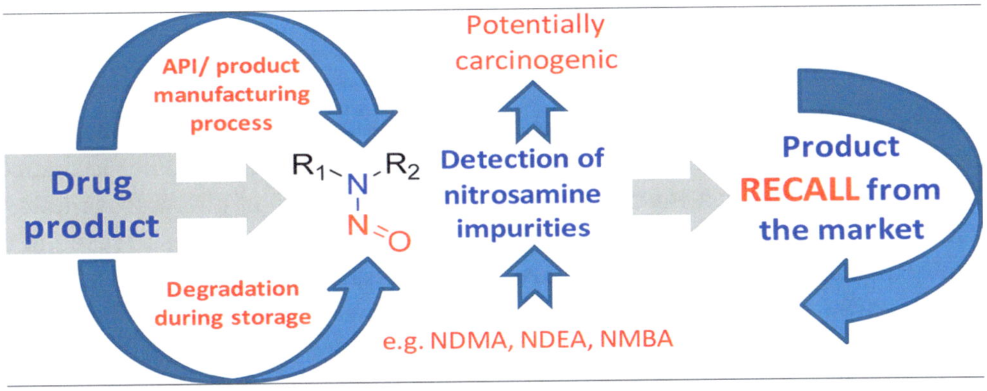

Figure 15.16. Examination of a drug recall and its implications.

Source: https://pubs.acs.org/cms/10.1021/acs.jmedchem.0c02120/asset/images/acs.jmedchem.0c02120.social.jpeg_v03.

The dynamic nature of these recalls underscores the importance of active regulatory oversight and transparency with the public. The ethical dimensions of drug recalls are multifaceted, calling for a critical examination of the roles and responsibilities of pharmaceutical companies in relation to regulatory agencies. During a recall, companies must balance the interests of business and public health. Ethical concerns are typically drawn about the timeliness of disclosures of risks, particularly in the case of financial consequences that can influence decision-making. In addition, the consequences of a recall can generate widespread public suspicion about pharmaceutical products, with far-reaching societal implications. As noted in the debate around neuroenhancement drugs (Lucidi et al., 2015), unease regarding the morality of drug development and marketing processes continues to spread. It becomes necessary for stakeholders like the public, HCPs, and regulatory agencies to provide a culture of responsibility and transparency to limit the effect of negative public opinion. Although questioning the ethicality of drug recalls is vital, they must be recognized for their regulatory role in respect to the public's health. Drug recalls serve as signals for potential deficiencies in the regulatory frameworks for assessing drug safety and efficacy. The growing number of drug recalls attests to the need for heightened caution and methodological rigor in post-market surveillance strategies. In the absence of robust mechanisms, frequent recalls have disastrous consequences for vulnerable groups, such as the elderly and children, which have been highlighted by research on the necessity of ethical controls in intervention policies (Griffiths et al., 2013). This implies that ongoing monitoring of existing regulatory practices should be conducted to ensure that consumer safety is in place, ultimately benefiting the pharmaceutical industry with a more stable environment (Figure 15.16).

15.6.3. Lessons Learned from Past Regulatory Failures

Analyzing past mistakes in the pharmaceutical industry shows what can be done to prevent similar problems now and in the future. Over time, the absence of strict controls has resulted in numerous safety problems, which has led people to doubt the health authorities. The Thalidomide tragedy in the late 1950s showed how not testing drugs enough could be very harmful to patients and their loved ones. As a result, regulators increased their efforts to ensure safety in clinical trials and after products are released by stressing the importance of thorough safety checks. They demonstrate that updating regulations is necessary following past issues to ensure that new drugs are both effective and safe.

Also, the progress in regulatory practices shows a continuous care for public health, which helps restore trust among consumers and HCPs. Another lesson from earlier mistakes is that regulations must be able to adapt to new scientific developments. The application of pharmacogenetics in clinical practice presents both new opportunities and challenges, prompting agencies to respond to changes that significantly impact patient care. It is apparent from literature that the main challenges in using pharmacogenetics are not due to ethical concerns, but to lack of funds in the healthcare system. If this is the case, clinicians may not be interested in using the latest methods. As mentioned in discussions about pharmacogenetic testing, introducing new technologies means regulators should consider the impact on both medical practice and patient outcomes. So, by making regulations flexible, we can ensure that the latest scientific advances are always included in the system. It is essential for regulatory bodies, researchers, and clinicians to collaborate in addressing the risks identified in previous regulatory failures. Recent studies have shown that clinicians' opinions about pharmacogenetics play a significant role in determining how these advances are incorporated into treatment plans. Learning about healthcare providers' opinions and concerns can improve the way regulations are made, which can boost the use of innovative therapies. It is crucial for regulatory agencies to communicate effectively with healthcare practitioners to ensure that the guidelines they develop are both accurate and practical in application. The approach taken by the organizations is aligned with Sage and Hammer's belief that competition and oversight in health care should be reconsidered. By paying attention to these collaborative aspects, regulatory bodies can ensure their guidelines are up to date and promote safety and effectiveness in the drugs available to the public, based on lessons learned from past mistakes (Figure 15.17).

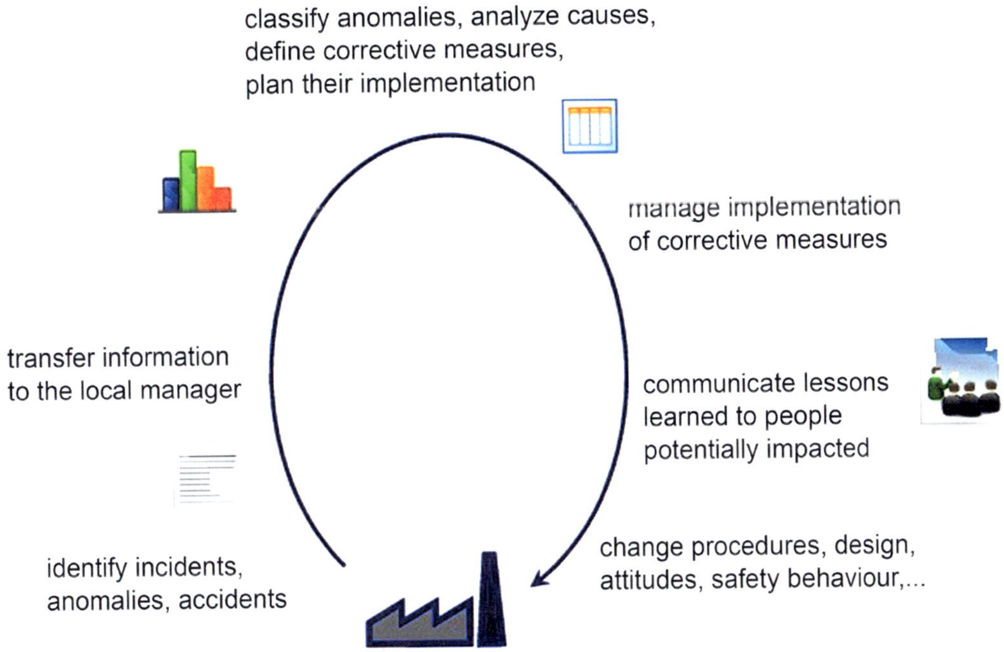
classify anomalies, analyze causes,
define corrective measures,
plan their implementation
manage implementation
of corrective measures
communicate lessons
learned to people
potentially impacted
change procedures, design,
attitudes, safety behaviour,...
identify incidents,
anomalies, accidents
transfer information
to the local manager

Figure 15.17. Lessons learned from past regulatory failures.

Source: https://governancepedia.com/wp-content/uploads/2025/01/Untitled-2025-01-01T085054.083.png.

Summary

To summarize the discussion on regulations and ethics in drug development, it is essential to recognize that regulations, public safety, and ethics are closely intertwined. Regulatory agencies, such as the US FDA, play a critical role in ensuring that drugs entering the market are both safe and effective for public consumption. Even so, the decisions made by these agencies are influenced by the values that exist in society. For instance, the FDA's regulatory stance on genetically modified organisms (GMOs) illustrates how neoliberal considerations can influence the review process, potentially sidelining ethical debates that demand public engagement during assessments. This highlights the importance of aligning regulatory practices with the ethical obligations of promoting public health and addressing societal and individual concerns related to emerging technologies (Meghani et al., 2014). Ethical review should continue even after a company starts operating in the market. It should be applied throughout the entire process of drug development, including the clinical research phases. If cost-effectiveness is considered in the ethical review of research, resources can be used more wisely, helping the healthcare system benefit society as much as possible. scholars that focusing on ethics in cost-effectiveness can help identify effective treatments more quickly and ensure that limited medical resources are distributed equitably. Thus, integrating cost considerations into the research protocols not only enhances the social value of research efforts but also promotes ethical stewardship regarding resource utilization (Briggs et al., 2016). A thorough examination of ethics can support the development of inventions that are both profitable and responsible. The discussion about the rules and ethics of drug development should always show a willingness to be open and involve everyone. To achieve this, it is essential to involve patients, researchers, and ethicists to ensure that the regulatory processes consider diverse perspectives. Because the medical and technological fields are constantly evolving, the ethical review of drugs must also change accordingly. Strong frameworks that involve the public and examine ethical issues in regulations can help connect science and societal values. By actively embodying these principles, regulatory bodies can foster trust and accountability, ensuring that the advancement of medical science does not come at the expense of ethical integrity or public concern (Meghani et al., 2014; Briggs et al., 2016).

Drug development and distribution are regulated by many rules that focus on both new ideas and keeping the public safe. Regulatory bodies, such as the FDA in the United States, play a pivotal role in overseeing the clinical trial process and evaluating new drugs before they reach the market. To confirm the safety and effectiveness of drugs, these agencies use strict procedures that involve randomized control trials and regularly check them after they are released. Even so, many people point out that the rules are either too strict or not detailed enough. As an illustration, strict regulations in the UK support ethical behavior, whereas the scattered rules in the USA sometimes lead to differences in the safety and effectiveness of drugs. Addressing these discrepancies is essential for fostering public trust while ensuring that innovative therapies are made available to patients promptly (Adamson et al., 2014). Considerations of ethics are crucial in the discussion of drug regulation, particularly in relation to informed consent and fairness in clinical trials. Since drug development is complicated these days, it is important to keep everything clear so that participants are aware of the possible risks and rewards of being involved. Ethical rules, for example, the Declaration of Helsinki, require strict monitoring of clinical trials to ensure the rights and welfare of patients are protected. Additionally, it is crucial to consider justice in the distribution of new therapies to patients, not just in relation to the individuals who participate in trials. Because vulnerable groups are at risk of exploitation, it is important to strengthen ethical guidelines. Ultimately, navigating these ethical imperatives is crucial for maintaining the integrity of clinical research and fostering a culture of accountability in pharmaceutical development (Atkins et al., 2011). Additionally, the pharmaceutical industry faces ongoing challenges due to the connection between following regulations and acting ethically. When drug development becomes more difficult, there is a greater chance of ethical problems that might make the public doubt the process. For example, when regulators want drug approval to occur quickly, it may lead to disagreements about the need to test drugs thoroughly. It is most evident in situations where providing patients with life-saving care takes precedence over conducting all possible evaluations. Recent public health emergencies have revealed that we should revisit our regulations to ensure that public health needs are met and that ethical drug testing is still conducted. Striking this balance will help cultivate a regulatory environment that safeguards patient welfare while promoting innovation in drug therapies (Adamson et al., 2014).

CLOSER LOOK

ELECTRONIC HEALTH RECORDS FOR CLINICAL RESEARCH (EHR4CR)

Electronic Health Records for Clinical Research (EHR4CR) represent a transformative approach to leveraging real-world clinical data for advancing medical research. Traditionally, clinical trials have faced significant challenges such as high costs, slow patient recruitment, and limited access to diverse populations. EHR4CR aims to overcome these barriers by utilizing data already captured during routine clinical care to support and accelerate the research process. This includes patient demographics, diagnoses, laboratory results, treatment histories, and outcomes—all stored digitally within EHR systems. By tapping into this rich data source, researchers can identify eligible trial participants more efficiently, design more relevant studies, and gain deeper insights into real-world treatment effects.

One of the key benefits of EHR4CR is its ability to streamline patient recruitment, a major bottleneck in clinical trials. Automated queries across multiple EHR systems can quickly screen large populations for eligibility criteria, significantly reducing time and labor. Furthermore, EHR4CR facilitates more representative sampling, improving the generalizability of trial results across diverse patient groups. Beyond recruitment, EHR data can also be used for long-term follow-up, safety monitoring, and comparative effectiveness studies without additional burden on patients or clinicians.

Despite its promise, EHR4CR also presents challenges. Data quality, standardization, and interoperability across different healthcare systems remain significant hurdles. Privacy concerns and regulatory compliance must be carefully managed to protect patient confidentiality. Nevertheless, advancements in health informatics, data anonymization, and federated data networks are addressing many of these concerns.

Overall, EHR4CR has the potential to reshape clinical research by making it more efficient, inclusive, and reflective of real-world clinical practice. As healthcare systems continue to digitize and integrate their data, EHR4CR stands as a powerful tool in bridging the gap between clinical care and scientific discovery, ultimately accelerating the development of safer and more effective treatments.

References

1. Brhlikova, P., Harper, I., Subedi, M., Bhattarai, S., Rawal, N., & Pollock, A. M. (2015). Aid conditionalities, international Good Manufacturing Practice standards and local production rights: a case study of local production in Nepal. *Globalization and Health*, *11*(1). https://doi.org/10.1186/s12992-015-0110-3Abraham, J., Bodewitz, H., Calnan, M., Hashem, F., Giddens, A., Habermas, J., et al. (2015). Trust, regulatory processes and NICE decision-making: Appraising cost-effectiveness models through appraising people and systems. https://core.ac.uk/download/30710015.pdf (accessed on 9 June 2025).
2. Abraham, J., et al. (2025). The sociology of pharmaceuticals: Progress and prospects. https://core.ac.uk/download/49001.pdf (accessed on 9 June 2025).
3. Altenstetter, C. (1995). Regulating healthcare technologies and medical supplies: A comparative overview. https://core.ac.uk/download/5079662.pdf (accessed on 9 June 2025).
4. Ankley, G. T., Carusi, A., Davies, M. R., et al. (2018). Harvesting the promise of AOPs: An assessment and recommendations. https://core.ac.uk/download/151211182.pdf (accessed on 9 June 2025).
5. Atkins, S., Bleakley, A., Bransford, C., Cave, J., Colliver, T., Donaldson, L., Dornan, T., et al. (2011). Preparedness is not enough: Understanding transitions as critically intensive learning periods. https://core.ac.uk/download/9346855.pdf (accessed on 9 June 2025).
6. Baltussen, R., Goetghebeur, M., Guindo, L. A., Kind, P., et al. (2012). From efficacy to equity: Literature review of decision criteria for resource allocation and healthcare decision-making. https://core.ac.uk/download/pdf/11485210.pdf (accessed on 9 June 2025).
7. Bedding, A. W., Choodari-Oskooei, B., Dimairo, M., Flight, L., et al. (2018). Adaptive designs in clinical trials: Why use them, and how to run and report them. https://core.ac.uk/download/154428378.pdf (accessed on 9 June 2025).
8. Berkman, B. E., & Gostin, L. O. (2007). Pandemic influenza: Ethics, law, and the public's health. https://core.ac.uk/download/70373887.pdf (accessed on 9 June 2025).
9. Birke, L., Boo, M. J., Buchanan-Smith, H. M., Butler, R., Calarco, M., Ehni, H., et al. (2011). Ethics, space, and somatic sensibilities: Comparing relationships between scientific researchers and their human and animal experimental subjects.
10. Bleich, A., Doron, A., Melamed, Y., et al. (2009). Ethical and scientific perspectives of placebo-controlled trials in schizophrenia. https://core.ac.uk/download/pdf/8706435.pdf (accessed on 9 June 2025).
11. Briggs, A., Fleischman, A., Rid, A., Paltiel, A. D., London, A. J., Garber, A. M., et al. (2016). Should research ethics encourage the production of cost-effective interventions? https://core.ac.uk/download/131207700.pdf (accessed on 9 June 2025).
12. Bultman, J., Kanywanyi, J. L., Maarifa, H., et al. (2012). Tanzania health insurance regulatory framework review. https://core.ac.uk/download/pdf/11307330.pdf (accessed on 9 June 2025).
13. Cockbain, J., & Sterckx, S. (2014). The UK National Health Service's 'innovation agenda': Lessons on commercialization and trust. https://core.ac.uk/download/55845652.pdf (accessed on 9 June 2025).
14. Coloma, P. M., Pane, J., Rebollo, I., et al. (2017). Evaluating the safety profile of non-

active implantable medical devices compared with medicines. https://core.ac.uk/download/154417147.pdf (accessed on 9 June 2025).

15. David, A. L. (2021). Ethical and regulatory considerations of placental therapeutics. https://core.ac.uk/download/388548075.pdf (accessed on 9 June 2025).

16. Drove, B., Gifford, K. L., Gonzalez-Meijome, J. M., et al. (2019). IMI–industry guidelines and ethical considerations for myopia control report. https://core.ac.uk/download/293867276.pdf (accessed on 9 June 2025).

17. Dugas, M., Ford, I., Kalra, D., et al. (2015). Using electronic health records to support clinical trials: A report on stakeholder engagement for EHR4CR. https://core.ac.uk/download/42366534.pdf (accessed on 9 June 2025).

18. Entorf, H., Fegert, J., & Kölch, M. (2025). Children in need of medical innovation. https://core.ac.uk/download/pdf/6569259.pdf; https://core.ac.uk/download/pdf/6336327.pdf (accessed on 9 June 2025).

19. Foit, L. (2022). The tin man needs a heart: A proposed framework for the regulation of bioprinter organs. https://core.ac.uk/download/519794716.pdf (accessed on 9 June 2025).

20. Frith, L., & Blyth, E. (2014). Assisted reproductive technology in the USA: Is more regulation needed? *Reproductive BioMedicine Online, 29*(4), 516–523. https://core.ac.uk/download/30730151.pdf (accessed on 9 June 2025).

21. Griffiths, M. D., Shonin, E., Slade, K., Van Gordon, W., et al. (2013). Mindfulness and other Buddhist-derived interventions in correctional settings: A systematic review. https://core.ac.uk/download/30639514.pdf (accessed on 9 June 2025).

22. Hammer, P. J., & Sage, W. M. (2002). A Copernican view of health care antitrust. https://core.ac.uk/download/62568344.pdf (accessed on 9 June 2025).

23. Hedgecoe, A. M. (2006). Context, ethics and pharmacogenetics. *Studies in History and Philosophy of Biological and Biomedical Sciences*, *37*(3), 566–582.

24. Horton, L. (1997). The United States Food and Drug Administration: Its role, authority, history, harmonization activities, and cooperation with the European Union. https://core.ac.uk/download/5079826.pdf (accessed on 9 June 2025).

25. Kanagarajah, A. (2024). AI-driven innovation in healthcare product development: Challenges and ethical implications. https://core.ac.uk/download/630299457.pdf (accessed on 9 June 2025).

26. Kesselheim, A. S., Riley, M. F., & Zettler, P. J. (2018). Implementing a public health perspective in FDA drug regulation. https://core.ac.uk/download/234561509.pdf (accessed on 9 June 2025).

27. Kunduru, A. R. (2023). Machine learning in drug discovery: A comprehensive analysis of applications, challenges, and future directions. https://core.ac.uk/download/613004960.pdf (accessed on 9 June 2025).

28. Lucidi, F., Mallia, L., & Zelli, A. (2015). The complexity of neuroenhancement and the adoption of a social cognitive perspective. https://core.ac.uk/download/54525558.pdf (accessed on 9 June 2025).

29. Lyon, A. R., López-Fernández, T., Couch, L. S., Asteggiano, R., Aznar, M. C., Bergler-Klein, J., Boriani, G., et al. (2022). 2022 ESC guidelines on cardio-oncology developed in collaboration with the European Hematology Association (EHA), the European Society for Therapeutic Radiology and Oncology (ESTRO), and the International Cardio-Oncology Society (IC-OS). *European Heart Journal, 43*, 4229–4361. https://doi.org/10.1093/eurheartj/ehac244.

30. Marks, M. (2022). Automating FDA regulation. https://core.ac.uk/download/491582957.pdf (accessed on 9 June 2025).

31. Meghani, Z. (2014). Risk assessment of genetically modified food and neoliberalism: An argument for democratizing the regulatory review protocol of the Food and Drug Administration. https://core.ac.uk/download/231877256.pdf (accessed on 9 June 2025).

32. N/A. (2006). New approaches to HIV prevention: Accelerating research and ensuring future access. https://core.ac.uk/download/71353396.pdf (accessed on 9 June 2025).

33. N/A. (2012). *Outlook Magazine*, Winter 2012. https://core.ac.uk/download/70380429.pdf (accessed on 9 June 2025).

34. OECD. (2021). Enhancing public trust in COVID-19 vaccination: The role of governments. OECD policy responses to coronavirus (COVID-19). https://doi.org/10.1787/eae0ec5a-en.

35. Oliveira, J. T. P. de. (2023). Programação de relatórios de dados clínicos para submissão regulamentar de ensaios clínicos de phase I. https://core.ac.uk/download/610601484.pdf (accessed on 9 June 2025).

36. Picciotto, S. (2000). Liberalization and democratization: The forum and the hearth in the era of cosmopolitan post-industrial capitalism. https://core.ac.uk/download/62568754.pdf (accessed on 9 June 2025).

37. Rosemann, A. (2014). Standardization as situation-specific achievement: Regulatory diversity and the production of value in intercontinental collaborations in stem cell medicine. https://core.ac.uk/download/30609220.pdf (accessed on 9 June 2025).

38. Santiago-Rodriguez, F. (2025). Facing the trial of internationalizing clinical trials to developing countries: Some evidence from Mexico. https://core.ac.uk/download/pdf/6941422.pdf (accessed on 9 June 2025).

39. Sokolić, D., Kaštelan Mrak, M., & Bodiroga Vukobrat, N. (2017). Personalized medicine industry model development. https://core.ac.uk/download/212453793.pdf (accessed on 9 June 2025).

40. Terzic, A., & Waldman, S. A. (2017). Process improvement for maximized therapeutic innovation outcome. https://core.ac.uk/download/155271556.pdf (accessed on 9 June 2025).

INDEX

D

I

K

L

M

N

R

S

T

U